Resistance to Targeted Anti-Cancer Therapeutics

Volume 7

Series Editor
Benjamin Bonavida
Department of Microbiology, Immunology, and Molecular Genetics
University of California at Los Angeles,
Los Angeles, CA, USA

More information about this series at http://www.springer.com/series/11727

For several decades, treatment of cancer consisted of chemotherapeutic drugs, radiation, and hormonal therapies. Those were not tumor specific and exhibited severe toxicities in many cases. But during the last several years, targeted cancer therapies have been developed. Targeted cancer therapies are drugs or other agents (e.g. antibodies) that block the growth and spread of cancer by interfering with specific gene products that regulate tumor cell growth and progression. Targeted cancer therapies are also sometimes called "molecularly targeted drugs." We have witnessed in the last decade a significant explosion in the development of targeted cancer therapies developed against various specific cancers. These include drugs/antibodies that interfere with cell growth signaling or tumor blood vessel development, promote the cell death of cancer cells, stimulate the immune system to destroy specific cancer cells and to deliver toxic drugs to cancer cells. One of the major problems that arise following treatment with both conventional therapies and targeted cancer therapies is the development of resistance, preexisting in a subset of cancer cells or cancer stem cells and/or induced by the treatments. Tumor cell resistance to therapies remains a major problem and several strategies are being considered to reverse the resistance by various manipulations.

Resistance to Targeted Anti-Cancer Therapeutics will focus on the basic and translational research behind the molecular mechanisms of resistance found in many kinds of anti-cancer therapeutics.

Benjamin Bonavida • Salem Chouaib
Editors

Resistance of Cancer Cells to CTL-Mediated Immunotherapy

Springer

Editors
Benjamin Bonavida
Department of Microbiology,
Immunology, and Molecular Genetics
University of California at Los Angeles
Los Angeles, CA, USA

Salem Chouaib
Institut Gustave Roussy
Villejuif, France

ISSN 2196-5501 ISSN 2196-551X (electronic)
Resistance to Targeted Anti-Cancer Therapeutics
ISBN 978-3-319-17806-6 ISBN 978-3-319-17807-3 (eBook)
DOI 10.1007/978-3-319-17807-3

Library of Congress Control Number: 2015940115

Springer Cham Heidelberg New York Dordrecht London

Printed on acid-free paper

Springer International Publishing AG Switzerland is part of Springer Science+Business Media (www.springer.com)

Preface

In 1909, Paul Ehrlich proposed that the immune system can recognize and destroy nascent tumor cells. A century later, this principle has been applied successfully for the treatment of patients with various cancers by the use of monoclonal antibodies, adoptively transferred T-cells, genetic amplification of T-cells bearing high affinity TCR, ADCs, CAR T-cells and check point blocking antibodies (see below). Immunotherapy against cancer has recently experienced significant translational clinical applications in the treatment of many cancer types. We witnessed a few decades ago the initial clinical application of T-cell-mediated immunotherapy, initially by the ex vivo culture and activation of cancer patients BPMCs with IL-2, to generate LAK cells and, subsequently, the culture and propagation of TILs from cancer tissues and their adoptive transfer into the patients. Subsequently, various modalities have been examined and applied in cancer, such as ex vivo DCs pulsed with tumor lysates or tumor peptides and administered into the patients with growth factors. In addition, several cancer vaccines have been developed. Further, targeting T-reg cells and MDCS resulted in enhancing the anti-tumor T-cell response. A number of successfully current immunotherapies in cancer patients, including check point targeted antibodies (e.g., anti-CTLA-4, PD-1, and PDL-1) and adoptive T-cell therapies (e.g., genetically transduced T-cell receptors and CARs), are reported to be clinically effective in the treatment of advanced cancers, many of which are resistant to conventional chemotherapy and radiation. The likelihood of responsiveness to these immunotherapies differs strongly depending on tumor type. Targeting check points resulted in significant responses in melanoma, renal cell carcinoma, and non-small cell lung cancer. For CARs, significant clinical responses have been achieved in lymphomas. All of the aforementioned is a testimony to the important role of immunotherapy mediated by T-cells and antibodies that have resulted in the new generation of targeted therapies and reduced toxicity encountered by conventional chemotherapy and radiotherapy. Several of the aforementioned immunotherapy strategies were effective in the treatment of drug-resistant tumor cells. However, there is still a subset of nonresponsive patients who have a cancer with either a naturally acquired resistance or an induced intrinsic resistance to such therapies.

The successful requirements for an adoptive and optimal T-cell response consist of three key elements: the ability to induce a T-cell response; the ability to infiltrate into the tumor microenvironment; and the ability to kill the tumor cells. Most anti-cancer cellular and humoral therapies have given little attention to the generally encountered tumor cell resistance to cytotoxic activities mediated by such therapies. In fact, tumor cells develop several mechanisms to escape tumor cell death. Tumor cell resistance may be responsible, in large part, for the fact that many cancer patients fail to respond to cytotoxic immunotherapy in the presence of anti-tumor cytotoxic T-effector cells and antibodies.

Clearly, one of the important, and not completely exploited, area in cancer immunotherapy is the underlying mechanisms of tumor cell resistance to CTL and antibody-mediated cytotoxicities. Several reported studies explored the underlying molecular bases of tumor cell resistance to CTL and shed new light on the improvement of current immunotherapy of cancer and that could significantly improve the clinical response. Resistance of Cancer Cells to CTL-Mediated Immunotherapy reviews, in large part, several of the mechanisms underlying the tumor cell resistance to CTL-Mediated cytotoxicity, and suggests several means to overcome the resistance by the use of combination treatments with agents targeting resistance in combination with CTL-Mediated immunotherapy. This volume comprises the contributions of leaders in the field, and provides numerous examples of molecular bases of CTL resistance. (While this volume does not cover the field in its entirety, due to the vast scope of the subject, subsequent volumes under consideration will cover other areas of CTL resistance in cancer and their clinical implications.)

This volume is divided into four parts. Part I, Factors Regulating Resistance to CTL Cytotoxicity, consists of five review chapters. Doctors Maccalli and colleagues reviewed "Resistance of Cancer Stem Cells to Cell-Mediated Immune Responses." It is clear that, in the majority of cancers, cancer stem cells (CSCs) are believed to be responsible, in large part, for tumor initiation, progression, metastasis, and resistance to cytotoxic therapies. CSCs have been reported to escape immune surveillance, though they exhibit antigenic molecules that can be targeted for immunotherapy, rescuing both the new growth and resistance to CTL-Mediated therapy. Doctors Dolstra and colleagues reviewed "Role of Co-inhibitory Molecules in Tumor Escape from CTL Attack." Tumor cells may express co-inhibitory molecules (CIMs) that can severely inhibit CD-8 T-cell cytotoxicity. These inhibitory molecules on the cancer cell surface, such as PDL-1, will inhibit CTL cytotoxic activity via interaction and cell signaling of PD-1 on the surface of CTL. In addition, CIMs such as CTLA-4, LAG-3, BTLA, Tim-3, and CD200R have been implicated in the inhibition of CTL functions. The authors have discussed the role each of the above CIMs and, as well, suggest various approaches to inhibit their activities and restore cytotoxic activity. Doctors Seliger and Bergner reviewed "Role of the Non-classical HLA Class I Antigens for Immune Escape." One of the mechanisms of tumor escape from immune surveillance is the overexpression of the non-classical class I HLA-G+ antigen that is often overexpressed in solid and hematopoietic tumors. This overexpression leads to its interaction with inhibitory receptors ILT2,

ILT4, and KIR2DL4. HLA-G+ tumors are associated with poor clinical outcomes. The inhibition of HLA-G can increase the sensitivity to tumor cells to CTL and NK cytotoxicities. The authors describe the role of HLA-G+ as a therapeutic target. Doctors Mami-Chouaib and colleagues reviewed "Integrins: Friends or Foes of Antitumor Cytotoxic T Lymphocyte Response." The authors describe the role of integrins and their ligands in the regulation of T-cell effector functions that result in CTL activation and triggering of their cytotoxic machinery. Of particular interest is the authors' description of the integrins CD103 and LFA-1 and their respective ligands, E-cadherin and ICAM-1, in the regulation of T-cell effector functions. Also discussed is the importance of integrin-antagonists in cancer immunotherapy. Doctors Noonan and Murphy reviewed "Cytotoxic T Lymphocytes and their Granzymes: An Overview." In addition to several immunotherapeutic strategies, including antibodies and adoptive transfer of CTLs, novel strategies are aimed at the cell death pathways including granzymes and death ligands (Fas-L TNFalpha TRAIL). In this review, examples of granzymes-mediated cell death using the prototype of granzyme-bound immunotoxin therapy are discussed. In addition, in this review, the authors discuss the initiation and the activation of the effector functions of CTL and how they can be used in cancer immunotherapy.

Part II, "Influence of the Tumor Microenvironment on the Resistance to CTL Cytotoxicity," consists of three review chapters. Doctors Chouaib and colleagues reviewed "Hypoxia: A Formidable Saboteur of the Anti-tumor Response." The tumor microenvironment (TME), in addition to modulating the anti-tumor response, fosters resistance of tumor cells to CTL cytotoxicity. This review emphasizes the influence of hypoxic stress that impacts angiogenesis, tumor progression, and immune tolerance. It includes a discussion on how hypoxia in TME protects tumor cells by modulation of various molecular signaling pathways in the tumor cells and rendering them viable, proliferative, and resistant to CTL. The authors suggest that hypoxia is a target for tumor reactivity to CTL. Doctors Mutis and colleagues reviewed "Mechanisms and Modulation of Tumor Microenvironment-Induced Immune Resistance." The authors discuss the mechanism by which the TME regulates the resistance of tumor cells to CTL cytotoxicity. The authors discuss the modulation of intrinsic, extrinsic, and granzyme/perforin-mediated pathways of apoptosis by the TME and have used multiple myeloma as a cancer model. As well, they discuss strategies to override the resistance of tumor cells to CTL-Mediated immunotherapies. Doctors Sandra Hodge and Greg Hodge reviewed "Evasion of Cytotoxic Lymphocyte and Pulmonary Macrophage Mediated Immune Responses in Lung Cancer." The authors discuss the regulation of tumor cell resistance to CTL cytotoxic therapy, and describe the resistance of lung cancer cells to granzyme B-mediated attack through the expression of a specific inhibitor (such as the intracellular serine protease inhibitor PI-9). PI-9 is expressed in CTLs and protects the tumor cells to killing by granzyme B. The authors cite studies that report that PI-9 expression positively correlated with cancer stage among patients with solid and hematologic malignancies, suggesting that targeting PI-9 may be a strategy to improve immunotherapy in lung cancers.

Part III, "Resistance to Death Ligands-Mediated Apoptosis and Sensitization" consists of four review chapters. Doctor Bonavida reviewed "Sensitization of Immune-Resistant Tumor Cells to CTL-Mediated Apoptosis via Interference at the Dysregulated NF-/Snail/YY1/PI3K/RKIP/PTEN Resistant Loop." He discusses the mechanisms by which tumor cells develop resistance to CTL-Mediated apoptosis via a dysregulated loop consisting of the NF-kB/Snail/YY1/RKIP/PTEN. This dysregulated loop further regulates cell growth, proliferation, MET, metastasis, and the resistance to both CTL and chemotherapeutic drugs. The role of each of the gene products in the loop and its direct involvement in the regulation of the above functions and, in particular, to CTL-Mediated apoptosis via death ligands (Fas-L, TNFa, DR4, and DR5) is discussed. Also discussed is the manner in which each of the gene products in the loop has potential for reversal of resistance as well as inhibition of tumor cell growth and metastasis. Several examples are provided with different agents that target different gene products of the loop and resulted in the reversal of resistance to CTL cytotoxicity. Doctors Zhang and colleagues reviewed "Overcoming Cancer Cell Resistance to Death Receptor Targeted Therapies." Targeting death receptors for cancer treatment has been explored in both the laboratory and in human clinical trials. Among the death ligands that are not toxic to normal tissues, TRAIL, is being investigated in clinical trials through the use of either recombinant TRAIL or agonist antibodies to TRAIL receptors DR4 and DR5. While these studies are ongoing clinically, both alone and in combination with conventional chemotherapy, it must be noted that many patient cancer cells are resistant to such therapies and require sensitizing agents that can be used in combination to reverse resistance. The authors discuss various approaches to reverse resistance. Doctors Chen and colleagues reviewed "Pancreatic Cancer Resistance to TRAIL Therapy: Regulators of the Death Inducing Signaling Complex." The authors discuss the resistance of pancreatic cancer to TRAIL-induced apoptosis. They have identified several factors in the death receptor activated DISC (which include FLIP, calmodulin, Src, and PARP-1) that contribute to the resistance of cancer cells to death receptor-mediated apoptosis. Also discussed are mechanisms that regulate the DISC that result in the resistance of TRAIL apoptosis. In addition, they suggest, for pancreatic cancer, various therapeutic targets for immunotherapy. Doctors Thiery and colleagues reviewed "Resistance of Carcinoma Cells to CTL-Mediated Immunotherapy." The authors discuss the role of EMT and cancer stemness in the resistance to both chemo and CTL-Mediated therapeutics. As well, they explored the immunological synapse and how it is affected by EMT and discuss the manner in which the inhibition of EMT can restore cytotoxic immune function.

Part IV, "Future Directions" consists of two chapter reviews. Doctors Kawakami and colleagues reviewed "Cancer Induced Immunosuppression and Its Modulation by Signal Inhibitors." The authors describe various signal-mediated pathways that regulate the immune response, and how signal inhibitors may enhance anti-tumor responses. The authors suggest personalized treatments (as the oncogenic signal activities are different for each cancer patient). They also consider and recommend personalized treatment for immunotherapy. Doctors Mehrotra and colleagues reviewed "Quality of CTL Therapies: A Changing Landscape." The authors discuss the various mechanisms by which tumor cells escape immune surveillance and discuss several strategies that they recommend be investigated in order to restore the immune functions and, in particular, the response of tumor cells to T-cellmediated therapy. This chapter also provides various challenges for consideration in the future.

Benjamin Bonavida
Salem Chouaib

Acknowledgements

The editors wish to acknowledge the significant and continuous help and assistance provided throughout the development of this book by Joy Evangeline Bramble, Emily Janakiram, and Michael Koy of Springer. In addition, the editors wish to acknowledge the excellent technical assistance of Kathy Nguyen in both the editing and finalization of the contents of this volume.

Contents

Part I
Factors Regulating Resistance to CTL Cytotoxicity

Chapter 1
Resistance of Cancer Stem Cells to Cell-Mediated Immune Responses

Veronica Catalano*, Cecilia Eleuteri*, Gaia Campoccia, Gianluca Giacobini, Mariangela Zane, Giorgio Stassi, Giorgio Parmiani, and Cristina Maccalli

Abstract In the past decades, the hierarchical organization of tumors, governed by Cancer Stem Cells (CSCs), have been reported with regard to several tumor types. Advances in sequencing technologies have demonstrated that diverse genetic CSCs subclones, derived from the branching evolution, compete with each other within the tumor mass, thereby contributing to the functional heterogeneity. It is becoming increasingly clear that epigenetic modifications and microenvironmental influences are important determinants of tumor fitness resulting in disease progression, recurrence and reduced patient survival. Therefore, more effective therapies will require gaining insights into the role of genetic and non-genetic influences in coordinating tumor maintenance.

CSCs are believed to be responsible for tumor initiation, progression and resistance to therapeutic agents. Therefore, CSC-targeted therapeutic interventions are desirable to achieve complete tumor eradication. Immunotherapy can represent a valuable treatment thanks to its antigen-specificity. The molecular and immunological characterizations, though still not definitive, of CSCs revealed their low efficiency in eliciting adaptive immune responses and the presence of features correlating with escape from immunosurveillance. Nevertheless, CSC-specific molecules may represent novel targets for immunotherapy and immunomodulatory agents may able to rescue their immunogenicity. This information might be exploited to design novel CSC-targeting therapies, possibly in association with inhibitors of

---

***No conflict statement:** "No potential conflicts of interest were disclosed."

V. Catalano • C. Eleuteri • M. Zane • G. Stassi
Department of Surgical and Oncological Sciences, University of Palermo, Palermo, Italy

G. Campoccia • G. Giacobini
Medical Oncology and Immunotherapy, University Hospital of Siena, V.le Bracci, 16, Siena 53100, Italy

G. Parmiani • C. Maccalli (✉)
Medical Oncology and Immunotherapy, University Hospital of Siena, V.le Bracci, 16, Siena 53100, Italy

NIBIT-Italian Network for Bio-therapy of Tumors, Siena, Italy
e-mail: crimaccalli@gmail.com

B. Bonavida, S. Chouaib (eds.), *Resistance of Cancer Cells to CTL-Mediated Immunotherapy*, Resistance to Targeted Anti-Cancer Therapeutics 7,
DOI 10.1007/978-3-319-17807-3_1

survival pathways and/or with differentiation agents and cytotoxic drugs. These therapeutic strategies are desirable in order to target the entire cancer and can represent a promising strategy to achieve complete tumor regression.

Keywords Cancer stem cells • Cancer stem cell markers • Signaling pathways of cancer stem cells • T cell responses • NK Cells • Immunomodulatory molecules • CSC-targeted therapies • Immune escape

Abbreviations

ABC	ATP-binding cassette
ADAM	A disintegrin and metalloprotease
APC	Adenomatosis polyposis coli
APCs	Antigen presenting cells
APM	Antigen processing machinery
B7-H1, 3, 4	B7 homolog family members
BMP	Bone morphogenetic protein
CEA	Carcino embryonic antigen
CK1	Casein kinase 1
COA-1	Colon antigen-1
CRC	Colorectal cancer
CSC	Cancer stem cells
CSL	CBF1/Su(H)/Lag-1
CXCR-4	C-X-C chemokine receptor type 4
EMT	Epithelial-to-mesenchymal transition
Ep-CAM	Epithelial cell adhesion molecule
EphB	Ephrin B
ESC	Embryonic stem cells
FZ	Frizzled
GBM	Glioblastoma multiforme
GDF-15	Growth differentiation factor 15
Gp100	Glycoprotein 100
GS	γ-Secretase
GSK3	Glycogen synthase kinase 3
Hh	Hedgehog
HLA	Human leukocyte antigen
IDO	Indoleamine 2,3-dioxigenase
IFN	Interferon
IL-10	Interleukin-10
IL-13α2	α2 chain of IL-13 receptor
IL-4	Interleukin-4
LRP	Low-density-lipoprotein-related protein5/6
M	Mastermind-like protein 1

MAA	Melanoma associated antigen
MAGE	Melanoma-associated antigen gene
MART-1	Melanoma antigen recognized by T cells
MDSC	Myeloid derived suppressor cell
Melan-A	Protein melan-A, *see also* MART-1
MHC	Major histocompatibility complex
MSC	Mesenchymal stem cell
MUC-1	Mucin 1
NKG2D	Natural killer group 2, member D
Notch-IC	Receptor intracellular domain
NY-ESO-1	New York esophagus 1 antigen
PD-1	Programmed cell death protein 1
PD-L1	Programmed death ligand 1
PGE2	Prostaglandin E2
PSA	Prostate specific antigen
PTCH	Patched
R	Recombining binding protein suppressor of hairless
Runx2	Runt-related transcription factor 2
SMO	Smoothened
STAT3	Signal transducer and activator of transcription 3
SVV-1	Survivin 1
TAA	Tumor associated antigen
TCF	T-cell factor-1
TGF-β1	Tumor growth factor beta 1
Treg	T regulatory cell

1.1 Introduction

According to the classical model of tumorigenesis, every cell of the body is equally susceptible to acquire an unlimited and uncontrolled proliferative potential, following genetic and epigenetic mutations. Clonal evolution of different subclones, dictated by environmental influences and continuing mutagenesis, explains the phenotypic differences observed in a tumor population [1]. Accumulating evidences suggest that tumor growth and progression are driven by a subset of cells with "stemness" properties, called cancer stem cells (CSCs). Located at the top of tumor hierarchy, these cells possess the long-life capacity to self-renew and generate the heterogeneous population of differentiated descendants, which constitute the tumor bulk [2]. The practical translation of this definition is their ability to generate a serially transplantable phenocopy of the original malignancy when injected into immuno-compromised mice [3].

From a clinical point of view, CSCs have been defined by multiple resistant mechanisms against anti-cancer therapies contributing to tumor recurrence and metastatic dissemination [4]. Similar to normal stem cells, CSCs were reported to shuttle between quiescence, slow-cycling and active states [5, 6]. Despite the loss of the CDK4/6 pathway regulation, the retention in a non-proliferating or G0 state, depends on the activation of p21 and p27 cell-cycle inhibitors, which block the transition from G1 to S-phase [7]. Interestingly, CSCs are stimulated to enter in a proliferative state in response to signals produced by the tumor microenvironment, such as the TGF-β family members which abrogate the p21 and p27 activation [8]. Although conventional cancer therapies are targeting the cell cycle and/or rapidly dividing cells, most patients relapse because of the quiescent regrowth of CSCs [9]. Complementary mechanisms responsible for chemoresistance are represented by high levels of anti-apoptotic factors (FLIP, BCL-2, Bcl-xl, IAP family members) [10], active DNA repair capacity [11], up-regulation of cell pumps such as the multidrug resistance transporter (MDR1) [4] and increased metabolic activity through ALDH1 [12]. By stabilizing the cysteine transporter subunit xCT and, thereby, regulating the intracellular levels of reduced glutathione (GSH), a primary intracellular antioxidant, CSCs are also able to protect themselves from ROS-inducing anticancer drugs [13]. Lastly, CSCs can be difficult to reach because they reside in a permissive environment that protects them from diverse genotoxic insults [14, 15].

In addition, to sustain CSCs functional traits [16, 17], the tumor microenvironment is also involved in the CSC generation through induction of "stemness" features into differentiated tumor cells [18, 19]. Along this line, HGF-producing myofibroblasts are able to provide a CSC phenotype to non-CSC, by reactivating the Wnt signaling pathway. These dedifferentiated cancer cells acquire the expression of stem cell-associated genes but also gain tumorigenic potential [20]. The unexpected plasticity of CSCs enables these cells to change their phenotype and to assume different functions and properties, including a stem cell state. Epithelial cells undergoing the epithelial-to-mesenchymal transition (EMT) lose polarity and cell-to-cell adhesion properties. However, they acquire a mesenchymal-like phenotype associated with increased motility, invasiveness and resistance to apoptosis [21]. CSCs can be also generated by inducting the EMT program, which stimulates the expression of CSCs markers and increases tumorigenic potential [22]. By either down-regulating "stemness"-repressed microRNAs [23, 24] or by inducing expression of Bmi-1 [25], EMT-inducing factors, like cytokines and hypoxia, stimulate the expression of transcription factors associated to self-renewal program.

Recent data show that cytokines secreted by the tumor microenvironment, including HGF, osteopontin and stromal-derived factor 1α, reprogram colorectal $CD44v6^-$ progenitors in metastatic stem cells by increasing the CD44v6 expression via the Wnt pathway activation. Survival analysis, conducted by using Kaplan-Meier curves, revealed that in patient cohorts, low levels of CD44v6 predict increased probability of disease-free survival. Importantly, the inhibition of phosphatidylinositol 3-kinase (PI3K) that selectively killed CD44v6 expressing CSCs has been shown to be effective in reducing the metastatic process initiated by CSCs, through the expression of CD44v6 [26].

These evidences underline the importance of studying the complex interplay between CSCs and the tumor microenvironment, which may lead to the identification of novel drug candidates.

It has been extensively demonstrated that the immune system plays a relevant role in the control of tumor growth; in fact, lost of immunity is associated with cancer risk, and on the other hand efficient systemic immune responses can lead to tumor killing [27, 28]. The interplay between tumor development and the immune system has been re-defined by a step-wise process that includes 3 different phases (3E), early elimination, equilibrium and escape [29]. The concept that the immune infiltrate at tumor site can have prognostic significance has been initially proposed by Mihm et al. [30] for melanoma; then it was extended to other neoplastic tissues and, more recently, it was quantitatively and molecularly defined leading to the development of the immunoscore as an efficient prognostic tool for solid tumors [31].

Despite the fact that in the last two decades a variety of molecular and regulatory features of tumor immunology have been extensively dissected, effective therapeutic vaccines for solid tumors have not yet been convincingly obtained; an overall 10–20 % of clinical responses have been observed. A possible explanation for these disappointing clinical results may lie in the failure to elicit effective and persistent immune responses by tumor vaccine in cancer patients. On the other hand, many factors can work in concert to inhibit anti-tumor immunity, including the release by tumor cells of suppressive cytokines/factors, the induction of regulatory T lymphocytes (Tregs) and/or myeloid derived suppressor cells (MDSCs) [32–34].

Moreover, the modulation by the complex interactions of co-stimulatory or negative regulatory molecules, defined as immune checkpoint molecules, on antigen presenting (APC)/tumor cells and on effector immune cells has been shown to play a key role in the regulation of anti-cancer immune responses [35]. The clinical development of immune-checkpoint blockade agents showed durable clinical responses and increase of survival for patients with solid tumors with different histological origins [36]. These evidences indicate that immunotherapy represents a promising treatment for cancer patients as it can induce efficient anti-tumor immune responses in these patients. Notably, the effectiveness of immunotherapy could be increased by targeting CSCs that represent the component of the tumor responsible of resistance to standard therapy, such as chemotherapy and radiotherapy, and to immunotherapy as well [11, 37–39].

The characterization of the immunological profile of CSCs and of the relationship between CSCs and anti-tumor immunity, thus, represent a relevant issue to design novel and more effective immunotherapy interventions for cancer patients.

1.2 CSCs Markers

CSCs are hypothesized to derive from normal stem cells through an aberrant step of differentiation or after a reprogrammed leading to a less differentiated status [3]. In light of this, it is possible to identify CSCs by using stemness characteristic markers, such as transcription factors acting during early embryogenesis, or genes involved in pluripotency maintenance. Similarly, cancer stem/progenitor cells can be recognized by following specific proteins that intervene in early organogenesis, from the three different germ layers.

In association with Oct4, Sox2 forms a trimeric complex involved in embryonic development. These markers are transcription factors that perform their function by binding to DNA and activating some important genes, such as *YES1*, *FGF4*, *UTF*, and *ZFP206*. Nanog is a transcription factor induced by Oct4 involved in stem cell self-renewal and pluripotency and hence, preventing differentiation. CSC identification can be obtained by following genes belonging to stem cell pathways, such as *Wnt*, *Hedgehog*, and *Notch* (classified also by EMT-inducing signaling pathways) (www.uniprot.org).

In proceeding with differentiation, embryonic stem cells undergo a phenotype change in their tissue destination. To analyze the differentiation towards each lineage, it is possible to use ectodermal (i.e., Notch, Nestin, p63), mesodermal (i.e., BMP4, Nodal, CD34, Cryptic), and endodermal (i.e., a-fetoprotein, beta-catenin, CXCR4, SOX17) markers. In relation to tissue differentiation and development, these marker classes belong to all cells with the same tissue derivation. For this reason, they are commonly used and constitute a simple screen panel for CSC characterization. Being that most markers are intracellular, they cannot be used for FACS sorting or beads separation. Hence, the challenge of many research groups is the identification of membrane markers that can be stable and specific to a definite pathology.

The cells with the capacity to efflux Hoechst 33342 vital dye, that were first identified in mouse bone marrow, are referred to as "side population" (SP) because they are composed of unstained cells in the left lower quadrant of a FACS profile [40]. SP has been used to isolate malignant cells since their ability to efflux dyes correlates to multidrug resistance mediated by the ABC transporters over-expression [41]. Moreover, these cell subsets are highly enriched for the capacity to initiate tumor formation upon serial transplantation and express stem-like genes [42].

The use of Hoechst dye to isolate stem-like cells has met with criticisms. In fact, this is a dynamic process, based on dye efflux, in which variables in staining times, dye and cellular concentrations can affect the SP phenotype. Since the DNA binding induced by Hoechst staining promotes a toxic effect in living cells, the SP cells, isolated through this method, may be a population able to resist the lethal effects rather than stem-like cells. Furthermore, flow cytometry gating strategies, used to define SP cells, cannot be associated with gating strategies involved in staining using other markers [43].

A similar method of characterization of CSCs is the analysis of the cell subset expressing an high Aldehyde Dehydrogenase (ALDH) activity, which is involved in early cellular differentiation, detoxification, and drug resistance, through the oxidation of intracellular aldehydes [44]. ALDH belongs to the oxidoreductase enzyme family and is highly expressed in stem and progenitor cells, thus it is used as a functional marker for CSC isolation from solid tumors (i.e., breast, lung, ovarian, prostate, head-neck, and thyroid cancer), as well as in multiple myelomas and acute leukemia [45]. Using the ALDEFLUOR™ assay, it is possible to isolate cancer stem and progenitor cells through cell sorting with a positive selection, without compromising their vitality.

In solid tumors, several cell surface markers are used to isolate cell subsets enriched with CSCs, such as CD44 [46–49], CD24 [57, 50], EpCAM [46, 51], THY1 (also called CD90) [52], and CD133 [51, 53–57].

CD133, also known as Prominin-1, is a pentaspan transmembrane glycoprotein originally identified as a marker for human $CD34^+$ hematopoietic stem and progenitor cells by Miraglia et al. [58]. It was recognized as an important marker in the identification and isolation of cell subsets with "stemness" properties in many tumor tissues, such as brain [55], kidney [59], prostate [56], hepatic [60], and colon [53, 57]. Nonetheless, the usage of CD133 as an identification and isolation marker in colon CSCs is controversial because its expression pattern is not completely elucidated. In line with this, $CD133^+$ and $CD133^-$ cell fractions have been reported to display similar "stemness" and differentiation potential, including the ability to generate tumors similar to the parental ones [61]. Kamper and colleagues explained the contradictions found in the literature by studying possible regulation mechanisms of epitope expression. CD133 is expressed in both CSCs and differentiated tumor cells. Whereas the CD133 mRNA and protein expression remained unchanged, differentiation led to down-regulation of the AC133 epitope, correlating with differential glycosylation and reduced antibody detection [62].

The CD133 polarized localization suggests its role in regulating proliferation but its functions remains still unclear. Recent studies highlight that CD133 could be involved in tumor angiogenesis since $CD133^+$ glioma cells have shown to produce vascular endothelial growth factors [63]. In the intestine, CD133 has been proposed as a stem cell marker susceptible to neoplastic transformation, being prone to activate Wnt signaling [64]. Therefore, it is important to note that CSC identification and isolation requires the use of more than one specific marker.

1.3 Survival Pathways in CSCs

The signaling pathways, which regulate normal stem cell self-renewal, lead to tumorigenesis when dysregulated; a comprehensive understanding of the pathways involved in development, "stemness" and apoptosis, is considered to be a very important goal in cancer therapy. The most important signaling pathways that regulate normal and cancer stem cell functions are: Notch, Wnt, BMP and Sonic-Hedgehog.

The Notch signaling pathway is evolutionarily conserved and has profound, context-dependent phenotypic consequences because it is involved in the maintenance of stem cells and in differentiation regulation. In both humans and rodents, the Notch genes encode four distinct members (from Notch1 to Notch4) of a transmembrane heterodimeric receptor family. In physiologic conditions, Notch ligands (Delta and Jagged) binding induces the Notch receptor intracellular domain (Notch-IC) release via a cascade of proteolytic cleavages catalyzed by a disintegrin and metalloprotease (ADAM) and γ-secretase (GS) proteases. Notch-IC translocates into the nucleus and modulates the gene expression by binding the transcription factor,

CBF1/Su(H)/Lag-1 (CSL), and recruiting co-activators, such as recombining binding protein suppressor of hairless (R) and mastermind-like protein 1 (M) [65] (Fig. 1.1a). The aberrant activation of this pathway contributes to tumorigenesis [66–70]. With the notable exception of epidermal keratinocytes where Notch-1

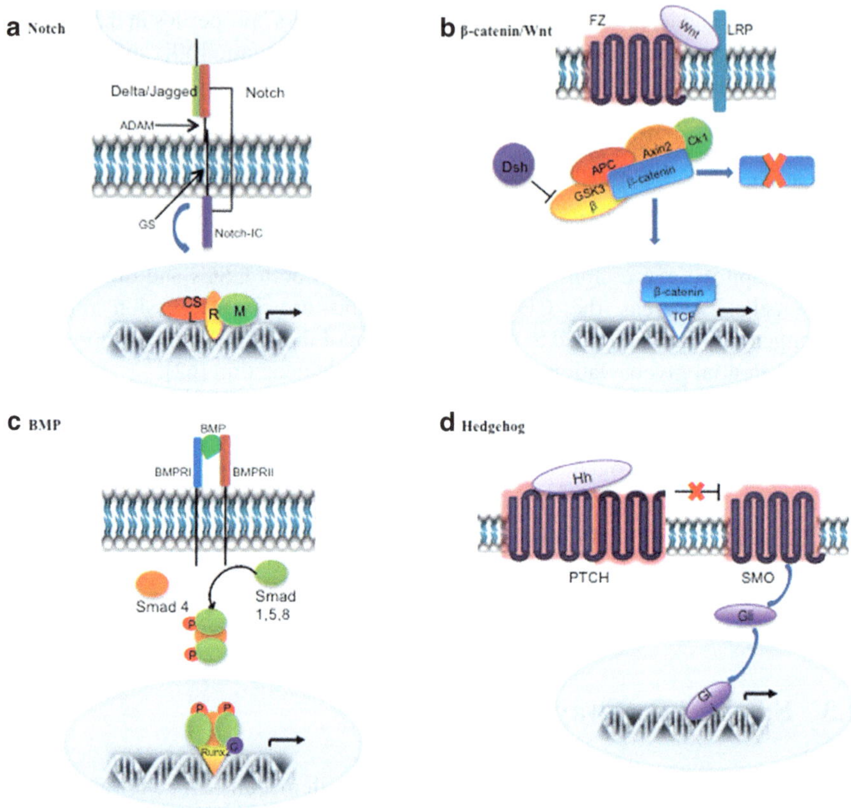

Fig. 1.1 Pathways involved in CSC survival and differentiation. (**a**) Notch signaling. Notch signaling relies on the activation of Notch receptors by Delta and Jagged ligands expressed in a neighbor cell. The release of Notch-IC, subsequent to the two proteolytic events catalyzed by ADAM and GS proteases, leads to the transcription of target genes by binding the transcription factor CSL and recruiting the co-activators R and M. (**b**) Canonical Wnt/β-catenin signaling. Wnt binds to FZ, which recruits LRP5/6 as co-factor and interacts with Dsh. β-catenin cytoplasmatic localization is regulated by a destruction complex formed by APC, Axin2, GSK3βCK1, which directs its degradation by ubiquitination. In presence of Wnt ligands, Dsh inhibits GSK3 and the destruction complex disassembles allowing β-catenin to shift to the nucleus. (**c**) BMP signaling. The heterodimerization of BMPR receptors induced by BMP proteins promotes the phosphorylation of SMAD 1,5,8 and their association with SMAD 4. The complex formed enters into the nucleus and stimulates the target genes' transcription aided by Runx2 and a cofactor (C). (**d**) Hedgehog signaling. Signaling by Hh depends on the interaction between the membrane proteins SMO and PTCH. When bound to Hh, PTCH does not repress SMO, which in turn activates GLI transcription factors

functions as a tumor suppressor [71], the inappropriate activation of the Notch pathway results in the stimulation of proliferation, restriction of differentiation and prevention of apoptosis in T-cell acute lymphoblastic leukemia [69], breast cancer [72, 73], melanoma [74], lung adenocarcinoma [75] and others. Therefore, a possible anticancer therapy goal may be the Notch signaling inhibition that is achieved at many different levels. It is possible to interfere with receptor activation by blocking ligand-induced conformational changes [76] and releasing the Notch-IC receptor by blocking the ADAM [77] or GS proteases cleavage [53, 65, 78]. In addition, Notch signaling could be inhibited by disrupting protein–protein interactions involved in nuclear events, including the assembly of co-activators [79, 80]. The γ-secretase inhibitors (GSIs) and monoclonal antibodies (mAbs), which block Notch receptors, are currently in the beginning stages of clinical trials [81, 82]. Moreover, mAbs that target Notch ligand Delta-like 4 have been shown to inhibit Notch signaling in endothelial cells by inducing disorganized angiogenesis [83]. In the platinum-resistant ovarian cancer, the inhibition of Notch signaling by a GSI and conventional Paclitaxel chemotherapy, synergistically reduced xenograft growth [84]. In intestinal crypts, where the staminal cell niche is located, Notch directs proliferation when Wnt signaling activity is high and promotes enterocyte differentiation when Wnt activity levels are reduced [85].

Wnt proteins constitute a family of signaling molecules that regulate cell-to-cell interactions during development. They are secreted glycoproteins that bind to the extra-cellular domain of the Frizzled (FZ) receptor, a seven-transmembrane protein that requires different co-receptors to mediate three different Wnt pathways:

(1) the canonical Wnt/β-catenin cascade; (2) the non canonical planar cell polarity (PCP) pathway; and (3) the Wnt/Ca^{2+} pathway.

In the canonical Wnt pathway, the co-factor low-density-lipoprotein-related protein5/6 (LRP5/6) interacts with the cytoplasmatic phosphoprotein Dishevelled (Dsh) [86]. This interaction causes an accumulation of β-catenin in the cytoplasm and its translocation into the nucleus, where it attracts, as co-activator, some transcription factors belonging to the T-cell factor-1 and lymphoid enhancing factor-1 TCF-1/LEF-1 family as well as regulating gene transduction. In the absence of Wnt ligands, a destruction complex formed by Axin2, adenomatosis polyposis coli (APC), glycogen synthase kinase 3 (GSK3) and casein kinase 1 (CK1), degrades β-catenin by targeting for ubiquitination. The canonical Wnt pathway activation produces the translocation of the negative Wnt regulator, Axin2, to the plasma membrane where it binds to the cytoplasmatic tail of LRP-5/6. Thus, Axin2 becomes de-phosphorylated and its stability is decreased. Moreover, Dsh inhibits the GSK3 activity of the destruction complex allowing the β-catenin accumulation in the nucleus (Fig. 1.1b) [85].

The Wnt canonical signaling is important in many developmental processes and in the regulation of self-renewal in normal and CSCs. In particular, the Wnt target gene *leucine-rich repeat-containing G protein-coupled receptor 5* (*Lgr5*) marks stem cells in multiple adult tissues and cancers [87]. A germline APC mutation is the genetic cause of a hereditary colorectal cancer syndrome called Familiar

Adenomatous Polyposis (FAP) [88, 89]. The cytoplasmatic interaction of APC with β-catenin provided the first connection between the Wnt pathway and human cancer [90, 91]. In intestinal epithelial cells in which APC is mutated, the constitutive β-catenin/TCF4 complex activates a genetic program within the crypt of stem/progenitor cells for the maintenance of cell proliferation [92]. In rare cases of colorectal cancer where APC is not mutated, Axin2 or β-catenin could be mutant [93, 94]. Loss-of-function mutations in Axin2 have been found in hepatocellular carcinomas whereas, oncogenic β-catenin mutations occur in a wide variety of solid tumors [95]. Concerning the colon cancer crypt, β-catenin induces the expression of EphB receptors which, interact with ephrin ligands inducing cells proliferation and thereby tumor progression [96, 97].

The non-canonical PCP pathway is one of the two Wnt pathways that does not involve β-catenin. After binding to Fz and its co-receptor (NRH1, Ryk, PTK7, or ROR2), the Wnt4, Wnt5a and Wnt11 ligands promote the pathway activation. These receptors form a complex inclusive of Dsh and Dishevelled-associated activator of morphogenesis 1 (DAAM1), which activate the small G-protein Rho and the Rho-associated kinase (ROCK), one of the cytoskeleton major regulators. The non-canonical Wnt pathway was shown to regulate both cell polarity and movements of dorsal mesodermal cells during neural tube closure [98]. ROCK activation has also been implicated in the cancer stem cells cytoskeleton organization and thereby in their migration and metastatis formation [99, 100].

The non-canonical Wnt signaling is reported to antagonize β-catenin-dependent transcription, suggesting an important anti-oncogenic effect [101]. However, a core PCP pathway scaffolding protein VANGL1 has been shown to promote metastasis in colon cancer. Moreover, it has been demonstrated that Wnt5a promotes mammosphere formation via a non-canonical mechanism which involves ROR2 as co-receptor [102].

The Wnt/Ca^{2+} pathway shares many components of the PCP pathway, but plays a different role in stimulating intracellular Ca^{2+} release by ER [103, 104]. The intracellular calcium accumulation activates several Ca^{2+} sensitive proteins, including protein kinase C [105] and calcium/calmodulin-dependent kinase II [106]. In melanomas, the activation of PKC as a result of the Wnt/Ca^{2+} pathway is involved in cell proliferation and metastasis. Thus, targeting this pathway could be relevant to cancer therapy [107].

The Bone morphogenetic protein 4 (BMP4) is able to activate a differentiation program and stimulate apoptosis in colon cancer stem cells. This reduces the β-catenin activation through inhibition of the PI3K/AKT pathway and up-regulation of the Wnt-negative modulators [108].

Bone Morphogenetic Proteins (BMPs) are secreted signaling molecules that comprise a subfamily of the TGF-β family. There are at least 20 structurally and functionally related BMPs, most of which play a role in embryogenesis and morphogenesis in various tissues and organs. BMP signaling depends on the heterodimerization of type I and II BMP receptors (BMPR) that lead to phosphorylation of the downstream molecules SMAD 1,5,8 and their association with SMAD 4. This complex translocates into the nucleus where it interacts with Runt-related transcription factor 2 (Runx2) and a cofactor (C) (Fig. 1.1c) [85]. Considering that BMP4 prevents cell proliferation and stimulates apoptosis by inducing the BAX expression and downregulating BCL-2 and Bcl-xL levels, the BMPR agonist could be useful in targeting cancer stem cells by activating a differentiation program and so potentiating the chemotherapy's cytotoxicity through BCL-2 negative inhibition in glioblastoma (GBM) [109]. It has recently been demonstrated that the BMP7 variant is a possible and innovative approach to the treatment of GBM since it decreases tumor growth in orthotopic mice models and stem cell markers expression, while enhancing differentiation markers expression [110].

The Hedgehog (Hh) signaling pathway plays very important functions in growth regulation, survival and fate during embryonic development and in the maintenance/repair of adult tissues. The Hh proteins initiate signaling by binding to the receptor Patched (PTCH). The subsequent receptor internalization alleviates the inhibitory effect of Patched on the 7-transmembrane protein Smoothened (SMO), which in turn activates the Hh pathway. Thus, the derepressed SMO activates GLI transcription factors, which translocate directly to the nucleus and drive the transcription of target genes (Fig. 1.1d) [111]. Deregulation of this pathway has been associated with tumorigenesis or tumor growth acceleration in a wide variety of tissues. Basal cell carcinoma, medulloblastoma, gastric cancer and pancreatic cancer bear mutations in components of the Hh pathway [112–116]. Moreover, the Hh pathway plays important roles in regulating self-renewal of normal and tumorigenic human mammary stem cells [117]. In GBM the treatment with an Hh pathway inhibitor, cyclopamine, caused a 40–60 % reduction in tumor growth and of the tumorigenic potential of CSCs [118].

Finally, it is demonstrated that, in the human pancreatic adenocarcinoma cell line, inhibiting the Hh pathway by cyclopamine, depressed tumor spheres self-renewal [119] and reversed gemcitabine resistance [120].

1.4 Immunological Profile of CSCs

The characterization of the immune profile of CSCs is complementary to their genomic/molecular assessment, and is mandatory to determine their susceptibility to innate and/or adaptive immune responses. Along this line, it is worthy to assess the expression of Tumor Associated Antigens (TAAs) and of the efficiency of their antigen processing and presentation by CSCs, as well as their expression profile of regulatory molecules of immune responses. Several groups have carried out studies in this field, however, thus far, this issue has not been clearly dissected.

The characterization of the immune profile of CSCs, including the expression of Major Histocompatibility Complex (MHC) class I and class II, of Antigen-Processing Machinery (APM) and of other immunologically relevant molecules has been determined in CSCs deriving from tumors with different histological origins, such GBM, melanoma and colorectal cancer (CRC) [121–124].

Low or negative expression of MHC class I and class II molecules is detected in these CSCs as compared with the autologous non-CSC counterpart of tumors [124, 125]. Moreover, low susceptibility of CSCs to IFN (α or γ) or de-methylating agent (5-Aza-2′-deoxycytidine), with some heterogeneity depending on the tissue origins, to increase the expression of MHC and APM molecules and of ligands of the receptor NKG2D (NKG2DLs) has been reported [124, 125]. Similar results are observed by Wu et al. [126], showing failure by GBM CSCs to express sufficient levels of MHC class I molecules and NK cell activatory ligands, leading to lack of susceptibility to NK-mediated lysis [126]. Along this line, melanoma-derived CSCs but not their autologous non-CSC counterparts have been found to be defective for MHC class I and class II molecules [122]. Taken together these evidences indicate that low efficiency in antigen processing and presentation of TAAs can occur in CSCs, revealing that these cells represent poor targets for cell-mediated immune responses (Fig. 1.2).

These observations are in line with the documentation that molecular defects can occur in MHC and APM molecules in bulk tumors with different tissue origins [127–130].

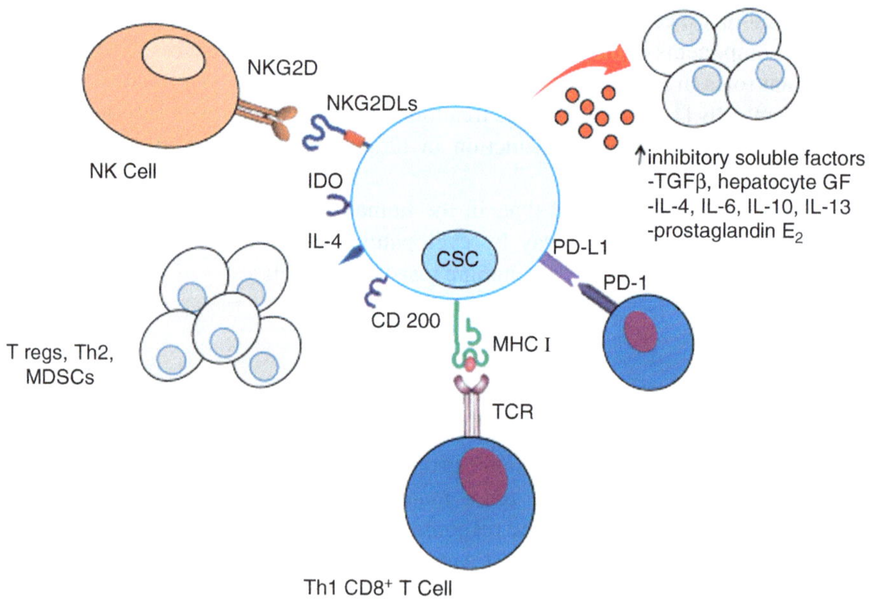

Fig. 1.2 The immunomodulatory activity of CSCs is regulated by the interaction of multiple stimulatory and inhibitory molecules. The expression or not of immune-related molecules, such as MHC molecules, NKG2DLs and other ligands of NK activatory receptors, can result in inducing or not efficient T cell-mediated responses against CSCs. On the other hand, negative immunomodulatory molecules such as PD-L1, CD200, IDO and IL-4 can suppress cell-mediated immunosurveillance. Soluble factors (TGFβ, hepatocyte GF, IL-4, IL-6, IL-10, IL-13 and prostaglandin E2) released by CSCs can inhibit effector functions and lead to the differentiation of immune cells with regulatory activity, T regulatory cells (Tregs) and myeloid-derived suppressor cells (MDSCs) or of Th2-type T cell responses

This immune profile of CSCs resembles that of the physiological normal stem cells. In fact, embryonic stem cells (ESCs) express low levels of classical antigen-presenting MHC class, no MHC class I and II molecules. Moreover, they express low levels or are negative for the ligands of activatory NK cell receptor (NKp44, NKp30, NKp46, and CD16) [131]. Similarly, normal heamatopoietic stem cells display down-regulation of MHC class I molecules [132] thus, suggesting that low MHC molecules expression is a common feature of "stemness" allowing their preservation and leading to the escape from cell-mediated immune responses. Non-classical MHC molecules, that can exert inhibitory signals (e.g. HLA-G), are commonly expressed at high levels by both ESCs and mesenchymal stem cells (MSCs) contributing to the evasion from recognition by T or NK cells [133–136].

1.5 Expression of TAAs by CSCs

During the neoplastic transformation the abnormal expression of some surface, nuclear or cytoplasmic molecules occur. These molecules can represent tumor-associated antigens (TAAs), that following their processing and presentation in association with MHC molecules, can elicit T lymphocyte-mediated anti-tumor responses. These TAAs can be classifies as following:

- *Differentiation TAAs*. Tumor cells share these antigens with normal cells of the same lineages, however, they are overexpressed in neoplastic cells. This group of TAAs has mainly been found in melanoma and melanocytes, e.g. MART-1/Melan-A, Gp100, and tyrosinase but also in other epithelial tissues such as the prostate specific antigen (PSA) found in prostate, CEA in CRC and MUC-1 in CRC, lung cancer, mammary cancer etc. [137].
- *Cancer-testis antigens* (CTAs), which represent tumor specific TAAs, since their expression in normal tissues is restricted to the testis and placenta. They include the MAGE family proteins (A1, -A2, -A3), NY-ESO-1, NA-17, LAGE, etc. [137].
- *Mutated TAAs*: they could arise from point mutations in oncogenes, tumor suppressor genes or genes involved in survival and proliferation pathways [138].

These molecules represent the potential targets of cancer immunotherapy and since their molecular identification, they have been exploited for several vaccine-based clinical studies for cancer patients. [139]. Targeting TAAs specifically expressed by CSCs could improve the efficacy of cancer vaccines and improve the induction of systemic T cell-mediated immune responses.

The characterization of molecularly known tumor antigens by CSCs has been the objects of a few studies, showing lack or limiting expression of these molecules. Failure in detecting either differentiation, such as MART-1, Gp100, or CT antigens, such as MAGE, NY-ESO-1, or IL-13Rα2 has been documented in CSC from melanoma, GBM or CRC [121–123]. On the other hand, NY-ESO1, Ep-CAM, CEA and SVV-1 were detected in CSCs either from melanoma or CRC, respectively (Table 1.1) [123, 140].

Table 1.1 Expression of TAAs by CSCs

TAA	Tumor type	TAA category	Expression in CSCs	Reference(s)
Survivin	CRC/GBM	Over-expressed antigen[a]	Yes	[121, 123]
Gp100	Melanoma/CRC/GBM	Differentiation antigen	Yes/no/no	[121, 123, 168]
MAGE	Melanoma/CRC/GBM	CT antigens	Yes/no/no	[121, 123, 169]
MART-1	Melanoma	Differentiation antigen	No	[122]
CEA	CRC	Differentiation antigen	Yes	[123]
MUC-1	Breast cancer	Over-expressed antigen	Yes	[170]
NY-ESO 1	CRC/CRC/GBM	CT antigens	Yes/no/no	[121, 123, 169]
HER2/neu	Breast cancer	Over-expressed antigen	No	[171]
COA-1	CRC	Over-expressed antigen	Yes	[123]
SOX-2	GBM	Over-expressed antigen	Yes	[121]
CD133	CRC/GBM	Over-expressed antigen	Yes	[172]
IL-13Rα2	GBM/CRC	Over-expressed antigen	Yes	[121, 123, 145]

[a]TAAs over-expressed in tumors

However, none of these TAAs are reported as eliciting efficient T cell-mediated responses against CSCs, suggesting that defective antigen processing and presentation of these antigens, as described in Sect. 1.4, and/or the lack of sufficient expression of these TAAs can prevent the activation of T cell immune responses and their exploitation as target for vaccine based-immunotherapy. Of note, circulating precursor effector cells recognizing a few of these antigens have been found in GBM, melanoma and CRC models, indicating that, though these TAA can elicit immune responses, they cannot be targeting CSCs (Table 1.1) [141–143].

Interestingly, T cell responses against the COA-1 antigen, which is expressed by CSCs, have been isolated in CRC patients, suggesting that this molecule may represent, al least for CRC, a valuable target molecule for T cell-mediated immune responses against CSCs (Table 1.1) [123].

Further efforts are needed to exploit the mutational profile of CSCs in order to identify candidate TAAs arising from somatic mutations in their genome and to validate their role as novel immunogenic CSC-associated target molecules for immunotherapy.

Although a definitive profile of TAAs expressed by CSCs has not been achieved yet, acquiring a comprehensive analysis of genetic, molecular and immunological features of CSCs may provide relevant information to identify novel highly immunogenic molecules for the specific targeting of CSCs.

1.6 Cell-Mediated Immune Responses Against CSCs and Immune Escape Mechanisms

The knowledge of immunological properties of CSCs in relationship with their tissue origins is still limited, however, several reports have shown their resistance to immune-mediated reactivity [124, 125]. Differential gene and protein expressions for some immunological-related molecules, such as down-modulation of molecules related to IFN signaling, cytokines, etc. or up-regulation of the AKT-STAT signal pathway, which was found to be involved in immune escape mechanisms [144], have been described in GBM-CSCs as compared with the differentiated non-CSC counterpart of tumors [121]. These evidences, together with that described in Sects. 1.4 and 1.5 indicate that CSCs deriving from solid tumors can indeed display peculiar biological properties and can behave differently from cells lacking the "stemness" function [124, 125].

Along with an increasing effort in characterizing immunological properties of CSCs, it comes clearer that CSCs can act as immunomodulators toward cell-mediated immune responses [124, 125]. Although some variability can occur depending on tissue origins and on the procedures for their in vitro isolation. GBM-CSCs display impairment of T cell proliferation and can induce a preferential selection/differentiation of Th2-type T cell responses following their co-culture in vitro with either autologous or allogeneic patient-derived peripheral blood lymphocytes [121].

On the other hand, CMV-specific T cells can recognize and kill brain-derived CSCs, indicating that strong immunogenic viral-derived epitopes can be presented in the HLA-restricted context by CSCs and can be recognized by T cells [145]. The evidence that $CD4^{+}CD56^{+}$ T cells with an Th2-associated cytokine profile represented the major subpopulation in tumor infiltrating lymphocytes of GBM patients was reported as result of local tumor suppression of immune responses [146]; thus, indicating that this mechanism might be driven by the presence of tumor cells with "stemness" properties. Along this line, the unsuccessful targeting of melanoma-derived CSCs by T lymphocytes recognizing melanoma-associated antigens (MAAs) has been also reported; this phenomenon is associated with negative or low levels of expression of MAA by CSCs, as discussed in Sect. 1.5 [122, 147].

Failure in successful anti-CSCs activity by the innate immune system has been documented in GBM and ovarian cancer, depending on low or negative expression of ligands for NK receptors and MHC class I molecules [126, 148]. Susceptibility to NK-mediated reactivity can be detected for CSCs from human CRC, primary oral squamous and ovarian carcinoma when the immune profile of these cells displays efficient expression of NK-receptor ligands and lack or low expression of MHC class I molecules [149–151], Similar observations have been reported for mouse prostate CSCs [152].

These evidences highlight the heterogeneity of CSCs in terms of the immunological profile and of their susceptibility to cell-mediated immune responses. The low expression of MHC molecules and APM by CSCs can be partially overcome by vaccine-based models using professional antigen-presenting cells (APCs) loaded with CSC lysates to elicit efficient cell-mediated immune responses, as shown in both human and mouse models [153–156].

Taken together, the observations discussed, thus far, corroborate the hypothesis that low efficiency by CSCs in antigen-processing and presentation, as well as low expression of TAAs and/or of ligands for activatory NK cell receptors can impair cell-mediated immune responses. In some cases, CSCs can be targeted by immune responses induced in vivo either by the vaccination with APC loaded with CSCs-derived TAAs or by the treatment with immunomodulatory agents (e.g. IFN-α) [126].

1.7 Immunoregulatory/Immune Escape Mechanisms Associated with CSCs

CSCs not only represent poor target cells for anti-tumor immune responses but they also display immune-regulatory properties. This indication originates from a variety of reports showing that these cells can secrete cytokines and soluble suppressive factors, such as Galectin-3, TGFβ, IL-10, IL-13, PGE2, PD-1, B7-H1, B7-H3, B7-H4, and GDF-15 [122, 157–161] (Table 1.2 and Fig. 1.2). The immunosuppressive

Table 1.2 Immunomodulatory molecules associated with CSCs

Molecule	CSCs	Non-CSC tumor	Normal stem cells	Reference(s)
IL-4	Over-expressed	Low levels	Not detected	[123]
IL-6	Over-expressed/ down-modulated	Expressed	Expressed	[122, 158, 159]
IL-10	Over-expressed/absent	Expressed	Expressed	[122, 158]
IL-13	Over-expressed/absent	Expressed	Expressed	[121, 122]
TGF-β1	Over-expressed/absent	Expressed	Expressed	[121, 122]
B7-H4	Over-expressed	Expressed	Expressed	[157]
PG2D	Expressed	Expressed	Expressed	[174]
GDF-15	Over-expressed	Not detected	Not detected	[159]
STAT3	Over-expressed	Expressed	Expressed	[158]
Galectin-3	Over-expressed	Expressed	Expressed	[122]
IDO	Over-expressed	Expressed	Expressed	[173], Unpublished results
CD200	Expressed	Expressed	Expressed	[165]

activity of cancer initiating cells has been recently described both in GBM and melanoma, showing that CSC-like cells can inhibit T cell activation and proliferation by the induction of Tregs [122, 158, 159]. Furthermore, B7-H1, B7-H4, PD-1 and PD-L1 can be detected on CSCs from both GBM and CRC; these molecules inhibit T cell activation and proliferation following their encountering with CSCs, with implication for cell-mediated immunesurveillance of tumors (Table 1.2 and Fig. 1.2) [121, 123].

Of note, the expression of B7 family members in brain tumor cells, including CSCs, has been related with their immunoresistance to T cell-mediated responses [157, 162]. CRC-CSCs express and secrete IL-4, with higher levels as compared with the autologous non-CSC tumor counterpart, which function is determinant for drug and apoptosis resistance and for the immune evasion of these cells [123, 163]. The membrane-associated IL-4 on CSCs predominantly exerts, by cell-to-cell contact, inhibition of T cell proliferation and of their anti-tumor activity (Table 1.2 and Fig. 1.2) [123]. Furthermore, the neutralization of this cytokine, by specific monoclonal antibodies, can restore T cell proliferation and anti-tumor activity [123]. In this model, soluble IL-4, though released by CRC-CSCs, leads only to partial in vitro inhibition of T cell reactivity [123]. Therefore, the blocking of IL-4 on CSCs can overcome at least one of the negative immunomodulatory activities of these cells and can rescue the activation and proliferation of both T and NK cells [123, 149]. These observations are in line with the demonstration that IL-4 signaling is a relevant key regulator for epithelial tumor behavior and lack of responsiveness to standard therapies [163, 164].

Moreover, CD200, a molecule that can block myeloid cell activities has been shown to be expressed by CSCs [165] while GBM-CSCs can evade from T cell recognition by the STAT3 pathway (Table 1.2 and Fig. 1.2) [158].

Despite the common feature of the immunosuppressive activity associated with CSCs, a variety of negative immunoregulatory signaling can be detected on these cells. Nevertheless, it appears clearly that these negative immune regulatory signals are not CSC-specific, but are shared with normal stem cells [166, 167]. Along this line, PGE2, acting by inhibiting macrophage and T cell activation, and indoleamine 2,3-dioxigenase (IDO) (Fig. 1.2), that depletes tryptophan preventing T cell activation and proliferation, are produced by CSCs to prevent immune reactivity and autoimmune diseases. Recently, the expression IDO has been found, following IFN-γ treatment, on CSCs from GBM and CRC and has been found as responsible for the inhibition of T cell proliferation following their coculture in vitro with autologous CSCs (*see* Table 1.2 and Maccalli et al., personal communication).

Taken together, the observations reported, thus far, indicate that CSCs indeed display a low immunogenic profile and immunomodulatory functions that are typical features of "stemness" functions. Thus, immune-escaped CSCs, with low immunological properties, can favour the propagation and accumulation of cancer cells and can evade immunosurveillance. These cells may represent the self-renewal reservoir of a tumor, allowing cancer cell survival and progression.

The immunological characterization of CSCs still needs to be fully elucidated, however, the available information can contribute in identifying novel strategies that can revert the immunomodulatory activity of these cells and can target CSCs, such as the usage of immune checkpoint blockade agents [35] in combination with vaccine-based immunotherapy.

1.8 Conclusions

Progress has been achieved in gaining the biological and immunological characterization of CSCs. Aberrantly expressed signaling pathways have been identified to be associated with CSCs and to confer their "stemness" properties and the ability to metastasize. In addition, these investigations have allowed the identification of markers that may be exploited to isolate ex vivo CSCs responsible for tumor initiation and propagation. Along this line, small agents are available to target CSCs that will be used soon for clinical studies.

Heterogeneity can be detected in CSCs isolated from different tumors depending on the genomic background and/or the histological origin, however, a common feature of these cells is their ability in evading cell-mediating immune responses. This characteristic is achieved by the expression and the activation in CSCs of a variety of immunomodulatory signaling pathways, thus leading to the impairment of cell-mediated immune responses specifically targeting CSCs (Fig. 1.2).

The immune privilege of CSCs can favor the survival of an immune-hidden reservoir of self-renewing cells that can warrant tumor propagation. Relevant implications are that the treatment with either a survival pathway inhibitor or differentiation-inducing small agents may be not sufficient for the complete CSC elimination. Therefore, the therapeutic combination of these agents with immunotherapy strategies is desirable. Novel immunotherapy strategies targeting CSCs should take into account the plasticity and heterogeneity of CSCs.

Further efforts are needed to fully dissect the relationship between CSCs and the innate/adaptive immune responses, however, the molecular identification of at least a few of the immunoregulatory molecules expressed by CSCs can enable to block these signaling pathways by the usage of appropriate immunomodulating agents (e.g. immune checkpoint blockade agents, inhibitory molecules).

Acknowledgements We thank Italian Alliance against Cancer and Italian Association for Cancer Research (AIRC) granted to G. Parmiani. AIRC and AIRC 5x1000 granted to G. Stassi. Thanks to Tatiana Terranova for collaborating in the editing.

References

1. Nowell PC. The clonal evolution of tumor cell populations. Science. 1976;194:23–8.
2. Clarke MF, Dick JE, Dirks PB, Eaves CJ, Jamieson CH, Jones DL, Visvader J, Weissman IL, Wahl GM. Cancer stem cells–perspectives on current status and future directions: AACR workshop on cancer stem cells. Cancer Res. 2006;66:9339–44.

3. Reya T, Morrison SJ, Clarke MF, Weissman IL. Stem cells, cancer, and cancer stem cells. Nature. 2001;414:105–11.
4. Dean M, Fojo T, Bates S. Tumour stem cells and drug resistance. Nat Rev Cancer. 2005;5:275–84.
5. Wilson A, Laurenti E, Oser G, van der Wath RC, Blanco-Bose W, Jaworski M, Offner S, Dunant CF, Eshkind L, Bockamp E, Lió P, Macdonald HR, Trumpp A. Hematopoietic stem cells reversibly switch from dormancy to self-renewal during homeostasis and repair. Cell. 2008;135:1118–29.
6. Fuchs E. The tortoise and the hair: slow-cycling cells in the stem cell race. Cell. 2009;137(5):811–9.
7. Sherr CJ. The Pezcoller lecture: cancer cell cycles revisited. Cancer Res. 2000;60:3689–95.
8. Siegel PM, Massague J. Cytostatic and apoptotic actions of TGF-beta in homeostasis and cancer. Nat Rev Cancer. 2003;3:807–21.
9. Soltanian S, Matin MM. Cancer stem cells and cancer therapy. Tumour Biol. 2011;3:425–40.
10. Liu G, Yuan X, Zeng Z, Tunici P, Ng H, Abdulkadir IR, Lu L, Irvin D, Black KL, Yu JS. Analysis of gene expression and chemoresistance of CD133+ cancer stem cells in glioblastoma. Mol Cancer. 2006;5:67.
11. Bao S, Wu Q, McLendon RE, Hao Y, Shi Q, Hjelmeland AB, Dewhirst MW, Bigner DD, Rich JN. Glioma stem cells promote radioresistance by preferential activation of the DNA damage response. Nature. 2006;444:756–60.
12. Ginestier C, Hur MH, Charafe-Jauffret E, Monville F, Dutcher J, Brown M, Jacquemier J, Viens P, Kleer CG, Liu S, Schott A, Hayes D, Birnbaum D, Wicha MS, Dontu G. ALDH1 is a marker of normal and malignant human mammary stem cells and a predictor of poor clinical outcome. Cell Stem Cell. 2007;1:555–67.
13. Ishimoto T, Nagano O, Yae T, Tamada M, Motohara T, Oshima H, Oshima M, Ikeda T, Asaba R, Yagi H, Masuko T, Shimizu T, Ishikawa T, Kai K, Takahashi E, Imamura Y, Baba Y, Ohmura M, Suematsu M, Baba H, Saya H. CD44 variant regulates redox status in cancer cells by stabilizing the xCT subunit of system xc(-) and thereby promotes tumor growth. Cancer Cell. 2011;19:387–400.
14. Hovinga KE, Shimizu F, Wang R, Panagiotakos G, Van Der Heijden M, Moayedpardazi H, Correia AS, Soulet D, Major T, Menon J, Tabar V. Inhibition of notch signaling in glioblastoma targets cancer stem cells via an endothelial cell intermediate. Stem Cells. 2010;28:1019–29.
15. Folkins C, Man S, Xu P, Shaked Y, Hicklin DJ, Kerbel RS. Anticancer therapies combining antiangiogenic and tumor cell cytotoxic effects reduce the tumor stem-like cell fraction in glioma xenograft tumors. Cancer Res. 2007;67:3560–4.
16. Cabarcas SM, Mathews LA, Farrar WL. The cancer stem cell niche–there goes the neighborhood? Int J Cancer. 2011;129(10):2315–27.
17. Calabrese C, Poppleton H, Kocak M, Hogg TL, Fuller C, Hamner B, Oh EY, Gaber MW, Finklestein D, Allen M, Frank A, Bayazitov IT, Zakharenko SS, Gajjar A, Davidoff A, Gilbertson RJ. A perivascular niche for brain tumor stem cells. Cancer Cell. 2007;11:69–82.
18. Scheel C, Weinberg RA. Phenotypic plasticity and epithelial-mesenchymal transitions in cancer and normal stem cells? Int J Cancer. 2011;129:2310–4.
19. Charles N, Ozawa T, Squatrito M, Bleau AM, Brennan CW, Hambardzumyan D, Holland EC. Perivascular nitric oxide activates notch signaling and promotes stem-like character in PDGF-induced glioma cells. Cell Stem Cell. 2010;6:141–52.
20. Vermeulen L, De Sousa E, Melo F, van der Heijden M, Cameron K, de Jong JH, Borovski T, Tuynman JB, Todaro M, Merz C, Rodermond H, Sprick MR, Kemper K, Richel DJ, Stassi G, Medema JP. Wnt activity defines colon cancer stem cells and is regulated by the microenvironment. Nat Cell Biol. 2010;12:468–76.
21. Mani SA, Guo W, Liao MJ, Eaton EN, Ayyanan A, Zhou AY, Brooks M, Reinhard F, Zhang CC, Shipitsin M, Campbell LL, Polyak K, Brisken C, Yang J, Weinberg RA. The epithelial-mesenchymal transition generates cells with properties of stem cells. Cell. 2008;133:704–15.

22. Morel AP, Lièvre M, Thomas C, Hinkal G, Ansieau S, Puisieux A. Generation of breast cancer stem cells through epithelial-mesenchymal transition. PLoS One. 2008;3:e2888.
23. Shimono Y, Zabala M, Cho RW, Lobo N, Dalerba P, Qian D, Diehn M, Liu H, Panula SP, Chiao E, Dirbas FM, Somlo G, Pera RA, Lao K, Clarke MF. Downregulation of miRNA-200c links breast cancer stem cells with normal stem cells. Cell. 2009;138(3):592–603.
24. Wellner U, Schubert J, Burk UC, Schmalhofer O, Zhu F, Sonntag A, Waldvogel B, Vannier C, Darling D, zur Hausen A, Brunton VG, Morton J, Sansom O, Schüler J, Stemmler MP, Herzberger C, Hopt U, Keck T, Brabletz S, Brabletz T. The EMT-activator ZEB1 promotes tumorigenicity by repressing stemness-inhibiting microRNAs. Nat Cell Biol. 2009;11:1487–95.
25. Yang MH, Hsu DS, Wang HW, Wang HJ, Lan HY, Yang WH, Huang CH, Kao SY, Tzeng CH, Tai SK, Chang SY, Lee OK, Wu KJ. Bmi1 is essential in Twist1-induced epithelial-mesenchymal transition. Nat Cell Biol. 2010;12:982–92.
26. Todaro M, Gaggianesi M, Catalano V, Benfante A, Iovino F, Biffoni M, Apuzzo T, Sperduti I, Volpe S, Cocorullo G, Gulotta G, Dieli F, De Maria R, Stassi G. CD44v6 is a marker of constitutive and reprogrammed cancer stem cells driving colon cancer metastasis. Cell Stem Cell. 2014;14:342–56.
27. Burnet FM. The concept of immunological surveillance. Prog Exp Tumor Res. 1970;13:1–27.
28. Thomas L. On immunosurveillance in human cancer. Yale J Biol Med. 1982;55:329–33.
29. Schreiber RD, Old LJ, Smyth MJ. Cancer immunoediting: integrating immunity's roles in cancer suppression and promotion. Science. 2011;331:1565–70.
30. Mihm Jr MC, Clemente CG, Cascinelli N. Tumor infiltrating lymphocytes in lymph node melanoma metastases: a histopathologic prognostic indicator and an expression of local immune response. Lab Invest. 1996;74:43–7.
31. Bindea G, Mlecnik B, Angell HK, Galon J. The immune landscape of human tumors: implications for cancer immunotherapy. Oncoimmunology. 2014;3:e27456. Epub 2014 Jan 3.
32. Fecci PE, Mitchell DA, Whitesides JF, Xie W, Friedman AH, Archer GE, Herndon 2nd JE, Bigner DD, Dranoff G, Sampson JH. Increased regulatory T-cell fraction amidst a diminished CD4 compartment explains cellular immune defects in patients with malignant glioma. Cancer Res. 2006;66:3294–302.
33. Cantini G, Pisati F, Mastropietro A, Frattini V, Iwakura Y, Finocchiaro G, Pellegatta S. A critical role for regulatory T cells in driving cytokine profiles of Th17 cells and their modulation of glioma microenvironment. Cancer Immunol Immunother. 2011;60:1739–50.
34. Gajewski T, Schreiber H, Fu YX. Innate and adaptive immune cells in the tumor microenvironment. Nat Immunol. 2013;14:1014–22.
35. Pardoll DM. The blockade of immune checkpoints in cancer immunotherapy. Nat Rev Cancer. 2012;12:252–64.
36. Naidoo J, Page DB, Wolchok JD. Immune checkpoint blockade. Hematol Oncol Clin North Am. 2014;28:585–600.
37. Dihen M, Clarke MF. Cancer stem cells and radiotherapy: new insights into tumor radioresistance. J Natl Cancer Inst. 2006;98:1755–7.
38. Irvin DK, Jouanneau E, Duvall G, Zhang XX, Zhai Y, Sarayba D, Seksenyan A, Panwar A, Black KL, Wheeler CJ. T cells enhance stem-like properties and conditional malignancy in gliomas. PLoS One. 2010;5:e10974.
39. Maugeri-Saccà M, Vigneri P, De Maria R. Cancer stem cells and chemosensitivity. Clin Cancer Res. 2011;17:4942–7.
40. Goodell MA, Brose K, Paradis G, Conner AS, Mulligan RC. Isolation and functional properties of murine hematopoietic stem cells that are replicating in vivo. J Exp Med. 1996;183:1797–806.
41. Hirschmann-Jax C, Foster AE, Wulf GG, Nuchtern JG, Jax TW, Gobel U, Goodell MA, Brenner MK. A distinct "side population" of cells with high drug efflux capacity in human tumor cells. Proc Natl Acad Sci U S A. 2004;101:14228–33.

42. Wu C, Wei Q, Utomo V, Nadesan P, Whetstone H, Kandel R, Wunder JS, Alman BA. Side population cells isolated from mesenchymal neoplasms have tumor initiating potential. Cancer Res. 2007;67:8216–22.
43. Wu C, Alman BA. Side population cells in human cancers. Cancer Lett. 2008;268:1–9.
44. Moreb JS, Ucar D, Han S, Amory JK, Goldstein AS, Ostmark B, Chang LJ. The enzymatic activity of human aldehyde dehydrogenases 1A2 and 2 (ALDH1A2 and ALDH2) is detected by Aldefluor, inhibited by diethylaminobenzaldehyde and has significant effects on cell proliferation and drug resistance. Chem Biol Interact. 2012;195:52–60.
45. Marcato P, Dean CA, Giacomantonio CA, Lee PW. Aldehyde dehydrogenase: its role as a cancer stem cell marker comes down to the specific isoform. Cell Cycle. 2011;10:1378–84.
46. Dalerba P, Dylla SJ, Park IK, Liu R, Wang X, Cho RW, Hoey T, Gurney A, Huang EH, Simeone DM, Shelton AA, Parmiani G, Castelli C, Clarke MF. Phenotypic characterization of human colorectal cancer stem cells. Proc Natl Acad Sci U S A. 2007;104:10158–63.
47. Li C, Heidt DG, Dalerba P, Burant CF, Zhang L, Adsay V, Wicha M, Clarke MF, Simeone DM. Identification of pancreatic cancer stem cells. Cancer Res. 2007;67:1030–7.
48. Du L, Wang H, He L, Zhang J, Ni B, Wang X, Jin H, Cahuzac N, Mehrpour M, Lu Y, Chen Q. CD44 is of functional importance for colorectal cancer stem cells. Clin Cancer Res. 2008;14:6751–60.
49. Wang YC, Yo YT, Lee HY, Liao YP, Chao TK, Su PH, Lai HC. ALDH1-bright epithelial ovarian cancer cells are associated with CD44 expression, drug resistance, and poor clinical outcome. Am J Pathol. 2012;180:1159–69.
50. Choi D, Lee HW, Hur KY, Kim JJ, Park GS, Jang SH, Song YS, Jang KS, Paik SS. Cancer stem cell markers CD133 and CD24 correlate with invasiveness and differentiation in colorectal adenocarcinoma. World J Gastroenterol. 2009;15:2258–64.
51. Chen Y, Yu D, Zhang H, He H, Zhang C, Zhao W, Shao RG. CD133(+)EpCAM(+) phenotype possesses more characteristics of tumor initiating cells in hepatocellular carcinoma Huh7 cells. Int J Biol Sci. 2012;8:992–1004.
52. Yang ZF, Ho DW, Ng MN, Lau CK, Yu WC, Ngai P, Chu PW, Lam CT, Poon RT, Fan ST. Significance of CD90+ cancer stem cells in human liver cancer. Cancer Cell. 2008;13:153–66.
53. Ricci-Vitiani L, Lombardi DG, Pilozzi E, Biffoni M, Todaro M, Peschle C, De Maria R. Identification and expansion of human colon-cancer-initiating cells. Nature. 2007;445:111–5.
54. Wakamatsu Y, Sakamoto N, Oo HZ, Naito Y, Uraoka N, Anami K, Sentani K, Oue N, Yasui W. Expression of cancer stem cell markers ALDH1, CD44 and CD133 in primary tumor and lymph node metastasis of gastric cancer. Pathol Int. 2012;62:112–9.
55. Singh SK, Hawkins C, Clarke ID, Squire JA, Bayani J, Hide T, Henkelman RM, Cusimano MD, Dirks PB. Identification of human brain tumour initiating cells. Nature. 2004;432:396–401.
56. Collins AT, Berry PA, Hyde C, Stower MJ, Maitland NJ. Prospective identification of tumorigenic prostate cancer stem cells. Cancer Res. 2005;65:10946–51.
57. O'Brien CA, Pollett A, Gallinger S, Dick JE. A human colon cancer cell capable of initiating tumour growth in immunodeficient mice. Nature. 2007;445:106–10.
58. Miraglia S, Godfrey W, Yin AH, Atkins K, Warnke R, Holden JT, Bray RA, Waller EK, Buck DW. A novel five-transmembrane hematopoietic stem cell antigen: isolation, characterization, and molecular cloning. Blood. 1997;90:5013–21.
59. Bussolati B, Bruno S, Grange C, Buttiglieri S, Deregibus MC, Cantino D, Camussi G. Isolation of renal progenitor cells from adult human kidney. Am J Pathol. 2005;166:545–55.
60. Yin S, Li J, Hu C, Chen X, Yao M, Yan M, Jiang G, Ge C, Xie H, Wan D, Yang S, Zheng S, Gu J. CD133 positive hepatocellular carcinoma cells possess high capacity for tumorigenicity. Int J Cancer. 2007;120:1444–50.
61. Shmelkov SV, Meeus S, Moussazadeh N, Kermani P, Rashbaum WK, Rabbany SY, Hanson MA, Lane WJ, St Clair R, Walsh KA, Dias S, Jacobson JT, Hempstead BL, Edelberg JM,

Rafii S. CD133 expression is not restricted to stem cells, and both CD133+ and CD133- metastatic colon cancer cells initiate tumors. J Clin Invest. 2008;118:2111–20.
62. Kemper K, Sprick MR, de Bree M, Scopelliti A, Vermeulen L, Hoek M, Zeilstra J, Pals ST, Mehmet H, Stassi G, Medema JP. The AC133 epitope, but not the CD133 protein, is lost upon cancer stem cell differentiation. Cancer Res. 2010;70:719–29.
63. Bauer N, Fonseca AV, Florek M, Freund D, Jászai J, Bornhäuser M, Fargeas CA, Corbeil D. New insights into the cell biology of hematopoietic progenitors by studying prominin-1 (CD133). Cells Tissues Organs. 2008;188:127–38.
64. Zhu L, Gibson P, Currle DS, Tong Y, Richardson RJ, Bayazitov IT, Poppleton H, Zakharenko S, Ellison DW, Gilbertson RJ. Prominin 1 marks intestinal stem cells that are susceptible to neoplastic transformation. Nature. 2009;457:603–7.
65. Takebe N, Nguyen D, Yang SX. Targeting notch signaling pathway in cancer: clinical development advances and challenges. Pharmacol Ther. 2014;141:140–9.
66. Miele L, Golde T, Osborne B. Notch signaling in cancer. Curr Mol Med. 2006;6:905–18.
67. Berman JN, Look AT. Targeting transcription factors in acute leukemia in children. Curr Drug Targets. 2007;8:727–37.
68. Koch U, Radtke F. Notch and cancer: a double-edged sword. Cell Mol Life Sci. 2007; 64:2746–62.
69. Roy M, Pear WS, Aster JC. The multifaceted role of Notch in cancer. Curr Opin Genet Dev. 2007;17:52–9.
70. Shih IeM, Wang TL. Notch signaling, gamma-secretase inhibitors, and cancer therapy. Cancer Res. 2007;67:1879–82.
71. Restivo G, Nguyen BC, Dziunycz P, Ristorcelli E, Ryan RJ, Özuysal ÖY, Di Piazza M, Radtke F, Dixon MJ, Hofbauer GF, Lefort K, Dotto GP. IRF6 is a mediator of Notch pro-differentiation and tumour suppressive function in keratinocytes. EMBO J. 2011;30: 4571–85.
72. Reedijk M, Odorcic S, Chang L, Zhang H, Miller N, McCready DR, Lockwood G, Egan SE. High-level coexpression of JAG1 and NOTCH1 is observed in human breast cancer and is associated with poor overall survival. Cancer Res. 2005;65:8530–7.
73. Dickson RB, Deb TB. EGF receptor in breast cancer chemoresistance. Adv Exp Med Biol. 2007;608:113–8.
74. Pinnix CC, Herlyn M. The many faces of Notch signaling in skin-derived cells. Pigment Cell Res. 2007;20:458–65.
75. Chen Y, De Marco MA, Graziani I, Gazdar AF, Strack PR, Miele L, Bocchetta M. Oxygen concentration determines the biological effects of NOTCH-1 signaling in adenocarcinoma of the lung. Cancer Res. 2007;67:7954–9.
76. Gordon WR, Vardar-Ulu D, Histen G, Sanchez-Irizarry C, Aster JC, Blacklow SC. Structural basis for autoinhibition of Notch. Nat Struct Mol Biol. 2007;14:295–300.
77. Brou C, Logeat F, Gupta N, Bessia C, LeBail O, Doedens JR, Cumano A, Roux P, Black RA, Israël A. A novel proteolytic cleavage involved in Notch signaling: the role of the disintegrin-metalloprotease TACE. Mol Cell. 2000;5:207–16.
78. Kopan R, Ilagan MX. Gamma-secretase: proteasome of the membrane? Nat Rev Mol Cell Biol. 2004;5:499–504.
79. Nam Y, Sliz P, Song L, Aster JC, Blacklow SC. Structural basis for cooperativity in recruitment of MAML coactivators to Notch transcription complexes. Cell. 2006;124:973–83.
80. Nam Y, Sliz P, Pear WS, Aster JC, Blacklow SC. Cooperative assembly of higher-order Notch complexes functions as a switch to induce transcription. Proc Natl Acad Sci U S A. 2007;104:2103–8.
81. Li K, Li Y, Wu W, Gordon WR, Chang DW, Lu M, Scoggin S, Fu T, Vien L, Histen G, Zheng J, Martin-Hollister R, Duensing T, Singh S, Blacklow SC, Yao Z, Aster JC, Zhou BB. Modulation of Notch signaling by antibodies specific for the extracellular negative regulatory region of NOTCH3. J Biol Chem. 2008;283:8046–54.
82. Schott AF, Landis MD, Dontu G, Griffith KA, Layman RM, Krop I, Paskett LA, Wong H, Dobrolecki LE, Lewis MT, Froehlich AM, Paranilam J, Hayes DF, Wicha MS, Chang JC.

Preclinical and clinical studies of gamma secretase inhibitors with docetaxel on human breast tumors. Clin Cancer Res. 2013;19:1512–24.
83. Ridgway J, Zhang G, Wu Y, Stawicki S, Liang WC, Chanthery Y, Kowalski J, Watts RJ, Callahan C, Kasman I, Singh M, Chien M, Tan C, Hongo JA, de Sauvage F, Plowman G, Yan M. Inhibition of Dll4 signalling inhibits tumour growth by deregulating angiogenesis. Nature. 2006;444:1083–7.
84. Groeneweg JW, DiGloria CM, Yuan J, Richardson WS, Growdon WB, Sathyanarayanan S, Foster R, Rueda BR. Inhibition of notch signaling in combination with Paclitaxel reduces platinum-resistant ovarian tumor growth. Front Oncol. 2014;4:171.
85. Medema JP, Vermeulen L. Microenvironmental regulation of stem cells in intestinal homeostasis and cancer. Nature. 2011;474:318–26.
86. He X, Semenov M, Tamai K, Zeng X. LDL receptor-related proteins 5 and 6 in Wnt/beta-catenin signaling: arrows point the way. Development. 2004;131:1663–77.
87. Barker N, van Es JH, Kuipers J, Kujala P, van den Born M, Cozijnsen M, Haegebarth A, Korving J, Begthel H, Peters PJ, Clevers H. Identification of stem cells in small intestine and colon by marker gene Lgr5. Nature. 2007;449:1003–7.
88. Kinzler KW, Nilbert MC, Su LK, Vogelstein B, Bryan TM, Levy DB, Smith KJ, Preisinger AC, Hedge P, McKechnie D, et al. Identification of FAP locus genes from chromosome 5q21. Science. 1991;253:661–5.
89. Nishisho I, Nakamura Y, Miyoshi Y, Miki Y, Ando H, Horii A, Koyama K, Utsunomiya J, Baba S, Hedge P. Mutations of chromosome 5q21 genes in FAP and colorectal cancer patients. Science. 1991;253:665–9.
90. Rubinfeld B, Souza B, Albert I, Müller O, Chamberlain SH, Masiarz FR, Munemitsu S, Polakis P. Association of the APC gene product with beta-catenin. Science. 1993;262: 1731–4.
91. Su LK, Vogelstein B, Kinzler KW. Association of the APC tumor suppressor protein with catenins. Science. 1993;262:1734–7.
92. van de Wetering M, de Lau W, Clevers H. WNT signaling and lymphocyte development. Cell. 2002;109(Suppl):S13–9.
93. Liu W, Dong X, Mai M, Seelan RS, Taniguchi K, Krishnadath KK, Halling KC, Cunningham JM, Boardman LA, Qian C, Christensen E, Schmidt SS, Roche PC, Smith DI, Thibodeau SN. Mutations in AXIN2 cause colorectal cancer with defective mismatch repair by activating beta-catenin/TCF signalling. Nat Genet. 2000;26:146–7.
94. Morin PJ, Sparks AB, Korinek V, Barker N, Clevers H, Vogelstein B, Kinzler KW. Activation of beta-catenin-Tcf signaling in colon cancer by mutations in beta-catenin or APC. Science. 1997;275:1787–90.
95. Reya T, Clevers H. Wnt signalling in stem cells and cancer. Nature. 2005;434:843–50.
96. Holmberg J, Genander M, Halford MM, Annerén C, Sondell M, Chumley MJ, Silvany RE, Henkemeyer M, Frisén J. EphB receptors coordinate migration and proliferation in the intestinal stem cell niche. Cell. 2006;125:1151–63.
97. Merlos-Suarez A, Batlle E. Eph-ephrin signalling in adult tissues and cancer. Curr Opin Cell Biol. 2008;20:94–200.
98. Veeman MT, Axelrod JD, Moon RT. A second canon. Functions and mechanisms of beta-catenin-independent Wnt signaling. Dev Cell. 2003;5:367–77.
99. Gaggioli C, Hooper S, Hidalgo-Carcedo C, Grosse R, Marshall JF, Harrington K, Sahai E. Fibroblast-led collective invasion of carcinoma cells with differing roles for RhoGTPases in leading and following cells. Nat Cell Biol. 2007;9:1392–400.
100. Sanz-Moreno V, Gaggioli C, Yeo M, Albrengues J, Wallberg F, Viros A, Hooper S, Mitter R, Féral CC, Cook M, Larkin J, Marais R, Meneguzzi G, Sahai E, Marshall CJ. ROCK and JAK1 signaling cooperate to control actomyosin contractility in tumor cells and stroma. Cancer Cell. 2011;20:229–45.
101. Dejmek J, Dejmek A, Säfholm A, Sjölander A, Andersson T. Wnt-5a protein expression in primary dukes B colon cancers identifies a subgroup of patients with good prognosis. Cancer Res. 2005;65:9142–6.

102. Many AM, Brown AM. Both canonical and non-canonical Wnt signaling independently promote stem cell growth in mammospheres. PLoS One. 2014;9:e101800.
103. Kohn AD, Moon RT. Wnt and calcium signaling: beta-catenin-independent pathways. Cell Calcium. 2005;38:439–46.
104. Slusarski DC, Pelegri F. Calcium signaling in vertebrate embryonic patterning and morphogenesis. Dev Biol. 2007;307:1–13.
105. Sheldahl LC, Slusarski DC, Pandur P, Miller JR, Kühl M, Moon RT. Dishevelled activates Ca2+ flux, PKC, and CamKII in vertebrate embryos. J Cell Biol. 2003;161:769–77.
106. Kuhl M, Sheldahl LC, Malbon CC, Moon RT. Ca(2+)/calmodulin-dependent protein kinase II is stimulated by Wnt and Frizzled homologs and promotes ventral cell fates in Xenopus. J Biol Chem. 2000;275:12701–11.
107. Dissanayake SK, Weeraratna AT. Detecting PKC phosphorylation as part of the Wnt/calcium pathway in cutaneous melanoma. Methods Mol Biol. 2008;468:57–72.
108. Lombardo Y, Scopelliti A, Cammareri P, Todaro M, Iovino F, Ricci-Vitiani L, Gulotta G, Dieli F, de Maria R, Stassi G. Bone morphogenetic protein 4 induces differentiation of colorectal cancer stem cells and increases their response to chemotherapy in mice. Gastroenterology. 2011;140:297–309.
109. Liu B, Chen Q, Tian D, Wu L, Dong H, Wang J, Ji B, Zhu X, Cai Q, Wang L, Zhang S. BMP4 reverses multidrug resistance through modulation of BCL-2 and GDNF in glioblastoma. Brain Res. 2013;1507:115–24.
110. Tate CM, Pallini R, Ricci-Vitiani L, Dowless M, Shiyanova T, D'Alessandris GQ, Morgante L, Giannetti S, Larocca LM, di Martino S, Rowlinson SW, De Maria R, Stancato L. A BMP7 variant inhibits the tumorigenic potential of glioblastoma stem-like cells. Cell Death Differ. 2012;19:1644–54.
111. Bijlsma MF, Spek CA, Peppelenbosch MP. Hedgehog: an unusual signal transducer. Bioessays. 2004;26:387–94.
112. Tostar U, Malm CJ, Meis-Kindblom JM, Kindblom LG, Toftgård R, Undén AB. Deregulation of the hedgehog signalling pathway: a possible role for the PTCH and SUFU genes in human rhabdomyoma and rhabdomyosarcoma development. J Pathol. 2006;208:17–25.
113. Taylor MD, Liu L, Raffel C, Hui CC, Mainprize TG, Zhang X, Agatep R, Chiappa S, Gao L, Lowrance A, Hao A, Goldstein AM, Stavrou T, Scherer SW, Dura WT, Wainwright B, Squire JA, Rutka JT, Hogg D. Mutations in SUFU predispose to medulloblastoma. Nat Genet. 2002;31:306–10.
114. Dahmane N, Lee J, Robins P, Heller P, Ruiz i Altaba A. Activation of the transcription factor Gli1 and the Sonic hedgehog signalling pathway in skin tumours. Nature. 1997;389: 876–81.
115. Han ME, Lee YS, Baek SY, Kim BS, Kim JB, Oh SO. Hedgehog signaling regulates the survival of gastric cancer cells by regulating the expression of Bcl-2. Int J Mol Sci. 2009;107:3033–43.
116. Thayer SP, di Magliano MP, Heiser PW, Nielsen CM, Roberts DJ, Lauwers GY, Qi YP, Gysin S, Fernández-del Castillo C, Yajnik V, Antoniu B, McMahon M, Warshaw AL, Hebrok M. Hedgehog is an early and late mediator of pancreatic cancer tumorigenesis. Nature. 2003;425(6960):851–6.
117. Liu S, Dontu G, Mantle ID, Patel S, Ahn NS, Jackson KW, Suri P, Wicha MS. Hedgehog signaling and Bmi-1 regulate self-renewal of normal and malignant human mammary stem cells. Cancer Res. 2006;66:6063–71.
118. Bar EE, Chaudhry A, Farah MH, Eberhart CG. Hedgehog signaling promotes medulloblastoma survival via Bc/II. Am J Pathol. 2007;170:347–55.
119. Huang FT, Zhuan-Sun YX, Zhuang YY, Wei SL, Tang J, Chen WB, Zhang SN. Inhibition of hedgehog signaling depresses self-renewal of pancreatic cancer stem cells and reverses chemoresistance. Int J Oncol. 2012;41:1707–14.
120. Yao J, An Y, Wie JS, Ji ZL, Lu ZP, Wu JL, Jiang KR, Chen P, Xu ZK, Miao Y. Cyclopamine reverts acquired chemoresistance and down-regulates cancer stem cell markers in pancreatic cancer cell lines. Swiss Med Wkly. 2011;141:w13208.

121. Di Tomaso T, Mazzoleni S, Wang E, Sovena G, Clavenna D, Franzin A, Mortini P, Ferrone S, Doglioni C, Marincola FM, Galli R, Parmiani G, Maccalli C. Immunobiological characterization of cancer stem cells isolated from glioblastoma patients. Clin Cancer Res. 2010;16:800–13.
122. Schatton T, Schütte U, Frank NY, Zhan Q, Hoerning A, Robles SC, Zhou J, Hodi FS, Spagnoli GC, Murphy GF, Frank MH. Modulation of T-cell activation by malignant melanoma initiating cells. Cancer Res. 2010;70:697–708.
123. Volonté A, Di Tomaso T, Spinelli M, Todaro M, Sanvito F, Albarello L, Bissolati M, Ghirardelli L, Orsenigo E, Ferrone S, Doglioni C, Stassi G, Dellabona P, Staudacher C, Parmiani G, Maccalli C. Cancer-initiating cells from colorectal cancer patients escape from T cell-mediated immunosurveillance in vitro through membrane-bound IL-4. J Immunol. 2014;192:523–32.
124. Maccalli C, Volontè A, Cimminiello C, Parmiani G. Immunology of cancer stem cells in solid tumours. A review. Eur J Cancer. 2014;50:649–55.
125. Maccalli C, De Maria R. Cancer stem cells: perspectives for therapeutic targeting. Cancer Immunol Immunother. 2015;64:91–7. Epub 2014 Aug 8.
126. Wu A, Wiesner S, Xiao J, Ericson K, Chen W, Hall WA, Low WC, Ohlfest JR. Expression of MHC I and NK ligands on human CD133+ glioma cells: possible targets of immunotherapy. J Neurooncol. 2007;83:121–31. Erratum in: J Neurooncol. 2007;83:133.
127. Ogino T, Wang X, Kato S, Miyokawa N, Harabuchi Y, Ferrone S. Endoplasmic reticulum chaperone-specific monoclonal antibodies for flow cytometry and immunohistochemical staining. Tissue Antigens. 2003;62:385–93.
128. Brantley EC, Nabors LB, Gillespie GY, Choi YH, Palmer CA, Harrison K, Roarty K, Benveniste EN. Loss of protein inhibitors of activated STAT-3 expression in glioblastoma multiforme tumors: implications for STAT-3 activation and gene expression. Clin Cancer Res. 2008;14:4694–704.
129. Pandha H, Rigg A, John J, Lemoine N. Loss of expression of antigen-presenting molecules in human pancreatic cancer and pancreatic cancer cell lines. Clin Exp Immunol. 2007; 148:127–35.
130. Johnsen A, France J, Sy MS, Harding CV. Down-regulation of the transporter for antigen presentation, proteasome subunits, and class I major histocompatibility complex in tumor cell lines. Cancer Res. 1998;58:3660–7.
131. Drukker M, Katz G, Urbach A, Schuldiner M, Markel G, Itskovitz-Eldor J, Reubinoff B, Mandelboim O, Benvenisty N. Characterization of the expression of MHC proteins in human embryonic stem cells. Proc Natl Acad Sci U S A. 2002;99:9864–9.
132. Le Blanc K, Tammik C, Rosendahl K, Zetterberg E, Ringdén O. HLA expression and immunologic properties of differentiated and undifferentiated mesenchymal stem cells. Exp Hematol. 2003;31:890–6.
133. Favier B, LeMaoult J, Carosella ED. Functions of HLA-G in the immune system. Tissue Antigens. 2007;69 Suppl 1:150–2.
134. Verloes A, Van de Velde H, LeMaoult J, Mateizel I, Cauffman G, Horn PA, Carosella ED, Devroey P, De Waele M, Rebmann V, Vercammen M. HLA-G expression in human embryonic stem cells and preimplantation embryos. J Immunol. 2011;186:2663–71.
135. Nasef A, Mathieu N, Chapel A, Frick J, François S, Mazurier C, Boutarfa A, Bouchet S, Gorin NC, Thierry D, Fouillard L. Immunosuppressive effects of mesenchymal stem cells: involvement of HLA-G. Transplantation. 2007;84:231–7.
136. Campoli M, Ferrone S. Tumor escape mechanisms: potential role of soluble HLA antigens and NK cells activating ligands. Tissue Antigens. 2008;72:321–34.
137. Novellino L, Castelli C, Parmiani G. A listing of human tumor antigens recognized by T cells: March 2004 update. Cancer Immunol Immunother. 2005;54:187–207.
138. Castle JC, Kreiter S, Diekmann J, Löwer M, van de Roemer N, de Graaf J, Selmi A, Diken M, Boegel S, Paret C, Koslowski M, Kuhn AN, Britten CM, Huber C, Türeci O, Sahin U. Exploiting the mutanome for tumor vaccination. Cancer Res. 2012;72:1081–91.

139. Parmiani G, Russo V, Maccalli C, Parolini D, Rizzo N, Maio M. Peptide-based vaccines for cancer therapy. Hum Vaccin Immunother. 2014;10:3175–8.
140. Gedye C, Quirk J, Browning J, Svobodová S, John T, Sluka P, Dunbar PR, Corbeil D, Cebon J, Davis ID. Cancer/testis antigens can be immunological targets in clonogenic CD133+ melanoma cells. Cancer Immunol Immunother. 2009;58:1635–46.
141. Nagorsen D, Scheibenbogen C, Letsch A, Germer CT, Buhr HJ, Hegewisch-Becker S, Rivoltini L, Thiel E, Keilholz U. T cell responses against tumor associated antigens and prognosis in colorectal cancer patients. J Transl Med. 2005;3:3–9.
142. Wheeler CJ, Black KL, Liu G, Mazer M, Zhang XX, Pepkowitz S, Goldfinger D, Ng H, Irvin D, Yu JS. Vaccination elicits correlated immune and clinical responses in glioblastoma multiforme patients. Cancer Res. 2008;68:5955–64.
143. Anichini A, Vegetti C, Mortarini R. The paradox of T-cell-mediated antitumor immunity in spite of poor clinical outcome in human melanoma. Cancer Immunol Immunother. 2004; 53:855–64.
144. Hamai A, Meslin F, Benlalam H, Jalil A, Mehrpour M, Faure F. ICAM-1 has a critical role in the regulation of metastatic melanoma tumor susceptibility to CTL lysis by interfering with PI3K/AKT pathway. Cancer Res. 2008;68:9854–64.
145. Brown CE, Starr R, Martinez C, Aguilar B, D'Apuzzo M, Todorov I, Shih CC, Badie B, Hudecek M, Riddell SR, Jensen MC. Recognition and killing of brain tumor stem-like initiating cells by CD8+ cytolytic T cells. Cancer Res. 2009;69:8886–93.
146. Waziri A, Killory B, Ogden III AT, Canoll P, Anderson RCE, Kent SC, Anderson DE, Bruce JN. Preferential in situ CD4+CD56+ T cell activation and expansion within human glioblastoma. J Immunol. 2008;180:7673–80.
147. Schatton T, Frank MH. Antitumor immunity and cancer stem cells. Ann N Y Acad Sci. 2009;1176:154–69.
148. Reim F, Dombrowski Y, Ritter C, Buttmann M, Häusler S, Ossadnik M, Krockenberger M, Beier D, Beier CP, Dietl J, Becker JC, Hönig A, Wischhusen J. Immunoselection of breast and ovarian cancer cells with trastuzumab and natural killer cells: selective escape of CD44high/CD24low/HER2low breast cancer stem cells. Cancer Res. 2009;69:8058–66.
149. Tallerico R, Todaro M, Di Franco S, Maccalli C, Garofalo C, Sottile R, Palmieri C, Tirinato L, Pangigadde PN, La Rocca R, Mandelboim O, Stassi G, Di Fabrizio E, Parmiani G, Moretta A, Dieli F, Kärre K, Carbone E. Human NK cells selective targeting of colon cancer-initiating cells: a role for natural cytotoxicity receptors and MHC class I molecules. J Immunol. 2013;190:2381–90.
150. Jewett A, Tseng HC, Arasteh A, Saadat S, Christensen RE, Cacalano NA. Natural killer cells preferentially target cancer stem cells; role of monocytes in protection against NK cell mediated lysis of cancer stem cells. Curr Drug Deliv. 2012;9:5–16.
151. Koh J, Lee SB, Park H, Lee HJ, Cho NH, Kim J. Susceptibility of CD24(+) ovarian cancer cells to anti-cancer drugs and natural killer cells. Biochem Biophys Res Commun. 2012; 427:373–8.
152. Jachetti E, Mazzoleni S, Grioni M, Ricupito A, Brambillasca C, Generoso L, Calcinotto A, Freschi M, Mondino A, Galli R, Bellone M. Prostate cancer stem cells are targets of both innate and adaptive immunity and elicit tumor-specific immune responses. Oncoimmunology. 2013;2(5):e24520. Epub 2013 Apr 16.
153. Pellegatta S, Poliani PL, Corno D, Menghi F, Ghielmetti F, Suarez-Merino B, Caldera V, Nava S, Ravanini M, Facchetti F, Bruzzone MG, Finocchiaro G. Neurospheres enriched in cancer stem-like cells are highly effective in eliciting a dendritic cell-mediated immune response against malignant gliomas. Cancer Res. 2006;66:10247–52.
154. Pellegatta S, Poliani PL, Corno D, Grisoli M, Cusimano M, Ubiali F, Baggi F, Bruzzone MG, Finocchiaro G. Dendritic cells pulsed with glioma lysates induce immunity against syngeneic intracranial gliomas and increase survival of tumor-bearing mice. Neurol Res. 2006; 28:527–31.
155. Xu Q, Liu G, Yuan X, Xu M, Wang H, Ji J, Konda B, Black KL, Yu JS. Antigen-specific T cell response from dendritic cell vaccination using cancer stem-like cell associated antigen. Stem Cells. 2009;27:1734–40.

156. Xu Q, Yuan X, Yu JS. Glioma stem cell research for the development of immunotherapy. Adv Exp Med Biol. 2012;746:216–25.
157. Yao Y, Wang X, Jin K, Zhu J, Wang Y, Xiong S, Mao Y, Zhou L. B7-H4 is preferentially expressed in non-dividing brain tumor cells and in a subset of brain tumor stem-like cells. J Neurooncol. 2008;89:121–9.
158. Wei J, Barr J, Kong L-Y, Wang Y, Wu A, Sharma AK, Gumin J, Henry V, Colman H, Sawaya R, Lang FF, Heimberger AB. Glioma-associated cancer-initiating cells induce immunosuppression. Clin Cancer Res. 2010;16:461–73.
159. Roth P, Junker M, Tritschler I, Mittelbronn M, Dombrowski Y, Breit SN. GDF-15 contributes to proliferation and immune escape of malignant gliomas. Clin Cancer Res. 2010;16:3851–9.
160. Shipitsin M, Campbell LL, Argani P, Weremowicz S, Bloushtain-Qimron N, Yao J, Nikolskaya T, Serebryiskaya T, Beroukhim R, Hu M, Halushka MK, Sukumar S, Parker LM, Anderson KS, Harris LN, Garber JE, Richardson AL, Schnitt SJ, Nikolsky Y, Gelman RS, Polyak K. Molecular definition of breast tumor heterogeneity. Cancer Cell. 2007;11:259–73.
161. Lottaz C, Beier D, Meyer K, Kumar P, Hermann A, Schwarz J, Junker M, Oefner PJ, Bogdahn U, Wischhusen J, Spang R, Storch A, Beier CP. Transcriptional profiles of CD133+ and CD133- glioblastoma-derived cancer stem cell lines suggest different cells of origin. Cancer Res. 2010;70:2030–40.
162. Parsa AT, Waldron JS, Panner A, Crane CA, Parney IF, Barry JJ, Cachola KE, Murray JC, Tihan T, Jensen MC, Mischel PS, Stokoe D, Pieper RO. Loss of tumor suppressor PTEN function increases B7-H1 expression and immunoresistance in glioma. Nat Med. 2007; 13:84–8.
163. Francipane MG, Alea MP, Lombardo Y, Todaro M, Medema JP, Stassi G. Crucial role of interleukin-4 in the survival of colon cancer stem cells. Cancer Res. 2008;68:4022–5.
164. Hallett MA, Venmar T, Fingleton B. Cytokine stimulation of epithelial cancer cells: the similar and divergent functions of IL-4 and IL-13. Cancer Res. 2012;72:6338–43.
165. Kawasaki BT, Farrar WL. Cancer stem cells, CD200 and immunoevasion. Trends Immunol. 2008;29:464–8.
166. Kim S-Y, Cho H-S, Yang S-H, Shin J-Y, Kim J-S, Lee S-T, Chu K, Roh JK, Kim SU, Park CG. Soluble mediators from human neural stem cells play a critical role in suppression of T-cell activation and proliferation. J Neurosci Res. 2009;87:2264–72.
167. Ljujic B, Milovanovic M, Volarevic V, Murray B, Bugarski D, Przyborski S, Arsenijevic N, Lukic ML, Stojkovic M. Human mesenchymal stem cells creating an immunosuppressive environment and promote breast cancer in mice. Sci Rep. 2013;3:2298.
168. Perego M, Tortoreto M, Tragni G, Mariani L, Deho P, Carbone A, Santinami M, Patuzzo R, Mina PD, Villa A, Pratesi G, Cossa G, Perego P, Daidone MG, Alison MR, Parmiani G, Rivoltini L, Castelli C. Heterogeneous phenotype of human melanoma cells with in vitro and in vivo features of tumor-initiating cells. J Invest Dermatol. 2010;130:1877–86.
169. Hirohashi Y, Torigoe T. Cytotoxic T lymphocytes. Sniping cancer stem cells. Oncoimmunology. 2012;1:123–5.
170. Engelmann K, Shen H, Finn OJ. MCF7 side population cells with characteristics of cancer stem/progenitor cells express the tumor antigen MUC1. Cancer Res. 2008;68:2419–26.
171. Ithimakin S, Day KC, Malik F, Zen Q, Dawsey SJ, Bersano-Begey TF, Quraishi AA, Ignatoski KW, Daignault S, Davis A, Hall CL, Palanisamy N, Heath AN, Tawakkol N, Luther TK, Clouthier SG, Chadwick WA, Day ML, Kleer CG, Thomas DG, Hayes DF, Korkaya H, Wicha MS. HER2 drives luminal breast cancer stem cells in the absence of HER2 amplification: implications for efficacy of adjuvant trastuzumab. Cancer Res. 2013;73:1635–46.
172. Hua W, Yao Y, Chu Y, Zhong P, Sheng X, Xiao B, Wu J, Yang B, Mao Y, Zhou L. The CD133+ tumor stem-like cell-associated antigen may elicit highly intense immune responses against human malignant glioma. J Neurooncol. 2011;105:149–57.
173. Meisel R, Zibert A, Laryea M, Göbel U, Däubener W, Dilloo D. Human bone marrow stromal cells inhibit allogeneic T-cell responses by indoleamine 2,3-dioxygenase-mediated tryptophan degradation. Blood. 2004;103:4619–21.
174. Harris SG, Padilla J, Koumas L, Ray D, Phipps RP. Prostaglandins as modulators of immunity. Trends Immunol. 2002;23:144–50.

Chapter 2
Role of Co-inhibitory Molecules in Tumor Escape from CTL Attack

Wieger J. Norde, Willemijn Hobo, and Harry Dolstra

Abstract The immune system can be a potent defense mechanism against cancer. Especially CD8⁺ cytotoxic T lymphocytes (CTL) have a great killing capacity towards tumor cells. However, their potential is often dampened by immune suppressive mechanisms in the tumor microenvironment. Co-inhibitory molecules (CIM) expressed by tumor cells, immune cells and stromal cells in the tumor milieu can severely hamper CD8⁺ T-cell responses against cancer cells. Today, a variety of co-inhibitory molecules, including PD-1, CTLA-4, LAG3, BTLA, Tim-3 and CD200R, have been implicated in tumor escape from CTL attack. Sustained signaling via these CIM can result in functional exhaustion of T-cells, a process in which the ability to proliferate, secrete cytokines and mediate lysis of tumor cells is sequentially lost. In this chapter, we discuss the influence of co-inhibitory pathways in suppressing CD8⁺ T-cell function in various immune settings. These include the natural immune surveillance by CTL against tumor cells, or in therapeutic settings like allogeneic stem cell transplantation or chimeric antigen receptor (CAR) T-cell therapy. In addition, we discuss exciting pre-clinical and clinical data of immunotherapeutic approaches interfering with negative co-signaling, either as monotherapy or in conjunction with vaccination strategies. Numerous studies indicate that co-inhibitory signaling limits the clinical benefit of current CTL-based therapies. Therefore, interference with CIM is an attractive immunotherapeutic intervention for cancer therapy.

Keywords Cytotoxic T-lymphocytes • Co-inhibitory molecules • Anti-tumor immunity • Tumor immune escape

---

No potential conflicts of interest were disclosed.

W.J. Norde • W. Hobo • H. Dolstra (✉)
Department of Laboratory Medicine – Laboratory of Hematology, Radboud University Nijmegen Medical Centre, Geert Grooteplein 8, P.O. Box 9101, 6500 HB Nijmegen, The Netherlands
e-mail: Harry.Dolstra@radboudumc.nl

B. Bonavida, S. Chouaib (eds.), *Resistance of Cancer Cells to CTL-Mediated Immunotherapy*, Resistance to Targeted Anti-Cancer Therapeutics 7,
DOI 10.1007/978-3-319-17807-3_2

Abbreviations

AB	Antibody
ACRBP	Acrosin binding protein
AG	Antigen
alloSCT	Allogeneic stem cell transplantation
AML	Acute myeloid leukemia
APC	Antigen-presenting cell
BMS	Bristol-Myers Squibb
BTLA	B- and T-lymphocyte attenuator
CAR	Chimeric antigen receptor
CAR-T	CAR-transduced T-cell
CCR7	C-C chemokine receptor type 7
CD	Cluster of differentiation
CD200R	CD200 Receptor
CD62L	CD62 ligand
CEA	Carcinoembryonic antigen
CIM	Co-inhibitory molecule
CIM-L	Co-inhibitory ligand
CIM-R	Co-inhibitory receptor
CLEC15A	C-type lectin domain family 15 member A
CLL	Chronic lymphoid leukemia
CML	Chronic myeloid leukemia
CMV	Cytomegalovirus
CSM-L	Co-stimulatory ligand
CSM-R	Co-stimulatory receptor
CTAG1B	Cancer/testis antigen 1B
CTL	Cytotoxic T-lymphocyte
CTLA-4	Cytotoxic T-lymphocyte-associated protein 4
DC	Dendritic cell
EBV	Epstein-Barr Virus
EMA	European Medicines Agency
Fc	Fragment crystallizable region
FDA	Food and Drug Administration
FoxP3	Forkhead box P3
gD	Herpes simplex virus glycoprotein D
GVHD	Graft-versus-host-disease
GVT	Graft-versus-tumor
Her-2	Human epidermal growth factor receptor 2
HIV	Human immunodeficiency virus
HLA	Human lymphocyte antigens
HVEM	Herpesvirus entry mediator
ICOS	Inducible T-cell costimulator
IFN-γ	Interferon gamma

Ig	Immunoglobulin
KLRG1	Killer cell lectin-like receptor G1
LAG3	Lymphocyte-activation gene 3
LIGHT	Lymphotoxin-like, exhibits inducible expression, and competes with herpes simplex virus glycoprotein D for HVEM, a receptor expressed by T lymphocytes
LT-α	Lymphotoxin-alpha
MAGE-A	Melanoma-associated antigen
MHC	Major histocompatibility complex
MiHA	Minor histocompatibility antigen
MM	Multiple myeloma
NK	Natural killer cell
NY-ESO-1	New York esophageal squamous cell carcinoma-1
PAP	Prostate acid phosphatase
PBMC	Peripheral blood mononuclear cells
PD-1	Programmed cell death 1
PD-1H	PD-1 homolog
PD-L1	Programmed death-ligand 1
PD-L2	Programmed death-ligand 2
pMHC	Peptide-MHC complex
siRNA	Small interfering RNA
SLAMf4	Signaling lymphocyte-activation molecule family member 4
TAA	Tumor-associated antigen
TCR	T-cell receptor
TCR-T	TCR-transduced T-cell
T_{EFF}	Effector T-cell
T_{EM}	Effector memory T-cell
Th1	Helper 1 T-cell
TIL	Tumor-infiltrating lymphocyte
Tim-3	T-cell immunoglobulin and mucin domain 3
Tim-4	T-cell immunoglobulin and mucin domain 4
T_N	Naïve T-cell
TNFR	Tumor necrosis factor receptor
T_{REG}	Regulatory T-cell
T_{SCM}	Stem cell memory T-cell
VISTA	V-domain Ig suppressor of T-cell activation
Wnt	Wingless-related integration site

2.1 Introduction

It is evident that both the innate and adaptive immune systems participate in the recognition and clearance of tumor cells by a process known as cancer immunosurveillance. In particular, tumor-reactive $CD8^+$ cytotoxic T-lymphocytes (CTL) are major effectors in the immune response against cancer cells. However, despite the powerful aspects of CTL-mediated immune reactions, too often tumor cells are able to evade immune recognition and destruction. Tumor cells exploit several mechanisms to escape from CTL-mediated immunity, such as disruption of antigen presentation, down-regulation of HLA molecules, recruitment of regulatory T-cells (T_{REG}) and myeloid-derived suppressor cells, as well as secretion of immune suppressive cytokines [1]. In the last decade, another powerful immune suppressive mechanism came into the limelight: the repressive action of co-inhibitory receptors [2].

2.2 CTL Activation

Activation of T-cells to become CTL effectors, initially requires two signals [3–5]. Firstly, the TCR-CD3 complex needs to interact with the cognate peptide presented in HLA molecules on dendritic cells (DC). However, whether or not the T-cell becomes activated, is predominantly dependent on signaling of either co-stimulatory molecules (CSM) or co-inhibitory molecules (CIM) upon ligation with their corresponding ligands expressed by the APC [6]. The balance between these positive and negative co-signals determines the functionality of T-cells during immunity and tolerance. The stimulatory signal is generally provided by CD28, expressed on the T-cell, interacting with its ligands CD80 and CD86 on the DC. In the absence of co-stimulation the T-cell will become functionally anergic, and thereby tolerant to the antigen, which is one of the physiological mechanisms involved in the elimination of self-reactive T-cells. In addition, ligation of CIM to their corresponding ligands on APC results in T-cell inhibition, and via this natural feedback loop, sustained T-cell activation is prevented and the effector T-cell response resolves. Therefore, the balance in positive and negative co-signals determines the activation state of the T cells during immunity and tolerance.

The kinetics and differentiation of CTL that constitute anti-tumor responses are divided in several stages [7]. First, the CD62L$^+$CCR7$^+$CD45RA$^+$ naive T-cells (T_N) encounter the antigen presented by DC. Due to the expression of the selectin CD62L and the chemokine receptor CCR7 these cells home to the secondary lymphoid organs. However, upon this stimulation by the DC, these T-cells clonally expand and loose the expression of CD62L, CCR7, CD28 and CD45RA, while upregulating activation markers such as CD45RO, CD69 and CD25. These effector T-cells (T_{EFF}) subsequently migrate to the target tissues, where they eradicate tumor cells. After the peak of the response, upon which most or all target cells have been destroyed, the contraction phase commences, and most tumor-reactive T-cells will undergo apoptosis. However, a minority of the T-cells will survive to become long-lived memory cells, either effector (T_{EM}) or central memory (T_{CM}). While the T_{EM} reside in the periphery and upon recall show a strong effector response, the T_{CM} have a strong proliferative property, regain expression of CD62L and CCR7, and migrate to the lymph nodes and BM, where they convey a lifelong memory against the antigen of their specificity. During all these activation and differentiation events, signaling through CSM and CIM has a great influence on the functional capacity and differentiation status of CTL.

2.3 Tumor-Associated Antigens

The immune system can harness a powerful attack against cancer cells. This can be done by cells from the innate immune system, such as NK cells that can attack tumor cells without prior sensitization [8]. Furthermore, the adaptive T-cell immune system has a great potential of recognizing and lysing tumor cells. This is mainly done by CTL, which recognize tumor-associated antigens (TAA) presented by the cancer cells. TAA are overexpressed, or ideally, solely expressed by tumor cells and consequently recognized as foreign, and an effective $CD8^+$ T-cell immune response can be constituted against these antigens. Different classes of TAA exist. One class of TAA is highly overexpressed differentiation genes, such as tyrosinase and gp100 in melanoma, proteins which are differentially expressed at low levels in healthy melanocytes [9].

Another class is the oncofetal antigens, like carcinoembryonic antigen (CEA), which are usually expressed only in the fetal stage, and therefore no immune tolerance against these TAA exists [10]. Furthermore, cancer-testis antigens, including MAGE-A, NY-ESO-1, ACRBP and CTAG1B, can be aberrantly expressed by tumor cells [11, 12]. Since these are also only expressed by fetal tissues and the immune-privileged testes, a prominent immune response can be observed against these TAA. Finally, new antigens caused by de novo mutations in the cancer cells can occur in any gene. Since these mutations result in a true novel epitope, a very strong CTL response can be elicited. Especially in cancers with a high mutation rate, such as melanoma and lung cancer, these novel TAA occur frequently [13].

Altogether, these TAA are the major target in natural $CD8^+$ T-cell tumor surveillance, and form an attractive field for immunotherapy, such as tumor infiltrating lymphocyte (TIL) infusion or DC vaccination loaded with TAA [14]. Vaccination with the most potent APC, i.e. DC, provides a great option for antigen-specific stimulation of tumor-reactive CTL [15]. Currently, DC vaccination is being performed in phase 3 clinical trials against four malignancies, including melanoma, prostate cancer, glioma and renal cell carcinomas [16]. In prostate cancer, vaccination is being performed against the prostate cancer-antigen prostate acid phosphatase (PAP) with the sipuleucel-T treatment [17]. In addition, vaccination with melanoma-antigens has reached promising results [18]. Several parameters of DC vaccination still need to be optimized, such as DC culture, choice of DC subpopulation, the method of loading of tumor antigens, choice of maturation stimuli, and method of administration to the patient [19]. However, in the majority of studies an increase in the median overall survival has been documented, underlining the potential of this therapy [16].

2.4 Allogeneic Stem Cell Transplantation

Another cancer immunotherapy, based on CTL recognition of antigens expressed on tumor cells, is allogeneic stem cell transplantation (alloSCT). This procedure can still be regarded as one of the most powerful cell-based immunotherapy to date, due to potent graft-versus-tumor (GVT) responses constituted by alloreactive T-cells [20]. These alloreactive $CD8^+$ T-cell responses eradicate the malignant cells upon recognition of polymorphic HLA-presented peptides, known as minor histocompatibility antigens (MiHA). AlloSCT greatly enhanced the cure rate for aggressive hematologic cancers, although many patients still fail to launch effective immune responses and develop relapsed disease. Moreover, a major drawback of alloSCT is the occurrence of graft-versus-host disease (GVHD), a potentially life-threatening complication predominantly caused by alloreactive T-cells recognizing healthy tissues, notably the skin, liver and gastrointestinal tract. Since hemato-restricted MiHA are solely expressed by the redundant patient hematopoietic system including the malignant counterparts, they hold the key to separate GVT from GVHD [21]. In fact, these MiHA are equally immunogenic as de novo TAA or viral epitopes, since the antigens are completely foreign to the donor immune system and immune tolerance has not been initiated. Therefore, alloSCT can be a very powerful and curative cancer immunotherapy.

2.5 Adoptive T-Cell Transfer

Adoptive transfer of CTL is an appealing means to prevent or treat relapse of the tumor cells, and so far various strategies have been exploited. Nevertheless, specificity is crucial to avoid systemic toxicity. One method to obtain sufficient numbers of T-cells reactive against a TAA or MiHA is via isolation of these cells from the effector repertoire of patients present, followed by a fast expansion protocol [22, 23]. Already in the 1980s, the first studies with tumor-reactive T-cells in mice were performed by the isolation of TIL and subsequent culture and administration, which resulted in remission of cancer [24]. This led to clinical trials in humans, and a response rate near 50 % or more has made TIL administration an established treatment option [25]. A different technique is the isolation and expansion of naive tumor-reactive T-cells from a healthy donor by ex vivo stimulation with peptide-presenting DC [26, 27]. However, this can be a time-consuming and laborious process, especially for overexpressed TAA. The feasibility of both approaches has been demonstrated by several groups [22, 23, 26–28]. Importantly, one phase I trial reported in five out of seven patients with relapsed leukemia a complete, but transient, remission upon adoptive transfer of MiHA-specific T-cells expanded from post-transplant recipient PBMC [28]. Unfortunately, the infused T-cells failed to persist in vivo, which might be due to their terminal $T_{EFF/EM}$ differentiation stage and, consequently, rapid exhaustion of these cells as a result of the extensive in vitro culture protocol. To prevent the exhaustion of these T-cells, a search for the T-cell type with the highest proliferative potential has led to the identification of the stem cell memory T-cell (T_{SCM}) [29, 30]. Although T_{SCM} have experienced antigen-stimulation, they resemble T_N in their expression of CD62L and their ability to differentiate into all other T-cell differentiation states. In addition, it was found that by inhibition of either the Akt or Wnt pathway in vitro, it is possible to generate high numbers of tumor-reactive T_{SCM} [30, 31]. Together with their proven excellent anti-tumor effects in murine models, this subtype of CTL holds great promise for future therapies [32].

A third way to efficiently generate high numbers of tumor-reactive CTL with high-affinity TCR is by gene transfer of the antigen-TCR α and β chains into donor T-cells [22, 33]. To prevent the induction of GVHD in patients treated with alloSCT, the TCR genes should preferentially be transferred into donor T-cells with a known specificity that does not recognize and target GVHD-tissues, such as virus-specific T-cells [34]. Another potential complication might be mispairing of the introduced and native TCR chains, thereby generating a new potentially harmful specificity [35]. Efforts are being made to prevent this mispairing, amongst which is the transfer of TCR α and β chains into γδ T-cells. Successful TCR gene transfer and resultant cytolytic competence has been demonstrated for both TAA and MiHA [36–39]. Importantly, with TCR gene transfer the complete MiHA-TCR is introduced into the donor T-cells, therefore matching of the HLA-restriction allele between recipient and donor is no longer required.

A novel therapeutic approach utilizing the power of CTL is chimeric antigen receptor (CAR) T-cells. These CAR consist of an antibody fragment recognizing a tumor antigen expressed on the surface of these T-cells. Ingeniously, to enable T-cell activation, this antibody fragment is coupled to the CD3 ξ-chain, leading to an intracellular activation cascaded upon recognition of the antigen [40]. This chimeric receptor combines the high avidity and specificity of antibodies with the activation of CTL, resulting in highly effective CTL responses. Second and third generation CAR have been engineered to express motives of CSM in the intracellular domain, such as CD28, 4-1BB and OX40. Thereby, in addition to the cytolytic capacity of CAR, also proliferation and survival are sustained. Impressive results have been obtained in clinical trials. Especially CAR recognizing CD19 developed by the June lab, have been able to efficiently lyse cancer cells in patients with high tumor burdens, and have resulted in cure of leukemia patients [41]. After this pioneering work in leukemia, other target antigens are currently being explored in different malignancies, making CAR therapy hold great promise for the future.

Nevertheless, despite the curative potential of the cellular therapies described afore, numerous studies have demonstrated that tumor cells explore immune suppressive mechanisms to dampen tumor-reactive CTL responses, resulting in suboptimal clinical efficacy. One of the pivotal mechanisms exploited by tumor cells is manipulation of CTL activation, either by enhancing CSM or interfering with CIM signaling. Tumor cells can evade immune control by down-regulating CSM such as CD80 and CD86, and up-regulating various co-inhibitory ligands, thereby limiting the therapeutic potential of current immunotherapies against cancer.

This chapter will address the role of CIM in tumor immune evasion from CTL attack, and discuss options to prevent T-cell inhibition without severe adverse effects. We will discuss the role of separate CIM involved in tumor escape from CTL, and subsequently elaborate on combinations of CIM in the tumor setting. Finally, the incorporation of CIM interference in near future anti-cancer immunotherapy will be discussed.

2.6 Co-inhibitory Molecules in Cancer

A variety of CIM have been implicated in cancer immune escape. Here, we discuss the CIM prominently involved in suppressing anti-tumor immunity.

2.6.1 PD-1

2.6.1.1 Expression and Function of PD-1

Programmed death 1 (PD-1; CD279) is an immunoreceptor and member of the B7/CD28 family [42]. In 1992, PD-1 was identified on hybridoma T-cells undergoing apoptosis and was believed to be a programmed cell death-induced gene [43]. Further characterization demonstrated that PD-1 is inducibly expressed on stimulated $CD8^+$ T-cells, $CD4^+$ T-cells, B cells and monocytes [44]. PD-1 binds two ligands, PD-L1 (B7-H1; CD274) and PD-L2 (B7-DC; CD273) [45]. While PD-L1 is expressed on various non-lymphoid tissues, PD-L2 expression is mainly restricted to APC, like DC and macrophages [46]. Furthermore, multiple tumor types express PD-L1 and its expression is elevated upon IFN-γ exposure [47]. PD-L1 molecules on tumor cells can deliver negative signals towards PD-1-expressing tumor-reactive CTL, thereby inhibiting anti-tumor immunity [48]. Indeed, PD-L1 expression has been associated with poor prognosis in solid tumors [47].

It has been demonstrated that PD-1 plays a crucial role in T-cell regulation in various immune responses such as peripheral tolerance, autoimmunity, infection and anti-tumor immunity [46]. High PD-1 expression on viral antigen-specific CTL in chronic viral infections was recognized as a hallmark for T-cell dysfunction upon antigen re-encounter [49]. This phenomenon, known as exhaustion, is characterized by the sequential loss of the ability to proliferate, secrete cytokines and kill target cells. Especially in HIV infection, T-cell impairment could be relieved by PD-1 blockade both in vitro and in animal models [50, 51]. It has also been shown that PD-1 strongly attenuates the downstream signaling of the TCR [52]. In an elegant model system, the influence of PD-1 ligation on T-cell triggering was investigated [53]. Engagement of PD-1 raises the threshold of T-cell stimulation by increasing the number of TCR/peptide-MHC complexes needed for activation. It has been reported that exhausted T-cells have elevated expression of multiple CIM and a distinct gene signature, different from anergic cells, resulting in changes in TCR and cytokine signaling pathways [54]. The importance of downstream PD-1 signaling was nicely demonstrated by the identification of an exhaustion-specific gene signature in HIV-specific T-cells [55].

2.6.1.2 PD-1 in Cancer

PD-1 has been shown to have a prominent suppressive function in anti-cancer immunity. Expression of its ligand PD-L1 on tumor cells conveys a negative signal to tumor-reactive T-cells [56]. In addition, PD-1-expressing TIL present in breast cancer tissue are associated with a poor prognosis [57]. Moreover, in melanoma was shown that PD-1$^+$ TIL were functionally impaired as compared to their PD-1-negative counterparts [58].

The involvement of PD-1 in alloSCT has been investigated both in mouse models and in the human setting. In a study investigating chronic myeloid leukemia (CML), using a retrovirus-induced CML model, it was demonstrated that tumor-specific T-cells can become exhausted [59]. In this model, consisting of PD-1$^+$ tumor-reactive T-cells and PD-L1$^+$ CML cells, exhaustion could be overcome by the administration of either PD-L1 antagonistic antibody or PD-1 deficient T-cells. In accordance, it was shown that the bulk T-cell population from CML patients exhibited increased expression of PD-1 [59]. Also, in the alloSCT setting, high PD-1 expression was observed on alloreactive CTL that specifically recognize hemato-restricted MiHA in myeloid leukemia patients [60]. Furthermore, proliferation of these PD-1$^+$ MiHA-specific CTL by stimulation with MiHA-loaded DC ex vivo was suboptimal, indicating dysfunctional CTL due to PD-1 signaling. Importantly, upon treatment with anti-PD-1 or anti-PD-L1 blocking antibodies ex vivo proliferation of the MiHA-specific CTL was reinvigorated.

These and many more studies have led to clinical trials exploring the potency of PD-1 blocking antibodies, putting the PD-1 pathway in the forefront of anti-tumor therapy. Three antagonistic anti-PD-1 antibodies are currently in advanced clinical trials, i.e. pidilizumab, nivolumab and pembrolizumab (formerly lambrolizumab) (Table 2.1). Furthermore, three anti-PD-L1 antibodies, BMS-936,559, MEDI4736, MPDL3280A and MSB0010718C, are being investigated inclinical trials (Table 2.1). In 2012, exciting reports on the use of the anti-PD-1 nivolumab and the anti-PD-L1 blocking antibody BMS-936,559 in patients with advanced malignancies were published [61, 62]. Response rates upon administration of anti-PD-1 to patients with solid tumors ranged from 18 % to 28 %, depending on tumor type. Importantly, responses were durable, with the majority of patients having responses for over a year. Notably, the therapy was relatively well tolerated and only for one patient a serious adverse event, inflammatory colitis, was reported [63]. Interestingly, also blocking the ligand, PD-L1, could induce durable tumor regression with an objective response rate of 6–17 %, with prolonged responses of over a year. The lack of strong toxic effects in this study provided promise that the PD-1 blockade might have a more subtle effect than the CTLA-4 blockade. This rendered anti-PD-1

Table 2.1 Blocking antibodies and fusion proteins targeting CIM in clinical trials

CIM	Name	Isotype	Company	Trial/approved
CD200	ALXN6000/ Samalizumab	IgG2/ G4—kappa, humanized	Alexion	Phase I/II
CTLA-4	Ipilimumab/Yervoy (MDX-010)	IgG1	BMS	FDA approved melanoma 2011; Canada and EU 2012
CTLA-4	Tremelimumab/ ticilimumab/ CP-675,206	Fully human IgG2	Pfizer	Clinical trials only
PD-1	Nivolumab/BMS-936558 (MDX-1106)	Fully human IgG4	BMS	Phase III multiple tumors
PD-1	Pidilizumab/CT-011	Humanized IgG1	CureTech/Teva	Phase II multiple tumors
PD-1	Pembrolizumab/ lambrolizumab/ MK-3475	Humanized IgG4	Merck	FDA approved sept 2014 melanoma
PD-L1	MPDL3280A	Engineered human IgG1	Roche/Genentech	Phase I/II
PD-L1	MEDI4736	Engineered human IgG1	MedImmune	Phase I
PD-L1	MSB0010718C	Fully human IgG1	Merck	
PD-L1	BMS-936,559	Fully human IgG4	BMS	Phase I
PD-L2	AMP-224	Rec fusion protein PD-L2/Fc	Amplimmune/ GlaxoSmithKline	
LAG3	BMS-986,016		BMS	Phase I
LAG3	IMP321	Rec fusion protein sLAG3/FC	Immutep	Phase I

IgG immunoglobulin G

antibodies as interesting candidates for cancer therapy and gave rise to more extensive trials. In 2013, the results were reported for the anti-PD-1 antibody pembrolizumab in melanoma [64]. In this more homogenous patient group, a response rate of 38 %, and even 52 % in the highest dose was obtained. As in the previous studies, most responses were durable. These exciting results have encouraged registration if these PD-1 blockers. On July 4th 2014, Ono Pharmaceutical and partner Bristol-Myers Squibb (BMS), gained approval in Japan for nivolumab [65]. Furthermore, Merck aims to receive the First US approval for pembrolizumab in melanoma on October 28th 2014. These approvals open up endless possibilities of using PD-1 antagonists against various malignancies, as well as combining anti-PD-1 antibodies with other treatment modalities.

2.6.2 CTLA-4

2.6.2.1 Expression and Function of CTLA-4

Cytotoxic T lymphocyte associated antigen-4 (CTLA-4; CD152), was the first identified CIM, and is partly similar to the co-signaling molecule CD28 [66]. While CD28 is constitutively expressed on the membrane of naïve T-cells, CTLA-4 is primarily localized in intracellular compartments and quickly translocates to the cell membrane upon T-cell activation. The inhibitory function of CTLA-4 was revealed in knockout mice, which showed multi-organ T-cell infiltration leading to lethal lymphoproliferative disease [67]. Like CD28, CTLA-4 has an extracellular domain containing the MYPPPY binding motif, enabling both receptors to interact with CD80 (B7-1) and CD86 (B7-2) expressed by APC. However, the binding affinity of CTLA-4 for these ligands is higher by a factor 10–100, thus outcompeting CD28 and thereby promoting immune inhibition [68].

As CTLA-4 is up-regulated upon TCR ligation, it plays an important role in attenuating effector T-cell activation and maintaining immune homeostasis and central tolerance. In addition, CTLA-4 signaling in immunosuppressive T_{REG} mediates the control of auto-reactive T-cells, as in vivo interference with CTLA-4 on these T-cells elicited pathological autoimmunity [69]. The effect of CTLA-4 interference could either be due to depletion and/or inhibition of T_{REG}. It was shown that T_{REG}-specific CTLA-4 deficiency resulted in down-regulation of CD80/CD86 on APC [70]. This can be explained by endocytosis of APC-derived CD80 and CD86 by T_{REG} [71]. Subsequently, the APC acquires a less stimulatory phenotype, resulting in a lasting inhibitory effect after CTLA-4 ligation. This concept has been investigated further in vivo. Here it was found that T_{REG} can reduce CD80/CD86 expression after encounter with a DC. When CTL are subsequently activated with these hypostimulatory DC, the effector T-cells display enhanced levels of T-cell immunoglobulin and mucin domain 3 (Tim-3) and PD-1. Via this mechanism, CTL function is indirectly attenuated via CTLA-4 signaling [72].

CTLA-4 as such is not a marker of exhausted cells, but elevated levels on viral antigen-specific T-cells correlated with their dysfunction in patients with chronic viral infections, which in turn could be restored by CTLA-4 blockade [73]. Also in metastatic melanoma, high expression of CTLA-4 was correlated to antigen-specific T-cell dysfunction [74]. Moreover, in various CD80 and CD86-positive tumor models, monotherapy with CTLA-4 blocking antibody resulted in elimination of established tumors and long-lasting antitumor immunity [75]. Interestingly, CTLA-4 also has an influence on the motility of CTL. After addition of a CTLA-4 antagonist in a mouse model, it was shown that CTL exhibited increased motility, indicating that CIM blockade does not only restore cytolytic activity, cytokine secretion and proliferation, but could also enhance CTL migration [76]. Although anti-CTLA-4 treatment works in vivo, CTLA-4 blockade in vitro has not been successful in reversing T-cell dysfunction. This can be due to limitations of the in vitro models, as CTLA-4 blockade may exert it's in vivo action via multiple immune mediators (e.g. effector T-cells, antibody responses, T_{REG}) [77].

All these preclinical findings have stimulated clinical exploration of anti-CTLA-4 blocking antibodies. At the moment, two blocking antibodies exist, ipilimumab and tremelimumab (Table 2.1). Most studies have been performed with ipilimumab in melanoma, and impressively, in these patients the median overall survival almost doubled [78]. In follow-up studies, the effects of CTLA-4 blockade were consistent [79] and in 2011, the FDA and EMA approved ipilimumab treatment for advanced melanoma, thereby paving the way for further exploration of therapies targeting CIM in cancer. Unfortunately, not all studies involving tremelimumab displayed a positive effect on overall survival [80]. Also, for both blocking antibodies, not all patients gained clinical benefit and individual responses are hard to predict. Furthermore, the occurrence of adverse toxic effects upon CTLA-4 blockade were a problem, even leading to death in some cases [80]. However, these were the pioneering studies involving CIM blockade, and by increased clinical awareness and protocols to tackle these immune related complications, severe adverse events have been decreased.

2.6.2.2 CTLA-4 in Stem Cell Transplantation

Experimental and clinical studies have demonstrated that co-inhibitory molecules hamper T-cell immunity against hematologic cancers in both the autologous and allogeneic settings. This might be due to native expression of CD80 and CD86 on hematologic tumor cells. CTLA-4:CD80/86 interactions also take place between T-cells and hematologic tumor cells. In multiple myeloma (MM) patients, CD86 but not CD80 was expressed by tumor cells, while CTLA-4 was up-regulated on T-cells, which led to anergy of tumor-specific T-cells [81]. Similar to these results, T-cells from chronic lymphocytic leukemia (CLL) patients responded to anti-CD3 activation by a decrease in CD28 and an increase in CTLA-4 expression, resulting in an inhibitory phenotype [82]. In addition to MM, also in acute myeloid leukemia (AML) cells tumor cells were demonstrated to have heterogeneous CD86 expression, but CD80 levels were generally low or absent [60, 83].

The alloreactive T-cell function after alloSCT is also strongly influenced by CIM. The importance of CTLA-4 in modulating allogeneic immune responses has been confirmed by association of certain CTLA-4 genotypes with overall survival and the incidence of leukemia relapse after alloSCT. It was demonstrated that CTLA-4 blockade shortly after alloSCT increased GVHD [84]. However, when anti-CTLA-4 was administered at later time-points after alloSCT, the GVT effect was boosted without signs of GVHD. In patients, ipilimumab administration at late time-points after alloSCT has been explored in one phase I trial [85]. Following a single infusion of the ipilimumab in 29 alloSCT patients with a recurrent or progressive hematological malignancy, three clinical responses were observed. Importantly, no induction or exacerbation of clinical GVHD was reported, although similar to other CTLA-4 blockade trials 14 % of the patients showed organ-specific immune-related adverse events. The lack of GVHD induction is likely attributed to the median interval of 1 year between the last donor T-cell infusion and ipilimumab administration. This provides a window for anti-tumor immunotherapy in the post-alloSCT setting and emphasizes the importance of appropriate timing of CIM blockade.

2.7 Combining PD-1 and CTLA-4 Blockade

It has been recognized that CTLA-4 and PD-1 exert their role in attenuating T-cell activation at different physiological locations and moments of the immune response. CTLA-4 is mostly involved in the inhibition of CTL priming in the lymph node, while PD-1 seems to limit T-cell proliferation and function in lymphoid tissues as well as in the periphery, i.e. at the tumor site. Therefore, the effects of concurrent PD-1 and CTLA-4 blockade are of great interest. In a mouse tumor model, it was demonstrated that double-positive $CD8^+$ TIL was more dysfunctional than either single PD-1 or CTLA-4 positive $CD8^+$ T-cells. In addition, double PD-1/CTLA-4 blockade led to reversal of TIL dysfunction and subsequent tumor rejection in the majority of mice [86]. Two studies which strengthen the idea of CTLA-4's role in T-cell priming versus PD-1's role in peripheral tolerance investigated the TCR repertoire [87, 88]. In patient who had received CTLA-4 blocking antibodies, an increased repertoire of TCR was observed. This indicates that at least part of the effect of CTLA-4 blockade is by an increase in T-cell priming. In contrast, in patients who had been treated with PD-1 blockade, this extended TCR repertoire was not observed, indicating that the clinical efficacy of this treatment is more likely due to reinvigoration of existing CTL responses.

These distinct roles of PD-1 and CTLA-4 warranted combined clinical trials to investigate whether administration of blocking both CIM would have an additive or a synergistic clinical effect. In the first study testing this hypothesis, in an impressive number of 65 % of patients clinical activity was observed, while these were patients with a very poor prognosis [89]. Also at the maximum dosages, 53 % of the patients fulfilled the criteria for the stringent objective responses, all with tumor reduction of 80 % or more. These impressive clinical responses were associated with in grade 3/4 adverse events in 53 % of the patients, which generally were reversible and were not more severe than observed with monotherapy. Also in follow-up data, it was shown that a group of 17 patients who received the optimum combination dose of anti-PD-1 and anti-CTLA-4 showed an overall survival rate of 94 % at 1 year and of 88 % at 2 years, exceeding by far the suboptimal responses typically observed in patients treated with either antibody alone [65]. These results are very promising for the future as optimal combinations of CIM blockade can yield very impressive clinical responses.

2.8 BTLA

2.8.1 Expression and Function of BTLA

B and T lymphocyte attenuator (BTLA), (CD272), is an inhibitory receptor with structural similarities to CTLA-4 and PD-1 [90]. BTLA is mainly expressed by immune cells, including T- and B-cells, DC and myeloid cells [91, 92]. In contrast to other B7/CD28 family members, BTLA binds a member of the tumor necrosis factor receptor (TNFR) superfamily, namely herpes virus entry mediator (HVEM) [93]. HVEM is part of an intricate signaling network as it has at least four additional binding partners that distinctively mediate T-cell responses: i.e. CD160, LIGHT (for lymphotoxin-like, exhibits inducible expression, and competes with HSV glycoprotein D for HVEM, a receptor expressed by T lymphocytes), lymphotoxin-α (LT-α) and herpes simplex virus glycoprotein D (gD) [94]. BTLA or CD160 signaling upon HVEM binding results in T-cell inhibition [93, 95]. Interestingly, naïve T-cells express both HVEM and BTLA, and these molecules form a T-cell intrinsic heterodimer complex [96]. Due to formation of this complex, HVEM is unavailable for extrinsic ligands, and no co-stimulatory signal is transduced. In humans, persistent expression of BTLA was observed on EBV- and CMV-specific $CD8^+$ T-cells, which negatively affected T-cell function [97, 98]. Furthermore, high BTLA expression correlated with impaired tumor-reactive T-cell function in melanoma patients [74, 97]. These tumor-specific T-cell responses could be restored in vitro by interference with the BTLA-HVEM pathway in combination with vaccination therapy. In addition, co-expression of BTLA, PD-1 and Tim-3 rendered melanoma-specific $CD8^+$ T-cells highly dysfunctional, which could be reversed by combined blockade of all three CIM [99]. In a mouse tumor vaccination model, blockade of the BTLA/CD160/HVEM pathway caused regression of large tumor masses [100]. These results show that in the right setting BTLA blockade can be of great significance, warranting evaluation of clinical effectiveness. In addition, the effect of a BTLA blocking antibody has been investigated on MiHA-specific T-cell functionality in samples from alloSCT patients [91]. As shown for PD-1, BTLA was also highly expressed on MiHA-specific CTL. Moreover, in the majority of the patients BTLA blockade resulted in increased outgrowth of MiHA-specific $CD8^+$ T-cells. Interestingly, in three patients BTLA blockade effects were more prominent than those of PD-1, indicating that BTLA has a non-redundant function to PD-1, and therefore it holds promise in cancer immunotherapies.

2.8.2 Tim-3

The co-signaling receptor Tim-3 is expressed on Th1 $CD4^+$ and $CD8^+$ T-cells, and is involved in co-inhibition. In mice, the interaction of Tim-3 with its ligand galectin-9 was demonstrated to prevent in autoimmune diseases and promote malignancies [101]. Furthermore, in HIV [102] and melanoma patients [103], dysfunctional CD8+ T-cells have been shown to co-express Tim-3. In this regard interference with Tim-3 signaling is an interesting treatment option, and enhanced tumor vaccine efficacy has been observed by Tim-3 blockade [104]. Interestingly, both Tim-3 and PD-1 were expressed on a subset of exhausted CD8+ T-cells in a murine AML model, and expression levels increased [105] during tumor progression [106]. While either Tim-3 or PD-L1 blockade alone was not sufficient to improve survival, the combination of the two antagonistic antibodies significantly decreased tumor burden and enhanced survival. Also, in a melanoma vaccination model, the vast majority of vaccination-induced CTL upregulated PD-1 and a minority also upregulated Tim-3. Levels of PD-1 and Tim-3 expression by CTL at the time of vaccine administration correlated inversely with their expansion potential in vivo. Importantly, dual blockade of PD-1 and Tim-3 enhanced the expansion and cytokine production of vaccine-induced CTL in vitro [107]. Also, combining Tim-3 blockade with activation of CD137, a co-stimulatory receptor, conveyed long term protection against ovarian carcinoma in a mouse model [108]. Finally, blocking of Tim-3 and its family member Tim-4 resulted in a better anti-tumor effect against murine melanoma. All these studies show that, although always in conjunction with another co-signaling molecule, Tim-3 can be involved in tumor evasion, making it an attractive partner in combinatorial blockade. In contrast, a stimulatory role for TIM-3 and galectin-9 has been reported in the interaction of CD8+ T-cells and DC [109]. This discrepancy might be explained by the findings that Tim-3 signaling enhances TCR stimulation [96]. T-cell exhaustion may be caused by prolonged TCR signaling via Tim-3, thereby prolonging the effector phase of T-cell activation at the expense of T-cell memory [110]. Therefore, depending on the setting, Tim-3 may act as either a co-stimulatory or a co-inhibitory receptor.

2.8.3 LAG3

Lymphocyte-activation gene 3 (LAG3; CD223) is a co-inhibitory receptor highly similar to CD4 and therefore also binds HLA class II molecules [111, 112]. LAG3 seems to be non-redundant from PD-1, as both are expressed on distinct populations CTL [113]. Recently, it was demonstrated that PD-1 and LAG3 act synergistically in the onset of autoimmune diseases and tumor escape in mice [114, 115]. In a leukemia model, PD-1 and CTLA-4 were blocked to reverse CTL tolerance. However, also blockade of LAG3 was necessary to fully restore CTL function [116]. Altogether, these results indicate that LAG3, like Tim-3, is a good candidate as an additive blocking target. At the moment, clinical trials are being performed with a blocking antibody and a soluble LAG3 fusion molecule (Table 2.1), and these studies have the potential to add LAG3 to the list of targets in cancer immunotherapy [117].

2.9 Other Co-inhibitory Players

In addition to the afore discussed molecules, other co-inhibitory players are being studied to characterize their contribution to functional suppression of tumor-reactive T-cell immunity.

In 2011, a new CIM highly similar to PD-1 was discovered by two groups: PD-1H (PD-1 homolog) or VISTA (V-domain Ig suppressor of T-cell activation) [105, 118]. This molecule is broadly expressed on hematopoietic cells and expression levels are further up-regulated on T-cells and APCs following activation. In in vitro studies the interaction with soluble VISTA-Ig fusion protein or VISTA$^+$ APC mediated the suppression of T-cell cytokine production and proliferation, which could be alleviated by blocking antibody treatment [118, 119]. Recently, it was also demonstrated that VISTA can enhance the conversion of naïve T-cells into FoxP3$^+$ T-cells [119]. In vivo, VISTA overexpression on tumor cells strongly hampered protective tumor-reactive T-cell responses. Importantly, VISTA blockade impaired the suppressive function and emergence of T_{REG}, as well as modulated the suppressive tumor micro-environment, thereby, promoting tumor-reactive T-cell immunity [120]. Interestingly, treatment with PD-1H blocking antibody prevented the induction of GVHD in murine alloSCT models, although the mechanism of action has not been elucidated [105]. These data illustrate that PD-1H/VISTA exerts both an immunoregulatory function in the tumor micro-environment, as well as a direct immunosuppressive action on anti-tumor T-cell responses, making it an interesting therapeutic target.

Killer cell lectin-like receptor G1 (KLRG1), also known as CLEC15A or MAFA, is an inhibitory receptor expressed on NK cells and subsets of CD4$^+$ and CD8$^+$ T-cells [121]. It has been demonstrated that interaction with its ligand E-cadherin results in the functional inhibition of KLRG1$^+$ NK cells, thereby preventing effective killing of tumor cells [122, 123]. In T-cells, KLRG1 expression has been mostly studied as a marker of terminal differentiation. KLRG1$^+$ antigen-experienced $T_{EFF/EM}$ cells exhibited preserved capacity to secrete cytokines upon antigen reencounter, but were incapable of proliferation [121]. Importantly, one study demonstrated that interference with KLRG1 signaling, by targeting of E-cadherin with a blocking antibody, results in enhanced TCR-induced proliferation of highly differentiated CD28$^-$CD27$^-$ CTL [124]. More studies are warranted to characterize the involvement of KLRG1 signaling in tumor immune escape and the potential of KLRG1 blockade for cancer immunotherapy.

2B4 (i.e. CD244, SLAMf4) is a member of the CD2 subset of the immunoglobulin superfamily, and is expressed on NK cells, monocytes, basophils and eosinophils. Furthermore, 2B4 expression is up-regulated on a subset of CD8$^+$ T-cells following activation [125, 126]. Its binding partner is CD48 [127]. Most functional studies have been performed with NK cells, where 2B4 was demonstrated to have both activating and inhibitory functions [128]. Interestingly, in a murine transplantation model, 2B4 expression was up-regulated on allograft-reactive CD8$^+$ T-cells, but not CD4$^+$ T-cells, following selective CD28 blockade [129]. Preservation of inhibitory signaling via CTLA-4 was required for the up-regulation of 2B4. Subsequent inhibitory signaling via 2B4 reduced expression levels of the co-stimulatory molecule ICOS, and mediated enhanced allograft survival. These results indicate that 2B4 is involved in the control of antigen-specific CTL functionality.

CD200 Receptor (CD200R) is an inhibitory receptor expressed by cells of myeloid and lymphoid origins, including NK cells and T-cells following activation [130]. Its ligand CD200 (OX2) is expressed by diverse cell types, including immune cells, neurons and epithelia. Importantly, overexpression of CD200 by tumor cells has been associated with progression of various solid and hematologic cancers [131]. In a murine leukemia model, CD200Fc suppressed $CD4^+$ and $CD8^+$ T-cell functionality, resulting in loss of protection from tumor growth [132]. Ex vivo studies with human CLL demonstrated that CD200 is involved in the functional suppression of CTL-mediated tumor killing and CD4-mediated suppression of CTL functionality, which could be reverted with CD200 blocking antibody or CD200 siRNA treatment [133]. In a murine model with $CD200^+$ human B-CLL, administration of CD200 blocking antibody resulted in restored T-cell proliferation and tumor control [134]. Moreover, patients with $CD200^+$ AML were found to have reduced numbers of functional NK cells [135], had significantly compromised Th1 memory and CTL memory responses [136], and showed increased numbers of $FoxP3^+$ T_{REG} [137]. CD200 blockade in vitro could recover NK cell and T-cell functionality [135, 136], and is therefore an attractive target for therapy. Interestingly, the first clinical results have already been reported about an anti-CD200 blocking antibody (Table 2.1) [138]. Although it was in a small cohort, promising results were obtained in a study with B-CLL and MM patients: 36 % of patients experienced at least a 10 % reduction in bulky disease and notably, one patient experienced a partial response with a maximum of 71 % reduction in bulky disease.

2.10 Future Prospects

Several therapeutic strategies are being developed to dampen the inhibitory signaling by CIM in order to optimize tumor-reactive CTL immunity (Fig. 2.1). The challenge of interference with immune checkpoints is to boost anti-tumor reactivity, while avoiding adverse events such as systemic toxicity. This can potentially be achieved by combining the alleviation of co-inhibition with other therapeutic options or optimal dosage and timing of antibody administration. Appealing combinations are the simultaneous targeting of multiple co-inhibitory receptors, co-stimulatory agonists in parallel with CIM antagonists, or incorporation in existing cellular therapies. For example, DC vaccination may be applied together with blocking antibodies against CIM to boost CTL-mediated anti-tumor immunity.

CAR T-cells are a promising treatment modality in cancer therapy. Although in second and third generation CAR T-cell constructs a strong co-stimulatory signal is incorporated in the form of CD28, 4-1BB and OX40 intracellular signaling domains, this powerful therapy also seems to be dampened by CIM [139, 140].

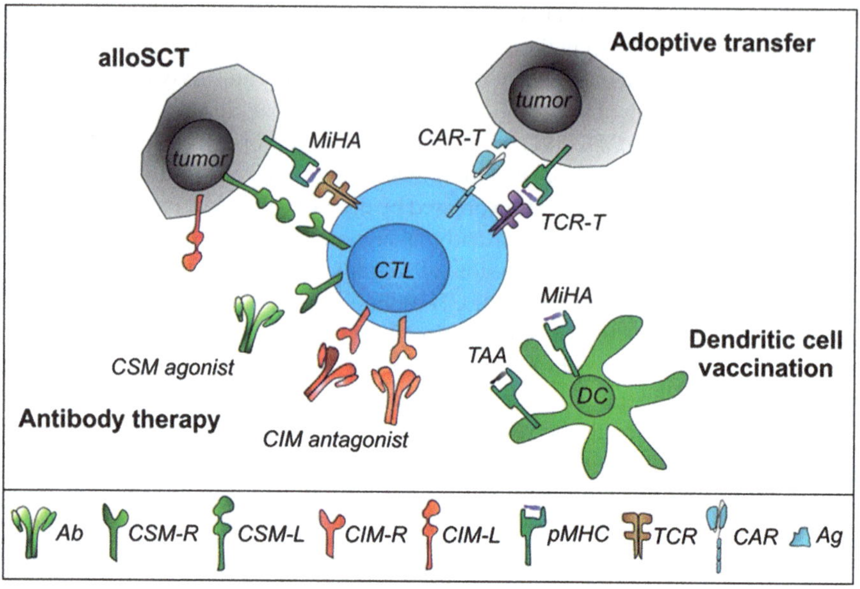

Fig. 2.1 To boost tumor-reactive T cell immunity different immunotherapeutic strategies can be exploited as monotherapy or in combination. First, co-inhibitory signaling pathways can be blocked with antagonistic antibodies to prevent and/or alleviate the functional impairment of CTLs. Furthermore, agonistic antibodies targeting co-stimulatory molecules can be applied to further augment CTL functionality. In addition, dendritic cell vaccination can be applied to provide efficient antigen presentation and strong stimulatory signals to tumor-reactive CTLs. Another strategy is the alloSCT in hematological malignancies, which can elicit powerful MiHA-reactive CTL responses. Finally, by adoptive transfer of highly potent TCR-transduced or CAR-transduced (stem-cell like) T cells direct attack of tumor cells can be provoked. The power of these immunotherapeutic approaches can be further intensified by combination with antibodies to interfere with co-inhibitory signaling pathways

In a murine tumor model with Her-2-specific CAR-T-cells, a significant increase in tumor growth inhibition was observed after PD-1 blockade [141]. In addition, the amount of immune suppressive myeloid derived suppressor cells was decreased upon PD-1 blockade, through a yet unknown mechanism. Therefore, CIM blockade in combination with CAR-T-cell therapy may improve the clinical efficacy of this novel therapy.

Although anti-CTLA-4 and anti-PD-1 monotherapies have shown very exciting results, toxic effects of blocking CIM may still be a problem. Approaches that concurrently deliver a tumor-antigen-specific stimulus may lead to less adverse events. These include combination therapies with treatment modalities such as immunomodulatory anti-cancer agents, vaccines, T_{REG} depletion or nanoparticles. Recently, another treatment modality in which an antigen-specific stimulation is combined with an intervention for co-inhibition was explored. PD-L1/L2 silenced MiHA-loaded DC boosted the expansion of MiHA-specific T-cells ex vivo [142], and following these promising results, a clinical trial combining DLI with vaccination of PD-L1/L2 silenced donor DC loaded with hemato-restricted MiHA will start. All clinical studies provide a platform for incorporating blockade of CIM as adjuvant therapy of choice in cancer patients, with numerous options for combination therapies. Importantly, the risk of breaking tolerance systemically by blockade of one CIM could be prevented by using lower levels of multiple blocking antibodies targeting different CIM simultaneously, since together these may boost immune responses in a non-redundant manner. This is stressed by the fact that exhausted T-cells are known to display multiple co-inhibitory receptors [143]. Notably, the impressive results obtained by combining blocking antibodies against PD-1 and CTLA-4 is a perfect example of harnessing the power of these two non-redundant immune checkpoints, and many more combinations need to be investigated in the clinical setting.

After identification of the role of CIM in $CD8^+$ T-cell functions, their significance on T-cell exhaustion was clearly established. However, with time, the notion of CIM as direct markers of dysfunction has been adjusted. Although their negative effect on T-cell functions is evident, expression as such does not qualify a T-cell as exhausted [144]. It has been shown that CIM, most notably PD-1, are also present on healthy cells [145] and that several CIM are up-regulated after T-cell activation [146, 147], while their expression had no direct effect on cytokine production by CTL. The activation-induced up-regulation indicated the physiological role of CIM as a negative feedback loop in CTL effector responses. Moreover, during T-cell differentiation most CIM are also up- or down-regulated [91, 146]. All these results indicate that, although on the whole T-cell population PD-1 expression can be an indicator for exhaustion, expression as such is not a marker of exhaustion on the individual T-cell level. Especially the fact that PD-1 can be an activation marker is demonstrated by a study investigating TIL in melanoma. Here it was shown that PD-1, LAG3 and Tim-3 are the identifying markers for tumor-reactive CTL [148]. The realization that not expression, but signaling via the CIM causes CTL dysfunction, has prompted the investigation of downstream signaling pathways and gene expression in impaired CTL. It was found that exhausted T-cells display a distinct gene signature, different from anergic cells, resulting in changes in TCR and cytokine signaling pathways [54]. Indeed, it was demonstrated that PD-1 downstream signaling results in an exhaustion gene signature in HIV-specific T-cells [55]. Further research into these mechanisms in CTL impairment in the tumor setting can yield novel targets to prevent or reverse exhaustion.

Altogether, CIM play a pivotal role in natural and therapeutic CTL-mediated immunity against cancers. With increasing knowledge of a growing number of CIM, novel mono- and combinatorial treatment options are becoming available. In the end, this can lead to optimized immunotherapy against cancers.

Acknowledgments This work was supported by grants from the Alpe d'HuZes foundation/Dutch Cancer Society (KWF 2011-5041) and (KWF 2012-5410).

References

1. Croci DO, Zacarias Fluck MF, Rico MJ, Matar P, Rabinovich GA, Scharovsky OG. Dynamic cross-talk between tumor and immune cells in orchestrating the immunosuppressive network at the tumor microenvironment. Cancer Immunol Immunother. 2007;56(11):1687–700.
2. Chen L. Co-inhibitory molecules of the B7-CD28 family in the control of T-cell immunity. Nat Rev Immunol. 2004;4(5):336–47.
3. Zang X, Allison JP. The B7 family and cancer therapy: costimulation and coinhibition. Clin Cancer Res. 2007;13(18 Pt 1):5271–9.
4. Greenwald RJ, Freeman GJ, Sharpe AH. The B7 family revisited. Annu Rev Immunol. 2005; 23:515–48.
5. Sharpe AH. Mechanisms of costimulation. Immunol Rev. 2009;229(1):5–11.
6. Carreno BM, Carter LL, Collins M. Therapeutic opportunities in the B7/CD28 family of ligands and receptors. Curr Opin Pharmacol. 2005;5(4):424–30.
7. Cui W, Kaech SM. Generation of effector CD8+ T cells and their conversion to memory T cells. Immunol Rev. 2010;236:151–66.
8. Marcus A, Gowen BG, Thompson TW, Iannello A, Ardolino M, Deng W, Wang L, Shifrin N, Raulet DH. Recognition of tumors by the innate immune system and natural killer cells. Adv Immunol. 2014;122:91–128.
9. Engelhard VH, Bullock TN, Colella TA, Sheasley SL, Mullins DW. Antigens derived from melanocyte differentiation proteins: self-tolerance, autoimmunity, and use for cancer immunotherapy. Immunol Rev. 2002;188:136–46.
10. Gameiro SR, Jammeh ML, Hodge JW. Cancer vaccines targeting carcinoembryonic antigen: state-of-the-art and future promise. Expert Rev Vaccines. 2013;12(6):617–29.
11. Meek DW, Marcar L. MAGE-A antigens as targets in tumour therapy. Cancer Lett. 2012;324(2):126–32.
12. Whitehurst AW. Cause and consequence of cancer/testis antigen activation in cancer. Annu Rev Pharmacol Toxicol. 2014;54:251–72.
13. Robbins PF, Lu YC, El-Gamil M, Li YF, Gross C, Gartner J, Lin JC, Teer JK, Cliften P, Tycksen E, Samuels Y, Rosenberg SA. Mining exomic sequencing data to identify mutated antigens recognized by adoptively transferred tumor-reactive T cells. Nat Med. 2013; 19(6):747–52.
14. Hinrichs CS, Rosenberg SA. Exploiting the curative potential of adoptive T-cell therapy for cancer. Immunol Rev. 2014;257(1):56–71.
15. Palucka K, Banchereau J. Cancer immunotherapy via dendritic cells. Nat Rev Cancer. 2012;12(4):265–77.
16. Anguille S, Smits EL, Lion E, van Tendeloo VF, Berneman ZN. Clinical use of dendritic cells for cancer therapy. Lancet Oncol. 2014;15(7):e257–67.
17. Westdorp H, Skold AE, Snijer BA, Franik S, Mulder SF, Major PP, Foley R, Gerritsen WR, de Vries IJ. Immunotherapy for prostate cancer: lessons from responses to tumor-associated antigens. Front Immunol. 2014;5:191.
18. Bol KF, Mensink HW, Aarntzen EH, Schreibelt G, Keunen JE, Coulie PG, de Klein A, Punt CJ, Paridaens D, Figdor CG, de Vries IJ. Long overall survival after dendritic cell vaccination in metastatic uveal melanoma patients. Am J Ophthalmol. 2014;158:939–47.
19. Tacken PJ, de Vries IJ, Torensma R, Figdor CG. Dendritic-cell immunotherapy: from ex vivo loading to in vivo targeting. Nat Rev Immunol. 2007;7(10):790–802.
20. Jenq RR, van den Brink MR. Allogeneic haematopoietic stem cell transplantation: individualized stem cell and immune therapy of cancer. Nat Rev Cancer. 2010;10(3):213–21.
21. Feng X, Hui KM, Younes HM, Brickner AG. Targeting minor histocompatibility antigens in graft versus tumor or graft versus leukemia responses. Trends Immunol. 2008;29(12): 624–32.
22. Bleakley M, Riddell SR. Exploiting T cells specific for human minor histocompatibility antigens for therapy of leukemia. Immunol Cell Biol. 2011;89(3):396–407.

23. Dudley ME, Wunderlich JR, Shelton TE, Even J, Rosenberg SA. Generation of tumor-infiltrating lymphocyte cultures for use in adoptive transfer therapy for melanoma patients. J Immunother. 2003;26(4):332–42.
24. Rosenberg SA, Spiess P, Lafreniere R. A new approach to the adoptive immunotherapy of cancer with tumor-infiltrating lymphocytes. Science. 1986;233(4770):1318–21.
25. Wu R, Forget MA, Chacon J, Bernatchez C, Haymaker C, Chen JQ, Hwu P, Radvanyi LG. Adoptive T-cell therapy using autologous tumor-infiltrating lymphocytes for metastatic melanoma: current status and future outlook. Cancer J. 2012;18(2):160–75.
26. Bleakley M, Otterud BE, Richardt JL, Mollerup AD, Hudecek M, Nishida T, Chaney CN, Warren EH, Leppert MF, Riddell SR. Leukemia-associated minor histocompatibility antigen discovery using T-cell clones isolated by in vitro stimulation of naive CD8+ T cells. Blood. 2010;115(23):4923–33.
27. Mutis T, Ghoreschi K, Schrama E, Kamp J, Heemskerk M, Falkenburg JH, Wilke M, Goulmy E. Efficient induction of minor histocompatibility antigen HA-1-specific cytotoxic T-cells using dendritic cells retrovirally transduced with HA-1-coding cDNA. Biol Blood Marrow Transplant. 2002;8(8):412–9.
28. Warren EH, Fujii N, Akatsuka Y, Chaney CN, Mito JK, Loeb KR, Gooley TA, Brown ML, Koo KK, Rosinski KV, Ogawa S, Matsubara A, Appelbaum FR, Riddell SR. Therapy of relapsed leukemia after allogeneic hematopoietic cell transplantation with T cells specific for minor histocompatibility antigens. Blood. 2010;115(19):3869–78.
29. Gattinoni L, Lugli E, Ji Y, Pos Z, Paulos CM, Quigley MF, Almeida JR, Gostick E, Yu Z, Carpenito C, Wang E, Douek DC, Price DA, June CH, Marincola FM, Roederer M, Restifo NP. A human memory T cell subset with stem cell-like properties. Nat Med. 2011; 17(10):1290–7.
30. Gattinoni L, Zhong XS, Palmer DC, Ji Y, Hinrichs CS, Yu Z, Wrzesinski C, Boni A, Cassard L, Garvin LM, Paulos CM, Muranski P, Restifo NP. Wnt signaling arrests effector T cell differentiation and generates CD8+ memory stem cells. Nat Med. 2009;15(7):808–13.
31. van der Waart A, van de Weem N, Maas F, Kramer C, Kester M, Falkenburg F, Schaap N, Jansen J, van der Voort R, Gattinoni L, Hobo W, Dolstra H. Inhibition of Akt-signaling promotes the generation of superior tumor-reactive T cells for adoptive immunotherapy. Blood. 2014;124:3490–500.
32. Gattinoni L, Klebanoff CA, Restifo NP. Paths to stemness: building the ultimate antitumour T cell. Nat Rev Cancer. 2012;12(10):671–84.
33. Heemskerk MH, Griffioen M, Falkenburg JH. T-cell receptor gene transfer for treatment of leukemia. Cytotherapy. 2008;10(2):108–15.
34. Heemskerk MH, Hoogeboom M, Hagedoorn R, Kester MG, Willemze R, Falkenburg JH. Reprogramming of virus-specific T cells into leukemia-reactive T cells using T cell receptor gene transfer. J Exp Med. 2004;199(7):885–94.
35. Bendle GM, Linnemann C, Hooijkaas AI, Bies L, de Witte MA, Jorritsma A, Kaiser AD, Pouw N, Debets R, Kieback E, Uckert W, Song JY, Haanen JB, Schumacher TN. Lethal graft-versus-host disease in mouse models of T cell receptor gene therapy. Nat Med. 2010;16(5):565. -70, 1p.
36. Morgan RA, Dudley ME, Wunderlich JR, Hughes MS, Yang JC, Sherry RM, Royal RE, Topalian SL, Kammula US, Restifo NP, Zheng Z, Nahvi A, de Vries CR, Rogers-Freezer LJ, Mavroukakis SA, Rosenberg SA. Cancer regression in patients after transfer of genetically engineered lymphocytes. Science. 2006;314(5796):126–9.
37. Heemskerk MH, Hoogeboom M, de Paus RA, Kester MG, van der Hoorn MA, Goulmy E, Willemze R, Falkenburg JH. Redirection of antileukemic reactivity of peripheral T lymphocytes using gene transfer of minor histocompatibility antigen HA-2-specific T-cell receptor complexes expressing a conserved alpha joining region. Blood. 2003;102(10):3530–40.
38. Johnson LA, Morgan RA, Dudley ME, Cassard L, Yang JC, Hughes MS, Kammula US, Royal RE, Sherry RM, Wunderlich JR, Lee CC, Restifo NP, Schwarz SL, Cogdill AP, Bishop RJ, Kim H, Brewer CC, Rudy SF, VanWaes C, Davis JL, Mathur A, Ripley RT, Nathan DA, Laurencot CM, Rosenberg SA. Gene therapy with human and mouse T-cell receptors

mediates cancer regression and targets normal tissues expressing cognate antigen. Blood. 2009;114(3):535–46.
39. Ochi T, Fujiwara H, Yasukawa M. Application of adoptive T-cell therapy using tumor antigen-specific T-cell receptor gene transfer for the treatment of human leukemia. J Biomed Biotechnol. 2010;2010:521248.
40. Curran KJ, Pegram HJ, Brentjens RJ. Chimeric antigen receptors for T cell immunotherapy: current understanding and future directions. J Gene Med. 2012;14(6):405–15.
41. Porter DL, Levine BL, Kalos M, Bagg A, June CH. Chimeric antigen receptor-modified T cells in chronic lymphoid leukemia. N Engl J Med. 2011;365(8):725–33.
42. Freeman GJ, Long AJ, Iwai Y, Bourque K, Chernova T, Nishimura H, Fitz LJ, Malenkovich N, Okazaki T, Byrne MC, Horton HF, Fouser L, Carter L, Ling V, Bowman MR, Carreno BM, Collins M, Wood CR, Honjo T. Engagement of the PD-1 immunoinhibitory receptor by a novel B7 family member leads to negative regulation of lymphocyte activation. J Exp Med. 2000;192(7):1027–34.
43. Ishida Y, Agata Y, Shibahara K, Honjo T. Induced expression of PD-1, a novel member of the immunoglobulin gene superfamily, upon programmed cell death. EMBO J. 1992;11(11): 3887–95.
44. Okazaki T, Honjo T. The PD-1-PD-L pathway in immunological tolerance. Trends Immunol. 2006;27(4):195–201.
45. Freeman GJ. Structures of PD-1 with its ligands: sideways and dancing cheek to cheek. Proc Natl Acad Sci U S A. 2008;105(30):10275–6.
46. Keir ME, Butte MJ, Freeman GJ, Sharpe AH. PD-1 and its ligands in tolerance and immunity. Annu Rev Immunol. 2008;26:677–704.
47. Gao Q, Wang XY, Qiu SJ, Yamato I, Sho M, Nakajima Y, Zhou J, Li BZ, Shi YH, Xiao YS, Xu Y, Fan J. Overexpression of PD-L1 significantly associates with tumor aggressiveness and postoperative recurrence in human hepatocellular carcinoma. Clin Cancer Res. 2009; 15(3):971–9.
48. Zhang C, Wu S, Xue X, Li M, Qin X, Li W, Han W, Zhang Y. Anti-tumor immunotherapy by blockade of the PD-1/PD-L1 pathway with recombinant human PD-1-IgV. Cytotherapy. 2008;10(7):711–9.
49. Velu V, Kannanganat S, Ibegbu C, Chennareddi L, Villinger F, Freeman GJ, Ahmed R, Amara RR. Elevated expression levels of inhibitory receptor programmed death 1 on simian immunodeficiency virus-specific CD8 T cells during chronic infection but not after vaccination. J Virol. 2007;81(11):5819–28.
50. Velu V, Titanji K, Zhu B, Husain S, Pladevega A, Lai L, Vanderford TH, Chennareddi L, Silvestri G, Freeman GJ, Ahmed R, Amara RR. Enhancing SIV-specific immunity in vivo by PD-1 blockade. Nature. 2009;458(7235):206–10.
51. Kaufmann DE, Walker BD. PD-1 and CTLA-4 inhibitory cosignaling pathways in HIV infection and the potential for therapeutic intervention. J Immunol. 2009;182(10):5891–7.
52. Boussiotis VA, Chatterjee P, Li L. Biochemical signaling of PD-1 on T cells and its functional implications. Cancer J. 2014;20(4):265–71.
53. Wei F, Zhong S, Ma Z, Kong H, Medvec A, Ahmed R, Freeman GJ, Krogsgaard M, Riley JL. Strength of PD-1 signaling differentially affects T-cell effector functions. Proc Natl Acad Sci U S A. 2013;110(27):E2480–9.
54. Wherry EJ, Ha SJ, Kaech SM, Haining WN, Sarkar S, Kalia V, Subramaniam S, Blattman JN, Barber DL, Ahmed R. Molecular signature of CD8+ T cell exhaustion during chronic viral infection. Immunity. 2007;27(4):670–84.
55. Quigley M, Pereyra F, Nilsson B, Porichis F, Fonseca C, Eichbaum Q, Julg B, Jesneck JL, Brosnahan K, Imam S, Russell K, Toth I, Piechocka-Trocha A, Dolfi D, Angelosanto J, Crawford A, Shin H, Kwon DS, Zupkosky J, Francisco L, Freeman GJ, Wherry EJ, Kaufmann DE, Walker BD, Ebert B, Haining WN. Transcriptional analysis of HIV-specific CD8+ T cells shows that PD-1 inhibits T cell function by upregulating BATF. Nat Med. 2010; 16(10):1147–51.

56. Iwai Y, Ishida M, Tanaka Y, Okazaki T, Honjo T, Minato N. Involvement of PD-L1 on tumor cells in the escape from host immune system and tumor immunotherapy by PD-L1 blockade. Proc Natl Acad Sci U S A. 2002;99(19):12293–7.
57. Muenst S, Soysal SD, Gao F, Obermann EC, Oertli D, Gillanders WE. The presence of programmed death 1 (PD-1)-positive tumor-infiltrating lymphocytes is associated with poor prognosis in human breast cancer. Breast Cancer Res Treat. 2013;139(3):667–76.
58. Ahmadzadeh M, Johnson LA, Heemskerk B, Wunderlich JR, Dudley ME, White DE, Rosenberg SA. Tumor antigen-specific CD8 T cells infiltrating the tumor express high levels of PD-1 and are functionally impaired. Blood. 2009;114(8):1537–44.
59. Mumprecht S, Schürch C, Schwaller J, Solenthaler M, Ochsenbein AF. Programmed death 1 signaling on chronic myeloid leukemia-specific T cells results in T-cell exhaustion and disease progression. Blood. 2009;114(8):1528–36.
60. Norde WJ, Maas F, Hobo W, Korman A, Quigley M, Kester MG, Hebeda K, Falkenburg JH, Schaap N, de Witte TM, van der Voort R, Dolstra H. PD-1/PD-L1 interactions contribute to functional T-cell impairment in patients who relapse with cancer after allogeneic stem cell transplantation. Cancer Res. 2011;71(15):5111–22.
61. Topalian SL, Hodi FS, Brahmer JR, Gettinger SN, Smith DC, McDermott DF, Powderly JD, Carvajal RD, Sosman JA, Atkins MB, Leming PD, Spigel DR, Antonia SJ, Horn L, Drake CG, Pardoll DM, Chen L, Sharfman WH, Anders RA, Taube JM, McMiller TL, Xu H, Korman AJ, Jure-Kunkel M, Agrawal S, McDonald D, Kollia GD, Gupta A, Wigginton JM, Sznol M. Safety, activity, and immune correlates of anti-PD-1 antibody in cancer. N Engl J Med. 2012;366(26):2443–54.
62. Brahmer JR, Tykodi SS, Chow LQ, Hwu WJ, Topalian SL, Hwu P, Drake CG, Camacho LH, Kauh J, Odunsi K, Pitot HC, Hamid O, Bhatia S, Martins R, Eaton K, Chen S, Salay TM, Alaparthy S, Grosso JF, Korman AJ, Parker SM, Agrawal S, Goldberg SM, Pardoll DM, Gupta A, Wigginton JM. Safety and activity of anti-PD-L1 antibody in patients with advanced cancer. N Engl J Med. 2012;366(26):2455–65.
63. Brahmer JR, Drake CG, Wollner I, Powderly JD, Picus J, Sharfman WH, Stankevich E, Pons A, Salay TM, McMiller TL, Gilson MM, Wang C, Selby M, Taube JM, Anders R, Chen L, Korman AJ, Pardoll DM, Lowy I, Topalian SL. Phase I study of single-agent anti-programmed death-1 (MDX-1106) in refractory solid tumors: safety, clinical activity, pharmacodynamics, and immunologic correlates. J Clin Oncol. 2010;28(19):3167–75.
64. Hamid O, Robert C, Daud A, Hodi FS, Hwu WJ, Kefford R, Wolchok JD, Hersey P, Joseph RW, Weber JS, Dronca R, Gangadhar TC, Patnaik A, Zarour H, Joshua AM, Gergich K, Elassaiss-Schaap J, Algazi A, Mateus C, Boasberg P, Tumeh PC, Chmielowski B, Ebbinghaus SW, Li XN, Kang SP, Ribas A. Safety and tumor responses with lambrolizumab (anti-PD-1) in melanoma. N Engl J Med. 2013;369(2):134–44.
65. Sheridan C. First PD-1 inhibitor breezes across finish line. Nat Biotechnol. 2014;32(9):847–8.
66. Brunet JF, Denizot F, Luciani MF, Roux-Dosseto M, Suzan M, Mattei MG, Golstein P. A new member of the immunoglobulin superfamily–CTLA-4. Nature. 1987;328(6127):267–70.
67. Tivol EA, Borriello F, Schweitzer AN, Lynch WP, Bluestone JA, Sharpe AH. Loss of CTLA-4 leads to massive lymphoproliferation and fatal multiorgan tissue destruction, revealing a critical negative regulatory role of CTLA-4. Immunity. 1995;3(5):541–7.
68. Peach RJ, Bajorath J, Brady W, Leytze G, Greene J, Naemura J, Linsley PS. Complementarity determining region 1 (CDR1)- and CDR3-analogous regions in CTLA-4 and CD28 determine the binding to B7-1. J Exp Med. 1994;180(6):2049–58.
69. Takahashi T, Tagami T, Yamazaki S, Uede T, Shimizu J, Sakaguchi N, Mak TW, Sakaguchi S. Immunologic self-tolerance maintained by CD25(+)CD4(+) regulatory T cells constitutively expressing cytotoxic T lymphocyte-associated antigen 4. J Exp Med. 2000;192(2):303–10.
70. Wing K, Onishi Y, Prieto-Martin P, Yamaguchi T, Miyara M, Fehervari Z, Nomura T, Sakaguchi S. CTLA-4 control over Foxp3+ regulatory T cell function. Science. 2008;322(5899):271–5.

71. Qureshi OS, Zheng Y, Nakamura K, Attridge K, Manzotti C, Schmidt EM, Baker J, Jeffery LE, Kaur S, Briggs Z, Hou TZ, Futter CE, Anderson G, Walker LS, Sansom DM. Trans-endocytosis of CD80 and CD86: a molecular basis for the cell-extrinsic function of CTLA-4. Science. 2011;332(6029):600–3.
72. Bauer CA, Kim EY, Marangoni F, Carrizosa E, Claudio NM, Mempel TR. Dynamic Treg interactions with intratumoral APCs promote local CTL dysfunction. J Clin Invest. 2014;124(6):2425–40.
73. Kaufmann DE, Kavanagh DG, Pereyra F, Zaunders JJ, Mackey EW, Miura T, Palmer S, Brockman M, Rathod A, Piechocka-Trocha A, Baker B, Zhu B, Le GS, Waring MT, Ahern R, Moss K, Kelleher AD, Coffin JM, Freeman GJ, Rosenberg ES, Walker BD. Upregulation of CTLA-4 by HIV-specific CD4+ T cells correlates with disease progression and defines a reversible immune dysfunction. Nat Immunol. 2007;8(11):1246–54.
74. Baitsch L, Baumgaertner P, Devevre E, Raghav SK, Legat A, Barba L, Wieckowski S, Bouzourene H, Deplancke B, Romero P, Rufer N, Speiser DE. Exhaustion of tumor-specific CD8(+) T cells in metastases from melanoma patients. J Clin Invest. 2011;121(6):2350–60.
75. Leach DR, Krummel MF, Allison JP. Enhancement of antitumor immunity by CTLA-4 blockade. Science. 1996;271(5256):1734–6.
76. Pentcheva-Hoang T, Simpson TR, Montalvo-Ortiz W, Allison JP. Cytotoxic T lymphocyte antigen-4 blockade enhances antitumor immunity by stimulating melanoma-specific T-cell motility. Cancer Immunol Res. 2014;2:970–80.
77. Fong L, Small EJ. Anti-cytotoxic T-lymphocyte antigen-4 antibody: the first in an emerging class of immunomodulatory antibodies for cancer treatment. J Clin Oncol. 2008;26(32): 5275–83.
78. Callahan MK, Wolchok JD, Allison JP. Anti-CTLA-4 antibody therapy: immune monitoring during clinical development of a novel immunotherapy. Semin Oncol. 2010;37(5):473–84.
79. Lipson EJ, Drake CG. Ipilimumab: an anti-CTLA-4 antibody for metastatic melanoma. Clin Cancer Res. 2011;17:6958–62.
80. Ribas A, Kefford R, Marshall MA, Punt CJ, Haanen JB, Marmol M, Garbe C, Gogas H, Schachter J, Linette G, Lorigan P, Kendra KL, Maio M, Trefzer U, Smylie M, McArthur GA, Dreno B, Nathan PD, Mackiewicz J, Kirkwood JM, Gomez-Navarro J, Huang B, Pavlov D, Hauschild A. Phase III randomized clinical trial comparing tremelimumab with standard-of-care chemotherapy in patients with advanced melanoma. J Clin Oncol. 2013;31(5):616–22.
81. Brown RD, Pope B, Yuen E, Gibson J, Joshua DE. The expression of T cell related costimulatory molecules in multiple myeloma. Leuk Lymphoma. 1998;31(3–4):379–84.
82. Frydecka I, Kosmaczewska A, Bocko D, Ciszak L, Wolowiec D, Kuliczkowski K, Kochanowska I. Alterations of the expression of T-cell-related costimulatory CD28 and downregulatory CD152 (CTLA-4) molecules in patients with B-cell chronic lymphocytic leukaemia. Br J Cancer. 2004;90(10):2042–8.
83. Costello RT, Mallet F, Sainty D, Maraninchi D, Gastaut JA, Olive D. Regulation of CD80/B7-1 and CD86/B7-2 molecule expression in human primary acute myeloid leukemia and their role in allogenic immune recognition. Eur J Immunol. 1998;28(1):90–103.
84. Blazar BR, Taylor PA, Panoskaltsis-Mortari A, Sharpe AH, Vallera DA. Opposing roles of CD28:B7 and CTLA-4:B7 pathways in regulating in vivo alloresponses in murine recipients of MHC disparate T cells. J Immunol. 1999;162(11):6368–77.
85. Bashey A, Medina B, Corringham S, Pasek M, Carrier E, Vrooman L, Lowy I, Solomon SR, Morris LE, Holland HK, Mason JR, Alyea EP, Soiffer RJ, Ball ED. CTLA4 blockade with ipilimumab to treat relapse of malignancy after allogeneic hematopoietic cell transplantation. Blood. 2009;113(7):1581–8.
86. Duraiswamy J, Kaluza KM, Freeman GJ, Coukos G. Dual blockade of PD-1 and CTLA-4 combined with tumor vaccine effectively restores T-cell rejection function in tumors. Cancer Res. 2013;73(12):3591–603.
87. Robert L, Tsoi J, Wang X, Emerson R, Homet B, Chodon T, Mok S, Huang RR, Cochran AJ, Comin-Anduix B, Koya RC, Graeber TG, Robins H, Ribas A. CTLA4 blockade broadens the peripheral T-cell receptor repertoire. Clin Cancer Res. 2014;20(9):2424–32.

88. Robert L, Harview C, Emerson R, Wang X, Mok S, Homet B, Comin-Anduix B, Koya RC, Robins H, Tumeh PC, Ribas A. Distinct immunological mechanisms of CTLA-4 and PD-1 blockade revealed by analyzing TCR usage in blood lymphocytes. Oncoimmunology. 2014;3:e29244.
89. Wolchok JD, Kluger H, Callahan MK, Postow MA, Rizvi NA, Lesokhin AM, Segal NH, Ariyan CE, Gordon RA, Reed K, Burke MM, Caldwell A, Kronenberg SA, Agunwamba BU, Zhang X, Lowy I, Inzunza HD, Feely W, Horak CE, Hong Q, Korman AJ, Wigginton JM, Gupta A, Sznol M. Nivolumab plus ipilimumab in advanced melanoma. N Engl J Med. 2013;369(2):122–33.
90. Watanabe N, Gavrieli M, Sedy JR, Yang J, Fallarino F, Loftin SK, Hurchla MA, Zimmerman N, Sim J, Zang X, Murphy TL, Russell JH, Allison JP, Murphy KM. BTLA is a lymphocyte inhibitory receptor with similarities to CTLA-4 and PD-1. Nat Immunol. 2003;4(7):670–9.
91. Hobo W, Norde WJ, Schaap N, Fredrix H, Maas F, Schellens K, Falkenburg JH, Korman AJ, Olive D, van der Voort R, Dolstra H. B and T lymphocyte attenuator mediates inhibition of tumor-reactive CD8+ T cells in patients after allogeneic stem cell transplantation. J Immunol. 2012;189(1):39–49.
92. Murphy TL, Murphy KM. Slow down and survive: enigmatic immunoregulation by BTLA and HVEM. Annu Rev Immunol. 2010;28:389–411.
93. Sedy JR, Gavrieli M, Potter KG, Hurchla MA, Lindsley RC, Hildner K, Scheu S, Pfeffer K, Ware CF, Murphy TL, Murphy KM. B and T lymphocyte attenuator regulates T cell activation through interaction with herpesvirus entry mediator. Nat Immunol. 2005;6(1):90–8.
94. Del Rio ML, Lucas CL, Buhler L, Rayat G, Rodriguez-Barbosa JI. HVEM/LIGHT/BTLA/CD160 cosignaling pathways as targets for immune regulation. J Leukoc Biol. 2010; 87(2):223–35.
95. Cai G, Anumanthan A, Brown JA, Greenfield EA, Zhu B, Freeman GJ. CD160 inhibits activation of human CD4+ T cells through interaction with herpesvirus entry mediator. Nat Immunol. 2008;9(2):176–85.
96. Cheung TC, Oborne LM, Steinberg MW, Macauley MG, Fukuyama S, Sanjo H, D'Souza C, Norris PS, Pfeffer K, Murphy KM, Kronenberg M, Spear PG, Ware CF. T cell intrinsic heterodimeric complexes between HVEM and BTLA determine receptivity to the surrounding microenvironment. J Immunol. 2009;183(11):7286–96.
97. Derre L, Rivals JP, Jandus C, Pastor S, Rimoldi D, Romero P, Michielin O, Olive D, Speiser DE. BTLA mediates inhibition of human tumor-specific CD8+ T cells that can be partially reversed by vaccination. J Clin Invest. 2010;120(1):157–67.
98. Serriari NE, Gondois-Rey F, Guillaume Y, Remmerswaal EB, Pastor S, Messal N, Truneh A, Hirsch I, van Lier RA, Olive D. B and T lymphocyte attenuator is highly expressed on CMV-specific T cells during infection and regulates their function. J Immunol. 2010;185(6): 3140–8.
99. Fourcade J, Sun Z, Pagliano O, Guillaume P, Luescher IF, Sander C, Kirkwood JM, Olive D, Kuchroo V, Zarour HM. CD8(+) T cells specific for tumor antigens can be rendered dysfunctional by the tumor microenvironment through upregulation of the inhibitory receptors BTLA and PD-1. Cancer Res. 2012;72(4):887–96.
100. Lasaro MO, Sazanovich M, Giles-Davis W, Mrass P, Bunte RM, Sewell DA, Hussain SF, Fu YX, Weninger W, Paterson Y, Ertl HC. Active immunotherapy combined with blockade of a coinhibitory pathway achieves regression of large tumor masses in cancer-prone mice. Mol Ther. 2011;19(9):1727–36.
101. Sakuishi K, Jayaraman P, Behar SM, Anderson AC, Kuchroo VK. Emerging Tim-3 functions in antimicrobial and tumor immunity. Trends Immunol. 2011;32(8):345–9.
102. Jones RB, Ndhlovu LC, Barbour JD, Sheth PM, Jha AR, Long BR, Wong JC, Satkunarajah M, Schweneker M, Chapman JM, Gyenes G, Vali B, Hyrcza MD, Yue FY, Kovacs C, Sassi A, Loutfy M, Halpenny R, Persad D, Spotts G, Hecht FM, Chun TW, McCune JM, Kaul R, Rini JM, Nixon DF, Ostrowski MA. Tim-3 expression defines a novel population of dysfunctional T cells with highly elevated frequencies in progressive HIV-1 infection. J Exp Med. 2008;205(12):2763–79.

103. Fourcade J, Sun Z, Benallaoua M, Guillaume P, Luescher IF, Sander C, Kirkwood JM, Kuchroo V, Zarour HM. Upregulation of Tim-3 and PD-1 expression is associated with tumor antigen-specific CD8+ T cell dysfunction in melanoma patients. J Exp Med. 2010; 207(10):2175–86.
104. Lee MJ, Woo MY, Heo YM, Kim JS, Kwon MH, Kim K, Park S. The inhibition of the T-cell immunoglobulin and mucin domain 3 (Tim3) pathway enhances the efficacy of tumor vaccine. Biochem Biophys Res Commun. 2010;402(1):88–93.
105. Flies DB, Wang S, Xu H, Chen L. Cutting edge: a monoclonal antibody specific for the programmed death-1 homolog prevents graft-versus-host disease in mouse models. J Immunol. 2011;187(4):1537–41.
106. Zhou Q, Munger ME, Veenstra RG, Weigel BJ, Hirashima M, Munn DH, Murphy WJ, Azuma M, Anderson AC, Kuchroo VK, Blazar BR. Coexpression of Tim-3 and PD-1 identifies a CD8+ T-cell exhaustion phenotype in mice with disseminated acute myelogenous leukemia. Blood. 2011;117(17):4501–10.
107. Fourcade J, Sun Z, Pagliano O, Chauvin JM, Sander C, Janjic B, Tarhini AA, Tawbi HA, Kirkwood JM, Moschos S, Wang H, Guillaume P, Luescher IF, Krieg A, Anderson AC, Kuchroo VK, Zarour HM. PD-1 and Tim-3 regulate the expansion of tumor antigen-specific CD8(+) T cells induced by melanoma vaccines. Cancer Res. 2014;74(4):1045–55.
108. Guo Z, Cheng D, Xia Z, Luan M, Wu L, Wang G, Zhang S. Combined TIM-3 blockade and CD137 activation affords the long-term protection in a murine model of ovarian cancer. J Transl Med. 2013;11:215.
109. Nagahara K, Arikawa T, Oomizu S, Kontani K, Nobumoto A, Tateno H, Watanabe K, Niki T, Katoh S, Miyake M, Nagahata S, Hirabayashi J, Kuchroo VK, Yamauchi A, Hirashima M. Galectin-9 increases Tim-3+ dendritic cells and CD8+ T cells and enhances antitumor immunity via galectin-9-Tim-3 interactions. J Immunol. 2008;181(11):7660–9.
110. Ferris RL, Lu B, Kane LP. Too much of a good thing? Tim-3 and TCR signaling in T cell exhaustion. J Immunol. 2014;193(4):1525–30.
111. Baixeras E, Huard B, Miossec C, Jitsukawa S, Martin M, Hercend T, Auffray C, Triebel F, Piatier-Tonneau D. Characterization of the lymphocyte activation gene 3-encoded protein. A new ligand for human leukocyte antigen class II antigens. J Exp Med. 1992;176(2):327–37.
112. Triebel F, Jitsukawa S, Baixeras E, Roman-Roman S, Genevee C, Viegas-Pequignot E, Hercend T. LAG-3, a novel lymphocyte activation gene closely related to CD4. J Exp Med. 1990;171(5):1393–405.
113. Grosso JF, Goldberg MV, Getnet D, Bruno TC, Yen HR, Pyle KJ, Hipkiss E, Vignali DA, Pardoll DM, Drake CG. Functionally distinct LAG-3 and PD-1 subsets on activated and chronically stimulated CD8 T cells. J Immunol. 2009;182(11):6659–69.
114. Okazaki T, Okazaki IM, Wang J, Sugiura D, Nakaki F, Yoshida T, Kato Y, Fagarasan S, Muramatsu M, Eto T, Hioki K, Honjo T. PD-1 and LAG-3 inhibitory co-receptors act synergistically to prevent autoimmunity in mice. J Exp Med. 2011;208(2):395–407.
115. Woo SR, Turnis ME, Goldberg MV, Bankoti J, Selby M, Nirschl CJ, Bettini ML, Gravano DM, Vogel P, Liu CL, Tangsombatvisit S, Grosso JF, Netto G, Smeltzer MP, Chaux A, Utz PJ, Workman CJ, Pardoll DM, Korman AJ, Drake CG, Vignali DA. Immune inhibitory molecules LAG-3 and PD-1 synergistically regulate T-cell function to promote tumoral immune escape. Cancer Res. 2012;72(4):917–27.
116. Berrien-Elliott MM, Jackson SR, Meyer JM, Rouskey CJ, Nguyen TL, Yagita H, Greenberg PD, DiPaolo RJ, Teague RM. Durable adoptive immunotherapy for leukemia produced by manipulation of multiple regulatory pathways of CD8+ T-cell tolerance. Cancer Res. 2013;73(2):605–16.
117. Wang-Gillam A, Plambeck-Suess S, Goedegebuure P, Simon PO, Mitchem JB, Hornick JR, Sorscher S, Picus J, Suresh R, Lockhart AC, Tan B, Hawkins WG. A phase I study of IMP321 and gemcitabine as the front-line therapy in patients with advanced pancreatic adenocarcinoma. Invest New Drugs. 2013;31(3):707–13.

118. Wang L, Rubinstein R, Lines JL, Wasiuk A, Ahonen C, Guo Y, Lu LF, Gondek D, Wang Y, Fava RA, Fiser A, Almo S, Noelle RJ. VISTA, a novel mouse Ig superfamily ligand that negatively regulates T cell responses. J Exp Med. 2011;208(3):577–92.
119. Lines JL, Pantazi E, Mak J, Sempere LF, Wang L, O'Connell S, Ceeraz S, Suriawinata AA, Yan S, Ernstoff MS, Noelle R. VISTA is an immune checkpoint molecule for human T cells. Cancer Res. 2014;74(7):1924–32.
120. Le Mercier I, Chen W, Lines JL, Day M, Li J, Sergent P, Noelle RJ, Wang L. VISTA regulates the development of protective antitumor immunity. Cancer Res. 2014;74(7):1933–44.
121. Voehringer D, Koschella M, Pircher H. Lack of proliferative capacity of human effector and memory T cells expressing killer cell lectinlike receptor G1 (KLRG1). Blood. 2002; 100(10):3698–702.
122. Ito M, Maruyama T, Saito N, Koganei S, Yamamoto K, Matsumoto N. Killer cell lectin-like receptor G1 binds three members of the classical cadherin family to inhibit NK cell cytotoxicity. J Exp Med. 2006;203(2):289–95.
123. Schwartzkopff S, Grundemann C, Schweier O, Rosshart S, Karjalainen KE, Becker KF, Pircher H. Tumor-associated E-cadherin mutations affect binding to the killer cell lectin-like receptor G1 in humans. J Immunol. 2007;179(2):1022–9.
124. Henson SM, Franzese O, Macaulay R, Libri V, Azevedo RI, Kiani-Alikhan S, Plunkett FJ, Masters JE, Jackson S, Griffiths SJ, Pircher HP, Soares MV, Akbar AN. KLRG1 signaling induces defective Akt (ser473) phosphorylation and proliferative dysfunction of highly differentiated CD8+ T cells. Blood. 2009;113(26):6619–28.
125. Garni-Wagner BA, Purohit A, Mathew PA, Bennett M, Kumar V. A novel function-associated molecule related to non-MHC-restricted cytotoxicity mediated by activated natural killer cells and T cells. J Immunol. 1993;151(1):60–70.
126. Boles KS, Stepp SE, Bennett M, Kumar V, Mathew PA. 2B4 (CD244) and CS1: novel members of the CD2 subset of the immunoglobulin superfamily molecules expressed on natural killer cells and other leukocytes. Immunol Rev. 2001;181:234–49.
127. Brown MH, Boles K, van der Merwe PA, Kumar V, Mathew PA, Barclay AN. 2B4, the natural killer and T cell immunoglobulin superfamily surface protein, is a ligand for CD48. J Exp Med. 1998;188(11):2083–90.
128. Laouar A, Manocha M, Wan M, Yagita H, van Lier RA, Manjunath N. Cutting edge: distinct NK receptor profiles are imprinted on CD8 T cells in the mucosa and periphery during the same antigen challenge: role of tissue-specific factors. J Immunol. 2007;178(2):652–6.
129. Liu D, Krummey SM, Badell IR, Wagener M, Schneeweis LA, Stetsko DK, Suchard SJ, Nadler SG, Ford ML. 2B4 (CD244) induced by selective CD28 blockade functionally regulates allograft-specific CD8+ T cell responses. J Exp Med. 2014;211(2):297–311.
130. Rijkers ES, de Ruiter T, Baridi A, Veninga H, Hoek RM, Meyaard L. The inhibitory CD200R is differentially expressed on human and mouse T and B lymphocytes. Mol Immunol. 2008;45(4):1126–35.
131. Stumpfova M, Ratner D, Desciak EB, Eliezri YD, Owens DM. The immunosuppressive surface ligand CD200 augments the metastatic capacity of squamous cell carcinoma. Cancer Res. 2010;70(7):2962–72.
132. Gorczynski RM, Chen Z, Hu J, Kai Y, Lei J. Evidence of a role for CD200 in regulation of immune rejection of leukaemic tumour cells in C57BL/6 mice. Clin Exp Immunol. 2001;126(2):220–9.
133. Wong KK, Khatri I, Shaha S, Spaner DE, Gorczynski RM. The role of CD200 in immunity to B cell lymphoma. J Leukoc Biol. 2010;88(2):361–72.
134. Kretz-Rommel A, Qin F, Dakappagari N, Ravey EP, McWhirter J, Oltean D, Frederickson S, Maruyama T, Wild MA, Nolan MJ, Wu D, Springhorn J, Bowdish KS. CD200 expression on tumor cells suppresses antitumor immunity: new approaches to cancer immunotherapy. J Immunol. 2007;178(9):5595–605.
135. Coles SJ, Wang EC, Man S, Hills RK, Burnett AK, Tonks A, Darley RL. CD200 expression suppresses natural killer cell function and directly inhibits patient anti-tumor response in acute myeloid leukemia. Leukemia. 2011;25(5):792–9.

136. Coles SJ, Hills RK, Wang EC, Burnett AK, Man S, Darley RL, Tonks A. Expression of CD200 on AML blasts directly suppresses memory T-cell function. Leukemia. 2012;26(9): 2148–51.
137. Coles SJ, Hills RK, Wang EC, Burnett AK, Man S, Darley RL, Tonks A. Increased CD200 expression in acute myeloid leukemia is linked with an increased frequency of FoxP3+ regulatory T cells. Leukemia. 2012;26(9):2146–8.
138. Mahadevan DLM, Whelden M, Faas SJ, Ulery TL, Kukreja A, Li L, Bedrosian CL, Heffner LT. First-in-human phase I dose escalation study of a humanized anti-CD200 antibody (Samalizumab) in patients with advanced stage B cell chronic lymphocytic leukemia (B-CLL) or multiple myeloma (MM). In: 2nd ASH Annu Meet Exposition 2012, Orlando, FL, 2012.
139. Morales-Kastresana A, Labiano S, Quetglas JI, Melero I. Better performance of CARs deprived of the PD-1 brake. Clin Cancer Res. 2013;19(20):5546–8.
140. John LB, Kershaw MH, Darcy PK. Blockade of PD-1 immunosuppression boosts CAR T-cell therapy. Oncoimmunology. 2013;2(10):e26286.
141. John LB, Devaud C, Duong CP, Yong CS, Beavis PA, Haynes NM, Chow MT, Smyth MJ, Kershaw MH, Darcy PK. Anti-PD-1 antibody therapy potently enhances the eradication of established tumors by gene-modified T cells. Clin Cancer Res. 2013;19(20):5636–46.
142. Hobo W, Maas F, Adisty N, de Witte T, Schaap N, van der Voort R, Dolstra H. siRNA silencing of PD-L1 and PD-L2 on dendritic cells augments expansion and function of minor histocompatibility antigen-specific CD8+ T cells. Blood. 2010;116(22):4501–11.
143. Blackburn SD, Shin H, Haining WN, Zou T, Workman CJ, Polley A, Betts MR, Freeman GJ, Vignali DA, Wherry EJ. Coregulation of CD8+ T cell exhaustion by multiple inhibitory receptors during chronic viral infection. Nat Immunol. 2009;10(1):29–37.
144. Speiser DE, Utzschneider DT, Oberle SG, Munz C, Romero P, Zehn D. T cell differentiation in chronic infection and cancer: functional adaptation or exhaustion? Nat Rev Immunol. 2014;14:768–74.
145. Duraiswamy J, Ibegbu CC, Masopust D, Miller JD, Araki K, Doho GH, Tata P, Gupta S, Zilliox MJ, Nakaya HI, Pulendran B, Haining WN, Freeman GJ, Ahmed R. Phenotype, function, and gene expression profiles of programmed death-1(hi) CD8 T cells in healthy human adults. J Immunol. 2011;186(7):4200–12.
146. Legat A, Speiser DE, Pircher H, Zehn D, Fuertes Marraco SA. Inhibitory receptor expression depends more dominantly on differentiation and activation than "exhaustion" of human CD8 T Cells. Front Immunol. 2013;4:455.
147. Haymaker C, Wu R, Bernatchez C, Radvanyi L. PD-1 and BTLA and CD8(+) T-cell "exhaustion" in cancer: "exercising" an alternative viewpoint. Oncoimmunology. 2012;1(5):735–8.
148. Gros A, Robbins PF, Yao X, Li YF, Turcotte S, Tran E, Wunderlich JR, Mixon A, Farid S, Dudley ME, Hanada K, Almeida JR, Darko S, Douek DC, Yang JC, Rosenberg SA. PD-1 identifies the patient-specific CD8(+) tumor-reactive repertoire infiltrating human tumors. J Clin Invest. 2014;124(5):2246–59.

Chapter 3
Role of the Non-classical HLA Class I Antigens for Immune Escape

Barbara Seliger and Simon Jasinski-Bergner

Abstract Tumors have developed different mechanisms to evade immune surveillance including alterations of classical and non-classical HLA class I antigens. The non-classical HLA-G antigen is often overexpressed in solid and hematopoietic tumors, thereby, creating a tolerogenic phenotype leading to an escape from T and NK cell-mediated immune responses by binding to the inhibitory receptors ILT2, ILT4 and KIR2DL4. Consequently, HLA-G$^+$ tumors are associated with disease progression and in some cases with a poor clinical outcome of patients. Furthermore, high levels of soluble HLA-G have often been detected in serum, plasma and malignant ascites of tumor patients, which also correlated with a poor patients' prognosis. Under physiologic conditions HLA-G expression is tightly controlled, limited to mainly immune privileged tissues/cells and could be regulated at the transcriptional, epigenetic as well as post-transcriptional levels. Recently, miRs regulating HLA-G expression have been identified, which could be used as tools for therapeutic intervention. Translational inhibition of HLA-G could reduce the immune escape of tumors, and increase the sensitivity to T cell- and/or NK cell-mediated cytotoxicity. However, the function of HLA-G expression is more complex, since next to trogocytosis a HLA-G-mediated inhibition of malignant hematopoietic cell proliferation was found mediated by an interaction of HLA-G with the ILT2 receptor involved in the negative signaling of B cell proliferation. Furthermore, HLA-G-regulating miRs also possess tumor suppressive activities by modulating apoptosis sensitivity and drug resistance. HLA-G exhibits a dual tumor type-dependent role by altering not only the immune surveillance, but rather also shaping the tumorigenic properties of tumor cells.

Keywords HLA-G • Classical HLA class I • Renal cell carcinoma • Tumor progression • Immune escape

---

No conflict statement: "No potential conflicts of interest were disclosed."

B. Seliger (✉) • S. Jasinski-Bergner
Institute of Medical Immunology, Martin Luther University Halle-Wittenberg,
Magdeburger Str. 2, 06112 Halle, Saale, Germany
e-mail: Barbara.Seliger@uk-halle.de

B. Bonavida, S. Chouaib (eds.), *Resistance of Cancer Cells to CTL-Mediated Immunotherapy*, Resistance to Targeted Anti-Cancer Therapeutics 7,
DOI 10.1007/978-3-319-17807-3_3

Abbreviations

β_2-m	β_2-Microglobulin
APC	Antigen presenting cells
APM	Antigen processing machinery
bp	Base pair
CLL	Chronic lymphatic leukemia
CTL	Cytotoxic T lymphocyte
DAC	Desoxyazacytidine
DC	Dendritic cells
GSN	Gelsolin
HLA	Human leukocyte antigen
IDO	Indolamine 2, 3-deoxygenase
IFN	Interferon
ILT	Immunoglobulin-like transcript
JAK	Janus kinase
LIF	Leukemia inhibitory factor
MDSC	Myeloid-derived suppressor cells
miR	MicroRNA
MMP	Matrix metalloproteinases
mTOR	Mammalian target of rapamycin
NK	Natural killer
PKC	Protein kinase C
RCC	Renal cell carcinoma
SNP	Single nucleotide polymorphism
TAM	Tumor associated macrophages
TAP	Transporter associated with antigen processing
TGF	Transforming growth factor
Treg	Regulatory T cell
TSA	Trichostatin A
UTR	Untranslated region

3.1 Introduction

Tumors could evade immune surveillance by multiple mechanisms including loss or downregulation of HLA class I antigens due to a reduced or impaired expression of various components of the antigen processing machinery (APM), loss of co-stimulatory molecules, expression of co-inhibitory molecules, such as B7-H1 and B7-H4 and of the non-classical antigens HLA-G and HLA-E as well as secretion of immune suppressive factors, like adenosine, indolamine 2,3-deoxygenase (IDO), IL-10 and transforming growth factor (TGF)-β. These different processes could result in impaired responses of immune effector cells and/or the induction of various immune suppressive cell subpopulations.

Since recent reports suggest an increased complexity regarding the activity of HLA-G in human tumors, this article will focus on the expression, function, regulation as well as on the clinical significance, but also on the non-immunologic activity of HLA-G both in solid tumors as well as in hematologic malignancies [1]. The diverse activities of HLA-G might be driven by the interaction of HLA-G with its receptors present on various immune cell types including NK, T, B and dendritic cells (DC) and phagocytes [2], thereby creating a negative signal that counteracts immune activation. This enables an evasion of HLA-G^+ tumor cells from the host immune surveillance. An increased knowledge of the molecular mechanisms of heterogeneous expression and regulation of HLA-G might help to develop therapeutic strategies to inhibit HLA-G expression [3, 4].

3.1.1 Features of HLA-G

In contrast to classical HLA class I molecules, HLA-G has a limited polymorphic diversity and is alternatively spliced leading to seven distinct protein isoforms encoding for four membrane-bound (HLA-G1, -G2, -G3, -G4) and three soluble HLA-G (sHLA-G, HLA-G5, -G6, -G7) molecules, respectively. The membrane-bound HLA-G1 variant represents a full length version of the molecule, while HLA-G2, HLA-G3 as well as HLA-G4 lack one or two exons. The HLA-G5-6 isoforms contain part of intron 4, while HLA-G7 contains a part of intron 2 harboring a stop codon, which leads to the loss of the membrane domain. In addition to sHLA-G5, -G6 and -G7, HLA-G1 also exists as a soluble molecule due to proteolytic cleavage by a matrix metalloprotease (MMP), in particular of MMP2, but not of MMP9 [5]. Like classical HLA-class I antigens, the non-classical HLA-G can form heterodimers with β_2-microglobulin (β_2-m), but also as homodimers- and tetramers, which are able to bind to receptors on T and NK cells, but dimers and tetramers exert a higher affinity. Both HLA-G1 and -G5 contain a peptide-binding region and could bind peptides originated from proteolysis of intracellular proteins. Thus, HLA-G is able to present antigenic peptides to T cells, which is important for monitoring an anti-tumoral defense.

Basal HLA-G expression is mainly restricted to immune-privileged organs, to cytotrophoblasts, pancreas, monocytes, erythroid and endothelial progenitors suggesting a tight regulation of HLA-G expression under physiologic conditions [6–9]. In addition, HLA-G expression could be found in different immune cell populations, like T cells, professional antigen presenting cells (APC) as well as mesenchymal stem cells. In this context it is noteworthy that the presence and absence of HLA-G in the physiologic context is independent of HLA class I antigen expression.

3.1.2 HLA-G and Immune Responses

HLA-G can bind to the leukocyte immunoglobulin-like receptors ILT-2 and ILT-4 expressed on B cells, T cells, NK cells, dendritic cells (DC), neutrophils and on KIR2DL4 on NK and T cells and on CD160 expressed on endothelial cells

(PMID: 16809620). This leads to a protection of cells from NK cell, T cell and neutrophil-mediated destruction [10] as well as impaired function of DC by binding ILT-2 and ILT-4 [11, 12]. HLA-G dimers consisting of HLA-G associated with β_2-m have been demonstrated to mainly exert an immune inhibitory function [13]. This tolerogenic activity is not only mediated by the interaction with its inhibitory receptor(s), but also by a synergy with other molecules e.g. IL-10 and IDO [14]. Furthermore, HLA-G-modified DC induces a tolerogenic potential by a selective increase in the expression of B7-1/CD80 [15]. In addition, β_2-m-free HLA-G could activate NK cells by increasing cytotoxicity and pro-inflammatory cytokine production [16]. HLA-G could also induce the frequency of myeloid-derived suppressor cells (MDSC) and shift cytokine production to a Th2 phenotype. In contrast, HLA-G monomers are mainly involved in non-immunologic functions.

3.1.3 Regulation of HLA-G Expression

Since physiologic HLA-G expression is very restricted in adults, HLA-G expression has to be tightly controlled. However, an aberrant expression is often found in pathophysiologic situations, such as tumors, viral infections, autoimmune diseases, inflammation as well as transplantations. HLA-G expression has been shown to be controlled at the epigenetic, transcriptional, posttranscriptional and posttranslational levels [17].

Epigenetic modifications mediated by DNA hypermethylation of the HLA-G promoter or hypoacetylation of the histones H3 and H4 are often associated with a lack of HLA-G expression. Repression or downregulation of HLA-G expression could be reverted by treatment with demethylating agents, like 5′aza-2′-deoxycytidine (DAC) or by inhibitors of histone deacetylases, e.g. trichostatin A (TSA), thereby directly inducing or enhancing HLA-G surface expression [18–20].

The analysis of the HLA-G promoter also suggested a transcriptional control, which is mediated by various unique regulatory elements including the cAMP response elements CRE to which the CREB1 transcription factor could bind [21], binding sites for the interferon regulatory factor (IRF), the heat shock factor (HSF-1) and the progesterone receptor [22, 23]. In addition, different negative regulatory sequences were identified, such as the Ras responsive element known to bind the Ras responsive element binding protein I (RREB-I), the GLI-3 factor and a LINE element [24, 25].

Environmental factors present in tumors as well as in placenta were able to modulate HLA-G expression. These include IL-10, IFN-γ, IFN-β, the leukemia inhibitory factor (LIF) [26], hormones like dexamethasone, hydrocortisone as well as progesterone, galectin-1, IDO and various stress conditions, like heat shock and hypoxia [27, 28]. Most of these molecules affect HLA-G gene expression transcriptionally and/or posttranscriptionally and were able to modulate HLA-G expression. Next to the transcriptional regulation, HLA-G expression is also often post-transcriptionally controlled, which could be mediated by mechanisms targeting the

3′ untranslated region (3′-UTR) that affect the mRNA stability and degradation of HLA-G. Recently, a number of HLA-G specific microRNAs (miRs) have been identified [29]. These include members of the miR-148 family, like miR-148a, miR-148b and miR-152, as well as miR-133a [30–32]. Recent data demonstrate that the G-protein coupled estrogen receptor reduced miR-148a expression and promotes HLA-G in breast cancer [33]. HLA-G can also undergo post-translational modifications. In particular, in trophoblasts HLA-G is highly glycosylated, while in an inflammatory microenvironment HLA-G could be also nitrated [34, 35]. Furthermore, HLA-G can form high molecular weight complexes due to ubiquination, which might have pathophysiologic relevance [36]. Concerning structural alterations/single nucleotide polymorphisms (SNPs) SNPs have been described in the 5′- and 3′-UTR of the HLA-G gene, which can modulate HLA-G expression under physiologic and pathophysiologic conditions.

So far, 33 SNPs have been identified in the 5′-UTR, which define at least eleven haplotypes [37, 38]. They have been shown to potentially modify methylated CpG oligonucleotides, thereby, influencing the transcriptionally activity of HLA-G. However, the impact of the HLA-G promoter polymorphisms in association with HLA-G expression has not yet been determined in detail. In contrast, SNPs identified in the 3′-UTR, in particular a 14 base pair (bp) insertion/deletion and 7 SNPs, which define at least 7 haplotypes, have been analyzed [39–41]. The presence and/or absence of the 14 bp SNP was directly associated with HLA-G expression under normal as well as pathophysiologic conditions [42]. Furthermore, HLA-G transcripts representing the 14 bp sequence are associated with reduced HLA-G mRNA expression and lower sHLA-G levels. HLA-G transcripts generated by the 14 bp alleles can be further processed by removing a 92 bp fragment containing the 14 bp sequence. These transcripts are more stable due to the AU-rich element within the 14 bp fragment. In addition, a 4 bp SNP was identified upstream of the AU-rich element, which could also influence HLA-G mRNA stability, since it affects the binding of the miR-148 family members. Thus, microenvironmental factors as well as the HLA-G polymorphisms are important regulators of HLA-G expression under physiologic and pathophysiologic conditions.

3.1.4 Pathophysiologic Expression of HLA-G in Human Tumors

HLA-G expression is upregulated in different pathophysiologic conditions including transplantation, inflammatory diseases and viral infections [43]. In addition, HLA-G could be expressed in both solid and hematopoietic tumor cells and has been extensively described [44–47]. HLA-G can be found in all types of cancer independent of their ectodermic, mesodermic or endodermic origin. However, the frequency of HLA-G positivity strongly varied from 20 to 90 % (Table 3.1). In addition, increased concentrations of sHLA-G isoforms have been detected in plasma and in malignant ascites of tumor patients. Until now, HLA-G expression has been

Table 3.1 Distinct frequency of HLA-G expression in different tumor types

Malignancy	Number and type of investigated samples	Used methods	Frequency in (%)	Reference(s)
Acute myeloid leukemia	99 sera	FC/ELISA	50.5 (FC) and 83 (ELISA)	[73, 81]
Acute lymphoblastic leukemia	25 sera	RT-PCR	100 (RT-PCR)	[68]
B-cell chronic lymphocytic leukemia	77 sera	FC	27.2 (FC) 36.7 (FC)	[53, 87]
Bladder transitional cell carcinoma	75 tumor lesions	IHC	68 (IHC)	[72]
Breast cancer	396 tumor lesions, 89 sera, 17 malignant ascites	IHC/ELISA/FC	52.7 (IHC), 59.6 (FC), 94.1 (ELISA)	[74, 76, 84, 86]
Breast ductal carcinoma	45 tumor lesions	IHC	62.2 (IHC)	[83]
Cervical cancer	119 tumor lesions, 152 sera	IHC/ELISA	45.4 (IHC), 90.1 (ELISA)	[89]
Colorectal cancer	181 sera	ELISA	76.8 (ELISA)	[70, 90]
Esophageal squamous cell carcinoma	60 tumor lesions, 118 sera	RT-PCR/ELISA	70 (RT-PCR), upregulated in sera	[70, 89]
Kazkh esophageal carcinoma	60 tumor lesions	IHC	75 (IHC)	[75, 88]
Gastric cancer	52 tumor lesions, 28 sera	IHC, ELISA	30.8 (IHC), 85.7 (ELISA)	[70, 82]
Glioblastoma	39 tumor lesions	IHC	64.1 (IHC)	[79]
Hepatocellular carcinoma	173 tumor lesions, 5 cell lines	IHC/WB	57.2 (IHC), 80 (WB)	[79]
Hodgkin's lymphoma	175 tumor lesions	IHC	54.3 (IHC)	[71]
Non-small lung cancer	43 sera	ELISA	51.2 (ELISA)	[70]
Lung cancer	136 sera	ELISA	40.4 (ELISA)	[85]
Ovarian serous carcinoma	74 tumor lesions, 24 malignant ascites	IHC/ELISA	60.8 (IHC), 100 (ELISA)	[86]
Ovarian carcinomas	137 tumor lesions	IHC	47.9 (IHC)	[52]
Renal cell carcinoma	146 tumor lesions, 16 sera	IHC/ELISA	48.6 (IHC), 100 (ELISA)	[69, 80]
Rectal cancer	484 tumor lesions	IHC	94 (IHC)	[51]
Testicular germ cell tumors	34 tumor lesions	IHC	20.6 (IHC)	[78]
Trophoblastic tumors	15 tumor lesions	IHC	93.3 (IHC)	[77]

IHC immunohistochemistry, *WB* western blot, *FC* flow cytometry analyzed in >1,000 tumor patients of distinct origin using antibodies recognizing membrane-bound and/or soluble HLA-G isoforms (Table 3.1). The frequency of HLA-G expression significantly varied between the tumor types analyzed. Furthermore, HLA-G expression was also detected in tumor-infiltrating immune cells as well as in regulatory T cells (Treg). HLA-G expressed or released by tumor associated macrophages (TAM) may interact with inhibitory receptors on NK cells, thereby, regulating the release of pro-angiogenic factors, which lead to the establishment of a tolerogenic microenvironment [48].

3.1.5 Clinical Significance of HLA-G in Solid and Hematopoietic Tumors

Relevance of HLA-G for tumor progression and survival of patients with solid tumors was found, since HLA-G expression has been shown to be associated with malignant transformation. High expression levels of membrane-bound HLA-G in solid tumors correlated with high histological grades, advanced clinical stages and worse patients' outcome. In addition, high levels of soluble HLA-G (sHLA-G) in plasma from patients were also associated with a poor prognosis [45, 46, 49, 50]. These data suggest a role of HLA-G in immune surveillance and progression of disease. Thus, HLA-G might have a clinical value in diagnosis, staging or prognosis of cancer. However, standardizing of HLA-G testing and analysis of large cohorts of solid tumor samples with known clinicopathologic parameters is required to use HLA-G as biomarker. Controversial to these findings HLA-G expression has recently also been shown to be associated with a better clinical outcome in rectal carcinoma and high grade ovarian cancer [51, 52].

In contrast to solid tumors, high levels of membrane-bound HLA-G was found in various B cell malignancies, which could be correlated with a good clinical outcome of multiple myeloma, non-Hodgkin-B lymphoma and chronic lymphoblastic leukemia (CLL) patients [53, 54]. The discrepancy of these results are so far not well understood, but might be explained by (1) distinct technologies and methods used for determination of HLA-G expression, (2) distinct guidance of the study and antibodies used and (3) the patients cohort analyzed, which might have received different treatment regimens e.g. tyrosine kinase inhibitors or chemotherapy and by (4) the presence of other immune modulatory molecules. However, another explanation might the interaction of HLA-G with its receptor expressed on hematopoietic malignant cells, which inhibits the proliferation and induces cell cycle arrest of B cell lymphoma, myeloma as well as B-CLL [55]. This is in line with an altered signal transduction found in malignant B cells upon interaction of HLA-G with the ILT-2 receptors, which was mediated by an increased phosphorylation of protein kinase C (PKC) and a decreased phosphorylation of AKT, mTOR, GSK-3β, c-Raf and FOX-O proteins [55]. Based on these results a dual role of HLA-G could be postulated, which dependent on the tumor type may enhance or inhibit tumor growth.

3.1.6 Modulation of HLA-G in Tumors

It has been shown that HLA-G could be upregulated by DAC and/or by different cytokines e.g. IFN-γ. A multicentric study recently demonstrated an upregulation of HLA-G by DAC and IFN-γ in glioblastoma [56]. Furthermore, both substances could also induce HLA-G expression in renal cell carcinoma [18]. Since tumor patients are treated with DAC and IFN-γ might be present in the microenvironment one might consider an impact of these substances on the HLA-G expression of tumors. Other factors of the tumor microenvironment like hypoxia and pH as well as hormones could alter HLA-G expression [28]. The modulation of HLA-G is dependent on HIF-1 stabilization and thus might control HLA-G expression in hypoxic tumors.

3.1.7 Altered Immune Response of HLA-G$^+$ Tumors

Despite high levels of immune cell infiltration tumors can evade immune surveillance, which based on the immune editing hypothesis consists of the three distinct processes (1) elimination, (2) equilibrium and (3) escape. Interestingly, HLA-G can interfere with each step: HLA-G impairs the elimination by inhibiting T and B cell proliferation, the cytotoxic activity of T and NK cells, antigen presentation of DCs as well as phagocytic activity of neutrophils. In addition, pro-inflammatory cytokines and immune suppressive factors present in the tumor microenvironment, like IFN-γ, IL-10 and IDO, could enhance HLA-G expression [57], thereby, affecting the equilibrium phase. In the evasion phase, tumors have also failed to express various immune modulatory molecules in the presence of enhanced HLA-G levels, thereby, gaining resistance to susceptibility of effector cells. Since tumors often create a hypoxic microenvironment and altered metabolism angiogenesis, invasion and metastasis formation are promoted in addition to induced HLA-G expression, which is associated with the secretion of high levels of IL-10 and IDO not only by tumor cells, but also by tumor-infiltrating leukocytes [27] and an increased frequency of Treg, and myeloid-derived suppressor cells (MDSC) [58, 59]. Recent data also emphasize an impact of the HLA-G conformation on the anti-tumor response, which could be altered by the tumor microenvironment [60]. In addition, sHLA-G plays a role in suppressing the functions of various immune competent cells. It could impair the chemoattraction of different immune cells, which is important for the modulation of immune responses in cancer, but also in other diseases [61]. After these different processes alter antitumor immune responses and lead not only to an expansion of tumor cells, but also to the inhibition of both innate and adaptive immune responses against the tumor. Such data have been recently obtained due to the development of a model using the murine receptor paired immunoglobulin-like receptor (PIR)–B to which human HLA-G binds [62] and which represents a homologue of the human ILT. Both human and murine HLA-G expressing tumor cells form tumors in immune competent mice, while treatment with HLA-G-specific antibodies led to reduced tumor formation. The role of HLA-G was demonstrated not only to negatively interfere with the innate and adaptive immune responses, but also to enhance the frequency of MDSC, Tregs and to induce a Th2 versus a Th1/TH17 phenotype.

3.1.8 Other Roles of HLA-G

Next to the distinct mechanisms and functions of HLA-G in the immunologic context described above, HLA-G plays a role in cell communications. It has been recently shown to act through trogocytosis, which allows the transfer of membrane proteins and fragments from one cell to the other. Interestingly, not only HLA-G, but also ILT-2 functions through trogocytosis [63]. Thus, trogocytosis might explain also the general inhibitory effect of HLA-G. HLA-G might also interact with other so far unknown receptors, thereby, mediating its activities. In addition, HLA-G is involved in cell proliferation and migration. Analysis of transfectants expressing the HLA-G homodimer resulted in the detection of a large set of differentially expressed genes including cytokines, but also pro-inflammatory and pro-angiogenic proteins [64] suggesting a role of HLA-G in angiogenesis and inflammation.

3.1.9 HLA-G as Therapeutic Target

Due to its immune suppressive function, HLA-G represents a suitable therapeutic target for transplantation, viral infection and tumors [65]. Interference with the HLA-G function might boost on one hand the anti-neoplastic potential of cytotoxic effectors, while on the other hand the activity of intrinsic immune suppressive cells. Indeed, synthetic HLA-G proteins could be used in therapy of transplantation [66]. Since downregulation of HLA-G transcripts or protein might affect cancer therapy, nanoparticles targeting HLA-G by RNA interference could be used in vivo [67]. Within the recent identification of HLA-G-specific miRs, the use of antagomiRs as modulators of HLA-G expression in tumors is postulated and should be further tested. Due to the advantage of its surface expression, one postulate is the use of a combination of HLA-G antibody with other cancer drugs to reach the tumor site in order to maximize the therapeutic effects and minimize the adverse side effects. Therefore, it is currently under investigation to control HLA-G expression for therapeutic purposes not only in the context of cancer immune therapy.

3.2 Conclusion

Membrane-bound and soluble HLA-G are important players for mounting immune tolerance in tumor patients and might serve as prognostic or therapeutic markers for malignancies.

Acknowledgements We would like to thank Sylvi Magdeburg for excellent secretarial help. The work was supported by a grant from the German Israeli Foundation (GIF) and the German Research Council GRK1591.

References

1. Rouas-Freiss N, Moreau P, LeMaoult J, Carosella ED. The dual role of HLA-G in cancer. J Immunol Res. 2014;2014:359748.
2. Yang Y, Chu W, Geraghty DE, Hunt JS. Expression of HLA-G in human mononuclear phagocytes and selective induction by IFN-gamma. J Immunol. 1996;156:4224–31.
3. Carosella ED, Favier B, Rouas-Freiss N, Moreau P, Lemaoult J. Beyond the increasing complexity of the immunomodulatory HLA-G molecule. Blood. 2008;111:4862–70.
4. Kochan G, Escors D, Breckpot K, Guerrero-Setas D. Role of non-classical MHC class I molecules in cancer immunosuppression. Oncoimmunology. 2013;2:e26491.
5. Rizzo R, Trentini A, Bortolotti D, Manfrinato MC, Rotola A, Castellazzi M, Melchiorri L, Di Luca D, Dallocchio F, Fainardi E, Bellini T. Matrix metalloproteinase-2 (MMP-2) generates soluble HLA-G1 by cell surface proteolytic shedding. Mol Cell Biochem. 2013;381:243–55.
6. Kovats S, Main EK, Librach C, Stubblebine M, Fisher SJ, DeMars R. A class I antigen, HLA-G, expressed in human trophoblasts. Science. 1990;248:220–3.
7. Le Discorde M, Moreau P, Sabatier P, Legeais JM, Carosella ED. Expression of HLA-G in human cornea, an immune-privileged tissue. Hum Immunol. 2003;64:1039–44.
8. Menier C, Rabreau M, Challier JC, Le Discorde M, Carosella ED, Rouas-Freiss N. Erythroblasts secrete the nonclassical HLA-G molecule from primitive to definitive hematopoiesis. Blood. 2004;104:3153–60.
9. Paul P, Rouas-Freiss N, Moreau P, Cabestre FA, Menier C, Khalil-Daher I, Pangault C, Onno M, Fauchet R, Martinez-Laso J, Morales P, Villena AA, Giacomini P, Natali PG, Frumento G, Ferrara GB, McMaster M, Fisher S, Schust D, Ferrone S, Dausset J, Geraghty D, Carosella ED. HLA-G, -E, -F preworkshop: tools and protocols for analysis of non-classical class I genes transcription and protein expression. Hum Immunol. 2000;61:1177–95.
10. Favier B, Lemaoult J, Lesport E, Carosella ED. ILT2/HLA-G interaction impairs NK-cell functions through the inhibition of the late but not the early events of the NK-cell activating synapse. FASEB J. 2010;24:689–99.
11. Gros F, Cabillic F, Toutirais O, Maux AL, Sebti Y, Amiot L. Soluble HLA-G molecules impair natural killer/dendritic cell crosstalk via inhibition of dendritic cells. Eur J Immunol. 2008;38:742–9.
12. LeMaoult J, Rouas-Freiss N, Carosella ED. Immuno-tolerogenic functions of HLA-G: relevance in transplantation and oncology. Autoimmun Rev. 2005;4:503–9.
13. Gonen-Gross T, Gazit R, Achdout H, Hanna J, Mizrahi S, Markel G, Horejsí V, Mandelboim O. Special organization of the HLA-G protein on the cell surface. Hum Immunol. 2003;64:1011–6.
14. Moreau P, Adrian-Cabestre F, Menier C, Guiard V, Gourand L, Dausset J, Carosella ED, Paul P. IL-10 selectively induces HLA-G expression in human trophoblasts and monocytes. Int Immunol. 1999;11:803–11.
15. Smith M, Bittner 4th JG, White S, Smith D, Horuzsko A. HLA-G-treated tolerogenic dendritic cells induce tolerogenic potential by increasing expression of B7-1 (CD80) molecules. Transplant Proc. 2008;40:1598–603.
16. Zhao L, Purandare B, Zhang J, Hantash BM. Beta2-Microglobulin-free HLA-G activates natural killer cells by increasing cytotoxicity and proinflammatory cytokine production. Hum Immunol. 2013;74:417–24.
17. Moreau P, Flajollet S, Carosella ED. Non-classical transcriptional regulation of HLA-G: an update. J Cell Mol Med. 2009;13:2973–89.

18. Dunker K, Schlaf G, Bukur J, Altermann WW, Handke D, Seliger B. Expression and regulation of non-classical HLA-G in renal cell carcinoma. Tissue Antigens. 2008;72:137–48.
19. Menendez L, Walker LD, Matyunina LV, Totten KA, Benigno BB, McDonald JF. Epigenetic changes within the promoter region of the HLA-G gene in ovarian tumors. Mol Cancer. 2008;7:43.
20. Suárez-Alvarez B, Rodriguez RM, Calvanese V, Blanco-Gelaz MA, Suhr ST, Ortega F, Otero J, Cibelli JB, Moore H, Fraga MF, López-Larrea C. Epigenetic mechanisms regulate MHC and antigen processing molecules in human embryonic and induced pluripotent stem cells. PLoS One. 2010;5:e10192.
21. Gobin SJ, Biesta P, de Steenwinkel JE, Datema G, van den Elsen PJ. HLA-G transactivation by cAMP-response element-binding protein (CREB). An alternative transactivation pathway to the conserved major histocompatibility complex (MHC) class I regulatory routes. J Biol Chem. 2002;277:39525–31.
22. Ibrahim EC, Morange M, Dausset J, Carosella ED, Paul P. Heat shock and arsenite induce expression of the nonclassical class I histocompatibility HLA-G gene in tumor cell lines. Cell Stress Chaperones. 2000;5:207–18.
23. Lefebvre S, Berrih-Aknin S, Adrian F, Moreau P, Poea S, Gourand L, Dausset J, Carosella ED, Paul P. A specific interferon (IFN)-stimulated response element of the distal HLA-G promoter binds IFN-regulatory factor 1 and mediates enhancement of this nonclassical class I gene by IFN-beta. J Biol Chem. 2001;276:6133–9.
24. Flajollet S, Poras I, Carosella ED, Moreau P. RREB-1 is a transcriptional repressor of HLA-G. J Immunol. 2009;183:6948–59.
25. Ikeno M, Suzuki N, Kamiya M, Takahashi Y, Kudoh J, Okazaki T. LINE1 family member is negative regulator of HLA-G expression. Nucleic Acids Res. 2012;40:10742–52.
26. Bamberger AM, Jenatschke S, Schulte HM, Löning T, Bamberger MC. Leukemia inhibitory factor (LIF) stimulates the human HLA-G promoter in JEG3 choriocarcinoma cells. J Clin Endocrinol Metab. 2000;85:3932–6.
27. González-Hernandez A, LeMaoult J, Lopez A, Alegre E, Caumartin J, Le Rond S, Daouya M, Moreau P, Carosella ED. Linking two immuno-suppressive molecules: indoleamine 2,3 dioxygenase can modify HLA-G cell-surface expression. Biol Reprod. 2005;73:571–8.
28. Mouillot G, Marcou C, Zidi I, Guillard C, Sangrouber D, Carosella ED, Moreau P. Hypoxia modulates HLA-G gene expression in tumor cells. Hum Immunol. 2007;68:277–85.
29. Castelli EC, Moreau P, Oya e Chiromatzo A, Mendes-Junior CT, Veiga-Castelli LC, Yaghi L, Giuliatti S, Carosella ED, Donadi EA. In silico analysis of microRNAS targeting the HLA-G 3′ untranslated region alleles and haplotypes. Hum Immunol. 2009;70:1020–5.
30. Jasinski-Bergner S, Mandelboim O, Seliger B. The role of MicroRNAs in the control of innate immune response in cancer. J Natl Cancer Inst. 2014;106(10). doi:10.1093/jnci/dju257.
31. Tan Z, Randall G, Fan J, Camoretti-Mercado B, Brockman-Schneider R, Pan L, Solway J, Gern JE, Lemanske RF, Nicolae D, Ober C. Allele-specific targeting of microRNAs to HLA-G and risk of asthma. Am J Hum Genet. 2007;81:829–34.
32. Wang X, Li B, Wang J, Lei J, Liu C, Ma Y, Zhao H. Evidence that miR-133a causes recurrent spontaneous abortion by reducing HLA-G expression. Reprod Biomed Online. 2012;25: 415–24.
33. Tao S, He H, Chen Q, Yue W. GPER mediated estradiol reduces miR-148a to promote HLA-G expression in breast cancer. Biochem Biophys Res Commun. 2014;451:74–8.
34. Díaz-Lagares A, Alegre E, LeMaoult J, Carosella ED, González A. Nitric oxide produces HLA-G nitration and induces metalloprotease-dependent shedding creating a tolerogenic milieu. Immunology. 2009;126:436–45.
35. McMaster M, Zhou Y, Shorter S, Kapasi K, Geraghty D, Lim KH, Fisher S. HLA-G isoforms produced by placental cytotrophoblasts and found in amniotic fluid are due to unusual glycosylation. J Immunol. 1998;160:5922–8.
36. Alegre E, Rebmann V, Lemaoult J, Rodriguez C, Horn PA, Díaz-Lagares A, Echeveste JI, González A. In vivo identification of an HLA-G complex as ubiquitinated protein circulating in exosomes. Eur J Immunol. 2013;43:1933–9.

37. Donadi EA, Castelli EC, Arnaiz-Villena A, Roger M, Rey D, Moreau P. Implications of the polymorphism of HLA-G on its function, regulation, evolution and disease association. Cell Mol Life Sci. 2011;68:369–95.
38. Hviid TV, Rizzo R, Melchiorri L, Stignani M, Baricordi OR. Polymorphism in the 5′ upstream regulatory and 3′ untranslated regions of the HLA-G gene in relation to soluble HLA-G and IL-10 expression. Hum Immunol. 2006;67:53–62.
39. Castelli EC, Mendes-Junior CT, Deghaide NH, de Albuquerque RS, Muniz YC, Simões RT, Carosella ED, Moreau P, Donadi EA. The genetic structure of 3′ untranslated region of the HLA-G gene: polymorphisms and haplotypes. Genes Immun. 2010;11:134–41.
40. Hviid TV, Hylenius S, Rørbye C, Nielsen LG. HLA-G allelic variants are associated with differences in the HLA-G mRNA isoform profile and HLA-G mRNA levels. Immunogenetics. 2003;55:63–79.
41. Rousseau P, Le Discorde M, Mouillot G, Marcou C, Carosella ED, Moreau P. The 14 bp deletion-insertion polymorphism in the 3′ UT region of the HLA-G gene influences HLA-G mRNA stability. Hum Immunol. 2003;64:1005–10.
42. Harrison GA, Humphrey KE, Jakobsen IB, Cooper DW. A 14 bp deletion polymorphism in the HLA-G gene. Hum Mol Genet. 1993;2:2200.
43. Morandi F, Pistoia V. Interactions between HLA-G and HLA-E in physiological and pathological conditions. Front Immunol. 2014;5:394.
44. Bukur J, Malenica B, Huber C, Seliger B. Altered expression of nonclassical HLA class Ib antigens in human renal cell carcinoma and its association with impaired immune response. Hum Immunol. 2003;64:1081–92.
45. Engels CC, Fontein DB, Kuppen PJ, de Kruijf EM, Smit VT, Nortier JW, Liefers GJ, van de Velde CJ, Bastiaannet E. Immunological subtypes in breast cancer are prognostic for invasive ductal but not for invasive lobular breast carcinoma. Br J Cancer. 2014;111:532–8.
46. Urosevic M, Kurrer MO, Kamarashev J, Mueller B, Weder W, Burg G, Stahel RA, Dummer R, Trojan A. Human leukocyte antigen G up-regulation in lung cancer associates with high-grade histology, human leukocyte antigen class I loss and interleukin-10 production. Am J Pathol. 2001;159:817–24.
47. Yan WH, Lin A, Chen BG, Luo WD, Dai MZ, Chen XJ, Xu HH, Li BL. Unfavourable clinical implications for HLA-G expression in acute myeloid leukaemia. J Cell Mol Med. 2008;12:889–98.
48. Rajagopalan S, Bryceson YT, Kuppusamy SP, Geraghty DE, van der Meer A, Joosten I, Long EO. Activation of NK cells by an endocytosed receptor for soluble HLA-G. PLoS Biol. 2006;4:e9.
49. Loumagne L, Baudhuin J, Favier B, Montespan F, Carosella ED, Rouas-Freiss N. In vivo evidence that secretion of HLA-G by immunogenic tumor cells allows their evasion from immunosurveillance. Int J Cancer. 2014;135:2107–17.
50. Rebmann V, Regel J, Stolke D, Grosse-Wilde H. Secretion of sHLA-G molecules in malignancies. Semin Cancer Biol. 2003;13:371–7.
51. Reimers MS, Engels CC, Putter H, Morreau H, Liefers GJ, van de Velde CJ, Kuppen PJ. Prognostic value of HLA class I, HLA-E, HLA-G and Tregs in rectal cancer: a retrospective cohort study. BMC Cancer. 2014;14:486.
52. Rutten MJ, Dijk F, Savci-Heijink CD, Buist MR, Kenter GG, van de Vijver MJ, Jordanova ES. HLA-G expression is an independent predictor for improved survival in high grade ovarian carcinomas. J Immunol Res. 2014;2014:274584.
53. Amiot L, LeFriec G, Sebti Y, Drenou B, Pangault C, Guilloux V, Leleu X, Bernard M, Facon T, Faucher R. HLA-G epression and lymphoproliferative disorders. Sem Cancer Biol. 2003;13:379–85.
54. Sebti Y, Le Maux A, Gros F, De Guibert S, Pangault C, Rouas-Freiss N, Bernard M, Amiot L. Expression of functional soluble human leucocyte antigen-G molecules in lymphoproliferative disorders. Br J Haematol. 2007;138:202–12.
55. Naji A, Menier C, Maki G, Carosella ED, Rouas-Freiss N. Neoplastic B-cell growth is impaired by HLA-G/ILT2 interaction. Leukemia. 2012;26:1889–92.

56. Wastowski IJ, Simões RT, Yaghi L, Donadi EA, Pancoto JT, Poras I, Lechapt-Zalcman E, Bernaudin M, Valable S, Carlotti Jr CG, Flajollet S, Jensen SS, Ferrone S, Carosella ED, Kristensen BW, Moreau P. Human leukocyte antigen-G is frequently expressed in glioblastoma and may be induced in vitro by combined 5-aza-2′-deoxycytidine and interferon-gamma treatments: results from a multicentric study. Am J Pathol. 2013;182:540–52.
57. Urosevic M, Dummer R. HLA-G and IL-10 expression in human cancer–different stories with the same message. Semin Cancer Biol. 2003;13:337–42.
58. Agaugué S, Carosella ED, Rouas-Freiss N. Role of HLA-G in tumor escape through expansion of myeloid-derived suppressor cells and cytokinic balance in favor of Th2 versus Th1/Th17. Blood. 2011;117:7021–31.
59. Gregori S, Tomasoni D, Pacciani V, Scirpoli M, Battaglia M, Magnani CF, Hauben E, Roncarolo MG. Differentiation of type 1 T regulatory cells (Tr1) by tolerogenic DC-10 requires the IL-10-dependent ILT4/HLA-G pathway. Blood. 2010;116:935–44.
60. Zilberman S, Schenowitz C, Agaugué S, Benoît F, Riteau B, Rouzier R, Carosella ED, Rouas-Freiss N, Menier C. HLA-G1 and HLA-G5 active dimers are present in malignant cells and effusions: the influence of the tumor microenvironment. Eur J Immunol. 2012;42:1599–608.
61. Morandi F, Rouas-Freiss N, Pistoia V. The emerging role of soluble HLA-G in the control of chemotaxis. Cytokine Growth Factor Rev. 2014;25:327–35.
62. Liang S, Baibakov B, Horuzsko A. HLA-G inhibits the functions of murine dendritic cells via the PIR-B immune inhibitory receptor. Eur J Immunol. 2002;32:2418–26.
63. Caumartin J, Favier B, Daouya M, Guillard C, Moreau P, Carosella ED, LeMaoult J. Trogocytosis-based generation of suppressive NK cells. EMBO J. 2007;26:1423–33.
64. Li C, Houser BL, Nicotra ML, Strominger JL. HLA-G homodimer-induced cytokine secretion through HLA-G receptors on human decidual macrophages and natural killer cells. Proc Natl Acad Sci U S A. 2009;106:5767–72.
65. Yan WH. HLA-G expression in cancers: potential role in diagnosis, prognosis and therapy. Endocr Metab Immune Disord Drug Targets. 2011;11:76–89.
66. LeMaoult J, Daouya M, Wu J, Loustau M, Horuzsko A, Carosella ED. Synthetic HLA-G proteins for therapeutic use in transplantation. FASEB J. 2013;27:3643–51.
67. Zidi IN, Ben Amor N. Nanoparticles targeting HLA-G for gene therapy in cancer. Med Oncol. 2012;29:1384–90.
68. Alkhouly N, Shehata I, Ahmed MB, Shehata H, Hassan S, Ibrahim T. HLA-G expression in acute lymphoblastic leukemia: a significant prognostic tumor biomarker. Med Oncol. 2013;30:460.
69. Bukur J, Rebmann V, Grosse-Wilde H, Luboldt H, Ruebben H, Drexler I, Sutter G, Huber C, Seliger B. Functional role of human leukocyte antigen-G up-regulation in renal cell carcinoma. Cancer Res. 2003;63:4107–11.
70. Cao M, Yie SM, Liu J, Ye SR, Xia D, Gao E. Plasma soluble HLA-G is a potential biomarker for diagnosis of colorectal, gastric, esophageal and lung cancer. Tissue Antigens. 2011;78:120–8.
71. Diepstra A, Poppema S, Boot M, Visser L, Nolte IM, Niens M, Te Meerman GJ, van den Berg A. HLA-G protein expression as a potential immune escape mechanism in classical Hodgkin's lymphoma. Tissue Antigens. 2008;71(3):219–26.
72. Gan LH, Huang LF, Zhang X, Lin A, Xu DP, Wang Q, Wang TJ, Yan WH. Tumor-specific upregulation of human leukocyte antigen-G expression in bladder transitional cell carcinoma. Hum Immunol. 2010;71:899–904.
73. Guo QY, Chen BG, Ruan YY, Lin A, Yan WH. HLA-G expression is irrelevant to prognosis in patients with acute myeloid leukemia. Leuk Res. 2011;35:1350–4.
74. He X, Dong DD, Yie SM, Yang H, Cao M, Ye SR, Li K, Liu J, Chen J. HLA-G expression in human breast cancer: implications for diagnosis and prognosis, and effect on allocytotoxic lymphocyte response after hormone treatment in vitro. Ann Surg Oncol. 2010;17:1459–69.
75. Hu J, Li L, Liu Y, Chen Y, Liu C, Liang W, Zhao J, Zou H, Cui X, Qi Y, Li L, Feng L. Overexpression of HLA-G is positively associated with Kazakh esophageal squamous cell carcinoma in Xinjiang. China Viral Immunol. 2013;26:180–4.

76. Jeong S, Park S, Park BW, Park Y, Kwon OJ, Kim HS. Human leukocyte antigen-G (HLA-G) polymorphism and expression in breast cancer patients. PLoS One. 2014;9:e98284.
77. Kalhor N, Ramirez PT, Deavers MT, Malpica A, Silva EG. Immunohistochemical studies of trophoblastic tumors. Am J Surg Pathol. 2009;33:633–8.
78. Karagöz B, Haholu A, Ozgün A, Bilgi O, Tunçel T, Emirzeoğlu L, Celik S, Demirel D. HLA-G in testicular germ cell tumors. Oncol Res Treat. 2014;37:245–8.
79. Kren L, Slaby O, Muckova K, Lzicarova E, Sova M, Vybihal V, Svoboda T, Fadrus P, Lakomy R, Vanhara P, Krenova Z, Sterba J, Smrcka M, Michalek J. Expression of immune-modulatory molecules HLA-G and HLA-E by tumor cells in glioblastomas: an unexpected prognostic significance? Neuropathology. 2011;31:129–34.
80. Li BL, Lin A, Zhang XJ, Zhang X, Zhang JG, Wang Q, Zhou WJ, Chen HX, Wang TJ, Yan WH. Characterization of HLA-G expression in renal cell carcinoma. Tissue Antigens. 2009;74:213–21.
81. Locafaro G, Amodio G, Tomasoni D, Tresoldi C, Ciceri F, Gregori S. HLA-G expression on blasts and tolerogenic cells in patients affected by acute myeloid leukemia. J Immunol Res. 2014;2014:636292.
82. Mohammadi S, Sulaiman S, Koon PB, Amani R, Hosseini SM. Association of nutritional status with quality of life in breast cancer survivors. Asian Pac J Cancer Prev. 2013;14:7749–55.
83. Ramos CS, Gonçalves AS, Marinho LC, Gomes Avelino MA, Saddi VA, Lopes AC, Simões RT, Wastowski IJ. Analysis of HLA-G gene polymorphism and protein expression in invasive breast ductal carcinoma. Hum Immunol. 2014;75:667–72.
84. Sayed D, Badr G, Maximous D, Mikhail NN, Abu-Tarboush F, Alhazza IM. HLA-G and its relation to proliferation index in detection and monitoring breast cancer patients. Tissue Antigens. 2010;75:40–7.
85. Schütt P, Schütt B, Switala M, Bauer S, Stamatis G, Opalka B, Eberhardt W, Schuler M, Horn PA, Rebmann V. Prognostic relevance of soluble human leukocyte antigen-G and total human leukocyte antigen class I molecules in lung cancer patients. Hum Immunol. 2010;71:489–95.
86. Singer G, Rebmann V, Chen YC, Liu HT, Ali SZ, Reinsberg J, McMaster MT, Pfeiffer K, Chan DW, Wardelmann E, Grosse-Wilde H, Cheng CC, Kurman RJ, Shih IM. HLA-G is a potential tumor marker in malignant ascites. Clin Cancer Res. 2003;9:4460–4.
87. Attia MA, Nosair NA, Gawally A, Eluagar G, Elshafey EM. HLA-G expression as prognostoc indicator in B cell chronic lmphatic leukemia. Acta Hemat. 2014;132:53–8.
88. Zheng J, Xu C, Chu D, Zhang X, Li J, Ji G, Hong L, Feng Q, Li X, Wu G, Du J, Zhao Q. Human leukocyte antigen G is associated with esophageal squamous cell carcinoma progression and poor prognosis. Immunol Lett. 2014;161:13–9.
89. Zheng N, Wang CX, Zhang X, Du LT, Zhang J, Kan SF, Zhu CB, Dong ZG, Wang LL, Wang S, Li W. Up-regulation of HLA-G expression in cervical premalignant and malignant lesions. Tissue Antigens. 2011;77:218–24.
90. Zhu CB, Wang CX, Zhang X, Zhang J, Li W. Serum sHLA-G levels: a useful indicator in distinguishing colorectal cancer from benign colorectal diseases. Int J Cancer. 2011;128: 617–22.

Chapter 4
Integrins: Friends or Foes of Antitumor Cytotoxic T Lymphocyte Response

Marie Boutet, Stephanie Cognac, and Fathia Mami-Chouaib

Abstract Elimination of cancer cells by the immune system requires the induction of a strong and durable antitumor cytotoxic T lymphocyte (CTL) response. Immunotherapy approaches aim at generating tumor-specific CTL capable of migrating to the tumor site and at optimizing their functional activities toward target cells. Unfortunately, clinical trials indicate that despite an increase in the frequency and reactivity of antitumor CD8$^+$ T lymphocytes, the efficacy of current immunotherapeutic strategies remains limited and rarely resulted in the eradication of malignant cells. Integrins and their ligands play critical roles in regulating T-cell effector functions, including adhesion to antigen presenting cells (APC), costimulation, migration to lymphoid organs and inflammatory sites, and extravasation. Although some of those are known to promote tumor cell proliferation and dissemination, others are required for T-lymphocyte homing and retention within the tumor microenvironment and for CTL activation and triggering of cytotoxic activity within a hostile ecosystem. In this chapter, we will briefly summarize findings involving integrins, in particular CD103 (α_E/β_7) and LFA-1 (α_L/β_2), and their respective ligands, E-cadherin and intercellular adhesion molecule 1 (ICAM-1), in regulating the effector phase of the antitumor T-cell response and we provide insights into the potential implication of their altered expression in tumor resistance to CTL-mediated cancer immunotherapy. The characterization of integrin-dependent pathways involved in the potentiation of antitumor CTL functions may lead to enhanced immune protection and improved cancer immunotherapy.

Keywords CTL • CD103 • E-cadherin • LFA-1 • ICAM-1 • Antitumor T-cell responses • Cancer immunotherapy

No conflict statement: No potential conflicts of interest were disclosed.

M. Boutet • S. Cognac • F. Mami-Chouaib (✉)
INSERM (Institut national de la Santé et de la Recherche médicale) Unité U753,
Team 1: Tumor Antigens and T-Cell Reactivity, Villejuif 94805, France

Gustave Roussy (Institut de Cancérologie Gustave Roussy),
Gustave Roussy. 114, rue Édouard Vaillant, Villejuif 94805, France

Université Paris-Sud, Orsay 91400, France
e-mail: fathia.mami-chouaib@gustaveroussy.fr

B. Bonavida, S. Chouaib (eds.), *Resistance of Cancer Cells to CTL-Mediated Immunotherapy*, Resistance to Targeted Anti-Cancer Therapeutics 7,
DOI 10.1007/978-3-319-17807-3_4

Abbreviations

APC	Antigen-presenting cell
CAF	Cancer-associated fibroblasts
ECM	Extracellular matrix
EMT	Epithelial-to-mesenchymal-transition
ICAM	Intercellular adhesion molecule
IS	Immune synapse
LFA	Leukocyte function-associated antigen
mAb	Monoclonal antibody
MTOC	Microtubule-organizing center
pMHC-I	Peptide-major histocompatibility complex class I
TAA	Tumor-associated antigen
TCR	T-cell receptor
TGF	Transforming growth factor.

4.1 Introduction

Over the last decade there have been significant advances in the field of tumor immunology and immunotherapy contributing to the validation of the concept of antitumor immune surveillance and leading to the development of novel therapies targeting tumor-specific processes in order to eliminate cancer cells. The generation of tumor-reactive cytotoxic T lymphocytes (CTL) from patients with various solid tumors had led to promising immunotherapeutic approaches, either by expanding the T cells in vitro before transferring them into patients [1] or by identifying the recognized tumor-associated antigens (TAA) which can then be used in vaccination trials such as in melanoma and lung cancer [2–4]. Unfortunately, clinical trials indicate that despite an increase in the frequency of tumor-specific $CD8^+$ T lymphocytes, the efficacy of current therapeutic vaccines remains limited and rarely resulted in the eradication of transformed cell [5]. Current studies are, therefore, focusing on a better understanding of the mechanisms of scarce tumor regressions [6, 7], the activation state of antitumor $CD8^+$ T cells and their capacity to migrate to the tumor site [8, 9]. Immunotherapy strategies have also benefited from the recent knowledge of the T-cell molecules involved in the regulation of antitumor CTL responses, leading to the development of monoclonal antibody (mAb)-based therapies against inhibitory receptors such as cytotoxic T-lymphocyte antigen 4 (CTLA-4) and programmed cell death protein 1 (PD-1), known to inhibit T-cell activities [10, 11]. However, although these treatments resulted in impressive survival responses in some cancers, including melanoma and lung cancer [12–14], a still are elevated fraction of cancer patients does not respond to these therapeutic interventions [15], indicating that these approaches alone cannot be a cure-all for the future.

It is now clear that multiple mechanisms inhibiting antitumor T-cell functions could be responsible for the failure of the immune system to destroy cancer cells [16, 17].

Overcoming these resistances needs a better understanding of the physiology of the tumor niche and the crosstalk between cancer cells and immune cells. Indeed, immunotherapy failures are likely due to diverse mechanisms related to the hostile microenvironment established by the tumor to suppress immune responses. In this regard, cancer cells frequently develop resistance to T-cell receptor (TCR)-mediated cytotoxic activity by using multiple strategies including loss of major histocompatibility complex (MHC) and adhesion molecules, such as the leukocyte function associated antigen-1 (LFA-1) ligand, intercellular adhesion molecule-1 (ICAM-1), resistance to the lytic granule exocytosis pathway and secretion of immunosuppressive factors, such as transforming growth factor-beta (TGF-β1) [18]. Defects in antigen processing molecules, such as proteasome or transporter associated with antigen processing (TAP) subunits, have also been described as a strategy used by malignant cells for countering the host CD8 T-cell immunity. TAP deficiencies have been observed in a wide variety of human cancers, including cervical carcinoma [19], head and neck cancer [20] and non-small cell lung carcinoma (NSCLC) [21], and are associated with tumor escape from the immune system control. In addition, factors that control the accumulation of immune cells at the tumor site are essential in controlling T-cell responses. Indeed, to destroy tumors, CTL must first be able to migrate to the tumor site, infiltrate the tumor tissue and interact with target cells to finally trigger tumor cell destruction. There is now overwhelming evidence indicating that chemokines and chemokine receptors regulate immunocompetent cell homing, retention and activation, and that some of them are able to induce changes in the tumor microenvironment that lead to a high infiltration by specific T lymphocytes (reviewed in [22]). However, previous studies have pointed toward a role of a dense and deregulated extracellular matrix (ECM) in controlling the distribution of T cells within the tumor and their capacity to interact with cancer cells [23]. Paradoxically, our group also pointed toward a role of TGF-β1, rather known for its immunosuppressive functions, in the induction of integrin α_E(CD103)β_7 (thereafter named CD103) on the tumor-infiltrating lymphocyte (TIL) surface to promote both cytokine secretion and cytotoxic activity toward autologous epithelial tumor cells lacking ICAM-1 [24, 25]. Thus, this integrin appears as a key player in CTL activation whose expression is probably adjusted by the tumor microenvironment not only to promote T-cell adhesion to target cells through its interaction with its ligand, the epithelial cell marker E-cadherin, but also to provide positive signals triggering CTL effector functions [26]. Here, we emphasize the role of integrins and their ligands in regulating the CTL-mediated antitumor response and we provide insights into their contribution to tumor growth, metastasis and escape from the T-cell immunity.

4.2 Integrins Are Major Regulators of T-Cell Functions

Integrins are heterodimeric cell adhesion receptors involved in cell–cell and cell-ECM adhesions [27]. Multiple integrins are expressed on T lymphocytes and play critical roles in regulating T-cell functions, including adhesion to antigen presenting cells (APC), costimulation, migration to lymphoid organs and inflammation sites, and extravasation [28, 29]. It is well known that interactions between lymphocytes and the vascular endothelium are essential for the recruitment of T cells to inflammatory tissues and achievement of efficient immune responses (Fig. 4.1). Diapedesis is a multistep process involving tethering and rolling of lymphocytes on endothelial cells and rapid activation of integrins, followed by firm arrest of the cells before extravasation into target tissues [30]. Integrins $\alpha_5\beta_1$, $\alpha_V\beta_3$ and $\alpha_2\beta_1$ and their respective ligands, collagen, fibronectin and vitronectin, play an important role in the migration of immune cells [31]. β_2 integrins LFA-1 (α_L/β_2 or CD11a/CD18) and Mac-1 ($\alpha_M\beta_2$), and $\alpha 4$ integrins such as VLA-4 ($\alpha_4\beta_1$) and $\alpha_4\beta_7$ are involved in the arrest of rolling leukocytes in blood vessels by binding to their respective available

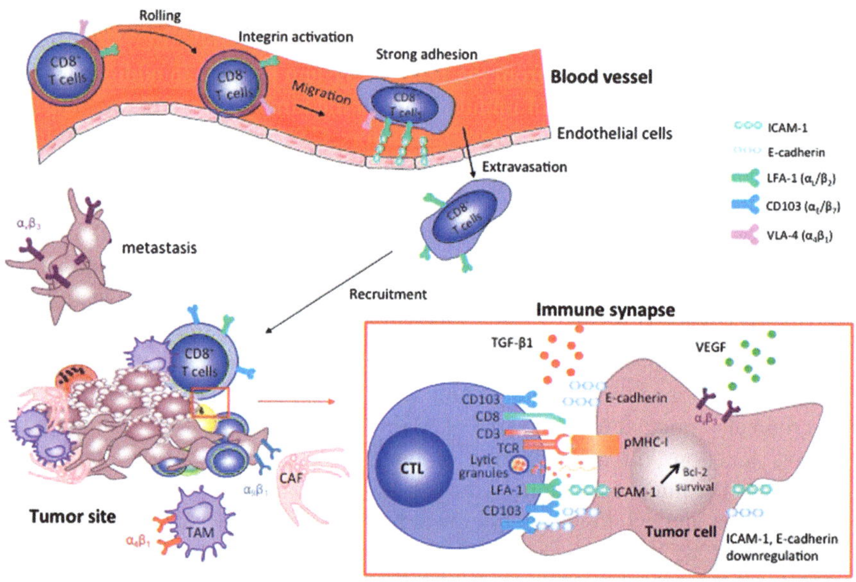

Fig. 4.1 Influence of integrin family members on antitumor T-cell responses. Leukocyte integrins $\alpha_L\beta_2$ and $\alpha_4\beta_1$ contribute to T-cell migration and recruitment at the tumor site. This multistep process is mediated by binding of integrins to their respective ligands on endothelial cells. T lymphocyte recruitment within a TGF-β1-rich tumor microenvironment results in decrease in LFA-1 expression and induction of CD103 integrin on activated tumor-specific $CD8^+$ T cells. The interaction of CD103 on TIL with E-cadherin on epithelial tumor cells promotes maturation of the immune synapse and triggers cytokine production and polarized exocytosis of cytotoxic granules leading to target cell lysis (*red outline*). However, TGF-β1 downregulates ICAM-1 expression on tumor cells and is also an important inducer of EMT, associated with a decrease in E-cadherin expression level, leading to cancer cell resistance to CTL-mediated killing. Moreover, integrins $\alpha_v\beta_3$, $\alpha_4\beta_1$ and $\alpha_9\beta_1$ confer tumor cell escape from the immune system by promoting angiogenesis, through VEGF production, and metastasis and inhibiting apoptosis of cancer cells such as by upregulating Bcl-2 expression. Others integrins, such as $\alpha_9\beta_1$ and $\alpha_4\beta_1$ on tumor cells, are involved in the recruitment of TAM and CAF at the tumor site, which also participate in the establishment of a protumoral microenvironment

ligands [32, 33]. The β_2 integrin LFA-1 plays also an essential role in TCR-dependent cytotoxicity by interacting with its cognate ligand, ICAM-1 (CD54), on target cells [34]. Indeed, tight adhesion between T cells and specific target cells is a prerequisite for effective CTL-mediated lysis. This adhesion can also be provided by the interaction of integrin CD103 ($\alpha_E\beta_7$) on $CD8^+$ T lymphocytes with its ligand, E-cadherin, on epithelial target cells [25]. The interaction of CD103 on tumor-specific TIL with E-cadherin on cancer cells is necessary for positioning the cytotoxic granules near the interface and their delivery into the target, leading to lysis of the target cell (Fig. 4.1).

Integrins transmit bidirectional signals including intracellular signals that initiate the so-called "inside-out" signaling and "outside-in" signals that are induced following the interaction between activated integrins and their ligands [35]. In T cells, the "inside-out" signaling is initiated by the T-cell receptor (TCR) or the chemokine receptor engagement resulting in clustering of individual integrin units and conformational changes in the integrin itself leading to a high increase in the affinity for its ligand. The "outside-in" signaling, triggered by the integrin-ligand binding, generates downstream signals that induce cell spreading, retraction, migration, proliferation, and survival. Studies indicated that the TCR engagement induces phosphorylation of signaling molecules, such as ZAP-70, which contribute to integrin activation [36]. Likewise, proinflammatory chemokines, such CXCL12 (SDF-1, stromal cell-derived factor 1), activate integrin LFA-1 and thus enhance the adhesion of T cells to dendritic cells (DC) [37]. It has been also reported that CCL25 (TECK) increases T-cell recruitment at inflammatory sites by enhancing $\alpha_4\beta_1$/VCAM-1 interaction [38]. Thus, besides their adhesion properties, integrins regulate multiple leukocyte functional responses resulting from outside-in signaling, including migration, proliferation, cytokine secretion, and degranulation [35].

4.3 CD103 Integrin: A Key Asset for CTL Functional Activities in Epithelial Tumors

CD103 integrin was initially detected on intestinal intraepithelial lymphocytes (IEL) [39, 40]. It is expressed at high levels on mucosal T lymphocytes, and is essential for $CD8^+$ T-cell functions within the gut epithelium [41]. Indeed, this integrin plays a major role in the retention of IEL in mucosal tissues by interacting with the extracellular domains 1 and 2 of its ligand, E-cadherin [42]. Consistently, experiments performed in α_E-subunit-deficient mice revealed a reduced number of T cells in mucosal tissues [43]. CD103 integrin is also found on mucosal mast cells and DC [44] as well as on $CD4^+$ and $CD8^+$ regulatory T cells [45]. $CD103^+$ DC have been reported to potentiate T-cell responses [46] and to prime $CD8^+$ T lymphocytes after vaccination [47]. Moreover, $CD103^+$ DC are involved in self or non-self antigen cross-presentation [48], gut homing [49] and Treg development [50]. It has been reported that $CD103^+$ Treg cells mediate immunosuppressive activities such as in the skin where they inhibit inflammation [51], and in graft-versus-host disease

(GVHD) where they contribute to preventing the disease [52]. CD103 also serves as a marker of tissue-resident memory (T_{RM}) T cells [53, 54], and accumulating evidence indicates that this integrin is directly involved in the intraepithelial retention of T_{RM} by modulating their capacity to exit non-lymphoid tissues [55].

Adhesiveness of CD103 to its ligand appeared to be regulated by "inside-out" signals, as CD103-expressing IEL have been shown to bind more avidly to E-cadherin after treatment with anti-CD3 mAb [42]. In addition, a role of CD103 in transmitting "outside-in" signaling has been reported, since anti-CD103 mAb increases T-cell proliferation in response to suboptimal concentrations of anti-CD3 [56, 57] and induce redirected lysis of Fc-receptor-bearing target cells [41, 58]. A role of CD103 in shaping leukocyte morphogenesis and motility has also been reported [59]. Moreover, this integrin has been associated with the cytotoxicity of $CD8^+$ T cells in GVHD [60, 61], allogeneic transplant rejection [62–64] and autoimmune diseases [65].

Importantly, studies have revealed the expression of CD103 on a large proportion of $CD8^+$ T cells infiltrating epithelial tumors, including bladder [66], colon [67], pancreas [68] and lung [25]. This integrin is induced on $CD8^+$ T lymphocytes upon TCR engagement and exposure to TGF-β1, abundant within the tumor microenvironment, through binding of NFAT-1 and Smad2/3 transcription factors to the promoter and enhancer elements of the *ITGAE* gene that encodes CD103 [69]. Thus, $CD8^+$ T lymphocytes expressing CD103 selectively expand within the lung tumor microenvironment, and the interaction of this integrin with E-cadherin on target cells plays an essential role in TCR-dependent cancer cell killing [25]. Indeed, CD103 is recruited at the immune synapse (IS) formed between CTL and epithelial tumor cells, and its interaction with E-cadherin is required for polarized exocytosis of lytic granules, specialized secretory lysosomes that contain perforin and granzymes, leading to target cell death. CD103 has a critical costimulatory function in antitumor CTL activation, and its ligation to E-cadherin triggers "outside-in" signals that promote phosphorylation of ERK1/2 kinases and phospholipase Cγ1 (PLCγ1) and lead to cytotoxic granule relocalization at the IS [26]. Moreover, the CD103-E-cadherin interaction potentiates cytokine production by activated CTL following stimulation with specific target cells and promotes attachment of T cells on epithelial tissues under conditions of vascular shear flow [24]. This integrin plays also a unique role in T-cell retention within epithelial tumors by a mechanism involving recruitment of CCR5 at the IS between TIL and specific target cells [70]. Together, these results emphasize a crucial role for $CD8^+/CD103^+$ T cells infiltrating human epithelial tumor lesions in the antitumor immune response and suggest their potential benefit in adoptive TIL transfer-based cancer immunotherapy.

4.4 Protumoral Effects of Certain Integrin Members

Solid tumors can express a variety of integrins that may be involved in their initiation, progression and metastasis. Indeed, tumor cells share the majority of integrins expressed on epithelial cells, the functions and expression levels of which could be modulated during tumor formation [71]. The cell–cell and cell-ECM adhesion proprieties of integrins are responsible for tumor cell migration and invasion. In this regard, integrins $\alpha_v\beta_3$, $\alpha_5\beta_1$, $\alpha_2\beta_1$ and $\alpha_v\beta_6$ as well as $\alpha_6\beta_4$, $\alpha_4\beta_1$ and $\alpha_V\beta_5$ have been extensively described for their contribution to tumor growth, angiogenesis and metastasis [72–76]. For instance, activation of integrin $\alpha_v\beta_3$ controls tumor angiogenesis and metastasis through continuous production of VEGF [77, 78]. Remarkably, it has been reported that $\alpha_v\beta_3$ antagonists, including specific mAb and RGD peptide mimetics, prevent tumor growth thus providing an effective antiangiogenic approach for cancer treatment [79, 80]. Another feature of integrins is their ability to regulate tumor cell survival and apoptosis. Indeed, by interacting with the ECM, integrins are capable of enhancing cell survival [81] through diverse mechanisms including Bcl-2 upregulation and activation of the PI3K-AKT pathway [82–84]. Moreover, adhesion of $\alpha_v\beta_3$ to vitronectin has been demonstrated to protect tumor cells from apoptosis enabling resistance to chemotherapeutic drugs [85]. Thus, by increasing survival, angiogenesis and metastatic potential, integrins are often associated with tumor progression and decreased survival of cancer patients [86, 87].

In addition to their direct impact on tumor cell behavior, integrins can also influence the migration and intratumoral functions of immunosuppressive cell subpopulations, such as tumor-associated macrophages (TAM), Treg and cancer-associated fibroblasts (CAF). In this context, $\alpha_4\beta_1$ integrin has been associated with recruitment of TAM at the tumor site where they participate to tumor growth by promoting the angiogenesis process [88]. More recently, it has been reported that the integrin $\alpha_9\beta_1$ on tumor cells promotes recruitment of CAF within the tumor microenvironment where they secrete growth factors, in particular osteopontin, a key mediator of tumor progression and metastasis [89]. Overall, integrins contribute to the proliferation, survival and migration not only of normal cells, but also of malignant cells [81].

4.5 Altered Expression of Integrins and Integrin Ligands Contributes to Tumor Escape from CTL Response

CTL are a key component of the adaptive immune response to tumors. Inadequate CD8 T-cell immunity is, at least in part, responsible for tumor growth. Cytotoxic activity proceeds through a multistep mechanism including interaction of the TCR with specific peptide-MHC class I (pMHC-I) complexes, integrin-mediated adhesion of CTL to target cells, polarization of the microtubule organizing center (MTOC) toward the cell–cell interface and relocalization of cytotoxic granules along the microtubules toward the MTOC [90]. Killing of target cells then occurs through the release of cytotoxic granule content in secretory clefts that provide a limited space in which cytolytic agents are kept concentrated without any bystander effect [91]. Upon T cell-target cell contact, remodeling of the actin cytoskeleton and rearrangement of cell surface receptors and cytoplasmic proteins result in the formation of a so-called IS [90, 92, 93]. TCR and associated signaling molecules are clustered at the center of the interface, the central supramolecular activation complex (cSMAC) [94], while adhesion molecules, such as integrin LFA-1, are localized at the peripheral (p)SMAC [95]. The interaction of LFA-1 on CTL with ICAM-1 on target cells plays a critical role in TCR-mediated lysis by directing the exocytosis of the cytotoxic granule content to the surface of target cells near the cSMAC [90, 96].

The involvement of integrin LFA-1 and its ligands ICAM-1 in the interaction between CTL and tumor cells has been widely documented [97, 98]. Binding of LFA-1 on CTL to ICAM-1 on target cells is a prerequisite for T-cell activation and for directing the release of cytotoxic granules into the target [34]. In addition to its well-documented role as an adhesion molecule, ICAM-1 might also function as a cell surface receptor capable of initiating intracellular molecular events that facilitate antigen presentation to T cells. Indeed, association of ICAM-1 with MHC-I proteins and subsequent engagement with LFA-1 leads to recruitment of MHC-I presenting molecules to the CTL-target cell contact zone and thus enhances recognition of pMHC-I complexes by specific TCR [99]. Moreover, in vivo experiments showed that increased expression of ICAM-1 in tumors results in an enhanced response to adoptive immunotherapy that is correlated with increased lymphocyte adhesion and enhanced cytotoxic activity of TIL [100, 101]. In contrast, LFA-1-deficient mice failed to reject immunogenic tumors demonstrating the pivotal role of LFA-1-ICAM-1 interaction in the antitumor T-cell response [102]. The LFA-1-ICAM-1 interaction also plays a major role in the generation of tumor-specific $CD8^+$ T cells capable of inhibiting tumor growth in vivo and maintaining long-term survival [97]. It has been demonstrated that ICAM-1 plays a critical role in the regulation of tumor susceptibility to CTL-mediated killing by interfering with activation of the PTEN/PI3K/AKT pathway, and ICAM-1 knockdown corresponds to a mechanism used by metastatic melanoma cells to escape from antitumor CTL responses [103]. It has been also shown that radiation induces enhancement of ICAM-1 expression on adenocarcinoma cells suggesting that low dose radiation may trigger the accumulation of LFA-1^+ CTL at the tumor site, thereby, promoting an antitumor immune response [104].

Thus far, the only reported ligand of CD103 is E-cadherin [42, 105]. E-cadherin is known to provide tumor suppressor function [106], and reduced expression of E-cadherin during cancer progression and metastatic invasion has been observed in many epithelial tumors [107, 108]. Lung cancers frequently express low levels of E-cadherin [25], and its knockdown may be associated with tumor escape from intraepithelial CTL responses. Indeed, the adhesive interaction between CD103 and its ligand plays a pivotal role in the retention of $CD8^+$ T cells in epithelial tissues [68, 109], thus providing a local adaptive immune response [110]. Our previous results indicated that loss of E-cadherin expression, such as using specific siRNA, abrogates TCR-mediated tumor cell killing by autologous $CD8^+CD103^+$ T cells. These results suggest that downregulation of E-cadherin during the epithelial tumor metastatic process could result in the inhibition of the local antitumor CTL response, suggesting a mechanism for immune selection of cancer cells with reduced E-cadherin expression.

Epithelial-to-mesenchymal transition (EMT) is a key process that contributes to tumor invasion, metastatic dissemination, and acquired resistance to therapy [111]. During EMT, the expression level of E-cadherin is decreased, whereas the N-cadherin and vimentin expression levels are increased. These events lead to an organized disassembly of epithelial cell–cell contacts and the acquisition of a mesenchymal motile phenotype allowing dissemination of tumor cells from the primary site [112, 113]. It has been shown that loss of E-cadherin expression by itself is sufficient to induce the entire process of EMT [114]. It has also been shown that the interaction of integrin $\alpha_1\beta_1$ with its ligand collagen type I leads to a decrease in E-cadherin expression [115]. This process is dependent on various integrin signaling pathways activated by Src, integrin-linked kinase (ILK), FAK or RhoGTPases [116]. ILK plays an important role in EMT, and its upregulation in tumor cells inhibits E-cadherin expression, thus promoting cancer cell invasion [117]. TGF-β is also an important factor in EMT by downregulating E-cadherin and inducing mesenchymal markers, such as Snail, slug or vimentin [118].

TGF-β1 is frequently described as an immunosuppressive cytokine used by cancer cells to escape from the immune system and CTL functions [18]. It is also a powerful tumor suppressor factor by inducing apoptosis of pre-malignant cells [119]. TGF-β is present in its inactivated form (latent TGF-β) within the tumor microenvironment, but it can be activated either by proteases (plasmin or matrix metalloproteases, MMP) or after interaction with α_v integrins. Members of the α_v integrin family and $\alpha_8\beta_1$ integrin bind directly to TGF-β through a RGD motif on the integrin, whereas $\alpha_v\beta_8$ needs MMP-1 to fully activate latent TGF-β [120–122]. Our previous data indicated that engagement of both the TGF-β1 receptor and TCR via an active form of TGF-β1 and the specific tumor pMHC-I complex, respectively, is required for CD103 expression on $CD3^+/CD8^+$ TIL. A variation in the density of $CD103^+$ TIL may reflect inter-patient variations in the intratumoral level of TGF-β1 or factors involved in its activation, such as α_V integrins, or the frequency of tumor antigen-specific T-cells. In contrast, secretion of TGF-β1 within the tumor microenvironment induces downregulation of LFA-1 and inhibition of integrin-dependent T-cell functions [123]. Moreover, it has been reported that TGF-β1 downregulates ICAM-1 expression on human cancer cells and inhibits CTL-mediated tumor cell killing [124]. These findings suggest that LFA-1 contributes to T-cell migration to the tumor site and that recruitment of T lymphocytes within a TGF-β1-rich ecosystem induces LFA-1 downregulation and CD103 induction on activated tumor-specific T cells thus insuring in situ CTL effector functions (Fig. 4.1). However, TGF-β1 is also involved in modulating E-cadherin expression on epithelial tumor cells thus conferring resistance to TIL-mediated cytotoxicity.

4.6 Conclusion

Multiple resistance mechanisms developed by the tumor to evade the immune system are far from having been all discovered. In this regard, integrins play an important role in tumor progression by promoting angiogenesis, metastasis and survival of malignant cells. One of the current approaches to prevent progression of solid tumors is to target integrins expressed on cancer cells. The design of integrin antagonists became an important tool in cancer immunotherapy. Clinical trials using specific mAbs, such as etaracizumab and Vitaxin targeting $\alpha_v\beta_3$ integrin, and RGD peptide mimetics are underway in cancer patients and showed encouraging results [125–127].

With regard to T cells, $CD8^+/CD103^+$ lymphocytes infiltrating the epithelial tumor lesions play a major role in antitumor CTL responses, and TIL expressing CD103 are associated with increased patient survival in ovarian cancer [128] and NSCLC (our group, manuscript submitted for publication). Thus, by characterizing $CD8^+/CD103^+$ TIL and identifying the molecular mechanisms involved in their retention within the tumor microenvironment and the signaling pathways associated with their activation and potentiation of TCR-mediated cytotoxic activities, we hope that manipulating this tumor-specific T-cell subpopulation will permit to improve cancer immunotherapy strategies.

Acknowledgements This work was supported by grants from the INSERM, the Institut National du Cancer (INCa), the Ligue contre le Cancer and the Fondation pour la Recherche Médicale (FRM).

MB is supported by a grant from Gustave Roussy (SIRIC SOCRATE) and SC is supported by a grant from the FRM.

References

1. Hinrichs CS, Rosenberg SA. Exploiting the curative potential of adoptive T-cell therapy for cancer. Immunol Rev. 2014;257:56–71.
2. Boon T. Tumor antigens recognized by cytolytic T lymphocytes: present perspectives for specific immunotherapy. Int J Cancer. 1993;54:177–80.
3. Rosenberg SA, Yang JC, Schwartzentruber DJ, Hwu P, Marincola FM, Topalian SL, Restifo NP, Dudley ME, Schwarz SL, Spiess PJ, Wunderlich JR, Parkhurst MR, Kawakami Y, Seipp CA, Einhorn JH, White DE. Immunologic and therapeutic evaluation of a synthetic peptide vaccine for the treatment of patients with metastatic melanoma. Nat Med. 1998;4:321–7.
4. Limacher JM, Spring-Giusti C, Bellon N, Ancian P, Rooke R, Bonnefoy JY. Therapeutic cancer vaccines in the treatment of non-small-cell lung cancer. Expert Rev Vaccines. 2013; 12:263–70.
5. Rosenberg SA, Yang JC, Restifo NP. Cancer immunotherapy: moving beyond current vaccines. Nat Med. 2004;10:909–15.
6. Germeau C, Ma W, Schiavetti F, Lurquin C, Henry E, Vigneron N, Brasseur F, Lethe B, De Plaen E, Velu T, Boon T, Coulie PG. High frequency of antitumor T cells in the blood of melanoma patients before and after vaccination with tumor antigens. J Exp Med. 2005; 201:241–8.
7. Lurquin C, Lethe B, De Plaen E, Corbiere V, Theate I, van Baren N, Coulie PG, Boon T. Contrasting frequencies of antitumor and anti-vaccine T cells in metastases of a melanoma patient vaccinated with a MAGE tumor antigen. J Exp Med. 2005;201:249–57.
8. Jackaman C, Bundell CS, Kinnear BF, Smith AM, Filion P, van Hagen D, Robinson BW, Nelson DJ. IL-2 intratumoral immunotherapy enhances CD8+ T cells that mediate destruction of tumor cells and tumor-associated vasculature: a novel mechanism for IL-2. J Immunol. 2003;171:5051–63.

9. Khawli LA, Hu P, Epstein AL. Cytokine, chemokine, and co-stimulatory fusion proteins for the immunotherapy of solid tumors. Handb Exp Pharmacol. 2008;181:291–328.
10. Korman AJ, Peggs KS, Allison JP. Checkpoint blockade in cancer immunotherapy. Adv Immunol. 2006;90:297–339.
11. Pardoll DM. The blockade of immune checkpoints in cancer immunotherapy. Nat Rev Cancer. 2012;12:252–64.
12. Simeone E, Ascierto PA. Immunomodulating antibodies in the treatment of metastatic melanoma: the experience with anti-CTLA-4, anti-CD137, and anti-PD1. J Immunotoxicol. 2012;9:241–7.
13. Hodi FS, O'Day SJ, McDermott DF, Weber RW, Sosman JA, Haanen JB, Gonzalez R, Robert C, Schadendorf D, Hassel JC, Akerley W, van den Eertwegh AJ, Lutzky J, Lorigan P, Vaubel JM, Linette GP, Hogg D, Ottensmeier CH, Lebbe C, Peschel C, Quirt I, Clark JI, Wolchok JD, Weber JS, Tian J, Yellin MJ, Nichol GM, Hoos A, Urba WJ. Improved survival with ipilimumab in patients with metastatic melanoma. N Engl J Med. 2010;363:711–23.
14. Champiat S, Ileana E, Giaccone G, Besse B, Mountzios G, Eggermont A, Soria JC. Incorporating immune-checkpoint inhibitors into systemic therapy of NSCLC. J Thorac Oncol. 2014;9:144–53.
15. Aerts JG, Hegmans JP. Tumor-specific cytotoxic T cells are crucial for efficacy of immunomodulatory antibodies in patients with lung cancer. Cancer Res. 2013;73:2381–8.
16. Gajewski TF, Meng Y, Harlin H. Immune suppression in the tumor microenvironment. J Immunother. 2006;29:233–40.
17. Gajewski TF, Woo SR, Zha Y, Spaapen R, Zheng Y, Corrales L, Spranger S. Cancer immunotherapy strategies based on overcoming barriers within the tumor microenvironment. Curr Opin Immunol. 2013;25:268–76.
18. Thomas DA, Massague J. TGF-beta directly targets cytotoxic T cell functions during tumor evasion of immune surveillance. Cancer Cell. 2005;8:369–80.
19. Einstein MH, Leanza S, Chiu LG, Schlecht NF, Goldberg GL, Steinberg BM, Burk RD. Genetic variants in TAP are associated with high-grade cervical neoplasia. Clin Cancer Res. 2009;15:1019–23.
20. Leibowitz MS, Andrade Filho PA, Ferrone S, Ferris RL. Deficiency of activated STAT1 in head and neck cancer cells mediates TAP1-dependent escape from cytotoxic T lymphocytes. Cancer Immunol Immunother. 2011;60:525–35.
21. Durgeau A, El Hage F, Vergnon I, Validire P, de Montpreville V, Besse B, Soria JC, van Hall T, Mami-Chouaib F. Different expression levels of the TAP peptide transporter lead to recognition of different antigenic peptides by tumor-specific CTL. J Immunol. 2011;187:5532–9.
22. Franciszkiewicz K, Boissonnas A, Boutet M, Combadiere C, Mami-Chouaib F. Role of chemokines and chemokine receptors in shaping the effector phase of the antitumor immune response. Cancer Res. 2012;72:6325–32.
23. Salmon H, Franciszkiewicz K, Damotte D, Dieu-Nosjean MC, Validire P, Trautmann A, Mami-Chouaib F, Donnadieu E. Matrix architecture defines the preferential localization and migration of T cells into the stroma of human lung tumors. J Clin Invest. 2012;122:899–910.
24. Franciszkiewicz K, Le Floc'h A, Boutet M, Vergnon I, Schmitt A, Mami-Chouaib F. CD103 or LFA-1 engagement at the immune synapse between cytotoxic T cells and tumor cells promotes maturation and regulates T-cell effector functions. Cancer Res. 2013;73:617–28.
25. Le Floc'h A, Jalil A, Vergnon I, Le Maux Chansac B, Lazar V, Bismuth G, Chouaib S, Mami-Chouaib F. Alpha E beta 7 integrin interaction with E-cadherin promotes antitumor CTL activity by triggering lytic granule polarization and exocytosis. J Exp Med. 2007;204:559–70.
26. Le Floc'h A, Jalil A, Franciszkiewicz K, Validire P, Vergnon I, Mami-Chouaib F. Minimal engagement of CD103 on cytotoxic T lymphocytes with an E-cadherin-Fc molecule triggers lytic granule polarization via a phospholipase Cgamma-dependent pathway. Cancer Res. 2011;71:328–38.

27. Barczyk M, Carracedo S, Gullberg D. Integrins. Cell Tissue Res. 2010;339:269–80.
28. Luo BH, Carman CV, Springer TA. Structural basis of integrin regulation and signaling. Annu Rev Immunol. 2007;25:619–47.
29. Denucci CC, Mitchell JS, Shimizu Y. Integrin function in T-cell homing to lymphoid and nonlymphoid sites: getting there and staying there. Crit Rev Immunol. 2009;29:87–109.
30. Springer TA. Traffic signals for lymphocyte recirculation and leukocyte emigration: the multistep paradigm. Cell. 1994;76:301–14.
31. Takada Y, Ye X, Simon S. The integrins. Genome Biol. 2007;8:215.
32. Constantin G, Majeed M, Giagulli C, Piccio L, Kim JY, Butcher EC, Laudanna C. Chemokines trigger immediate beta2 integrin affinity and mobility changes: differential regulation and roles in lymphocyte arrest under flow. Immunity. 2000;13:759–69.
33. Laudanna C, Alon R. Right on the spot. Chemokine triggering of integrin-mediated arrest of rolling leukocytes. Thromb Haemost. 2006;95:5–11.
34. Anikeeva N, Somersalo K, Sims TN, Thomas VK, Dustin ML, Sykulev Y. Distinct role of lymphocyte function-associated antigen-1 in mediating effective cytolytic activity by cytotoxic T lymphocytes. Proc Natl Acad Sci U S A. 2005;102:6437–42.
35. Abram CL, Lowell CA. The ins and outs of leukocyte integrin signaling. Annu Rev Immunol. 2009;27:339–62.
36. Goda S, Quale AC, Woods ML, Felthauser A, Shimizu Y. Control of TCR-mediated activation of beta 1 integrins by the ZAP-70 tyrosine kinase interdomain B region and the linker for activation of T cells adapter protein. J Immunol. 2004;172:5379–87.
37. Laudanna C, Kim JY, Constantin G, Butcher E. Rapid leukocyte integrin activation by chemokines. Immunol Rev. 2002;186:37–46.
38. Parmo-Cabanas M, Garcia-Bernal D, Garcia-Verdugo R, Kremer L, Marquez G, Teixido J. Intracellular signaling required for CCL25-stimulated T cell adhesion mediated by the integrin alpha4beta1. J Leukoc Biol. 2007;82:380–91.
39. Kilshaw PJ, Murant SJ. A new surface antigen on intraepithelial lymphocytes in the intestine. Eur J Immunol. 1990;20:2201–7.
40. Cerf-Bensussan N, Begue B, Gagnon J, Meo T. The human intraepithelial lymphocyte marker HML-1 is an integrin consisting of a beta 7 subunit associated with a distinctive alpha chain. Eur J Immunol. 1992;22:885.
41. Roberts K, Kilshaw PJ. The mucosal T cell integrin alpha M290 beta 7 recognizes a ligand on mucosal epithelial cell lines. Eur J Immunol. 1993;23:1630–5.
42. Higgins JM, Mandlebrot DA, Shaw SK, Russell GJ, Murphy EA, Chen YT, Nelson WJ, Parker CM, Brenner MB. Direct and regulated interaction of integrin alphaEbeta7 with E-cadherin. J Cell Biol. 1998;140:197–210.
43. Schon MP, Arya A, Murphy EA, Adams CM, Strauch UG, Agace WW, Marsal J, Donohue JP, Her H, Beier DR, Olson S, Lefrançois L, Brenner MB, Grusby MJ, Parker CM. Mucosal T lymphocyte numbers are selectively reduced in integrin alpha E (CD103)-deficient mice. J Immunol. 1999;162:6641–9.
44. Sung SS, Fu SM, Rose Jr CE, Gaskin F, Ju ST, Beaty SR. A major lung CD103 (alphaE)-beta7 integrin-positive epithelial dendritic cell population expressing Langerin and tight junction proteins. J Immunol. 2006;176:2161–72.
45. Annacker O, Coombes JL, Malmstrom V, Uhlig HH, Bourne T, Johansson-Lindbom B, Agace WW, Parker CM, Powrie F. Essential role for CD103 in the T cell-mediated regulation of experimental colitis. J Exp Med. 2005;202:1051–61.
46. Heath WR, Carbone FR. Dendritic cell subsets in primary and secondary T cell responses at body surfaces. Nat Immunol. 2009;10:1237–44.
47. Li L, Kim S, Herndon JM, Goedegebuure P, Belt BA, Satpathy AT, Fleming TP, Hansen TH, Murphy KM, Gillanders WE. Cross-dressed CD8alpha+/CD103+ dendritic cells prime CD8+ T cells following vaccination. Proc Natl Acad Sci U S A. 2012;109:12716–21.
48. Bedoui S, Whitney PG, Waithman J, Eidsmo L, Wakim L, Caminschi I, Allan RS, Wojtasiak M, Shortman K, Carbone FR, Brooks AG, Heath WR. Cross-presentation of viral and self antigens by skin-derived CD103+ dendritic cells. Nat Immunol. 2009;10:488–95.

49. Jaensson E, Uronen-Hansson H, Pabst O, Eksteen B, Tian J, Coombes JL, Berg PL, Davidsson T, Powrie F, Johansson-Lindbom B, Agace WW. Small intestinal CD103+ dendritic cells display unique functional properties that are conserved between mice and humans. J Exp Med. 2008;205:2139–49.
50. Coombes JL, Siddiqui KR, Arancibia-Carcamo CV, Hall J, Sun CM, Belkaid Y, Powrie F. A functionally specialized population of mucosal CD103+ DCs induces Foxp3+ regulatory T cells via a TGF-beta and retinoic acid-dependent mechanism. J Exp Med. 2007;204: 1757–64.
51. Suffia I, Reckling SK, Salay G, Belkaid Y. A role for CD103 in the retention of CD4 + CD25+ Treg and control of Leishmania major infection. J Immunol. 2005;174:5444–55.
52. Zhao D, Zhang C, Yi T, Lin CL, Todorov I, Kandeel F, Forman S, Zeng D. In vivo-activated CD103 + CD4+ regulatory T cells ameliorate ongoing chronic graft-versus-host disease. Blood. 2008;112:2129–38.
53. Sheridan BS, Lefrancois L. Regional and mucosal memory T cells. Nat Immunol. 2011; 12:485–91.
54. Jiang X, Clark RA, Liu L, Wagers AJ, Fuhlbrigge RC, Kupper TS. Skin infection generates non-migratory memory CD8+ T(RM) cells providing global skin immunity. Nature. 2012; 483:227–31.
55. Zhang N, Bevan MJ. Transforming growth factor-beta signaling controls the formation and maintenance of gut-resident memory T cells by regulating migration and retention. Immunity. 2013;39:687–96.
56. Cepek KL, Shaw SK, Parker CM, Russell GJ, Morrow JS, Rimm DL, Brenner MB. Adhesion between epithelial cells and T lymphocytes mediated by E-cadherin and the alpha E beta 7 integrin. Nature. 1994;372:190–3.
57. Sarnacki S, Begue B, Buc H, Le Deist F, Cerf-Bensussan N. Enhancement of CD3-induced activation of human intestinal intraepithelial lymphocytes by stimulation of the beta 7-containing integrin defined by HML-1 monoclonal antibody. Eur J Immunol. 1992;22: 2887–92.
58. Hadley GA, Bartlett ST, Via CS, Rostapshova EA, Moainie S. The epithelial cell-specific integrin, CD103 (alpha E integrin), defines a novel subset of alloreactive CD8+ CTL. J Immunol. 1997;159:3748–56.
59. Schlickum S, Sennefelder H, Friedrich M, Harms G, Lohse MJ, Kilshaw P, Schon MP. Integrin alpha E(CD103)beta 7 influences cellular shape and motility in a ligand-dependent fashion. Blood. 2008;112:619–25.
60. El-Asady R, Yuan R, Liu K, Wang D, Gress RE, Lucas PJ, Drachenberg CB, Hadley GA. TGF-{beta}-dependent CD103 expression by CD8(+) T cells promotes selective destruction of the host intestinal epithelium during graft-versus-host disease. J Exp Med. 2005;201:1647–57.
61. Liu K, Anthony BA, Yearsly MM, Hamadani M, Gaughan A, Wang JJ, Devine SM, Hadley GA. CD103 deficiency prevents graft-versus-host disease but spares graft-versus-tumor effects mediated by alloreactive CD8 T cells. PLoS One. 2011;6:e21968.
62. Hadley GA, Charandee C, Weir MR, Wang D, Bartlett ST, Drachenberg CB. CD103+ CTL accumulate within the graft epithelium during clinical renal allograft rejection. Transplantation. 2001;72:1548–55.
63. Feng Y, Wang D, Yuan R, Parker CM, Farber DL, Hadley GA. CD103 expression is required for destruction of pancreatic islet allografts by CD8(+) T cells. J Exp Med. 2002;196: 877–86.
64. Yuan R, El-Asady R, Liu K, Wang D, Drachenberg CB, Hadley GA. Critical role for CD103 + CD8+ effectors in promoting tubular injury following allogeneic renal transplantation. J Immunol. 2005;175:2868–79.
65. Oshitani N, Watanabe K, Maeda K, Fujiwara Y, Higuchi K, Matsumoto T, Arakawa T. Differential expression of homing receptor CD103 on lamina propria lymphocytes and association of CD103 with epithelial adhesion molecules in inflammatory bowel disease. Int J Mol Med. 2003;12:715–9.

66. Cresswell J, Wong WK, Henry MJ, Robertson H, Neal DE, Kirby JA. Adhesion of lymphocytes to bladder cancer cells: the role of the alpha(E)beta(7) integrin. Cancer Immunol Immunother. 2002;51:483–91.
67. Quinn E, Hawkins N, Yip YL, Suter C, Ward R. CD103+ intraepithelial lymphocytes—a unique population in microsatellite unstable sporadic colorectal cancer. Eur J Cancer. 2003;39:469–75.
68. French JJ, Cresswell J, Wong WK, Seymour K, Charnley RM, Kirby JA. T cell adhesion and cytolysis of pancreatic cancer cells: a role for E-cadherin in immunotherapy? Br J Cancer. 2002;87:1034–41.
69. Mokrani M, Klibi J, Bluteau D, Bismuth G, Mami-Chouaib F. Smad and NFAT pathways cooperate to induce CD103 expression in human CD8 T lymphocytes. J Immunol. 2014; 192:2471–9.
70. Franciszkiewicz K, Le Floc'h A, Jalil A, Vigant F, Robert T, Vergnon I, Mackiewicz A, Benihoud K, Validire P, Chouaib S, Combadière C, Mami-Chouaib F. Intratumoral induction of CD103 triggers tumor-specific CTL function and CCR5-dependent T-cell retention. Cancer Res. 2009;69:6249–55.
71. Hehlgans S, Haase M, Cordes N. Signalling via integrins: implications for cell survival and anticancer strategies. Biochim Biophys Acta. 2007;1775:163–80.
72. Vogetseder A, Thies S, Ingold B, Roth P, Weller M, Schraml P, Goodman SL, Moch H. Alphav-integrin isoform expression in primary human tumors and brain metastases. Int J Cancer. 2013;133:2362–71.
73. McCabe NP, De S, Vasanji A, Brainard J, Byzova TV. Prostate cancer specific integrin alphavbeta3 modulates bone metastatic growth and tissue remodeling. Oncogene. 2007;26: 6238–43.
74. Desgrosellier JS, Cheresh DA. Integrins in cancer: biological implications and therapeutic opportunities. Nat Rev Cancer. 2010;10:9–22.
75. Weis SM, Cheresh DA. AlphaV integrins in angiogenesis and cancer. Cold Spring Harb Perspect Med. 2011;1:a006478.
76. Slack-Davis JK, Atkins KA, Harrer C, Hershey ED, Conaway M. Vascular cell adhesion molecule-1 is a regulator of ovarian cancer peritoneal metastasis. Cancer Res. 2009;69: 1469–76.
77. Lorger M, Krueger JS, O'Neal M, Staflin K, Felding-Habermann B. Activation of tumor cell integrin alphavbeta3 controls angiogenesis and metastatic growth in the brain. Proc Natl Acad Sci U S A. 2009;106:10666–71.
78. De S, Razorenova O, McCabe NP, O'Toole T, Qin J, Byzova TV. VEGF-integrin interplay controls tumor growth and vascularization. Proc Natl Acad Sci U S A. 2005;102:7589–94.
79. Brooks PC, Stromblad S, Klemke R, Visscher D, Sarkar FH, Cheresh DA. Antiintegrin alpha v beta 3 blocks human breast cancer growth and angiogenesis in human skin. J Clin Invest. 1995;96:1815–22.
80. Drake CJ, Cheresh DA, Little CD. An antagonist of integrin alpha v beta 3 prevents maturation of blood vessels during embryonic neovascularization. J Cell Sci. 1995;108(Pt 7): 2655–61.
81. Cabodi S, del Pilar Camacho-Leal M, Di Stefano P, Defilippi P. Integrin signalling adaptors: not only figurants in the cancer story. Nat Rev Cancer. 2010;10:858–70.
82. Griffiths GS, Grundl M, Leychenko A, Reiter S, Young-Robbins SS, Sulzmaier FJ, Caliva MJ, Ramos JW, Matter ML. Bit-1 mediates integrin-dependent cell survival through activation of the NFkappaB pathway. J Biol Chem. 2011;286:14713–23.
83. Aoudjit F, Vuori K. Integrin signaling inhibits paclitaxel-induced apoptosis in breast cancer cells. Oncogene. 2001;20:4995–5004.
84. Matter ML, Ruoslahti E. A signaling pathway from the alpha5beta1 and alpha(v)beta3 integrins that elevates bcl-2 transcription. J Biol Chem. 2001;276:27757–63.
85. Uhm JH, Dooley NP, Kyritsis AP, Rao JS, Gladson CL. Vitronectin, a glioma-derived extracellular matrix protein, protects tumor cells from apoptotic death. Clin Cancer Res. 1999;5: 1587–94.

86. Bates RC. The alphaVbeta6 integrin as a novel molecular target for colorectal cancer. Future Oncol. 2005;1:821–8.
87. Hazelbag S, Kenter GG, Gorter A, Dreef EJ, Koopman LA, Violette SM, Weinreb PH, Fleuren GJ. Overexpression of the alpha v beta 6 integrin in cervical squamous cell carcinoma is a prognostic factor for decreased survival. J Pathol. 2007;212:316–24.
88. Jin H, Su J, Garmy-Susini B, Kleeman J, Varner J. Integrin alpha4beta1 promotes monocyte trafficking and angiogenesis in tumors. Cancer Res. 2006;66:2146–52.
89. Ota D, Kanayama M, Matsui Y, Ito K, Maeda N, Kutomi G, Hirata K, Torigoe T, Sato N, Takaoka A, Chambers AF, Morimoto J, Uede T. Tumor-alpha9beta1 integrin-mediated signaling induces breast cancer growth and lymphatic metastasis via the recruitment of cancer-associated fibroblasts. J Mol Med. 2014;92:1271–81.
90. Stinchcombe JC, Bossi G, Booth S, Griffiths GM. The immunological synapse of CTL contains a secretory domain and membrane bridges. Immunity. 2001;15:751–61.
91. Stinchcombe JC, Griffiths GM. Secretory mechanisms in cell-mediated cytotoxicity. Annu Rev Cell Dev Biol. 2007;23:495–517.
92. Griffiths GM, Tsun A, Stinchcombe JC. The immunological synapse: a focal point for endocytosis and exocytosis. J Cell Biol. 2010;189:399–406.
93. Stinchcombe JC, Majorovits E, Bossi G, Fuller S, Griffiths GM. Centrosome polarization delivers secretory granules to the immunological synapse. Nature. 2006;443:462–5.
94. Monks CR, Freiberg BA, Kupfer H, Sciaky N, Kupfer A. Three-dimensional segregation of supramolecular activation clusters in T cells. Nature. 1998;395:82–6.
95. Huppa JB, Davis MM. T-cell-antigen recognition and the immunological synapse. Nat Rev Immunol. 2003;3:973–83.
96. Kuhn JR, Poenie M. Dynamic polarization of the microtubule cytoskeleton during CTL-mediated killing. Immunity. 2002;16:111–21.
97. Jenkinson SR, Williams NA, Morgan DJ. The role of intercellular adhesion molecule-1/LFA-1 interactions in the generation of tumor-specific CD8+ T cell responses. J Immunol. 2005;174:3401–7.
98. Yasuda M, Tanaka Y, Tamura M, Fujii K, Sugaya M, So T, Takenoyama M, Yasumoto K. Stimulation of beta1 integrin down-regulates ICAM-1 expression and ICAM-1-dependent adhesion of lung cancer cells through focal adhesion kinase. Cancer Res. 2001;61:2022–30.
99. Lebedeva T, Dustin ML, Sykulev Y. ICAM-1 co-stimulates target cells to facilitate antigen presentation. Curr Opin Immunol. 2005;17:251–8.
100. Sartor WM, Kyprianou N, Fabian DF, Lefor AT. Enhanced expression of ICAM-1 in a murine fibrosarcoma reduces tumor growth rate. J Surg Res. 1995;59:66–74.
101. Turner J, Rhee JG, Fabian DF, Lefor AT. Expression of ICAM-1 enhances in vivo lymphocyte adhesion in a murine fibrosarcoma. J Surg Oncol. 1997;66:39–44.
102. Schmits R, Kundig TM, Baker DM, Shumaker G, Simard JJ, Duncan G, Wakeham A, Shahinian A, van der Heiden A, Bachmann MF, Ohashi PS, Mak TW, Hickstein DD. LFA-1-deficient mice show normal CTL responses to virus but fail to reject immunogenic tumor. J Exp Med. 1996;183:1415–26.
103. Hamai A, Benlalam H, Meslin F, Hasmim M, Carre T, Akalay I, Janji B, Berchem G, Noman MZ, Chouaib S. Immune surveillance of human cancer: if the cytotoxic T-lymphocytes play the music, does the tumoral system call the tune? Tissue Antigens. 2010;75:1–8.
104. Hareyama M, Imai K, Oouchi A, Takahashi H, Hinoda Y, Tsujisaki M, Adachi M, Shonai T, Sakata K, Morita K. The effect of radiation on the expression of intercellular adhesion molecule-1 of human adenocarcinoma cells. Int J Radiat Oncol Biol Phys. 1998;40:691–6.
105. Corps E, Carter C, Karecla P, Ahrens T, Evans P, Kilshaw P. Recognition of E-cadherin by integrin alpha(E)beta(7): requirement for cadherin dimerization and implications for cadherin and integrin function. J Biol Chem. 2001;276:30862–70.
106. Frixen UH, Behrens J, Sachs M, Eberle G, Voss B, Warda A, Lochner D, Birchmeier W. E-cadherin-mediated cell-cell adhesion prevents invasiveness of human carcinoma cells. J Cell Biol. 1991;113:173–85.

107. Vleminckx K, Vakaet Jr L, Mareel M, Fiers W, van Roy F. Genetic manipulation of E-cadherin expression by epithelial tumor cells reveals an invasion suppressor role. Cell. 1991;66: 107–19.
108. Berx G, Cleton-Jansen AM, Nollet F, de Leeuw WJ, van de Vijver M, Cornelisse C, van Roy F. E-cadherin is a tumour/invasion suppressor gene mutated in human lobular breast cancers. EMBO J. 1995;14:6107–15.
109. Kilshaw PJ, Higgins JM. Alpha E: no more rejection? J Exp Med. 2002;196:873–5.
110. Kilshaw PJ, Karecla P. Structure and function of the mucosal T-cell integrin alpha E beta 7. Biochem Soc Trans. 1997;25:433–9.
111. Tiwari N, Gheldof A, Tatari M, Christofori G. EMT as the ultimate survival mechanism of cancer cells. Semin Cancer Biol. 2012;22:194–207.
112. Thiery JP, Sleeman JP. Complex networks orchestrate epithelial-mesenchymal transitions. Nat Rev Mol Cell Biol. 2006;7:131–42.
113. Nieto MA. The ins and outs of the epithelial to mesenchymal transition in health and disease. Annu Rev Cell Dev Biol. 2011;27:347–76.
114. Thiery JP, Acloque H, Huang RY, Nieto MA. Epithelial-mesenchymal transitions in development and disease. Cell. 2009;139:871–90.
115. Koenig A, Mueller C, Hasel C, Adler G, Menke A. Collagen type I induces disruption of E-cadherin-mediated cell-cell contacts and promotes proliferation of pancreatic carcinoma cells. Cancer Res. 2006;66:4662–71.
116. Canel M, Serrels A, Frame MC, Brunton VG. E-cadherin-integrin crosstalk in cancer invasion and metastasis. J Cell Sci. 2013;126:393–401.
117. Matsui Y, Assi K, Ogawa O, Raven PA, Dedhar S, Gleave ME, Salh B, So AI. The importance of integrin-linked kinase in the regulation of bladder cancer invasion. Int J Cancer. 2012;130:521–31.
118. Derynck R, Akhurst RJ. Differentiation plasticity regulated by TGF-beta family proteins in development and disease. Nat Cell Biol. 2007;9:1000–4.
119. Guasch G, Schober M, Pasolli HA, Conn EB, Polak L, Fuchs E. Loss of TGFbeta signaling destabilizes homeostasis and promotes squamous cell carcinomas in stratified epithelia. Cancer Cell. 2007;12:313–27.
120. Horiguchi M, Ota M, Rifkin DB. Matrix control of transforming growth factor-beta function. J Biochem. 2012;152:321–9.
121. Worthington JJ, Fenton TM, Czajkowska BI, Klementowicz JE, Travis MA. Regulation of TGFbeta in the immune system: an emerging role for integrins and dendritic cells. Immunobiology. 2012;217:1259–65.
122. Henderson NC, Arnold TD, Katamura Y, Giacomini MM, Rodriguez JD, McCarty JH, Pellicoro A, Raschperger E, Betsholtz C, Ruminski PG, Griggs DW, Prinsen MJ, Maher JJ, Iredale JP, Lacy-Hulbert A, Adams RH, Sheppard D. Targeting of alphav integrin identifies a core molecular pathway that regulates fibrosis in several organs. Nat Med. 2013;19: 1617–24.
123. Sela U, Mauermann N, Hershkoviz R, Zinger H, Dayan M, Cahalon L, Liu JP, Mozes E, Lider O. The inhibition of autoreactive T cell functions by a peptide based on the CDR1 of an anti-DNA autoantibody is via TGF-beta-mediated suppression of LFA-1 and CD44 expression and function. J Immunol. 2005;175:7255–63.
124. Sawada T, Kimura K, Nishihara T, Onoda N, Teraoka H, Yamashita Y, Yamada N, Yashiro M, Ohira M, Hirakawa K. TGF-beta1 down-regulates ICAM-1 expression and enhances liver metastasis of pancreatic cancer. Adv Med Sci. 2006;51:60–5.
125. Gutheil JC, Campbell TN, Pierce PR, Watkins JD, Huse WD, Bodkin DJ, Cheresh DA. Targeted antiangiogenic therapy for cancer using Vitaxin: a humanized monoclonal antibody to the integrin alphavbeta3. Clin Cancer Res. 2000;6:3056–61.
126. McNeel DG, Eickhoff J, Lee FT, King DM, Alberti D, Thomas JP, Friedl A, Kolesar J, Marnocha R, Volkman J, Zhang J, Hammershaimb L, Zwiebel JA, Wilding G. Phase I trial of a monoclonal antibody specific for alphavbeta3 integrin (MEDI-522) in patients with

advanced malignancies, including an assessment of effect on tumor perfusion. Clin Cancer Res. 2005;11:7851–60.
127. Hersey P, Sosman J, O'Day S, Richards J, Bedikian A, Gonzalez R, Sharfman W, Weber R, Logan T, Buzoianu M, Hammershaimb L, Kirkwood JM. A randomized phase 2 study of etaracizumab, a monoclonal antibody against integrin alpha(v)beta(3), + or − dacarbazine in patients with stage IV metastatic melanoma. Cancer. 2010;116:1526–34.
128. Webb JR, Milne K, Watson P, Deleeuw RJ, Nelson BH. Tumor-infiltrating lymphocytes expressing the tissue resident memory marker CD103 are associated with increased survival in high-grade serous ovarian cancer. Clin Cancer Res. 2014;20:434–44.

Chapter 5
Cytotoxic T Lymphocytes and Their Granzymes: An Overview

Janis Noonan and Brona M. Murphy

Abstract There is considerable evidence that the immune system armed with deadly cytotoxic T lymphocytes (CTLs) has the proclivity to destroy cancer cells. Based on these findings, a number of cancer immunotherapies have been designed, each utilising a different approach to acquire their lethal skills. However, despite the sound rationale underlying CTL-based immunotherapies, treatment resistance remains a galling obstacle. This review provides an overview of the molecular events that inspired the development of CTL-based immunotherapies and explains some of the mechanisms by which these treatments unfortunately fail.

Keywords Cytotoxic T lymphocytes • Granzymes • T cell receptor • Apoptosis • Antigens

Abbreviations

APCs	Antigen presenting cells
CTLA-4	Cytotoxic T lymphocyte antigen 4
CTLs	Cytotoxic T lymphocytes
GzmA	Granzyme A
GzmB	Granzyme B
GzmH	Granzyme H
GzmK	Granzyme K
GzmM	Granzyme M
IFN-γ	Interferon-γ
IS	Immunological synapse
MHC	Major histocompatibility complex

Conflict of interest: The authors declare no conflict of interest.

J. Noonan • B.M. Murphy (✉)
Centre for Systems Medicine, Department of Physiology and Medical Physics, Royal College of Surgeons in Ireland, 31A York Street, Dublin 2, Ireland
e-mail: bronamurphy@rcsi.ie

B. Bonavida, S. Chouaib (eds.), *Resistance of Cancer Cells to CTL-Mediated Immunotherapy*, Resistance to Targeted Anti-Cancer Therapeutics 7,
DOI 10.1007/978-3-319-17807-3_5

PD-1 Programmed death-1
TCR T cell receptor
TNF Tumour necrosis factor

5.1 Introduction

Our understanding of the immune system and its involvement in cancer prevention and development has greatly evolved over the last century, from Ehrlich's first conception of cancer immune-surveillance to Burnet and Thomas' reformulation of his theory to the current concept of cancer immune-editing. Nowadays, it is generally accepted that by monitoring, targeting and destroying transformed cells, the immune system can function as an extrinsic tumour suppressor mechanism when intrinsic mechanisms fail. While both innate and adaptive immune responses are considered necessary for efficient cancer immunotherapy, the recognition and destruction of transformed cells relies largely on the lethal talents of cytotoxic T lymphocytes (CTLs). It is thanks to the tremendous progress that has been made in unveiling the molecular basis of CTL killer activity that new and promising therapies have emerged, such as vaccination, the adoptive transfer of tumour specific T lymphocytes, the delivery of agonist and antagonist antibodies, and the administration of granzyme-based immunotoxins. Herein, we will describe the maturation, activation and effector functions of CTLs that underlie the rationale for utilising these anti-cancer therapies. In particular, we will emphasise the role of CTLs in cancer immune-surveillance and describe some of the mechanisms by which cancer cells can evade this process, leading ultimately to cancer immune-escape.

5.2 Origin and Maturation of Cytotoxic T Lymphocytes

CTLs are the killer arm of T cells or T lymphocytes, a type of white blood cell belonging to the adaptive immune system. Like all mature blood lineages, they originate from hematopoietic stem cells, which reside almost exclusively in adult bone marrow. These precursors then enter the thymus, where T lymphocyte maturation and development occur. During their migration from the thymic cortex into the medulla, developing T lymphocytes (thymocytes) are subjected to a number of sequential signals that essentially educate them to distinguish between healthy 'self' and 'non-self', a process which in turn bestows central tolerance upon the immune system.

At the core of this 'education' lies the T cell receptor (TCR), which is responsible for recognizing and binding antigenic peptides displayed on the surface of antigen presenting cells (APCs) by major histocompatibility complex (MHC) molecules. TCRs are heterodimers composed mostly of α and β chains, both of which are encoded by pre-existing variable (V), diverse (D) and joining (J) gene segments.

Different combinations of these gene segments underlie the diverse recognition spectrum of mature T lymphocytes and give rise to a flexible immune system capable of identifying foreign invaders, such as viruses and bacteria, as well as transformed tumour cells. The TCR α chain is comprised of V and J segments only, while the TCR β chains contains all three V, D and J segments. Rearrangement of these segments is accomplished by a coordinated set of reactions, beginning with the cleavage of DNA within well-conserved recombination signal sequences (RSSs) by lymphocyte-specific recombination-activating genes (RAG1 and RAG2), and ending with the reassembly of these segments using common DNA repair mechanisms. Further TCR diversity is introduced through various deletions and insertions at gene segment junctions, a process known as junctional diversification. Together with V(D)J recombination, this gives rise to a repertoire of T lymphocytes, each with its own receptor that is structurally organised to respond to a different antigen.

To ensure these receptors are 'sensible' they undergo the life and death tests of positive and negative selection. Positive selection, which is primarily mediated by thymic epithelial cells, ensures that randomly generated TCRs are able to interact with 'self' peptides bound to either Class I or Class II 'self' MHC molecules. In this case, high affinity interactions generate a strong TCR signal that results in thymocyte survival, while the rest die by 'neglect' via apoptosis. In contrast, the process of negative selection, which is mediated largely by bone marrow-derived APCs, namely macrophages and dendritic cells, ensures that those thymocytes that bind too strongly to 'self' peptides bound to 'self' MHC molecules die by apoptosis. As a result of these life and death processes, the repertoire of T lymphocytes leaving the thymus is restricted to interactions with 'self' MHC molecules and tolerant to 'self' antigens.

The majority of developing T lymphocytes that survive the thymic selection process develop into α:β TCR expressing cells, while the rest give rise to a small population of T lymphocytes comprised of γ and δ chains. If this selection process goes awry, autoreactive T lymphocytes escape into the circulation, which may result in autoimmunity if peripheral tolerance mechanisms also fail to censor these 'self' harming cells. An equally dire outcome may arise if thymocytes gain oncogenic mutations that result in various forms of T lymphocytic leukemia.

During the maturation process, T lymphocytes also develop other specific cell surface markers, such as CD4 and CD8, which are considered T lymphocyte co-receptors since they 'co-recognize' the TCR ligands; CD4 recognises antigens bound to MHC class II molecules while CD8 recognises those bound to MHC class I. When T lymphocyte progenitors first enter the thymus from the bone marrow they are double negative for CD4 and CD8; however, following productive V(D)J recombination and functional generation of the TCR-β chain, thymocytes committed to the α:β lineage start to express CD8 and then CD4, forming a pool of double positive ($CD4^{+}CD8^{+}$) cells; these occupy much of the thymic cortex while they wait for their TCR α chains to be rearranged. Given their distinct ability to recognise either MHC class I or II molecules, it is not surprising that CD4 and CD8 play a fundamental role in the positive selection process of α:β TCR expressing thymocytes fated for survival. Those that do mature beyond the negative selection process leave the thymus and enter the periphery as single positive CD4⁺ or CD8⁺ cells, although double positive CD4⁺CD8⁺ T cells have also been described in pathological conditions and in healthy individuals [1, 2]. The expression of CD4 or CD8 on mature yet naïve α:β TCR expressing cells reflects their eventual effector function; CD4⁺ cells are mostly programmed to become cytokine-secreting helper T cells, while CD8⁺ cells are programmed to become CTLs that monitor the body, ready to destroy anything considered to be a threat to the host.

One of the early hypotheses of immune-surveillance postulated that our immune systems survey our bodies for tumours, similar to the way it scans for invading foreign pathogens. However, this theory was largely abandoned following a number of studies carried out in the 1970s that demonstrated the rate of spontaneous tumour growth in nude mice, which lack a thymus and thus possess significantly less T lymphocytes, was similar to that of their immune-competent littermates [3, 4]. We now know that nude mice retain some functional CTLs and a normal or even elevated level of natural killer (NK) cells, a type of cytotoxic lymphocyte critical to innate immunity; this almost certainly explains why these athymic animals do not show an increased incidence of spontaneous tumours. Improved mouse models of immune-deficiency have since provided the first real evidence that an intact immune system can help defend against the formation of tumour cells. For example, mice deficient in RAG2, which is needed for the rearrangement of TCR gene segments and thus the maturation of T lymphocytes, demonstrate more susceptibility to carcinogen-induced sarcomas and spontaneous epithelial tumours compared to age-matched wild-type controls [5]. While this study supports, in principle, the concept of immune-surveillance, it was also the first to highlight the paradoxical role the immune system can play in tumour cell destruction and development. Critically, the authors observed that tumour cells developing in the presence of an intact immune system are less immunogenic than those developing in immune-deficient hosts. In other words, the immune system favours the eventual outgrowth of tumours that are more adept at escaping immune detection. This finding helped to pave the way for the coining of a new hypothesis, that of 'cancer immune-editing', which emphasises the dual role of the immune system in cancer suppression and promotion [6]. Schreiber et al. [6] have since divided this process into three distinct phases, termed "elimination", "equilibrium", and "escape". Although the underlying molecular mechanisms driving these three phases have yet to be fully elucidated, we do know that one of the first responses of the immune system is to activate our T lymphocytes and arm them with effective killing machinery.

5.3 Activation of Cytotoxic T Lymphocytes

Our understanding of the mechanisms underlying CTL activation and antigen recognition has grown exponentially in recent years and this understanding has led to exciting advancements in the field of autoimmunity and cancer immunology. Briefly, as mentioned above, CD4⁺ and CD8⁺ T cells recognise antigens bound to

MHC class II and I molecules, respectively; these antigens represent a 'sampling' of cellular proteins that are brought to the surface of APCs by MHC-derived molecules. Once there, they are presented to naïve CTL precursor cells, which then scan for cellular alterations using their specific TCR. It was once thought that MHC molecules only presented antigens that were of intracellular origin; however, an alternative cross-presentation pathway also exists, whereby APCs such as dendritic cells internalise exogenous antigens bound to MHC class I molecules [7]. This process of antigen presentation occurs in the secondary lymphoid tissues and is necessary for naïve T cells to gain effector function.

An effective CTL immune response, which is mainly derived from naïve $CD8^+$ T cells, can be divided into three phases: priming, contraction, and memory formation. The priming phase follows the initial recognition of a foreign antigen and leads to extensive proliferation and expansion of that specific T cell; these develop into effector CTLs that travel to the site of infection and eliminate the infected or altered cell by inducing apoptosis and secreting effector cytokines. During the contraction phase, approximately 95 % of these CTLs are subjected to activation-induced cell death (AICD), making them short lived effector cells, while the remainder become long lived memory cells that are maintained at stable levels for years; this allows for a swift recall of the CTL response should the same antigen be encountered again.

Three signalling events are basically required for the expansion, differentiation and cytolytic activity of antigen-specific CTLs. The first, provided by the abovementioned TCR-antigen-MHC complex, takes place in the context of an immunological synapse (IS) and leads to $CD8^+$ T cell proliferation and differentiation. In this case, TCR signalling, which requires CD8 and the associated common CD3 signalling chain [8], results in the phosphorylation of the Src kinases, Lck and Fyn [9], which in turn initiate phosphorylation of the immunoreceptor tyrosine based activation motifs (ITAMs) in the CD3 complex [10] and recruitment of ζ-associated protein of 70 kDa (ZAP-70) [11]. ZAP-70 is activated by Lck and goes on to phosphorylate the adaptor protein LAT, resulting in the assembly of a 'proximal signalling complex', consisting of the adaptors Grb2, GADS and SLP-76, the guanine nucleotide exchange factor, Vav1, the Tec kinases, Itk and Txk/Rlk, and the phospholipase, PLCγ [8, 12]. Other drivers of activation include phosphoinositide 3-kinase (PI3K), which leads to activation of pyruvate dehydrogenase kinase (PDK) and subsequent activation of the Akt/PKB signalling pathway [13]; this ultimately triggers further signalling pathways, including those of NFκB, FoxO and mTOR [14, 15]. TCR-induced increases in intracellular calcium via PLCγ-mediated generation of the second messengers IP3 and DAG, as well as activation of MAPK pathways, are also critical for the activation of naïve CTL precursors [8].

Co-stimulatory molecules provide the second signalling event required to activate efficient cytolytic function. Indeed, evidence from the last decade has revealed that the ultimate fate of the T lymphocyte response, i.e. tolerance versus immunity, is dependent upon the balance of co-stimulatory and co-inhibitory signals received. The immunoglobulin (Ig) superfamily member, CD28, has long been considered the main co-stimulatory receptor involved in this process; it is constitutively expressed on naïve T lymphocytes and binds two ligands, B7-1 (CD80) and B7-2 (CD86), expressed on APCs [16–18]. Through the modification and amplification of TCR signalling, CD28 has been shown to have a broad impact on CTL function, including activation [19], differentiation [20], proliferation and survival [21], tolerance [22], memory [23], upregulation of metabolic activity [24], and upregulation of IL-2 expression [25]. Similarly, the co-stimulatory molecule, 4-1BB (CD137), a member of the tumour necrosis factor (TNF) receptor superfamily that is inducibly expressed on activated $CD8^+$ T cells, plays a crucial role in $CD8^+$ T cell proliferation [26], upregulation of anti-apoptotic genes [27, 28], prevention of AICD [29], augmentation of cytotoxicity, and production of type 1 cytokines such as IL-2, TNF-α and interferon-γ (IFN-γ) [30]. CD40, a co-stimulatory TNF family member that is expressed on APCs is involved in the priming of CTL responses [31, 32] and in the induction of IL-12, a known amplifier of CTL responses [33, 34]. Most of the evidence suggests that these molecules provide the majority of co-stimulatory signals needed for optimal $CD8^+$ T cell expansion and survival in vivo. Additional co-stimulatory molecules include the TNF receptor family members, OX-40, herpesvirus entry mediator (HVEM), glucocorticoid-induced tumour necrosis factor receptor (GITR), CD30, and CD27, as well as the B7 family member, inducible co-stimulator (ICOS). In the absence of such signals, $CD8^+$ T cells remain unresponsive or become actively tolerant to antigens.

In order to keep T cell activation in check and 'fine tune' the CTL response co-stimulation must be countered by co-inhibitory signals. Cytotoxic T lymphocyte antigen 4 (CTLA-4), a homologue of CD28, is the best described co-inhibitory molecule. In contrast to CD28 that is constitutively expressed on $CD8^+$ T cells, CTLA-4 expression is rapidly upregulated following $CD8^+$ T cell activation; the level of expression and recruitment to the IS is dependent upon the intensity of the TCR signal [35]. Like CD28, it binds B7-1 and B7-2, although its affinity for these ligands is 20–100 times higher [36]. Thus, small amounts of CTLA-4 can effectively out-compete CD28 ligand binding, leading to attenuation of the CTL response. CTLA-4 binding to B7-1 and B7-2 has also been shown to cause transendocytosis of these co-stimulatory ligands, resulting in their degradation inside CTLA-4 expressing cells [37]. Furthermore, various studies have demonstrated that reverse signalling through B7-1 and B7-2 on APCs can result in the production of indoleamine 2,3-dioxygenase (IDO), an enzyme that degrades tryptophan into by-products that inhibit $CD8^+$ T cell proliferation [38–41]. Recruitment of inhibitory proteins to the IS has also been highlighted as a mechanism of CTLA-4 action [42–44], as has reduction in the dwell time between $CD8^+$ T cells and APCs [45]. Other co-inhibitory molecules include programmed death-1 (PD-1), B7-H4, lymphocyte activating gene 3 (LAG3), T cell immunoglobulin and mucin domain containing 3 (Tim3), and CD200 receptor. Ultimately, co-inhibitory signals lead to inhibition of $CD8^+$ T cell cycle progression, survival pathways and IL-2 production.

The third signal required for the successful development of CTLs comes from pro-inflammatory cytokines such as IL-12 and IFN-α/β, released by directly activated APCs [46]. Studies have shown that $CD8^+$ T cells that expand in the absence of this third signal show poor survival, do not develop cytolytic function in vitro

[47] or in vivo [48, 49], and fail to generate a responsive memory population [46]. In other words, it appears that inflammatory cytokines underlie the immunological decision to either enforce tolerance or to produce an effective cytolytic response. Cytokine-driven chromatin remodelling seems to play an important role in the molecular mechanisms responsible for the effects of IL-12 and IFN-α/β [47–50]. Indeed, it has been demonstrated that IL-12 and IFN-α influence the expression of a variety of proteins in CD8$^+$ T cells; Agarwal et al. [50] reported that IL-12 and IFN-α regulate approximately 350 genes in common, many of which are involved in the cytolytic functions of CTLs, such as granzymes, FasL and IFNγ, as well as others involved in proliferation and co-stimulation, such as OX-40 and 4-1BB. IL-12, in particular, has been shown to promote the differentiation of effector CD8$^+$ T cells [47]. For example, Joshi et al. [51] demonstrated that IL-12-induced elevation of the transcription factor, T-bet, in responding CD8$^+$ T cells enforces an effector CTL phenotype [51], which seems to be linked to mammalian target of rapamycin (mTOR) activity [52]. Furthermore, Lee et al. [53] reported that IL-12 priming induces IL-10 expression from activated CD8$^+$ T cells, which functionally mediates the memory-generating effect of IL-12 by enhancing the survival of activated CD8$^+$ T cells. In addition, IFN-α/β signalling has been implicated in pre-sensitising naïve CTL precursor cells for the rapid acquisition of effector function upon antigen exposure [54]. More recently, it was demonstrated that sustained IL-2 signalling through the IL-2 receptor, CD25, prolongs the division of activated CD8$^+$ T cells, a signalling event that is maintained by IL-12 and type 1 IFN [55]. Countless studies have reported on the role of IL-2 in CTL activation and response, especially with regards to memory formation and CTL proliferation. Upon their initial activation, CD8$^+$ T cells are known to produce a burst of IL-2 that coincides with their extensive proliferation; however, upon the acquisition and demonstration of cytolytic activity, IL-2 production ceases and CD8$^+$ T cells are unable to proliferate in response to subsequent stimulation [56]. During this period, they must rely upon the 'help' of CD4$^+$ T cells, one of the main producers of IL-2 in the body. CD4$^+$ T cells also secrete IL-21, which is reportedly necessary for sustaining long-term effector function of CTLs, particularly during chronic viral infection when IL-2 production is decreasing [57]. A recent study also highlights the 'help' provided by IL-21-secreting CD4$^+$ T cells in promoting the survival of CD8$^+$ T cells under IL-2 deprivation [58]. Such studies enforce the importance of inflammatory cytokines in driving maximal activation of the CTL response. They also emphasise the requirement of CD4$^+$ helper T cells for CD8$^+$ T cell priming, effector function, as well as the development of CTL memory. Besides their secretion of IL-2 and IL-21, these cells provide helper affects by directly inducing CD40 co-stimulation [59] and by indirectly activating APCs through CD40–CD40L interactions [31, 60]. Of course, it must also be mentioned that a small subset of highly differentiated CD4$^+$ T cells acquire cytolytic activity, thus making them CD4$^+$ CTLs.

One of the main turning points in the field of cancer immunology was the identification of antigens expressed on the surface of naturally occurring tumours, along with the finding that cancer patients can produce T lymphocytes that are capable of both recognising and reacting to these antigens. We now know that CTLs can elicit an immune response to antigens with high tumour specificity, such as those derived from mutated genes, those encoded by cancer germ-line genes, and those of viral origin, as well as antigens with low tumour specificity (tumour-associated antigens), such as differentiation antigens and those arising from the overexpression of a particular protein. Current immunotherapy strategies in development and undergoing a clinical trial assessment owe their rationale and continuing success to both our growing understanding of the mechanisms involved in antigen recognition and TCR activation, such as those described above, as well as the identification of these vital tumour antigens. To date, there are three main immunotherapeutic strategies that have emerged as a result of such knowledge: adoptive T cell transfer, vaccination, and the delivery of antibodies that enhance the anti-tumour immune response. The former involves the isolation of tumour-specific T lymphocytes from the patient or a donor, which are then expanded ex vivo before being re-infused back into the body. This approach has seen particular success in melanoma and viral-based malignancies [61, 62], prompting attempts to utilise this method in a broader range of cancers. Furthermore, to enhance the efficacy of this approach, genetic engineering of antigen receptors on ex vivo-expanded T lymphocytes, mainly the TCR and the chimeric antigen receptor (CAR) has also been employed. For a summary of the available clinical data, see a recent review by Kershaw et al. [63]. Agonist and antagonist antibodies that target co-stimulatory and co-inhibitory molecules, respectively, have also been developed to enhance the anti-tumour response of the immune system. This approach is based on the finding that tumour cells can evade immune-surveillance by down-regulating co-stimulatory molecules, like CD80 and CD86, or by contrast, up-regulating co-inhibitory molecules, like CTLA-4 and PD-1 [64]. To date, there are two FDA approved drugs for the treatment of melanoma that are based on targeting these co-inhibitory molecules: Ipilimumab, which blocks CTLA-4, and Keytruda, an inhibitor of PD-1. Due to their success, these drugs are now in clinical trials for other types of cancer. Finally, promising pre-clinical and clinical data have emerged from new cancer vaccination therapies that employ the use of TAAs, such as CD47 and MUC1, respectively, to elicit an immune response predominated by CTLs [65, 66]. Furthermore, the potential synergy of combining vaccination with antibodies against CTLA-4 and PD-1 has also been realised. A recent study by Duraiswamy et al. [67] demonstrated that dual blockade of these co-inhibitory molecules along with tumour vaccination led to remarkable tumour rejection in mice as a result of enhanced CTL activity.

While each of these therapies adopts a different approach to induce an efficacious CTL immune response, their success relies on one common theme: the ability of CTLs to kill infected and transformed cells. Above, we have described the mechanism by which CTLs can identify these harmful cells, now we will venture to explain the process by which CTLs can kill them, and how, even when a CTL response has been elicited, tumour cells can fight back to suppress the immune response once again.

5.4 Effector Mechanisms of Cytotoxic T Lymphocytes

CTLs display their lethal talents by programming target cells to undergo apoptosis by one of at least two main effector mechanisms: death receptor ligand binding and granzyme release from specialised secretory lysosomes. Both mechanisms require cell–cell contact and can be executed within minutes of antigen recognition. The former requires the presence of death receptors on the surface of target cells and the presence of their cognate ligands on the surface of CTLs, e.g. Fas, TNF and TNF-related apoptosis-inducing ligand (TRAIL). Upon ligand-receptor binding, activation of the extrinsic apoptotic pathway is triggered and cell death occurs via the classical caspase cascade. IFN-γ secretion by CTLs, which occurs so long as TCR stimulation continues, also contributes to this event by boosting the level of Fas and MHC class I on target cells, thereby enhancing both the potential of CTLs to recognise foreign antigens and to kill tumour cells. From here-on, we will focus on the second and foremost effector mechanism of CTLs, which relies on the polarised release of cytotoxic molecules into the intercellular space and the formation of pores in the target cell; this is a tightly regulated process, designed to prevent CTLs from accidentally killing themselves as well as healthy neighbouring cells.

It takes approximately 5–8 days after antigen recognition for naïve CTL precursor cells to differentiate, proliferate and migrate to the appropriate target site. It is while these cells are differentiating into effector CTLs that pore-forming perforin and cell death-inducing granzymes are synthesised and stored. Perforin, a 67 kDa protein, is first synthesised as an inactive precursor protein in the endoplasmic reticulum (ER), then modified in the Golgi apparatus by the addition of glycans, and finally packaged into specialised secretory lysosomes as an active protein. Upon its release into the synaptic cleft, the high extracellular concentration of Ca^{2+} as well as the neutral pH of the extracellular environment promotes the binding of perforin to the target cell membrane [68], where monomers polymerise to form a range of pores, approximately 120–170 Å in diameter [69]; these in turn facilitate the delivery of granzymes in the cytoplasm. A recent study by Lopez et al. [70] demonstrated that the influx of Ca^{2+} into isolated human lymphocytes is followed by the exocytosis of perforin and the formation of pores in target cells in as little as 30 s; using time-lapse microscopy, these authors demonstrated that the initiation of pore repair occurs 20 s later and is completed within 80 s. Importantly, this short window is sufficient time for lethal amounts of granzymes to be delivered into the target cell. These particular conditions of high Ca^{2+} concentration and neutral pH, which are found in the extracellular environment but not in the secretory lysosomes, help explain why perforin doesn't subject CTLs to self-imposed toxicity.

There are 5 known human granzymes: granzyme A (GzmA), GzmB, GzmH, GzmK, and GzmM; and 11 known mice granzymes: GrzA-G and GzmK-N. The five human granzymes share an amino acid sequence homology of approximately 40 %, are structurally related to the trypsin-chymotrypsin serine protease family, and have an active catalytic site made up of key residues corresponding to histidine, serine and aspartic acids. The genes encoding these human granzymes have been mapped to different chromosomal loci, with *GzmA* and *K*, both tryptases, found on chromosome 5, *GzmB*, an aspase, and *H*, a chymase, found on chromosome 14, and *GzmM*, a metase, found on chromosome 19 [71]. Granzymes make up approximately 90 % of the secretory lysosomal mass. These proteases are expressed with a signal sequence that first directs them to the ER, where cleavage of the signal peptide produces an inactive proenzyme. Then a mannose-6-phosphate tag is added to them in the Golgi apparatus, which subsequently directs them to secretory lysosomes, where they are proteolytically activated by the lysosomal cysteine protease, cathepsin C [72]. Alternate mechanisms for granzyme activation within secretory lysosomes likely exist as well, given that some granzyme activity can be observed in CTLs derived from cathepsin C-deficient mice [73]. Within the secretory lysosomes, granzymes and perforin are found in the electron-dense central core, bound to a chondroitin sulphate proteoglycan, serglycin; this complex is thought to prevent both the oligomerisation of perforin and the diffusion of granzymes inside CTLs, while also concentrating the granzymes prior to their secretion. As with perforin, the acidic pH of secretory lysosomes keeps the proteolytic activity of granzymes at bay, although, should they leak out into the cytosol, CTLs are further protected by their intracellular expression of serine protease inhibitors, serpins [74].

Once inside the cytoplasm of target cells, each granzyme has distinct methods of promoting cell death. Thus, a cohort of cell death pathways are activated at once, which in turn enhances both the speed and efficiency of the cell death process. The ability of granzymes to act on different substrates also enhances the probability of malignant cells dying by CTLs since it ensures cell death can still occur even if one pathway to death becomes blocked. For a disease such as cancer in which apoptotic dysfunction is a major molecular hallmark, this capability of CTLs is a particularly exploitable trait.

GrzA and GrzB are the best described granzymes, with GrzB considered the most potent inducer of apoptosis and, thus, the main effector of immune-surveillance. Consequently, GzmB has received a great deal of attention with regards to developing an immunotoxin for cancer therapy. GzmB induces apoptosis by two main pathways; the first is mediated through the direct activation of caspases like -3, -7, -8, and 10, and the second is arbitrated through the cleavage of Bid [75, 76]. Caspases convey the apoptotic signal in a proteolytic cascade, beginning with the initiator caspases like -8 and -10 and ending with the executioner caspases like -3 and -7; these then propel the apoptotic signal forward by cleaving several downstream death substrates like the inhibitor of caspase-activated DNase (ICAD), poly(ADP ribose) polymerase (PARP), and the nuclear-envelope intermediate-filament protein, lamin B. These, in turn, are responsible for most of the morphological hallmarks of apoptosis, such as DNA fragmentation and membrane blebbing. Besides direct cleavage, executioner caspases can also be activated by GzmB-induced cleavage of Bid. This pathway is associated with the Bcl-2 family of proteins that govern the integrity of the outer mitochondrial membrane; briefly, cleavage of Bid by GzmB results in its truncated form, tBid, migrating to the outer mitochondrial membrane, where it promotes the release of caspase activators, like cytochrome c and SMAC/DIABLO. The presence of cytochrome c in the cytosol is necessary for the subsequent formation of the apoptosome and the downstream activation of caspase-3, while SMAC/DIABLO promotes caspase activation by inhibiting inhibitors of apoptosis (IAP) family proteins. In the presence of perforin, GzmB has also been shown to accumulate in the nucleus of target cells, where it can directly cleave substrates involved in the maintenance of DNA, like ICAD and PARP, thereby resulting in DNA fragmentation and cell death in a caspase-independent manner [77]. Similarly, GzmB can cleave cytoskeletal alpha-tubulin in a caspase-independent manner, which likely incapacitates target cells during CTL-mediated killing [78]. Lastly, the induction of reactive oxygen species (ROS) from caspase-dependent nicotinamide adenine dinucleotide phosphate (NADPH) oxidase activation has been implicated in GzmB-induced death [79]. Thus, GzmB not only has the propensity to induce cell death but it can do so at multiple levels of the apoptotic pathway.

Of course, should CTLs or GzmB-based immunotoxin therapy be successfully delivered into targeted malignant cells, these cells still have ways of preventing their demise. In such cases, immune-surveillance leads to immune-escape and subsequently to tumour development. For example, a number of GzmB-specific serpins that inhibit its activity, such as PI-9 and SPI-6, have been detected at high concentrations in tumour cells resistant to CTL-induced death [80–84]. While this may act as an obstacle to GzmB-mediated therapy, the potential use of these serpins as biomarkers for early-stage carcinomas should not go unrecognised. On the other hand, enhanced PI-9 expression has been linked to poor clinical prognosis in a number of cancer types, including large cell lymphoma [85], nasopharyngeal carcinoma [86], melanoma [87], and lung cancer [88], which may in turn be useful for predicting treatment outcome to GzmB-based therapies. Despite these serpin setbacks, GzmB is still an attractive molecule for targeted cancer treatment. In 2012, Losasso et al. [89] used computational approaches to identify GzmB mutations that affect their binding to PI-9 without significantly disturbing their enzymatic activity; in this study, the R201K mutation emerged as a particularly promising candidate for anti-tumour immunotherapy. In agreement with this finding, Schiffer et al. [90] recently reported on the anti-tumour efficacy of the R201k GzmB mutant in an in vitro and in vivo models of classical Hodgkin lymphoma; these authors used a cytolytic fusion protein technique against the Hodgkin-selective receptor, CD30, to target abnormal cells exclusively. Alternatively, down-regulation of PI-9 expression and activity in target cells has been proposed as a treatment option to overcome GzmB resistance [91]. While both approaches have great clinical potential, their success is, however, dependent upon enhanced PI-9 expression being the mechanism of cancer immune-escape. Combinatorial drug therapies have also received some positive results. Chuang et al. [92] used a perforin-CCAAT/enhancer binding protein delta (CEBPD) pro-drug to enhance levels of pro-caspase-8 and combined it with a perforin-GzmB pro-drug to activate caspase-8 and caspase-3; used together, these drugs displayed an additive effect on triggering the apoptotic pathway in prostate cancer cells [92]. Another combination therapy with potential clinical value is GzmB and ABT-737 [93]; the latter acts as an antagonist of the anti-apoptotic protein, Bcl-2, which is frequently overexpressed in cancer cells. Given that GzmB preferentially activates the mitochondrial pathway to cell death, an event that is prevented by Bcl-2, the combination of ABT-737 and GzmB may have the proclivity to sensitise Bcl-2 overexpressing cells to GzmB-induced death. Yet, one could argue on the necessity of pairing this enzyme with a selective inhibitor of Bcl-2 given its propensity to elicit multiple pathways to death. In particular, this argument may be strengthened by the findings that CTLs can overcome Bcl-2 overexpression to kill target cells [94, 95], presumably through the actions of alternative granzymes.

Unlike GzmB, GzmA induces single-stranded DNA damage rather than DNA fragmentation [96], while the cell death pathway evoked by GzmA culminates without caspase involvement and without cleavage of important caspase substrates, like ICAD [97]. Instead, this pathway to death is characterised by damage to the inner mitochondrial membrane, leading to the lethal production of ROS. Martinvalet et al. [98] provided some insight into how GzmA can accomplish this feat; their work revealed that GzmA-mediated generation of ROS leads to the induction of cell death by rapidly penetrating the mitochondrial matrix to cleave components of the electron transport chain, namely the NADH dehydrogenase (ubiquinone) Fe-S protein 3 (NDUFS3). This process of ROS production has been postulated to mediate the subsequent translocation of the ER-associated complex, SET, to the nucleus, where it induces DNA damage through single-stranded nicking [99]. Other targets of GzmA include lamins, which play a role in maintaining the structural integrity of the nuclear membrane [100], and linker histone H1, which affects chromatin organisation. A second cell death pathway evoked by GzmA that challenges these above-mentioned findings was recently described by Susanto et al. [101]; these authors used time-lapse microscopy to demonstrate that GzmA can induce a novel form of cell death characterised by a writhing "worm-like" morphology that they termed "athetosis". In contrast to previous findings, this study found that GzmA-mediated cell death was dependent upon an intact actin cytoskeleton and occurred in the absence of early mitochondrial damage and ROS production and without the distinct apoptotic feature of membrane blebbing. Their data further indicate that mitochondrial damage occurs late in the GzmA-mediated cell death process, downstream of actin cytoskeletal alterations. While certainly intriguing, additional experiments are required to validate their findings, particularly with regards to identifying GzmA substrates linked to the actin cytoskeleton. Their study does, however, support the notion that GzmA acts as a back-up cell death mechanism should the GzmB pathway to death become blocked, as demonstrated by the fact that apoptosis was induced far more than athetosis in wild-type cytotoxic lymphocytes. This suggests that GzmA-mediated cell death may be occurring at a slower pace than that of GzmB, presumably due to the ability of GzmB to rapidly activate several caspases. Thus, it may be that although GzmA contributes to the overall cell death process by targeting the actin cytoskeleton and generating ROS, ultimately the cells die by GzmB since this granzyme completes its pathway to death first. This would also explain the dominant apoptotic phenotype that is observed following CTL treatment.

To date, no intracellular inhibitor of human GzmA has been uncovered; although recently, Kaiserman et al. [102] identified Serpinb6b as a fast and efficient inhibitor of mouse GzmA. On the one hand, this indicates a possible functional divergence between the two species that may affect consistencies in research findings but it also highlights a potential clinical benefit of using GzmA-based therapies to treat cancer. Without risk of inhibition, GzmA-induced toxicity could provide an essential and uninterrupted pathway to tumour cell death. Or perhaps even better, the combined treatment of GzmA and GzmB could deliver a faster induction of tumour cell death driven mostly by GzmB but reinforced by GzmA should PI-9 expression become up-regulated or caspase-mediated cell death become blocked. In accordance with this, cells demonstrating resistance to caspase-mediated cell death, including Bcl-2 overexpressing cells, remain sensitive to apoptosis by GzmA but not GzmB [99].

However, despite the multitude of evidence indicating a role for GzmA in targeted cell death, there are many reports and suppositions that GzmA is not cytotoxic at all. The fact that human GzmA has no known intracellular inhibitor is one of the leading arguments in support of this theory. Rather, two human extracellular inhibitors of GzmA, pancreatic secretory trypsin inhibitor and serpin antithrombin III (serpinC1), have been identified, which helps to strengthen the notion that GzmA is primarily involved in the regulation of inflammation rather than cytotoxicity. Support for this theory was recently helped along by Kaiserman et al. [102]; they assessed the cytotoxicity of human and mouse GzmA and found a fivefold increase in the cytotoxicity of mouse GzmA compared to human. And yet, the EC_{50} (650 nM) was still an order of magnitude higher than that of mouse GzmB and two orders of magnitude higher than that of human GzmB. As mentioned by the authors, based on these figures alone, it is difficult to see how GzmA could function as a dedicated cytotoxin or, indeed, as a back-up to GzmB. Interestingly, Martinvalet et al. [103] found that purified human GzmA was barely active in killer cell assays while the recombinant form expressed in bacteria was cytolytic at high nanomolar concentrations and demonstrated comparable activity to GzmB; this study highlights the importance of enzyme preparation when reporting on findings from GzmA-related studies. It also proposes the possibility that purified native material potentially has reduced cytotoxicity because it contains mostly pro-enzyme not yet activated. Alternatively, the native enzyme preparation could contain an inhibitor that hasn't been identified to date. Lastly, given the above-mentioned differences in mouse and human GzmA, caution is essential when drawing conclusions from knockout mouse models or mouse models of disease. More studies on humanised cancer mouse models are needed to validate the physiological relevance of GzmA before its cytotoxic potential is cast aside.

A similar caution was recently provided by de Poot and Bovenschen [104] in their review of GzmM following findings that mouse and human GzmM display divergent and species-specific substrate specificities. The cell death pathway activated by GzmM is not completely understood, and like GzmA, there is much in the way of contradictory findings. While several studies have observed that GzmM induces apoptosis without evoking DNA fragmentation, mitochondrial perturbation, and caspase activation [105, 106], there is an equal amount of studies that have found the opposite to be true [107, 108]. Still, several intracellular substrates of human GzmM have been identified, some of which overlap with those of other granzymes. GzmM substrates include: components of the cytoskeleton such as ezrin and α-tubulin [109]; ICAD and PARP [110]; surviving [111]; nucleophosmin [106]; FADD [108]; and the DNA topology enzyme, topoisomerase II alpha [107]. A particularly interesting substrate of GzmM, and one with great clinical potential, was identified by Mahrus et al. [112], namely, the specific GzmB serpin inhibitor, PI-9. Cleavage of PI-9 by GzmM renders this serpin functionally inactive, leaving GzmB free to induce apoptotic cell death. Given the role of PI-9 in tumour resistance to GzmB-mediated therapy, a GzmM and GzmB combination therapy approach might enable CTLs to overcome this immune-escape mechanism. However, to substantiate this supposition, more work needs to be carried out in humanised mouse models, especially given the fact that PI-9 inhibition of GzmB occurs at a faster rate than its cleavage by GzmM [112]. Unfortunately, another challenge that may supersede this exciting clinical possibility comes from the discovery of GzmM specific serpins. Both extracellular, SerpinA1 and SerpinA3, and intracellular, SPI-CI and SerpinB4, serpins have been identified to date [112–114]. SerpinB4, in particular, has been shown to inhibit GzmM activity, while overexpression of SerpinB4 in tumour cells prevents GzmM-induced and NK-cell mediated cell death [114]. Thus, upregulation of GzmM specific serpins likely represents another mechanism by which tumour cells can escape death.

Far less is known about the function and molecular mechanisms of GzmK and GzmH. GzmK shares some similarities with GzmA in that they are both tryptases that can cause ROS generation, single-stranded DNA nicking, SET cleavage, and the induction of caspase-independent cell death [115]. This has led to suggestions that GzmK acts as a back-up or fail-safe mechanism for GzmA. Still, GzmK substrates that don't overlap with those of GzmA have also been identified, such as p53 and Bid [116, 117], which contends with this belief. GrzH demonstrates death-inducing similarities with GzmB, such as loss of plasma membrane potential, chromatin condensation, DNA damage, phosphatidylserine exposure, and Bid-dependent mitochondrial damage [118]. However, as with GzmA and M, these findings have been widely contradicted by other studies. For example, Fellows et al. [119] found that GzmH induces cell death independent of Bid and caspase activity and with a transient production of ROS. A study by Ewena et al. [120] recently aimed to clarify these disparities; their findings indicate that GzmH only weakly processes Bid and only at high concentrations and after a long exposure time, which suggests that this process is not central to the death-inducing capabilities of GzmH. Instead, their findings suggest that Bax and/or Bak are central mediators of GzmH-mediated cell death, although it remains unclear as to how these proteins are activated. Interestingly, they did find that GzmH, like GzmB, can directly cleave ICAD, while overexpression of Bcl-2 also significantly affected target cell death. However, unlike GzmB, they found no evidence that GzmH promotes the activation of caspases; rather, they found that the presence of caspase-3 enhanced the killing ability of GzmH without being necessary for it to occur. This caspase-independent form of cell death produced by both GzmK and GzmH might prove vital to the future development of granzyme-based immunotoxins for the treatment of cancers in which caspase inhibitors like XIAP are highly expressed.

5.5 Extracellular Roles of Granzymes

It is only in recent years that research has turned away from solely concentrating on the intracellular roles of granzymes. Now, evidence is mounting in favour of alternative perforin-independent extracellular functions that granzymes play in inflammation and extracellular matrix remodelling. How these relate to their ability to kill cancer cells has yet to be fully clarified. It is widely known that inflammation promotes tumorigenesis and yet GzmA, in particular, has been demonstrated to influence the production and processing of certain inflammatory cytokines. One can only conclude from this that the extracellular roles of granzymes might counter their intracellular tumour-cell-death promoting roles, and lead instead to tumour growth and invasion. Indeed, extracellular matrix remodelling by GzmB has been implicated in the invasion of cancer cells in urothelial carcinoma [121]. This of course fits in with Schreiber's theory of cancer immuno-editing in which the immune system promotes both host protection and tumour development. The precise timing and/or mechanism by which the immune system begins to favour one over the other needs to be elucidated to ensure CTL-based immunotherapies don't worsen rather than help the problem.

5.6 Concluding Remarks

Thanks to the remarkable unveiling of the mechanisms involved in CTL activation and tumour antigen recognition, promising therapies like vaccination, the adoptive transfer of tumour specific T lymphocytes, and the delivery of antibodies that enhance the anti-tumour immune response are now in development and undergoing clinical trial assessment, with some already FDA approved. Furthermore, due to the elucidation of the cell death pathways elicited by granzymes, administration of granzyme-based immunotoxin therapy is another avenue proving to be a potential clinical contender. Such findings and developments have validated the long-standing theory that the immune system can survey our bodies for tumours similar to the way it scans for foreign invading bodies. However, presently, it is far from being a curative treatment option. Serpin setbacks, poor reactivity of T lymphocytes against TAAs, immunosuppressive features of tumour cells, and severe side effects associated with some immunotherapy drugs have dampened the initial enthusiasm for immunotherapy-based treatments. Many of these obstacles have been addressed in this ever-advancing field, leading in turn to modification of established treatment strategies. Time will tell if they stand a chance in ensuring that tumour immune-surveillance leads only to tumour immune-elimination and never to tumour-immune escape.

References

1. Nascimbeni M, Shin EC, Chiriboga L, Kleiner DE, Rehermann B. Peripheral CD4+CD8+ T cells are differentiated effector memory cells with antiviral functions. Blood. 2004;104(2):478–86.
2. Parel Y, Chizzolini C. CD4+ CD8+ double positive (DP) T cells in health and disease. Autoimmun Rev. 2004;3(3):215–20.
3. Rygaard J, Povlsen CO. The mouse mutant nude does not develop spontaneous tumours. An argument against immunological surveillance. Acta Pathol Microbiol Scand B Microbiol Immunol. 1974;82:99–106.
4. Stutman O. Tumor development after 3-methylcholanthrene in immunologically deficient athymic-nude mice. Science. 1974;183:534–6.
5. Shankaran V, Ikeda H, Bruce AT, White JM, Swanson PE, Old LJ, Schreiber RD. IFNgamma and lymphocytes prevent primary tumour development and shape tumour immunogenicity. Nature. 2001;410:1107–11.
6. Schreiber RD, Old LJ, Smyth MJ. Cancer immunoediting: integrating immunity's roles in cancer suppression and promotion. Science. 2011;331:1565–70.
7. Joffre JP, Segura E, Savina A, Amigorena S. Cross-presentation by dendritic cells. Nat Rev Immunol. 2012;12:557–69.
8. Kannan A, Huang W, Huang F, August A. Signal transduction via the T cell antigen receptor in naïve and effector/memory T cells. Int J Biochem Cell Biol. 2012;44:2129–34.
9. Salmond RJ, Filby A, Qureshi I, Caserta S, Zamoyska R. T-cell receptor proximal signaling via the Src-family kinases, Lck and Fyn, influences T-cell activation, differentiation, and tolerance. Immunol Rev. 2009;228:9–22.
10. van der Merwe PA, Dushek O. Mechanisms for T cell receptor triggering. Nat Rev Immunol. 2011;11:47–55.
11. Wang H, Kadlecek TA, Au-Yeung BB, Sjölin Goodfellow HE, Hsu LY, Freedman TS, Weiss A. ZAP-70: An Essential Kinase in T-cell Signaling. Cold Spring Harb Perspect Biol. 2010;2(5):a002279.
12. Schouppea E, Overmeirea EV, Laouia D, Keirssea J, Van Ginderachtera JA. Modulation of CD8+ T-cell activation events by monocytic and granulocytic myeloid-derived suppressor cells. Immunobiology. 2013;218(11):1385–91.
13. Fayard E, Moncayo G, Hemmings BA, Hollander GA. Phosphatidylinositol 3-kinase signaling in thymocytes: the need for stringent control. Sci Signal. 2010;3:re5.
14. Sheppard K, Kinross KM, Solomon B, Pearson RB, Phillips WA. Targeting PI3 kinase/AKT/mTOR signaling in cancer. Crit Rev Oncog. 2012;17(1):69–95.
15. Waickman AT, Powell JD. Mammalian target of rapamycin integrates diverse inputs to guide the outcome of antigen recognition in T cells. J Immunol. 2012;188:4721–9.
16. Linsley PS, Clark EA, Ledbetter JA. T-cell antigen CD28 mediates adhesion with B cells by interacting with activation antigen B7/BB-1. Proc Natl Acad Sci U S A. 1990;87(13):5031–5.
17. Freeman GJ, Gribben JG, Boussiotis VA, Ng JW, Restivo Jr VA, Lombard LA, Gray GS, Nadler LM. Cloning of B7-2: a CTLA-4 counter-receptor that costimulates human T cell proliferation. Science. 1993;262(5135):909–11.
18. Azuma M, Ito D, Yagita H, Okumura K, Phillips JH, Lanier LL, Somoza C. B70 antigen is a second ligand for CTLA-4 and CD28. Nature. 1993;366(6450):76–9.
19. Riley JL, June CH. The CD28 family: a T-cell rheostat for therapeutic control of T-cell activation. Blood. 2005;105:13–21.
20. de Jong R, Stokkers P, Lamme E, Kool JM, Borst F, Brouwer M, Miedema F, van Lier RA. Regulation of T-cell differentiation by CD2 and CD28 accessory molecules. Immunology. 1991;74(2):175–82.

21. Boise LH, Minn AJ, Noel PJ, June CH, Accavitti MA, Lindsten T, Thompson CB. CD28 costimulation can promote T cell survival by enhancing the expression of Bcl-XL. Immunity. 1995;3(1):87–98.
22. Bour-Jordan H, Esensten JH, Martinez-Llordella M, Penaranda C, Stumpf M, Bluestone JA. Intrinsic and extrinsic control of peripheral T-cell tolerance by costimulatory molecules of the CD28/B7 family. Immunol Rev. 2011;24:180–205.
23. Boesteanu AC, Katsikis PD. Memory T cells need CD28 costimulation to remember. Semin Immunol. 2009;2:69–77.
24. Wahl DR, Byersdorfer CA, Ferrara JLM, Opipari AW, Glick GD. Distinct metabolic programs in activated T cells: opportunities for selective immunomodulation. Immunol Rev. 2012;249:104–15.
25. Thomas RM, Gao L, Wells AD. Signals from CD28 induce stable epigenetic modification of the IL-2 promoter. J Immunol. 2005;174:4639–46.
26. Shuford WW, Klussman K, Tritchler DD, Loo DT, Chalupny J, Siadak AW, Brown TJ, Emswiler J, Raecho H, Larsen CP, Pearson TC, Ledbetter JA, Aruffo A, Mittler RS. 4-1BB costimulatory signals preferentially induce CD8+ T cell proliferation and lead to the amplification in vivo of cytotoxic T cell responses. J Exp Med. 1997;186:47–55.
27. Laderach D, Movassagh M, Johnson A, Mittler RS, Galy A. 4-1BB co-stimulation enhances human CD8(+) T cell priming by augmenting the proliferation and survival of effector CD8(+) T cells. Int Immunol. 2002;14(10):1155–67.
28. Stärck L, Scholz C, Dörken B, Daniel PT. Costimulation by CD137/4–1BB inhibits T cell apoptosis and induces Bcl-xL and c-FLIPshort via phosphatidylinositol 3-kinase and AKT/ protein kinase B. Eur J Immunol. 2005;35:1257–66.
29. Hurtado JC, Kim YJ, Kwon BS. Signals through 4-1BB are costimulatory to previously activated splenic T cells and inhibit activation-induced cell death. J Immunol. 1997;158: 2600–9.
30. Wen Y, Bukczynski J, Watts T. 4-1BB ligand-mediated costimulation of human T cells induces CD4 and CD8 T cell expansion, cytokine production and the development of cytolytic effector function. J Immunol. 2002;168:4897.
31. Schoenberger SP, Toes RE, van der Voort EI, Offringa R, Melief CJ. T-cell help for cytotoxic T lymphocytes is mediated by CD40–CD40L interactions. Nature. 1998;393:480–3.
32. Ridge JP, Di Rosa F, Matzinger P. A conditioned dendritic cell can be a temporal bridge between a CD4+ T-helper and a T-killer cell. Nature. 1998;393:474–8.
33. O'Sullivan B, Thomas R. CD40 and dendritic cell function. Crit Rev Immunol. 2003; 23(1–2):83–107.
34. Disis ML, Bernhard H, Jaffee EM. Use of tumour-responsive T cells as cancer treatment. Lancet. 2009;373:673–83.
35. Egen JG, Kuhns MS, Allison JP. CTLA-4: new insights into its biological function and use in tumor immunotherapy. Nat Immunol. 2002;3(7):611–8.
36. Sansom DM. CD28, CTLA-4 and their ligands: who does what and to whom? Immunology. 2000;101(2):169–77.
37. Qureshi OS, Zheng Y, Nakamura K, Attridge K, Manzotti C, Schmidt EM, Baker J, Jeffery LE, Kaur S, Briggs Z, Hou TZ, Futter CE, Anderson G, Walker LS, Sansom DM. Trans-endocytosis of CD80 and CD86: a molecular basis for the cell-extrinsic function of CTLA-4. Science. 2011;29(332):600–3.
38. Grohmann U, Orabona C, Fallarino F, Vacca C, Calcinaro F, Falorni A, Candeloro P, Belladonna ML, Bianchi R, Fioretti MC, Puccetti P. CTLA-4-Ig regulates tryptophan catabolism in vivo. Nat Immunol. 2002;3:1097–101.
39. Fallarino F, Grohmann U, Hwang KW, Orabona C, Vacca C, Bianchi R, Belladonna ML, Fioretti MC, Alegre ML, Puccetti P. Modulation of tryptophan catabolism by regulatory T cells. Nat Immunol. 2003;4:1206–12.
40. Munn DH, Shafizadeh E, Attwood JT, Bondarev I, Pashine A, Mellor AL. Inhibition of T cell proliferation by macrophage tryptophan catabolism. J Exp Med. 1999;189:1363–72.

41. Mellor AL, Chandler P, Baban B, Hansen AM, Marshall B, Pihkala J, Waldmann H, Cobbold S, Adams E, Munn DH. Specific subsets of murine dendritic cells acquire potent T cell regulatory functions following CTLA4-mediated induction of indoleamine 2,3 dioxygenase. Int Immunol. 2004;16:1391–401.
42. Chuang E, Fisher TS, Morgan RW, Robbins MD, Duerr JM, Vander Heiden MG, Gardner JP, Hambor JE, Neveu MJ, Thompson CB. The CD28 and CTLA-4 receptors associate with the serine/threonine phosphatase PP2A. Immunity. 2000;13:313–22.
43. Parry RV, Chemnitz JM, Frauwirth KA, Lanfranco AR, Braunstein I, Kobayashi SV, Linsley PS, Thompson CB, Riley JL. CTLA-4 and PD-1 receptors inhibit T cell activation by distinct mechanisms. Mol Cell Biol. 2005;25:9543–53.
44. Marengère LE, Waterhouse P, Duncan GS, Mittrücker HW, Feng GS, Mak TW. Regulation of T cell receptor signaling by tyrosine phosphatase SYP association with CTLA-4. Science. 1996;272:1170–3.
45. Schneider H, Smith X, Liu H, Bismuth G, Rudd CE. CTLA-4 disrupts ZAP70 microcluster formation with reduced T cell/APC dwell times and calcium mobilization. Eur J Immunol. 2008;38:40–7.
46. Kratkya W, Reis e Sousab C, Oxeniusa A, Spörria R. Direct activation of antigen-presenting cells is required for CD8+ T-cell priming and tumor vaccination. Proc Natl Acad Sci. 2011;108(42):17414–9.
47. Curtsinger JM, Mescher MF. Inflammatory cytokines as a third signal for T cell activation. Curr Opin Immunol. 2010;22(3):333–40.
48. Schmidt CS, Mescher MF. Peptide Ag priming of naive, but not memory, CD8 T cells requires a third signal that can be provided by IL-12. J Immunol. 2002;168(11):5521–9.
49. Schmidt CS, Mescher MF. Adjuvant effect of IL-12: conversion of peptide antigen administration from tolerizing to immunizing for CD8+ T cells in vivo. J Immunol. 1999;163: 2561–7.
50. Agarwal P, Raghavan A, Nandiwada SL, Curtsinger JM, Bohjanen PR, Mueller DL, Mescher MF. Gene regulation and chromatin remodeling by IL-12 and type I IFN in programming for CD8 T cell effector function and memory. J Immunol. 2009;183:1695–704.
51. Joshi NS, Cui W, Chandele A, Lee HK, Urso DR, Hagman J, Gapin L, Kaech SM. Inflammation directs memory precursor and short-lived effector CD8(+) T cell fates via the graded expression of T-bet transcription factor. Immunity. 2007;27(2):281–95.
52. Rao RR, Li Q, Odunsi K, Shrikant PA. The mTOR kinase determines effector versus memory CD8+ T cell fate by regulating the expression of transcription factors T-bet and Eomesodermin. Immunity. 2010;32(1):67–78.
53. Lee JB, Lee KA, Chang J. Phenotypic changes induced by IL-12 priming regulate effector and memory CD8 T cell differentiation. Int Immunol. 2007;19(9):1039–48.
54. Marshall HD, Prince AL, Berg LJ, Welsh RM. IFN-alpha beta and self-MHC divert CD8 T cells into a distinct differentiation pathway characterized by rapid acquisition of effector functions. J Immunol. 2010;185(3):1419–28.
55. Starbeck-Miller GR, Xue HH, Harty JT. IL-12 and type I interferon prolong the division of activated CD8 T cells by maintaining high-affinity IL-2 signaling in vivo. J Exp Med. 2013;211(1):105–20.
56. Deeths MJ, Kedl RM, Mescher MF. CD8+ T cells become nonresponsive (anergic) following activation in the presence of costimulation. J Immunol. 1999;163(1):102–10.
57. Frohlich A, Kisielow J, Schmitz I, Freigang S, Shamshiev AT, Weber J, Marsland BJ, Oxenius A, Kopf M. IL-21R on T cells is critical for sustained functionality and control of chronic viral infection. Science. 2009;324:1576–80.
58. Khattar M, Miyahara Y, Schroder PM, Xie A, Chen W, Stepkowski SM. Interleukin-21 is a critical regulator of CD4 and CD8 T cell survival during priming under interleukin-2 deprivation conditions. PLoS One. 2014;9(1):e85882.
59. Bennett SR, Carbone FR, Karamalis F, Flavell RA, Miller JF, Heath WR. Help for cytotoxic-T-cell responses is mediated by CD40 signalling. Nature. 1998;393:478–80.

60. Umeshappa CS, Xie Y, Xu S, Nanjundappa RH, Freywald A, Deng Y, Ma H, Xiang J. Th cells promote CTL survival and memory via acquired pMHC-I and endogenous IL-2 and CD40L signaling and by modulating apoptosis-controlling pathways. PLoS One. 2013;8(6): e644787.
61. Dudley ME, Yang JC, Sherry R, Hughes MS, Royal R, Kammula U, Robbins PF, Huang J, Citrin DE, Leitman SF, Wunderlich J, Restifo NP, Thomasian A, Downey SG, Smith FO, Klapper J, Morton K, Laurencot C, White DE, Rosenberg SA. Adoptive cell therapy for patients with metastatic melanoma: evaluation of intensive myeloablative chemoradiation preparative regimens. J Clin Oncol. 2008;26:5233–9.
62. Heslop HE, Slobod KS, Pule MA, Hale GA, Rousseau A, Smith CA, Bollard CM, Liu H, Wu MF, Rochester RJ, Amrolia PJ, Hurwitz JL, Brenner MK, Rooney CM. Long-term outcome of EBV-specific T-cell infusions to prevent or treat EBV-related lymphoproliferative disease in transplant recipients. Blood. 2010;115:925–35.
63. Kershaw MH, Westwood JA, Slaney CY, Darcy PK. Clinical application of genetically modified T cells in cancer therapy. Clin Transl Immunol. 2014;3:e16.
64. Driessens G, Kline J, Gajewski TF. Costimulatory and coinhibitory receptors in anti-tumor immunity. Immunol Rev. 2009;229(1):126–44.
65. Tseng D, Volkmer JP, Willingham SB, Contreras-Trujillo H, Fathman JW, Fernhoff NB, Seita J, Inlay MA, Weiskopf K, Miyanishi M, Weissman IL. Anti-CD47 antibody-mediated phagocytosis of cancer by macrophages primes an effective antitumor T-cell response. Proc Natl Acad Sci U S A. 2013;110(27):11103–8.
66. Nemunaitis J, Bedell C, Klucher K, Vo A, Whiting S. Phase 1 dose escalation of ONT-10, a therapeutic MUC1 vaccine, in patients with advanced cancer. J Immunother Cancer. 2013;1 Suppl 1:240.
67. Duraiswamy J, Kaluza KM, Freeman GJ, Coukos G. Dual blockade of PD-1 and CTLA-4 combined with tumor vaccine effectively restores T cell rejection function in tumors. Cancer Res. 2013;73(12):3591–603.
68. Voskoboinik I, Thia MC, Fletcher J, Ciccone A, Browne K, Smyth MJ, Trapani JA. Calcium-dependent plasma membrane binding and cell lysis by perforin are mediated through its C2 domain: a critical role for aspartate residues 429, 435, 483, and 485 but not 491. J Biol Chem. 2005;280:8426–34.
69. Law RHP, Lukoyanova N, Voskoboinik I, Caradoc-Davies TT, Baran K, Dunstone MA, D'Angelo ME, Orlova EV, Coulibaly F, Verschoor S, Browne KA, Ciccone A, Kuiper MJ, Bird PI, Trapani JA, Saibil HR, Whisstock JC. The structural basis for membrane binding and pore formation by lymphocyte perforin. Nat Lett. 2010;468:447–51.
70. Lopez JA, Susanto O, Jenkins MR, Lukoyanova N, Sutton VR, Law RH, Johnston A, Bird CH, Bird PI, Whisstock JC, Trapani JA, Saibil HR, Voskoboinik I. Perforin forms transient pores on the target cell plasma membrane to facilitate rapid access of granzymes during killer cell attack. Blood. 2013;121(14):2659–68.
71. Chowdhury D, Lieberman J. Death by a thousand cuts: granzyme pathways of programmed cell death. Annu Rev Immunol. 2008;26:389–420.
72. Kummer JA, Kamp AM, Citarella F, Horrevoets AJ, Hack CE. Expression of human recombinant granzyme A zymogen and its activation by the cysteine proteinase cathepsin C. J Biol Chem. 1996;271:9281–6.
73. Sutton VR, Waterhouse NJ, Browne KA, Sedelies K, Ciccone A, Anthony D, Koskinen A, Mullbacher A, Trapani JA. Residual active granzyme B in cathepsin C-null lymphocytes is sufficient for perforin-dependent target cell apoptosis. J Biol Chem. 2007;176:425–33.
74. Kaiserman D, Bird PI. Control of granzymes by serpins. Cell Death Differ. 2010;17: 586–95.
75. Afonina IS, Cullen SP, Martin SJ. Cytotoxic and non-cytotoxic roles of the CTL/NK protease granzyme B. Immunol Rev. 2010;235:105–16.
76. Waterhouse NJ, Sedelies KA, Browne KA, Wowk ME, Newbold A, Sutton VR, Clarke CJ, Oliaro J, Lindemann RK, Bird PI, Johnstone RW, Trapani JA. A central role for bid in granzyme B-induced apoptosis. J Biol Chem. 2005;280(6):4476–82.

77. Thomas DA, Du C, Xu M, Wang X, Ley TJ. DFF45/ICAD can be directly processed by granzyme B during the induction of apoptosis. Immunity. 2000;12(6):621–32.
78. Adrain C, Duriez PJ, Brumatti G, Delivani P, Martin SJ. The cytotoxic lymphocyte protease, granzyme B, targets the cytoskeleton and perturbs microtubule polymerization dynamics. J Biol Chem. 2006;281:8118–25.
79. Aguiló JI, Anel A, Catalán E, Sebastián A, Acín-Pérez R, Naval J, Wallich R, Simon MM, Pardo J. Granzyme B of cytotoxic T cells induces extramitochondrial reactive oxygen species production via caspase-dependent NADPH oxidase activation. Immunol Cell Biol. 2010;88(5):545–54.
80. Ray M, Hostetter DR, Loeb CR, Simko J, Craik CS. Inhibition of granzyme B by PI-9 protects prostate cancer cells from apoptosis. Prostate. 2012;72(8):846–55.
81. Bladergroen BA, Meijer CJ, ten Berge RL, Hack CE, Muris JJ, Dukers DF, Chott A, Kazama Y, Oudejans JJ, van Berkum O, Kummer JA. Expression of the granzyme B inhibitor, protease inhibitor 9, by tumor cells in patients with non-Hodgkin and Hodgkin lymphoma: a novel protective mechanism for tumor cells to circumvent the immune system? Blood. 2002;99(1): 232–7.
82. Bots M, van Bostelen L, Rademaker MT, Offringa R, Medema JP. Serpins prevent granzyme-induced death in a species-specific manner. Immunol Cell Biol. 2006;84(1);79–86.
83. Medema JP, de Jong J, Peltenburg LT, Verdegaal EM, Gorter A, Bres SA, Franken KL, Hahne M, Albar JP, Melief CJ, Offringa R. Blockade of the granzyme B/perforin pathway through overexpression of the serine protease inhibitor PI-9/SPI-6 constitutes a mechanism for immune escape by tumors. Proc Natl Acad Sci U S A. 2001;98:11515–20.
84. Rousalova I, Krepela E, Prochazka J, Cermak J, Benkova K. Expression of proteinase inhibitor-9/serpinB9 in non-small cell lung carcinoma cells and tissues. Int J Oncol. 2010;36: 275–83.
85. ten Berge RL, Oudejans JJ, Ossenkoppele GJ, Meijer CJLM. ALK-negative systemic anaplastic large cell lymphoma: differential diagnostic and prognostic aspects–a review. J Pathol. 2003;200(1):4–15.
86. Oudejans JJ, Harijadi H, Kummer JA, Tan IB, Bloemena E, Middeldorp JM, Bladergroen B, Dukers DF, Vos W, Meijer CJ. High numbers of granzyme B/CD8-positive tumour-infiltrating lymphocytes in nasopharyngeal carcinoma biopsies predict rapid fatal outcome in patients treated with curative intent. J Pathol. 2002;198(4):468–75.
87. van Houdt IS, Oudejans JJ, van den Eertwegh AJ, Baars A, Vos W, Bladergroen BA, Rimoldi D, Muris JJ, Hooijberg E, Gundy CM, Meijer CJ, Kummer JA. Expression of the apoptosis inhibitor protease inhibitor 9 predicts clinical outcome in vaccinated patients with stage III and IV melanoma. Clin Cancer Res. 2005;11:6400–07.
88. Soriano C, Mukaro V, Hodge G, Ahern J, Holmes M, Jersmann H, Moffat D, Meredith D, Jurisevic C, Reynolds PN, Hodge S. Increased proteinase inhibitor-9 (PI-9) and reduced granzyme B in lung cancer: mechanism for immune evasion? Lung Cancer. 2012;77(1): 38–45.
89. Losasso V, Schiffer S, Barth S, Carloni P. Design of human granzyme B variants resistant to serpin B9. Proteins. 2012;80(11):2514–22.
90. Schiffer S, Hansen HP, Hehmann-Titt G, Huhn M, Fischer R, Barth S, Thepen T. Efficacy of an adapted granzyme B-based anti-CD30 cytolytic fusion protein against PI-9-positive classical Hodgkin lymphoma cells in a murine model. Blood Cancer J. 2013;3(3):e106.
91. Jiang X, Ellison SJ, Alarid ET, Shapiro DJ. Interplay between the levels of estrogen and estrogen receptor controls the level of the granzyme inhibitor, proteinase inhibitor 9 and susceptibility to immune surveillance by natural killer cells. Oncogene. 2007;26:4106–14.
92. Chuang CH, Wang WJ, Li CF, Ko CY, Chou YH, Chuu CP, Cheng TL, Wang JM. The combination of the prodrugs perforin-CEBPD and perforin-granzyme B efficiently enhances the activation of caspase signaling and kills prostate cancer. Cell Death Dis. 2014;5(5):e1220.
93. Sutton VR, Sedelies K, Dewson G, Christensen ME, Bird PI, Johnstone RW, Kluck RM, Trapani JA, Waterhouse NJ. Granzyme B triggers a prolonged pressure to die in Bcl-2

overexpressing cells, defining a window of opportunity for effective treatment with ABT-737. Cell Death Dis. 2012;3(7):e344.
94. Davis JE, Sutton VR, Smyth MJ, Trapani JA. Dependence of granzyme B-mediated cell death on a pathway regulated by Bcl-2 or its viral homolog, BHRF1. Cell Death Differ. 2000;7:973–83.
95. Goping IS, Sawchuk T, Rieger A, Shostak I, Bleackley RC. Cytotoxic T lymphocytes overcome Bcl-2 inhibition: target cells contribute to their own demise. Blood. 2008;111(4):2142–51.
96. Beresford PJ, Zhang D, Oh DY, Fan Z, Greer EL, Russo ML, Jaju M, Lieberman J. Granzyme A activates an endoplasmic reticulum-associated caspase-independent nuclease to induce single-stranded DNA nicks. J Biol Chem. 2001;276:43285–93.
97. Beresford PJ, Xia Z, Greenberg AH, Lieberman J. Granzyme A loading induces rapid cytolysis and a novel form of DNA damage independently of caspase activation. Immunity. 1999;10(5):585–94.
98. Martinvalet D, Dykxhoorn DM, Ferrini R, Lieberman J. Granzyme A cleaves a mitochondrial complex I protein to initiate caspase-independent cell death. Cell. 2008;133(4):681–92.
99. Martinvalet D, Zhu P, Lieberman J. Granzyme A induces caspase-independent mitochondrial damage, a required first step for apoptosis. Cell. 2005;22(3):355–70.
100. Zhang D, Beresford PJ, Greenberg AH, Lieberman J. Granzymes A and B directly cleave lamins and disrupt the nuclear lamina during granule-mediated cytolysis. Proc Natl Acad Sci U S A. 2001;98:5746–51.
101. Susanto O, Stewart SE, Voskoboinik I, Brasacchio D, Hagn M, Ellis S, Asquith S, Sedelies KA, Bird PI, Waterhouse NJ, Trapani JA. Mouse granzyme A induces a novel death with writhing morphology that is mechanistically distinct from granzyme B-induced apoptosis. Cell Death Differ. 2013;20:1183–93.
102. Kaiserman D, Stewart SE, Plasman K, Gevaert K, Van Damme P, Bird PI. Identification of Serpinb6b as a species-specific mouse granzyme A inhibitor suggests functional divergence between human and mouse granzyme A. J Biol Chem. 2014;289(13):9408–17.
103. Martinvalet D, Walch M, Jensen DK, Lieberman J. Response: granzyme A: cell death-inducing protease, pro-inflammatory agent, or both? Blood. 2009;114:3969–70.
104. de Poot SA, Bovenschen N. Granzyme M: behind enemy lines. Cell Death Differ. 2014;21(3):359–68.
105. Kelly JM, Waterhouse NJ, Cretney E, Browne KA, Ellis S, Trapani JA, Smyth MJ. Granzyme M mediates a novel form of perforin-dependent cell death. J Biol Chem. 2004;279(21):22236–42.
106. Cullen SP, Afonina IS, Donadini R, Lüthi AU, Medema JP, Bird PI, Martin SJ. Nucleophosmin is cleaved and inactivated by the cytotoxic granule protease granzyme M during natural killer cell-mediated killing. J Biol Chem. 2009;284(8):5137–47.
107. de Poot SA, Lai KW, van der Wal L, Plasman K, Van Damme P, Porter AC, Gevaert K, Bovenschen N. Granzyme M targets topoisomerase II alpha to trigger cell cycle arrest and caspase-dependent apoptosis. Cell Death Differ. 2014;21:416–26.
108. Wang S, Xia P, Shi L, Fan Z. FADD cleavage by NK cell granzyme M enhances its self-association to facilitate procaspase-8 recruitment for auto-processing leading to caspase cascade. Cell Death Differ. 2012;19(4):605–15.
109. Bovenschen N, de Koning PJ, Quadir R, Broekhuizen R, Damen JM, Froelich CJ, Slijper M, Kummer JA. NK cell protease granzyme M targets alpha-tubulin and disorganizes the microtubule network. J Immunol. 2008;180(12):8184–91.
110. Lu H, Hou Q, Zhao T, Zhang H, Zhang Q, Wu L, Fan Z. Granzyme M directly cleaves inhibitor of caspase-activated DNase (CAD) to unleash CAD leading to DNA fragmentation. J Immunol. 2006;177(2):1171–8.
111. Hu D, Liu S, Shi L, Li C, Wu L, Fan Z. Cleavage of survivin by granzyme M triggers degradation of the survivin-X-linked inhibitor of apoptosis protein (XIAP) complex to free caspase activity leading to cytolysis of target tumor cells. J Biol Chem. 2010;285(24):18326–35.

112. Mahrus S, Kisiel W, Craik CS. Granzyme M is a regulatory protease that inactivates proteinase inhibitor 9, an endogenous inhibitor of granzyme B. J Biol Chem. 2004;279: 54275–82.
113. Bots M, Kolfschoten IG, Bres SA, Rademaker MT, de Roo GM, Krüse M, Franken KL, Hahne M, Froelich CJ, Melief CJ, Offringa R, Medema JP. SPI-CI and SPI-6 cooperate in the protection from effector cell-mediated cytotoxicity. Blood. 2005;105(3):1153–61.
114. de Koning PJ, Kummer JA, de Poot SA, Quadir R, Broekhuizen R, McGettrick AF, Higgins WJ, Devreese B, Worrall DM, Bovenschen N. Intracellular serine protease inhibitor SERPINB4 inhibits granzyme M-induced cell death. PLoS One. 2011;6(8):e22645.
115. Zhao T, Zhang H, Guo Y, Zhang Q, Hua G, Lu H, Hou Q, Liu H, Fan Z. Granzyme K cleaves the nucleosome assembly protein SET to induce single-stranded DNA nicks of target cells. Cell Death Differ. 2007;14:489–99.
116. Hua G, Wang S, Zhong C, Xue P, Fan Z. Ignition of p53 bomb sensitizes tumor cells to granzyme K-mediated cytolysis. J Immunol. 2009;182:2152–9.
117. Zhao T, Zhang H, Guo Y, Fan Z. Granzyme K directly processes bid to release cytochrome c and endonuclease G leading to mitochondria-dependent cell death. J Biol Chem. 2007; 282:12104–11.
118. Hou Q, Zhao T, Zhang H, Lu H, Zhang Q, Sun L, Fan Z. Granzyme H induces apoptosis of target tumor cells characterized by DNA fragmentation and Bid-dependent mitochondrial damage. Mol Immunol. 2008;45:1044–55.
119. Fellows E, Gil-Parrado S, Jenne DE, Kurschus FC. Natural killer cell-derived human granzyme H induces an alternative, caspase-independent cell-death program. Blood. 2007;110: 544–52.
120. Ewena CL, Kanea KP, Bleackley RP. Granzyme H induces cell death primarily via a Bcl-2-sensitive mitochondrial cell death pathway that does not require direct Bid activation. Mol Immunol. 2013;54(3–4):309–18.
121. D'Eliseo D, Pisu P, Romano C, Tubaro A, De Nunzio C, Morrone S, Santoni A, Stoppacciaro A, Velotti F. Granzyme B is expressed in urothelial carcinoma and promotes cancer cell invasion. Int J Cancer. 2010;127(6):1283–94.

Part II
Influence of the Tumor Microenvironment on the Resistance to CTL Cytotoxicity

Chapter 6
Hypoxia: A Formidable Saboteur of the Anti-tumor Response

Meriem Hasmim, Yosra Messai, Stéphane Terry, Bassam Janji, Muhammad Zaeem Noman, and Salem Chouaib

Abstract The tumor microenvironment (TME) promotes neoplastic transformation, supports tumor growth and invasion, protects the tumor from host immunity and fosters therapeutic resistance. It is well established that tumor stroma components are engaged in an active and complex molecular cross-talk that has serious implications for immunological recognition of tumor cells in shaping the microenvironment. In this regard, a common feature of solid tumors and one of the hallmarks of the TME is at present attracting a particular and increased attention in the field of cancer immunology since hypoxic stress impacts angiogenesis, tumor progression and immune tolerance. In this chapter, we will discuss how tumors use hypoxic stress to their own advantage by activating key biochemical and cellular pathways that are important in their progression and survival and how hypoxic stress induces tumor target adaptation that compromises the effectiveness of CTL activity. In this respect, modulating hypoxia may be a good strategy to control tumor progression at different fronts.

Keywords CTL • Hypoxia • HIF • Hypoxic stress • Tumor microenvironment • Resistance to cytotoxic effectors

Abbreviations

CSC Cancer stem cells
CTL Cytotoxic T lymphocytes
EMT Epithelial-to-mesenchymal transition

No conflict statement: No potential conflicts of interest were disclosed.

M. Hasmim • Y. Messai • S. Terry • M.Z. Noman • S. Chouaib (✉)
INSERM U753, Gustave Roussy Campus, 114 rue Edouard Vaillant, 94805 Villejuif, France
e-mail: salem.chouaib@gustaveroussy.fr

B. Janji
Laboratory of Experimental Hemato-Oncology, Centre de Recherche Public de la Santé (CRP-Santé), 84, Val Fleuri, 1526 Luxembourg, Luxembourg

B. Bonavida, S. Chouaib (eds.), *Resistance of Cancer Cells to CTL-Mediated Immunotherapy*, Resistance to Targeted Anti-Cancer Therapeutics 7,
DOI 10.1007/978-3-319-17807-3_6

HIF	Hypoxia-inducible factor
MDSC	Myeloid-derived suppressive cells
TAM	Tumor-associated macrophages
TGF-β	Transforming growth factor-β
Treg	T regulatory cells

6.1 The CTL in the Context of Microenvironmental Hypoxia

Multiple efforts have been made to develop cancer immunotherapy strategies because of their unique capacity to distinguish between normal cells and neoplastic cells. The identification of tumor-associated antigens (TAAs) recognized by specific cytotoxic T lymphocytes (CTL) within solid tumors argues in favor of a role of the immune system in controlling tumor progression and has made possible their use in vaccination trials, mainly in melanoma and lung cancer [1, 2]. However, positive clinical results have been scarce most likely because of the weak immunogenicity of these TAA, the low frequency of tumor-specific T lymphocyte precursors and the resistance of tumor cells to CTL attack [3]. Therefore, the development of more efficient therapeutic vaccines inducing strong and long-lasting CTL responses still requires improved strategies to increase CTL recruitment at the tumor site and potentiate their cytotoxic activity, and sensitization of cancer cells to CTL-mediated killing. The ultimate goal of most cancer immunotherapy strategies is to induce a strong CTL response. The prevailing view is that induced CTL will eradicate tumor cells. However, this view has been seriously challenged by clinical observations showing that even if a strong and sustained cytotoxic response are induced, complex issues, due to an unfavorable tumor microenvironment resulting in an impaired lymphocyte migration and recruitment, tumor evasion and selection of immuno-resistant tumor cell variants remain [4]. Despite the significant progress during the last decade in antitumor immunotherapy and cancer vaccine approaches, there is still a need for more effective treatments to maximize cancer patients survival rates. In this regard, novel strategies for tumor target selection, vaccine design and immunostimulatory intervention are being developed in the context of the tumor microenvironment.

The restricted view of tumor progression as a multistep process as defined by the accumulation of mutations in cancer cells has largely ignored the substantial contribution of the tumor microenvironment to malignancy. It has been less than two decades since researchers have included the tumor ecosystem in their analysis of cancer development. Indeed, it is now well admitted that the environment of a tumor is an integral part of its physiology, structure and function. Its role during the initiation and progression of carcinogenesis is presently considered to be of critical importance [5], both for better understanding of the fundamental cancer biology and for exploiting this source of relatively new knowledge to improve molecular diagnostics and therapeutics.

It is now well established that the dynamic and reciprocal interactions between tumor cells, metabolites and a variety of cells from the tumor microenvironment orchestrate several events, which are critical for tumor evolution toward metastasis. In this context, many cellular and molecular elements of the tumor ecosystem are emerging as attractive targets for therapeutic approaches. Among these targets, hypoxia, which is a hallmark of solid tumors, is strongly associated with the advanced disease stage and the poor clinical outcome [6]. These are, in part, due to inappropriate local immune reaction and resistance of hypoxic tumor cells to cytotoxic treatments. In fact, most human tumors develop a pathophysiological microenvironment during growth, characterized by an irregular microvascular network and regions of chronically and transiently hypoxic cells [7]. It has become clear that hypoxia plays a crucial role in tumor promotion and immune escape by conferring tumor resistance [8], immunosuppression [9–11] and tumor heterogeneity [12], which contribute to the generation of diverse cancer invasion programs and enhanced stroma plasticity [8, 13]. Accumulating evidence indicates that tumor stroma components, including hypoxia, are engaged in an active molecular crosstalk that has serious implications for immunological recognition of target cells. Therefore, it is crucial to elucidate the effect of hypoxia on shaping the immune and the tumor cells within the tumor milieu and its functional consequences on the antitumor immune response.

6.2 Hypoxia as a Major Component of the Tumor Microenvironment

Oxygen (O2) is one of the most important elements necessary to sustain life of aerobic organisms. In fact, oxygen is essential for aerobic respiration and robust mitochondrial generation of ATP as well as to perform other critical biological processes [14]. Oxygen homeostasis is, therefore, a critical component of many physiologic and pathologic processes. Hypoxia is an oxygen deprivation condition in which tissues are inadequately oxygenated. While ambient air is 21 % O2, the majority of healthy tissues has access to 2–9 % O2. Hypoxia is therefore defined as less than 2 % O2 [15]. Hypoxia is frequently encountered in both healthy and disease states. Physiological hypoxia is associated with a range of normal processes including fetal development, adaptation to altitude, and wound healing. The presence of physiologic hypoxic microenvironments has been observed in a range of tissues including the retina, medulla of the kidney, epidermis of the skin, thymus, hypoxic niches within the bone marrow, and even regions within the spleen. Pathologic states of hypoxia are associated with intense inflammation such as within arthritic joints, atherosclerotic plaques and domains within solid tumors, which can modulate the responses of infiltrating cells including T lymphocytes. Thus, an insufficient oxygen supply in cells or tissues is also a prominent feature of a number of pathological conditions including ischemic cardiovascular disease, myocardial infarction, stroke, obesity, etc. [16]. In solid tumors, hypoxia is a major microenvironmental component (Fig. 6.1). In order to protect themselves from hypoxia, cells have developed an adaptive molecular response involving a transcriptional program regulated by the hypoxia-inducible factors (HIFs). HIF is a dimeric protein composed of an oxygen-sensitive alpha subunit (HIF-1α, HIF-2α or HIF-3α) and an

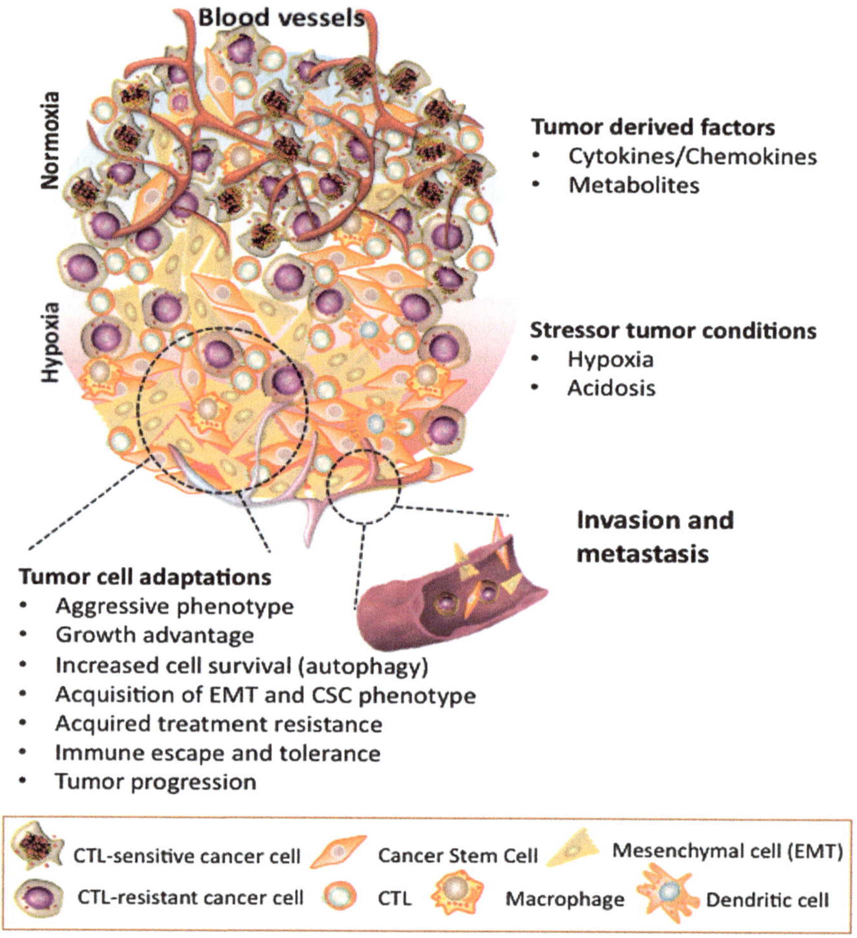

Fig. 6.1 Hypothetical model of conditioning tumor cells and the subsequent tumor evolution by the tumor microenvironment. Immune pressure and hypoxic stress shape tumor stroma and facilitate malignant progression through induction of tumor cell plasticity and the subsequent aggressive tumor phenotype. Under a favorable tumor microenvironment (normoxia), tumor cells are eliminated by CTLs. However, in a more hostile and stressor tumor microenvironment (i.e., hypoxic, immunosuppressive cytokines, acidosis), resistant tumor subtypes are generated by several intrinsic and/or microenvironmental mechanisms such as immune or stromal pressure, EMT, stemness, and morphological change. Upon acquisition of an aggressive phenotype, tumor resistant variants expand and invade surrounding tissue. Hypoxic stress induces protective autophagy in tumor cells and plays a determinant role in shaping tumor stroma and regulating the cross-talk between the tumor infiltrating lymphocytes and stromal cells. Adapted from *Chouaib et al., Crit Rev Immunol 2014*

oxygen-insensitive beta subunit (HIF-1β/ARNT). Each subunit contains basic helix-loop-helix-PAS (bHLH-PAS) domains that mediate heterodimerization and DNA binding. In the presence of oxygen, HIF-1α is hydroxylated on proline residues 402 and/or 564 by the prolyl hydroxylase domain protein 2 (PHD2), resulting in the interaction of HIF-1α with the von Hippel–Lindau (VHL) tumor suppressor protein. VHL recruits an ubiquitin ligase that targets HIF-1α for proteasomal degradation. Under hypoxic conditions, PHD2-dependent hydroxylation is inhibited leading to a rapid accumulation of HIF-1α and its dimerization with HIF-1β. HIF-1 then binds to the core DNA binding sequence 50-RCGTG-30 (R, purine (A or G)) in the promoter region of target genes, recruits co-activators and activates transcription (Fig. 6.2). In addition to PHD2-dependent hydroxylation of proline residues, oxygen-dependent hydroxylation of asparagine-803 by the factor inhibiting HIF-1 (FIH-1) blocks the interaction of HIF-1α with the co-activators P300/CBP under normoxic conditions. Both PHD2 and FIH-1 use oxygen and α-ketoglutarate as substrates and generate CO2 and succinate as by-products of the hydroxylation reaction. Their activities are therefore inhibited under hypoxic conditions. Similar to HIF-1α, HIF-2α is also regulated by oxygen-dependent hydroxylation. HIF-1α and HIF-2α are structurally similar in DNA binding and dimerization domains but differ in their transactivation domains. Consequently, they share overlapping target

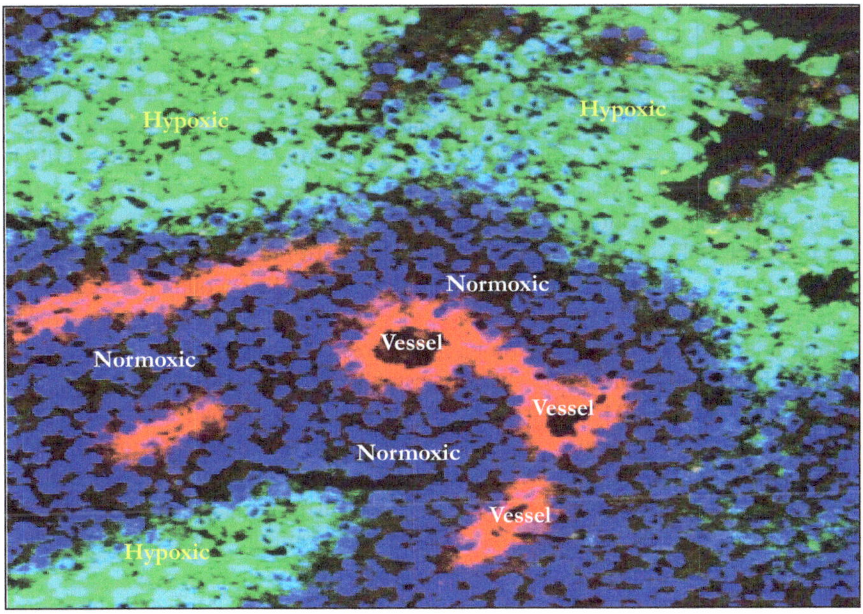

Fig. 6.2 Hypoxic and normoxic areas in solid B16-F10 tumors. Confocal microscopy analysis of hypoxic areas (pimonidazole staining, *green*), blood vessels (CD31 staining, *red*), and nuclei (ToPro, *blue*) in B16-F10 melanoma engrafted tumor sections. Adapted from *Noman et al., Cancer Res 2011*

genes in addition to the regulation by each of a set of unique targets. The genes induced by hypoxia-dependent HIF-1α and HIF-2α play important roles in the metabolism, pH regulation, cell survival, and angiogenesis. Homozygous mice for a null allele at the locus encoding HIF-1α and HIF-2α die at embryonic days 10.5 and 12.5, respectively [17], confirming the critical role of HIF's in vertebrate evolution. More recently, the conditional knockout of HIF-1α in specific types of cells has demonstrated important roles in adipogenesis, chondrogenesis, hematopoiesis, etc. [16]. Hypoxia was also demonstrated to have an important impact on immune functions. In fact, HIF-1α was shown to play an active role in the regulation of neutrophil survival, macrophage survival and differentiation, dendritic cell function and T-cell differentiation [18]. In addition, prolonged exposure of T cells to a hypoxic environment, both under physiologic and pathologic conditions, suggested that their role is likely influenced both by hypoxia exposure and modulation of HIF.

6.3 Hypoxic Stress and T Cells

6.3.1 Hypoxia Interferes with the CTL Response

The HIF stabilization in T cells is not exclusively dependent on decreased oxygen since oxygen-independent inducers of HIF have been identified in T cells. Antibody-mediated TCR/CD3 engagement results in HIF-1α stabilization via the PI3K/mTOR pathway leading to increased HIF-1α protein synthesis [19]. TCR-activated T cells also increased HIF-1α mRNA synthesis by mechanisms involving protein kinase C and Ca(2+)/calcineurin [20]. TCR-mediated HIF-1 stabilization can be further enhanced under hypoxic conditions [21]. Independently of TCR stimulation, HIF-1α mRNA is augmented when T cells are cultured in the presence of TGF-β or IL-6 alone and the combination of the two further enhanced HIF-1α mRNA levels [22]; the IL-6 and TGF-B-dependent regulations of HIF-1α mRNA involve STAT3 [22].

It is now admitted that in physiologic conditions, cells encounter oxygen levels that do not exceed 20–40 mmHg. $CD8^+$ T cells from lymphoid organs (spleen, lymph nodes) were found to harbor pimonidazole staining, indicating a hypoxic state within these organs [23]. This suggests that $CD8^+$ T cells could be found in hypoxic tissue zones. Moreover, $CD8^+$ (and $CD4^+$) T cells were found in hypoxic adipose tissues of obese mice [24]. Whether these hypoxic levels are comparable to those found in tumors has not been evaluated. Instead, $CD8^+$T cells have been found to localize to hypoxic tumors [25]; however, their distribution inside the tumors, i.e. whether $CD8^+$ T cells are inside or outside the intra-tumoral hypoxic zones, is not clearly elucidated.

The effects of hypoxia on the cytotoxic functions of $CD8^+$ T cells have been analyzed by several groups. A study by Caldwell et al. revealed that hypoxic stress potentiated the lytic capacities of $CD8^+$ T cells [26]. The authors have shown that culturing mouse splenocytes under hypoxic conditions (2.5 % pO2) induced a delay in $CD8^+$ T cell development as compared to normoxia but increased the cytolytic activity of developed CD8⁺ T cells. These CD8⁺ T cells displayed higher cell surface density of CD25, TCR/CD3 complexes and LFA-1 molecules. More recently, deletion of *Vhl* in CD8⁺ T cells, which resulted in constitutive expression of HIF-1 and HIF-2, delayed CD8⁺ T cell differentiation into effector cells but increased their cytotoxic functions which correlated with an increased expression of granzyme B [27]. These increased effector capacities were dependent on HIF-1 and HIF-2 and resulted in a better ability to inhibit tumor growth in mice.

HIF-1 was also shown to control the expression of *GZMD*, *E*, and *F* genes [28]. Whether HIF factors were able to directly regulate the expression of granzymes genes is not documented. In normoxic conditions, the effector CD8⁺ T lymphocytes were found to have constitutive levels of HIF-1 as compared to naïve CD8⁺ T cells due to activation of the mTORC pathway [28]. If they were cultured under hypoxia (1 % pO2), their HIF-1 levels increased more along with perforin expression. Targeting HIF-1β in effector CD8⁺ T cells decreased the expression of perforin but perforin is not a direct target gene of HIF-1 [28]. These results illustrate the in vitro effects of hypoxia on CD8⁺ T cell activity and suggest that hypoxic stress increases lytic functions of these cells but decreases their proliferative and differentiating capacities.

In mice challenged with tumors, hypoxic tumors were described to induce the upregulation of the costimulatory receptor CD137 at the surface of tumor-infiltrating CD8⁺ T cells in a HIF-1-dependent manner. The ligation of CD137 by agonistic antibodies increased CD8⁺ T cell activity based on in vitro increased production of IFNγ and TNFα by CD137⁺ CD8⁺ T cells and on in vivo decrease in tumor growth [25]. However, the beneficial effects of CD137 upregulation on tumor progression were found to be tumor specific since spontaneous breast carcinoma were resistant to anti-CD137 immunotherapy. Moreover, antigenic stimulation of T cells was necessary for optimal upregulation of CD137 by hypoxia, implying that, in antigenic loss variant tumors, the hypoxia-induced upregulation of CD137 may be impaired.

Therefore CD8⁺ T cells facing hypoxic conditions do not lose their cytolytic properties and even seem to be more lytic due to their upregulation of cytotoxic proteins, TCR, and adhesion molecules.

On the other hand, the effect of hypoxia on cytokine production by CD8⁺ T cells is less well determined. In vitro cultured hypoxic CD8⁺ T cells secreted less IFN-γ and less IL-2 [26]. In vitro-activated CD8⁺ T cells with constitutive HIF-1 did not alter their IFN-γ production [28]. *Vhl*-deficient CD8⁺ T cells isolated from mice expressed more IFN-γ and TNF [27]. This diversity in culture conditions and in the activation of the hypoxic signalization (hypoxia, antigenic stimulation, or VHL deletion) could have different impacts on cytokine production by CD8⁺ T cells, making it difficult to draw definite conclusions.

6.3.2 Hypoxic Stress Impacts Immune Suppression

Increasing evidence demonstrates that tumor hypoxia impacts the anti-tumor immune response by promoting local immunosuppression and inhibiting immune killing functions. Macrophages, T regulatory (Treg) cells, and myeloid-derived suppressor cells (MDSC) are the most studied immunosuppressive cells within the tumor microenvironment, and the role of tumor hypoxia in their recruitment and immunosuppressive functions is becoming evident (Fig. 6.3). Within the tumoral tissue, macrophages differentiate into tumor-associated macrophages (TAM) with the expression of TAM markers such as CD206 [29]. The exposure of TAM to tumor-derived cytokines such as IL-4 and IL-10 is able to convert them into polarized type II or M2 macrophages with immune-suppressive activities and resulting in tumor progression [29]. TAM are found to be preferentially located in tumor hypoxic areas, where they accumulate HIF-1 and HIF-2 [30]. The relative contribution of HIF-1 and HIF-2 in the regulation of gene expression in TAM is not yet completely elucidated. Besides studies reporting a role of HIF-1 and HIF-2 in the promotion of macrophage angiogenic properties [31, 32], HIF-1α was also reported to be crucial for macrophage-mediated inhibition of T cells in hypoxic conditions [33].

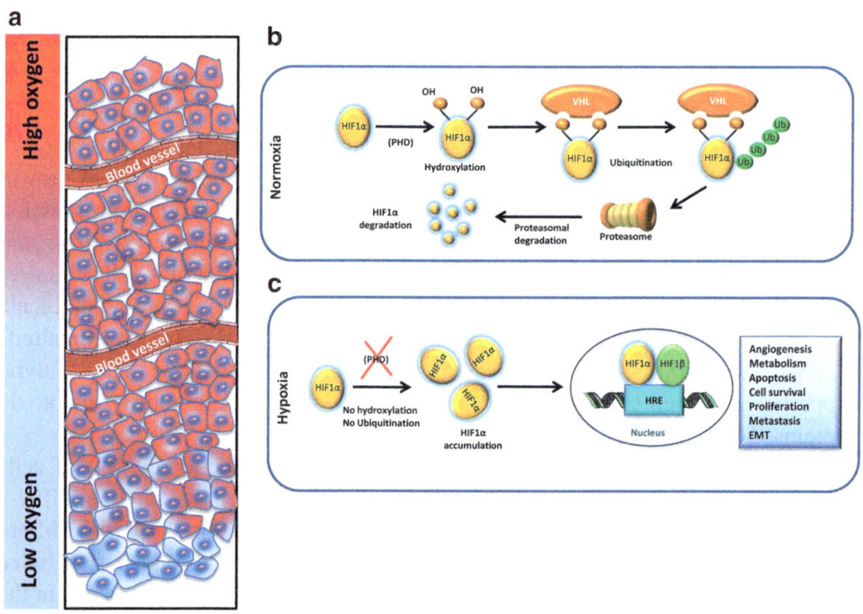

Fig. 6.3 Schematic overview of normoxic and hypoxic regulation of HIF1α. (**a**) Solid tumors contain areas of variable oxygen concentrations. Tumor cells closest to a perfused blood vessel have relatively high O2 concentrations (normoxic cells, highlighted in *red*). The O2 concentrations decline as distance from the vessel increases (hypoxic cells, highlighted in *blue*). (**b**) In normoxia, HIF1α is hydroxylated by prolyl hydroxylases (PHDs), resulting in its interaction with the von Hippel–Lindau tumor suppressor protein (VHL), which recruits an E3 ubiquitin-protein ligase that subsequently catalyzes polyubiquitination of HIF-1α, thereby targeting it for proteasomal degradation (**c**) Under hypoxic conditions, hydroxylation is inhibited and HIF-1α rapidly accumulates, dimerizes with HIF-1β and binds to the HRE (hypoxia response elements) in target genes. HIF1 thereby controls several important processes in tumor biology. Adapted from *Noman et al., CRI 2011*

In hypoxic areas of tumors, TAM also up-regulate the expression of the MMP-7 protein in hypoxic areas of tumors [34]. MMP-7 is known to cleave the Fas ligand from neighbouring cells, making tumor cells less responsive to lysis by NK and T cells [35].

MDSCs have also been demonstrated to directly promote immune tolerance [36]. In tumor bearing hosts, tumor-derived factors such as VEGF, GM-CSF, prostaglandins favour the accumulation of MDSCs in tumoral tissues and secondary lymphoid organs [37]. In these sites, MDSCs induce T cell anergy, restrain the effector phase of the $CD8^+$ T cell, and can promote antigen-specific T reg proliferation [37, 38]. HIF-1α has been directly shown to regulate the function and differentiation of MDSC within the hypoxic tumor microenvironment [39]. In this regard, our laboratory has recently shown that tumoral MDSC upregulate the expression of PD-L1 in a HIF-1-dependent manner through direct binding to the *Pd-l1* promoter. PDL-1-positive MDSC decrease effector functions of $CD8^+$ and $CD4^+$ T cells via secretion of immunosuppressive cytokines such as IL-6 and IL-10 [11]. A cross-talk between MDSC and macrophages has also been reported, proposing that MDSC down-regulate IL-12 production by macrophages and increase their own production of IL-10 in response to signals from macrophages. This interaction between MDSC and macrophages polarizes classically activated (M1) macrophages toward a type 2 immunosuppressive phenotype and accentuates the M2 phenotype of M2 macrophages, which is likely to establish an environment that skew $CD4^+$ and $CD8^+$ T cell immunity toward a tumor-promoting type 2 response [40].

Under hypoxic stress and in the presence of TGF-β, $CD4^+$ T cells upregulate Foxp3 through direct binding of HIF-1 to the Foxp3 promoter region, inducing Treg formation [41]. Tumor hypoxia also attracts Treg inside the tumor bed by impacting the cytokinic profile inside the microevironment. Facciabene et al. have recently reported that hypoxic stress increases the expression and secretion of CCL28 by tumor cells [9]. CCL28 act as a chemoattractant for Treg cells, whose immunosuppressive functions on $CD8^+$ T cells are well documented. We have also provided evidence that hypoxic stress, by inducing the embryonic factor Nanog in tumor cells, activates the expression and secretion of the immunosuppressive TGF-β by tumor cells by a mechanism involving at least the direct binding of Nanog to the TGF-B promoter. Targeting Nanog in tumor cells decreases TGF-β and reverses the intra-tumoral immune cell infiltrate by increasing $CD8^+$ T cells and decreasing macrophages and Treg numbers [10]. These findings connect stem-cell-associated factors with inhibition of the immune response in the hypoxic tumor environment.

Metabolic factors are also involved in hypoxia-mediated immunosuppression. Tissue hypoxia increases the local concentration of extracellular adenosine that acts on $CD8^+$ (and $CD4^+$) T cell A2A adenosine receptors (A2AR) causing intracellular AMPc accumulation and subsequent inhibition of activated T cells. The use of A2AR antagonists or genetic depletion of A2AR in mice challenged with tumors is able to inhibit or delay tumor growth [42].

6.3.3 Hypoxia Influences Tumor Vessel Normalization and T Cell Migration

Tumor vasculature is structurally and functionally abnormal due to the disequilibrium between pro- and anti-angiogenic factors within the tumors. Tumor vessels are leaky and tortuous with inadequate pericyte coverage and with absence or insufficient basal membrane support [7]. Blood flow is impaired resulting in decreased oxygen supply creating a hypoxic tumor microenvironment enriched with VEGF and other growth factors that, besides enhancing tumor progression and angiogenesis, modulate immune infiltration. Indeed, CCL2 released by tumor cells attract monocytes that differentiate into macrophages within the tumoral tissue [43]. Cancer cells that overexpress TGF-β are associated with increased TAM and decreased tumor-infiltrating dendritic cells in their microenvironment [44]. TGF-β is also involved in tumor recruitment of Treg cells via regulation of CCL22 production by tumor cells [45]. Within tumors, TAM are preferentially located in hypoxic zones of the tumors where they polarize to a an M2-like immunosuppressive phenotype. Tumor hypoxia induces tumor cells to secrete CCL28 which are chemoattractants for Treg cells [9]. Tumor hypoxia induces the expression by tumor cells of transcription factors such as Nanog which, via the direct activation of TGF-β expression in tumor cells, favors tumor infiltration by macrophages and Treg to the detriment of $CD8^+$ T cells [10]. In addition, the tumor microenvironment affects the cell adhesion molecule expression profile of the tumor endothelium which is implicated in the preferential infiltration of tumors by immunosuppressive cells. For example, ICAM-1, VCAM-1, or CLEVER-1 expressions on tumor vessels have been involved in the preferential trans-endothelial migration of Treg cells [46]. On the other hand, infiltrating anti-tumor T cells remain segregated at the tumor periphery. Margin et al., using adoptive transfer of GFP-labeled anti-tumor $CD8^+$ T cells into mice bearing tumors, have shown that $CD8^+$ T cells are located at the periphery of tumors [47], which are the less hypoxic zones. Blohm et al. have also shown that transferred anti-tumor $CD8^+$ T cells were at the merges of the tumor and excluded from the central avascular areas which were mostly colonized by $Gr1^+$ cells [48] (Fig. 6.4).

Targeting tumor angiogenesis using anti-angiogenic therapies results in a window whereby tumor vessels are "normalized" with increased vessel perfusion and decreased hypoxia, a concept proposed by Jain [7]. This normalization associates with better infiltration of drugs and anti-tumor immune cells. Recently, Collet et al. have shown that the use of tumor cells expressing a hypoxia-driven soluble VEGF-R2 leads to vessel normalization, improved oxygenation of tumors, and tumor growth inhibition [49], reflecting the prominent contribution of hypoxia to tumor progression. In a spontaneous model of insulinoma, deletion of the *Rgs5* gene results in normal vascular architecture in the tumoral tissue as compared to wild type mice, with reduced vessel leakiness, improved oxygenation, and clearly increased anti-tumor T cell infiltration following adoptive transfer [50]. Overexpression of the histidine-rich glycoprotein (HRG) in tumor cells reduces

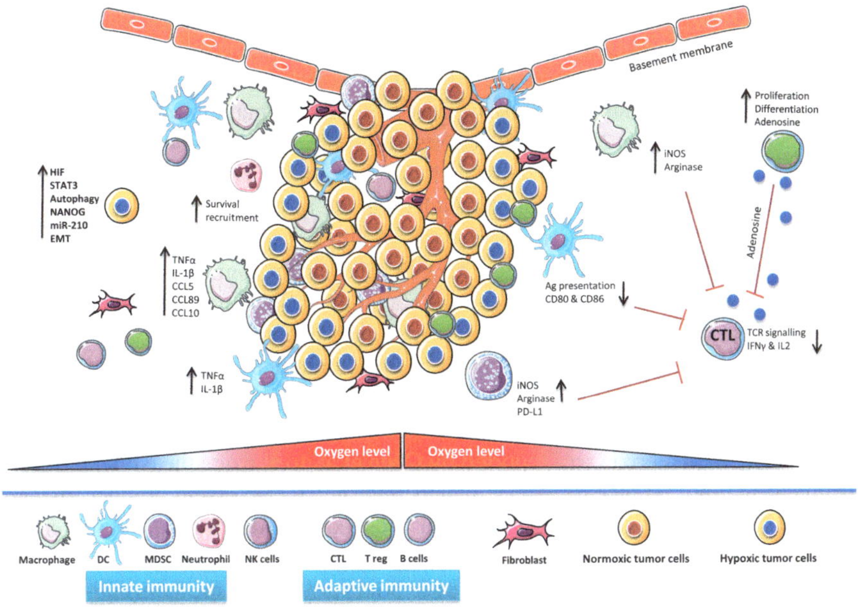

Fig. 6.4 Influence of Hypoxia on the tumor cells and on innate and adaptive immune systems. Diverse effects of hypoxia on innate immune system (Macrophage, DC, MDSC, NK and neutrophil) and adaptive immune system (CTL, T reg and B cells). In general, hypoxia amplifies the activity of innate immune cells while suppressing the response of the adaptive immune system. *DC* dendritic cells, *MDSC* myeloid derived suppressor cells, *NK* natural killer cells, *CTL* cytotoxic T lymphocyte, *T reg* T regulatory cells. Adapted from *Noman et al., CRI 2011*

tumor growth and induces vessel normalization, which associates with a skewing of TAM to M1-like macrophages and an increased dendritic cell recruitment [51]. The use of anti-angiogenic therapy to normalize tumor vessels also decreases immunosuppressive cell infiltration by reducing MDSC recruitment within the tumor bed and polarizing TAM to an M1-like phenotype [52].

6.4 Hypoxic Stress and Tumor Target Plasticity

6.4.1 Tumor Cell Heterogeneity: Cancer Stem Cells

Tumor growth is dependent on the presence of a subpopulation with stem-like properties called cancer stem cells (CSCs) within the tumor [53]. CSC are in an undifferentiated state, undergo self-renewal, and when implanted in immunodeficient mice are able to develop tumors and to re-establish the bulk tumoral heterogeneity [54]. CSC also have the property to resist conventional anti-tumor therapies [55], which makes them a probable cause of tumor recurrences after treatment.

Therefore, their eradication in the tumor is a therapeutic challenge that justifies a better understanding of their emergence and persistence in the tumoral tissue. In this regard, hypoxia and HIFs have been described to induce tumor cell dedifferentiation towards an immature phenotype and similarly to maintain tumor cells with stem-cell properties [12]. Several reports show the role of hypoxia and HIFs in promoting a stem-like phenotype through the expression of embryonic transcription factors such as OCT4, SOX2, and NANOG that are required for self-renewal maintenance in stem cells or the activation of the Notch- signaling pathway that regulates cell self-renewal and differentiation [12]. A study from Jogi et al. has shown that culturing neuroblastoma cells under hypoxia led to an increase of neural crest gene expression and a decrease of neuron lineage marker expression [56]. In glioblastoma, Mc Cord et al. have reported that glioblastoma neurospheres under hypoxia show an increased proportion of $CD133^+$ stem-like cells and the induction of embryonic markers such as OCT4 and SOX2. This was associated with a selective increase of HIF-2α [57]. Hypoxia was reported by Chen et al. to activate the Notch signaling pathway in lung adenocarcinoma, which revealed to be essential since using a Notch-signaling inhibitor under hypoxia induced cell death [58]. However, the Notch pathway can also promote cell differentiation in keratinocytes and certain neural stem cells [59, 60]. This ability of hypoxia to increase the stem cell-like subset inside a tumor cell population reflects the plasticity of the CSC compartment and the role of micro-environmental stimuli in shaping this particular subset.

Some of the effects of hypoxia on tumor cell differentiation are directly mediated by the HIFs. Li et al. reported that targeting HIF-1α and HIF-2α in $CD133^+$ glioma stem cells decreased their survival and their tumorigenic and angiogenic potentials [61]. They also reported a preferential expression of HIF-2α in $CD133^+$ glioma stem cells whereas HIF-1α was present in both the stem and non-stem tumor cells and it needed more severe hypoxia to be stabilized. Another study using human neuroblastoma cells also found a selective expression of HIF-2α in an immature cell subset, with the induction of differentiation when targeting HIF-2α [62]. Overexpression of HIF-2α in non-glioma stem cells was sufficient to induce a stem-cell like phenotype (sphere forming ability, and larger tumors after mice engraftment) [63]. HIF-2 was also shown to directly activate the expression of SOX2 [64]. At a clinical level, HIF-2α expression in patients correlated with poorer prognosis. These findings support a preferential targeting of HIF-2α for selective eradication of CSC without adverse effects on normal progenitor cells. HIF-1α is not outdone since a recent study by Wang et al. using human leukemia showed a selective activation of HIF-1α in CSC under normoxic conditions due to VHL deficiency, and that blocking HIF-1α activity was able to eliminate leukemia stem cells without affecting the normal hematopoietic stem cells [65]. Our laboratory has identified HIF-1 as the inducer of NANOG expression under hypoxic stress in non small cell lung carcinoma and in B16-F10 melanoma cells, and NANOG contributed to the acquisition of stem-cell like features under hypoxic stress [10, 66]. These studies and others describe the effects of hypoxia in converting differentiated cancer cells into stem-like cancer cells via the expression of embryonic factors or the induction of stem cell properties. The tumoral expression of transcription factors associated with stemness may also lead to tumor target resistance to CTL-mediated lysis. Our group has identified hypoxia-induced NANOG as a critical molecule involved in resistance to CTL-mediated lysis in an HIF-1-dependent manner and by a mechanism involving STAT3. Indeed, hypoxia-induced NANOG was found to be implicated in the phosphorylation of STAT3 under hypoxic stress and, thereby, in its translocation to the nucleus [66]. Of note, the constitutive expression of NANOG in cervical cancer cells also mediates resistance to lysis by CTL by a mechanism involving Akt [67].

6.4.2 Tumor Cell Heterogeneity: Circulating Tumor Cells

Circulating tumor cells (CTCs) are rare isolated cells that have shed from a primary tumor into the vasculature and invade surrounding tissues through lymphatic and blood vessels. CTCs are therefore believed to be responsible for dissemination from a primary tumor to reach distant sites forming metastases. The presence of CTCs was associated with tumor progression and metastatic disease in several epithelial tumors and they could be used as strong prognostic and predictive markers for patient's clinical outcome and survival [68]. Although the relationship between CTCs and tumor hypoxia has not been fully investigated, it is evident that the hypoxic tumor microenvironment contributes both directly and indirectly to increased metastases by regulating the number of genes. Kallergi and colleagues showed that metastatic breast cancer patients's CTCs express VEGF both at the mRNA and protein levels. More interestingly, double and triple staining experiments on CTCs showed that VEGF co-expressed with HIF-1α and VEGF2 [69]. In another study, Eliane et al., using the human triple negative breast cancer cell line MDA-MB-231, generated orthotopic xenografts in mice that produced CTCs and resulted in lung metastases. These xenografts were found to be profoundly hypoxic and produced CTCs that were captured and cultured. They examined the response of CTCs and parental MDA-MB-231 cells to hypoxia (O2 levels of 0.2 %) and compared the ability of both cell types to develop tumor xenografts in vivo. These CTCs demonstrated an altered response to hypoxia compared with the parental MDA-MB-231 cells from which they were derived and a greater aggression in vivo [70].

It is still unclear whether the hypoxia-driven CTCs resistant phenotype (EMT and CSC like) helps these cells evade the immune system. However, given that CTCs express EMT and CSC markers, both involved in a decreased sensitivity to cytotoxic immune effectors, one could expect that CTC are resistant to cell-mediated cell death as compared to the primary tumor from which they originate. Interestingly, Steiner et al showed that several CTCs exhibited mutations in key genes such as *KRAS* or *TP53* that could not be detected in the tumor. Gene expression analyses revealed both a pronounced upregulation of CD47 as a potential immune-escape mechanism and a significant down-regulation of several other pathways. This study suggests that upregulated immune-escape pathway, may be responsible for survival of CTCs in the circulation [71]. Moreover, as EMT and CTCs emergence are an interrelated process and as almost all CTCs express EMT markers, it is strongly suggested that CTCs are resistant tumor cells to T cell-mediated lysis. CTCs are reported to express survivin [72, 73], an anti-apoptotic protein that confers resistance to cytotoxic therapies and cytotoxic effectors [74]. Survivin expression in CTC may, thus, promote immune escape. Whether CTCs can resist the immune system by using the above mentioned pathways is a very interesting and unknown question. The identification of CTCs-immune-escape mechanisms as potential targets to disrupt the metastatic cascade in cancer is critical and a better understanding of the interaction between CTCs, CTLs and their microenvironment may provide new antitumoral targeted therapies.

6.4.3 Tumor Plasticity: Epithelial-to-Mesenchymal Transition

Epithelial-to-mesenchymal transition (EMT) is a complex biological process in which polarized epithelial cells lose their epithelial properties while gaining phenotypic properties of mesenchymal cells. These include a down-regulation of the epithelial (E)-cadherin expression and tight junctional proteins such as occludins, and increased expression levels of the mesenchymal cytoskeleton component, vimentin, and/or neuronal (N)-cadherin. This phenotypic conversion generally correlates with increased resistance to cell death, and enhanced migratory and invasive properties. In many types of tumors, EMT is believed to be an important step toward local invasion and subsequent tumor dissemination through lymphatic or hematogenous spread, thus allowing tumor progression. Moreover, EMT may be important in the initiation or maintenance of a subpopulation of cancer stem cells [75]. Accumulating evidence now suggests that HIF factors can directly stimulate the expression of several E-box binding transcription factors (TFs) known to regulate EMT including (SNAIL, SLUG, TWIST), and the pivotal roles of these factors have been demonstrated in cancer cells from various tissues [76]. In addition, hypoxic conditions can sustain major EMT-inducing pathways such as transforming growth factor-β, nuclear factor kappaB and Notch signaling pathways. This clearly establishes a link between hypoxia and the induction of EMT and/or maintenance of a mesenchymal phenotype. EMT can also provide cancer cells with the capacity to escape immune surveillance. Thus, immunosuppression was induced in melanoma cells transduced with SNAIL in a manner that seems to rely on inhibition of dendritic cell maturation and concomitant expansion of a population of Treg-like $CD4^+$ Foxp3+, which can result in inhibition of the cytotoxic T lymphocytes (CTL) lysis activity toward the cancer cells [77]. In line with this finding, we provided evidence that introduction of SNAIL in mammary carcinoma cells induces resistance to CTL-mediated lysis [78]. In addition, acquisition of the EMT phenotype in the cells was associated with stem-like properties and activation of autophagy. In this respect, we found that this observed autophagic state was responsible, at least in part, for the reduced susceptibility to CTL-mediated lysis. Our most recent analyses also identified the WISP2 (WNT-1-inducible signaling pathway protein 2), KLF-4, miR-7 and TGF-beta signaling as part of a regulatory network controlling EMT and stem-cell properties in breast cancer cells, that may be responsible for promoting reduced susceptibility to CTL-mediated lysis [79]. Although the link between hypoxia and EMT has been established, the precise molecular network and pathways in place have yet to be fully characterized. Clearly, future studies should explore further the potential relationships between these events and immune surveillance during cancer progression.

6.5 Hypoxic Stress Impairs Tumor Target Susceptibility Through Different Mechanisms

6.5.1 Hypoxia Confers Resistance to Tumor Targets Against Effector Cell-Mediated Killing

Several reports have clearly demonstrated that the hypoxic tumor microenvironment favours the emergence of tumor variants with increased metastatic and invasive potentials [80]. HIF's, mostly HIF-1α, play a central protective role under hypoxic conditions [81, 82]. As the hypoxic tumor variants are resistant to radiotherapy and chemotherapy, one might postulate that the exposure to low levels of oxygen may lead to adaptive responses allowing tumor cells to escape from immune surveillance. Fink and colleagues reported the inhibition of Natural Killer (NK) cytotoxicity toward liver cell lines under hypoxic conditions [83]. Hypoxia contributes to tumor cell shedding of MHC class I chain-related molecule (MIC) through a mechanism involving impaired nitric oxide (NO) signalling [84]. Thus, hypoxia is able to confer tumoral cell resistance to effector cell cytotoxicity.

Since hypoxia is a common feature of solid tumors and one of the hallmarks of tumor microenvironment, we asked whether hypoxia confers tumor resistance to CTL-mediated killing. We have shown that hypoxic exposure of tumor cells (lung cancer, melanoma and breast cancer) inhibits the CTL clone-induced autologous target cell lysis [85]. Such inhibition correlates with HIF-1α induction. While hypoxia had no effect on p53 accumulation, it induced the phosphorylation of STAT3 in tumor cells by a mechanisms at-least in part, involving VEGF secretion. Interestingly, the observed lysis inhibition was not associated with an alteration of CTL reactivity and tumor cell recognition indicating that tumor-induced priming of the autologous CTL clone was not affected after exposure of tumor target cells to hypoxia.

STAT3 contributes to malignant transformation and progression by regulating genes involved in proliferation, survival, self-renewal, invasion, angiogenesis and immune evasion [86, 87]. STAT3 is a critical modulator of the cross-talk between tumor and immune cells within the solid tumor microenvironment [88]. A STAT3 small molecule inhibitor has been reported to reverse immune tolerance in malignant glioma patients [89]. Another STAT3 inhibitor, sunitinib, positively changed the immunosuppressive phenotype in RCC tumors [90]. More interestingly, sunitinib malate, a receptor tyrosine kinase inhibitor, could reverse MDSC-mediated immune suppression and modulate the tumor microenvironment by increasing higher percentage and infiltration of CD8 and CD4 cells, thereby improving the efficacy of immune-based therapies [91].

While numerous findings provided compelling evidence that a causal relationship exists between the signal transducer and activator of transcription (STAT3) activation and HIF-1α dependent angiogenesis, their relationship in regulating tumor cell susceptibility to CTL-mediated specific lysis under hypoxic conditions is not yet known [8]. Interestingly, gene silencing of STAT3 by siRNA resulted in HIF-1α inhibition and a significant restoration of target cell susceptibility to CTL-induced killing under hypoxic conditions by a mechanism involving, at least in part, the down-regulation of AKT phosphorylation. Moreover, knock down of HIF-1α resulted in the restoration of target cell lysis under hypoxic conditions. This was further supported by DNA microarray analysis whereby STAT3 inhibition resulted in a partly reversal of the hypoxia-induced gene expression profile [85].

These above results suggest a new role for hypoxia-dependent activation of STAT3 in tumor resistance to the immune system [85]. The proposed role for STAT3 suggests that the effect of hypoxic induction of STAT3 extends beyond its critically important role in controlling cell survival and apoptosis. This points to the potential role of STAT3 in tumor adaptation induced by hypoxia. Our data suggested a new role for hypoxia-dependent induction of HIF-1 and activation of STAT3 in tumor resistance to the immune system [85]. Our studies have demonstrated that the concomitant hypoxic induction of pSTAT3 and HIF-1α are functionally linked to the alteration of NSCLC target susceptibility to CTL-mediated killing. This emphasizes that a better understanding of the tumor behavior and its interplay with the killer cells in the context of the complexity and plasticity of an hypoxic microenvironment will be a critical determinant in a rational approach to tumor immunotherapy. Although resistance of tumor targets to killer cells is likely to be regulated by multiple factors [92], we believe that the hypoxic microenvironment is a key determinant involved in the control of target sensitivity to CTL-mediated lysis. Therefore, the possibility that novel approaches targeting HIF-1α and STAT3 with potent small molecule drugs, being actively developed, may provide an exciting novel approach for cancer immunotherapy.

6.5.2 *Hypoxia-Induced Autophagy Renders Tumor Cells Resistant to Anticancer Therapies Including Effector Cell-Mediated Killing*

It is now well established that hypoxia, through HIF induction, regulates a plethora of genes involved in several biological processes to allow survival and to re-establish a normal oxygen supply. Thus, autophagy is an important pathway activated under hypoxic stress allowing tumor cell adaptation and survival by acting as a catabolic process crucial for cellular homeostasis and maintenance of cell integrity [93, 94]. It is also well established that autophagy can act as either a tumor suppressor or a tumor promoter. The different roles of autophagy in cancer cells seem to depend on the tumor type, stage, and genetic context. Indeed, autophagy clearly suppresses the initiation and development of tumors [95], however, it is considered as a key survival pathway in response to stress, and many established tumors require autophagy to survive.

Briefly, autophagy is a degradation mechanism of cell components which allows the recycling of essential amino acids, nucleotides, and fatty acids necessary for energy and macromolecule biosynthesis [96, 97]. The autophagic degradation process occurs in double-membrane vesicles called autophagosomes. These autophagosomes sequester organelles damaged proteins and cytoplasmic contents to deliver them to lysosomes for degradation [98].

The mechanisms by which hypoxia activates the autophagy pathway in cancer cells are currently well defined. Briefly, HIF-1 induces the expression of the atypical BH3-only proteins the Bcl-2/E1B 19 kDa-interacting protein 3 (BNIP3/BNIP3L) which are capable of triggering autophagy by displacing Beclin1 from Bcl-2/Beclin1 or Bcl-XL/Beclin1 complexes. Subsequently, free Beclin1 can thus induce autophagy (Fig. 6.5) [99, 100]. Recently it has been shown that, in several human cancer cell lines, hypoxia increased the transcription of the essential autophagy genes, namely, the microtubule-associated protein 1 light chain 3beta (*MAP1LC3B*) and autophagy-related gene 5 (*ATG5*) through the transcription factors ATF4 and CHOP, respectively, which are regulated by the PKR-like ER kinase (PERK, also known as EIF2AK3). MAP1LC3B and ATG5 are not required for the initiation of autophagy but mediate phagophore expansion and autophagosome formation which are the major steps in the autophagy flux. It has been proposed that the transcriptional induction of MAP1LC3B replenished MAP1LC3B protein that was turned over during extensive hypoxia-induced autophagy. Furthermore, pharmacological inhibition of autophagy sensitized human tumor cells to hypoxia, reduced the fraction of viable hypoxic tumor cells, and sensitized xenografted human tumors to irradiation. Therefore, UPR is an important mediator of the hypoxic tumor microenvironment and that it contributes to resistance to treatment through its ability to facilitate autophagy [101]. Autophagy is not only involved in tumor resistance to irradiation but also plays a critical role in chemo- and immune-therapy [102]. Collectively, these studies strongly argue that autophagy is an important mediator of the hypoxic tumor microenvironment and that it contributes to resistance to treatment.

The relationship between hypoxic stress, autophagy and specific cell-mediated cytotoxicity remains unknown. We have shown that hypoxia-induced resistance of lung tumor to CTL-mediated lysis was associated with autophagy induction in target cells. In turn, this correlated with STAT3 phosphorylation on tyrosine 705 residue (pSTAT3) and HIF-1α accumulation. Inhibition of autophagy by siRNA targeting of either beclin1 or Atg5 resulted in impairment of pSTAT3 (via inhibition of Src kinase) and restoration of hypoxic tumor cell susceptibility to CTL-mediated lysis. Autophagy-induced pSTAT3 and pSrc regulation appeared to involve the Ubiquitin Proteasome System (UPS) and p62/SQSTM1.

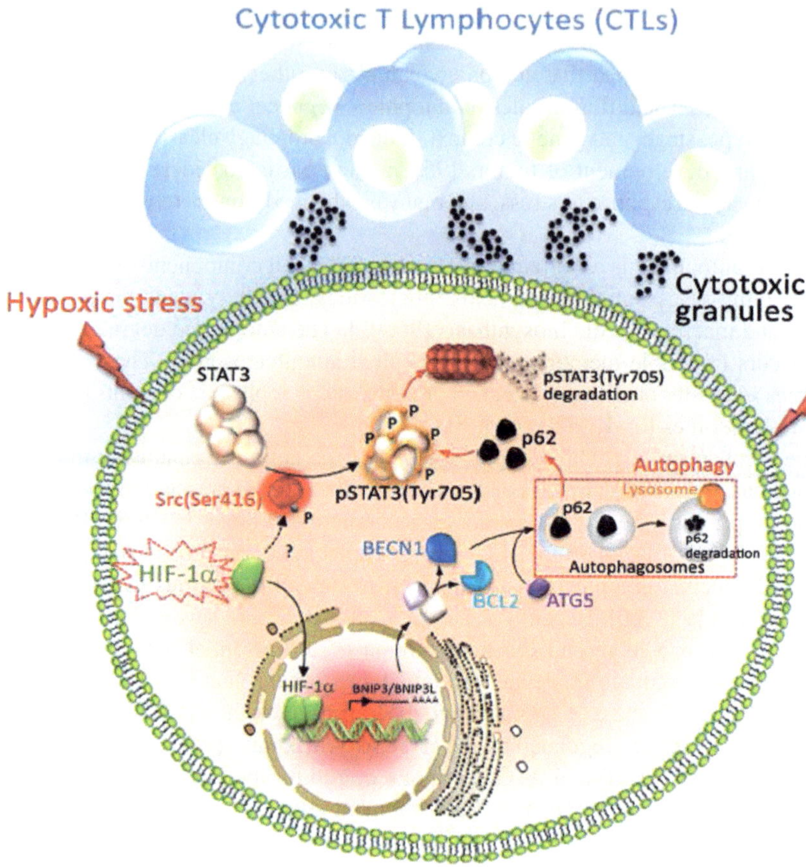

Fig. 6.5 Model of pSTAT3 regulation by hypoxia-induced autophagy in tumor cells. Hypoxic stress leads to the accumulation of HIF-1a. By an as yet undefined mechanism, HIF-1a increases the level of phospho-Src, which subsequently phosphorylates STAT3 at the Tyr705 residue. As HIF-target gene products, BNIP3 and BNIP3L are transcriptionally upregulated and compete with the BECN1-BCL2 complex. This competition releases BECN1 from the complex and then activates the autophagic machinery by recruiting several autophagic proteins including ATG5. As an autophagic substrate, SQSTM1/p62 is degraded in the autophagosomes following their fusion with lysosomes. In view of the fact that SQSTM1/p62 is involved in targeting pSTAT3 to the UPS, its degradation leads to the accumulation of pSTAT3 in cells. In autophagy-defective cells, SQSTM1/p62 is no longer degraded, and its accumulation accelerates the UPS-dependent degradation of pSTAT3. Adapted from *Noman et al., Autophagy 2012*

6.5.3 Blocking Hypoxia-Induced Autophagy in Tumors Promotes Regression

Of more interest, in vivo experiments using B16F10 melanoma tumor cells indicated that depletion of beclin1 resulted in an inhibition of B16F10 tumor growth and increased tumor apoptosis. Moreover, in vivo inhibition of autophagy by hydroxychloroquine (HCQ) in B16F10 tumor bearing mice and mice vaccinated with the TRP2 peptide dramatically increased tumor growth inhibition. Collectively, the current study establishes a novel functional link between hypoxia-induced autophagy and the regulation of antigen specific T cell lysis and points to a major role of autophagy in the control of in vivo tumor growth [8]. Beside its function as a protein degradation process, recent evidence points for a novel role of autophagy in innate and adaptive immunites [103]. Indeed, the autophagy pathway can modulate key steps in the development of adaptive immunity. In this context, it has been proposed that autophagy regulates the development and survival of lymphocytes as well as the modulation of antigen processing and presentation [104]. Autophagy induction in target cells also increases their potential to serve as immunogens for dendritic cell cross-presentation to $CD8^+$ T cells. Furthermore, the autophagy pathway can also modulate the selection and survival of some $CD4^+$ T cells in the thymus [105]. However, much still remains to be learned about the relationship between hypoxia-induced autophagy and the tumor immunotherapy. Obviously, targeting autophagy in hypoxic tumor cells may have a major impact on the cancer immunotherapy.

6.5.4 Role of Hypoxia-Regulated MicroRNA's in the Fine Tuning of the Hypoxic Response

MicroRNA's (miRNA's) are about 18–24 nucleotides, small non-coding RNAs. They negatively regulate mRNA expression by repressing translation or directly cleaving the targeted mRNA [106]. Over the past few years, the role of miRNA has expanded from their functions in the development of round worms to ubiquitous regulator implicated in several critical processes, including proliferation, cell death and differentiation, metabolism and, importantly, tumorigenesis [107].

Hypoxia, as an essential component of the tumor microenvironment, is capable of stabilizing transcription factor HIF-1α which, in turn, is capable of regulating its target genes (classical pathway of response to hypoxia), but also a lot of microRNA's (new pathways of response to hypoxia). These microRNA's regulated by hypoxia are known as Hypoxia regulated microRNA's (HRM). These HRM are capable of repressing the expression of different target genes, thereby, influencing important processes in tumor development like angiogenesis, cell survival and cell death [108, 109]. Recently it has been shown that certain HRM are capable of affecting HIF1α expression [110]. Among these HRM, miR-210 is the only miRNA consistently upregulated in both normal and transformed hypoxic cells and it is also generally recognized as a robust HIF target [111]. Mir-210 has been considered as an in vivo marker of tumor hypoxia [112]. Mir-210 has been correlated positively to poor patient's prognosis in head and neck cancers and mir-210 has been detected in the serum of breast cancer patients [113–115]. Mir-210 also participates in the hypoxic response of endothelial and neuronal cells [116]. MiR-210 has been frequently reported as the master regulator of the tumor hypoxic response [108, 109].

However, a significant number of additional miRNAs have also been linked to the cellular response to hypoxia. Although the role of miR-210 in tumorigenesis, angiogenesis, mitochondrial metabolism, cell survival and DNA repair has been well characterized [108, 109], its role in the immune response remains unknown. Of particular interest is its role in the regulation of tumor susceptibility to antigen specific killer cells.

We have reported the definition of miR-210 as a microRNA regulated by hypoxia in lung cancer and melanoma, documenting its involvement in blunting the susceptibility of tumor cells to lysis by antigen-specific cytotoxic T lymphocytes (CTL). MiR-210 was induced in the hypoxic zones of human tumor tissues. Its attenuation in hypoxic cells significantly restored susceptibility to autologous CTL-mediated lysis, independent of tumor cell recognition and CTL reactivity. A comprehensive approach using transcriptome analysis, argonaute protein immunoprecipitation and luciferase reporter assays revealed that the genes *PTPN1*, *HOXA1* and *TP53I11* were miR-210 target genes regulated in hypoxic cells. In support of their primary importance in mediating the immunosuppressive effects of miR-210, coordinate silencing of PTPN1, HOXA1 and TP53I11 dramatically decreased tumor cell susceptibility to CTL-mediated lysis. These findings show how miR-210 induction links hypoxia to immune escape from CTL-mediated lysis, by providing a mechanistic understanding of how this miRNA mediates immunosuppression in oxygen-deprived regions of tumors where cancer stem-like cells and metastatic cellular behaviors are known to evolve. More importantly, the increased expression of miR-210 also correlates with the improved survival of transplanted mesenchymal stem cells (MSC) in a rat model. By downregulating caspase-8-associated protein 2 (CASP8-AP2), a pro-apoptotic regulator of Fas-mediated apoptosis, miR-210 protects MSC from cell death. At last mir-210 is capable of regulating several cellular processes by regulating the expression of genes involved in angiogenesis, cell cycle, cell survival and tumor initiation [111]. In summary, miR-210 plays a crucial role in mediating the cellular response to hypoxia resulting in a better adaptation of hypoxic cells to the tumor microenvironment. Manipulating miR-210 within the tumor microenvironment may therefore lead to novel diagnostic and therapeutic approaches.

The mechanisms depicted in III, IV, and V sections are summarized in Fig. 6.3.

6.6 Targeting Hypoxia to Improve Current Immunotherapy Approaches

Immunotherapeutic strategies aimed at triggering or enhancing anti-tumor immunity are at present disappointing due to diverse tumor escape mechanisms from immunosurveillance [117, 118]. It has been well established now that tumor-derived changes to the patient's immune system may influence anti-cancer responses and favour tumor growth. There are increasing indications that tumor stroma including hypoxia plays a crucial role in the control of immune protection and contains many overlapping mechanisms to maintain tumor functional disorder and evasion of antigenic-specific immunotherapy. Therefore, in parallel to the efforts oriented towards the identification of potential candidate antigens for vaccination, closer attention should be paid to the complexity of the tumour ecosystem in deviating the functions of tumour infiltrating cells. It seems obvious that more could be achieved by combining therapies that tackle malignancies from multiple angles, with the tumor microenvironment conditioned to support a powerful effector arm generated by immunotherapy. Tumor immunotherapy in the clinic has not taken it into account the hypoxic microenvironment and its impact on the therapeutic outcome. Because hypoxia-inducible factor (HIF) was recently shown to regulate the tumorigenic capacity of tumor and cancer stem cells under hypoxic conditions [61], further investigation is required to demonstrate if HIF-1 is prevalent enough in human cancer to be a general target. A number of anticancer drugs have been shown to inhibit HIF's, which interfere with a range of processes including HIF-1α mRNA production (e.g. aminoflavone), HIF-1α protein synthesis (e.g. rapamycin), HIF-1α protein stabilization (e.g. HSP90 inhibitors, pleurotin), HIF-1α/HIF-1β dimerization (e.g. acriflavine), HIF-DNA binding (e.g. echinomycin), HIF transactivation (e.g. bortezomib), HIF-1α protein expression (e.g. wortmannin), and HIF-1α activity (bortezomib) [18, 119]. However, none of these drugs have been shown to specifically target HIF-1α. We believe that pharmacologic manipulation of hypoxic signaling will result in increased effector T cells, improve vaccine efficacy, and in general improving anti-tumoral immunotherapy. Whether the suppression of hypoxia may be a promising strategy that is selective for facilitating immunotherapeutic efficacy in cancer patients is at present being investigated.

6.7 Conclusion

Hypoxia is a key component of the tumor microenvironment and represents a well admitted source of therapeutic failure in clinical oncology. Accumulating data suggest that a hypoxic microenvironment promotes the acquisition of tumor resistance to cell death and protects cancer cells from antitumor immune attack by multiple overlapping mechanisms. The tremendous progress in our knowledge of the molecular mechanisms underlying tumor hypoxia will certainly provide new opportunities to better understand and target the tumor microenvironment. At present, one challenge in cancer immunology is how to shape the microenvironment to promote T cell trafficking and overcome immunosuppression. We believe that a better knowledge of the key suppressive mechanisms associated with the hypoxic tumor microenvironment should provide the means to tailor treatments and develop new combinatorial therapeutic strategies. Therefore, targeting tumor hypoxia and its associated pathways should be a new strategy to better control the emergence of resistant tumor variants and ensure more effective cancer therapies. We believe that a better knowledge of the key suppressive mechanisms associated with the hypoxic tumor microenvironment should provide the means to tailor treatments and develop new combinatorial therapeutic strategies for immunotherapy.

Acknowledgments The authors are supported by the Ligue contre le Cancer; Institut National du Cancer (INCa); Association de Recherche sur le Cancer (ARC) and INSERM.

References

1. Cormier JN, Salgaller ML, Prevette T, Barracchini KC, Rivoltini L, Restifo NP, Rosenberg SA, Marincola FM. Enhancement of cellular immunity in melanoma patients immunized with a peptide from MART-1/Melan A. Cancer J Sci Am. 1997;3:37–44.
2. Jorritsma A, Schumacher TN, Haanen JB. Immunotherapeutic strategies: the melanoma example. Immunotherapy. 2009;1:679–90.
3. Yasumoto K, Hanagiri T, Takenoyama M. Lung cancer-associated tumor antigens and the present status of immunotherapy against non-small-cell lung cancer. Gen Thorac Cardiovasc Surg. 2009;57:449–57.
4. Chouaib S, Janji B, Tittarelli A, Eggermont A, Thiery JP. Tumor plasticity interferes with anti-tumor immunity. Crit Rev Immunol. 2014;34:91–102.
5. Laconi E. The evolving concept of tumor microenvironments. Bioessays. 2007;29:738–44.
6. Harris AL. Hypoxia—a key regulatory factor in tumour growth. Nat Rev Cancer. 2002;2: 38–47.
7. Jain RK. Normalization of tumor vasculature: an emerging concept in antiangiogenic therapy. Science. 2005;307:58–62.
8. Noman MZ, Messai Y, Carre T, Akalay I, Meron M, Janji B, Hasmim M, Chouaib S. Microenvironmental hypoxia orchestrating the cell stroma cross talk, tumor progression and antitumor response. Crit Rev Immunol. 2011;31:357–77.
9. Facciabene A, Peng X, Hagemann IS, Balint K, Barchetti A, Wang LP, Gimotty PA, Gilks CB, Lal P, Zhang L, Coukos G. Tumour hypoxia promotes tolerance and angiogenesis via CCL28 and T(reg) cells. Nature. 2011;475:226–30.
10. Hasmim M, Noman MZ, Messai Y, Bordereaux D, Gros G, Baud V, Chouaib S. Cutting edge: Hypoxia-induced Nanog favors the intratumoral infiltration of regulatory T cells and macrophages via direct regulation of TGF-beta1. J Immunol. 2013;191:5802–6.
11. Noman MZ, Desantis G, Janji B, Hasmim M, Karray S, Dessen P, Bronte V, Chouaib S. PD-L1 is a novel direct target of HIF-1alpha, and its blockade under hypoxia enhanced MDSC-mediated T cell activation. J Exp Med. 2014;211:781–90.
12. Keith B, Simon MC. Hypoxia-inducible factors, stem cells, and cancer. Cell. 2007;129: 465–72.
13. Chouaib S, Messai Y, Couve S, Escudier B, Hasmim M, Noman MZ. Hypoxia promotes tumor growth in linking angiogenesis to immune escape. Front Immunol. 2012;3:21.
14. Ruthenborg RJ, Ban JJ, Wazir A, Takeda N, Kim JW. Regulation of wound healing and fibrosis by hypoxia and hypoxia-inducible factor-1. Mol Cells. 2014;37:637–43.
15. Shay JE, Celeste SM. Hypoxia-inducible factors: crosstalk between inflammation and metabolism. Semin Cell Dev Biol. 2012;23:389–94.
16. Semenza GL. Hypoxia-inducible factors in physiology and medicine. Cell. 2012;148: 399–408.
17. Iyer NV, Kotch LE, Agani F, Leung SW, Laughner E, Wenger RH, Gassmann M, Gearhart JD, Lawler AM, Yu AY, Semenza GL. Cellular and developmental control of O2 homeostasis by hypoxia-inducible factor 1 alpha. Genes Dev. 1998;12:149–62.
18. Scholz CC, Taylor CT. Targeting the HIF pathway in inflammation and immunity. Curr Opin Pharmacol. 2013;13:646–53.
19. Nakamura H, Makino Y, Okamoto K, Poellinger L, Ohnuma K, Morimoto C, Tanaka H. TCR engagement increases hypoxia-inducible factor-1 alpha protein synthesis via rapamycin-sensitive pathway under hypoxic conditions in human peripheral T cells. J Immunol. 2005; 174:7592–9.

20. Lukashev D, Caldwell C, Ohta A, Chen P, Sitkovsky M. Differential regulation of two alternatively spliced isoforms of hypoxia-inducible factor-1 alpha in activated T lymphocytes. J Biol Chem. 2001;276:48754–63.
21. Makino Y, Nakamura H, Ikeda E, Ohnuma K, Yamauchi K, Yabe Y, Poellinger L, Okada Y, Morimoto C, Tanaka H. Hypoxia-inducible factor regulates survival of antigen receptor-driven T cells. J Immunol. 2003;171:6534–40.
22. Dang EV, Barbi J, Yang HY, Jinasena D, Yu H, Zheng Y, Bordman Z, Fu J, Kim Y, Yen HR, Luo W, Zeller K, Shimoda L, Topalian SL, Semenza GL, Dang CV, Pardoll DM, Pan F. Control of T(H)17/T(reg) balance by hypoxia-inducible factor 1. Cell. 2011;146:772–84.
23. Ohta A, Diwanji R, Kini R, Subramanian M, Sitkovsky M. In vivo T cell activation in lymphoid tissues is inhibited in the oxygen-poor microenvironment. Front Immunol. 2011;2:27.
24. Rausch ME, Weisberg S, Vardhana P, Tortoriello DV. Obesity in C57BL/6J mice is characterized by adipose tissue hypoxia and cytotoxic T-cell infiltration. Int J Obes (Lond). 2008;32:451–63.
25. Palazon A, Martinez-Forero I, Teijeira A, Morales-Kastresana A, Alfaro C, Sanmamed MF, Perez-Gracia JL, Penuelas I, Hervas-Stubbs S, Rouzaut A, de Landázuri MO, Jure-Kunkel M, Aragonés J, Melero I. The HIF-1alpha hypoxia response in tumor-infiltrating T lymphocytes induces functional CD137 (4-1BB) for immunotherapy. Cancer Discov. 2012;2:608–23.
26. Caldwell CC, Kojima H, Lukashev D, Armstrong J, Farber M, Apasov SG, Sitkovsky MV. Differential effects of physiologically relevant hypoxic conditions on T lymphocyte development and effector functions. J Immunol. 2001;167:6140–9.
27. Doedens AL, Phan AT, Stradner MH, Fujimoto JK, Nguyen JV, Yang E, Johnson RS, Goldrath AW. Hypoxia-inducible factors enhance the effector responses of CD8(+) T cells to persistent antigen. Nat Immunol. 2013;14:1173–82.
28. Finlay DK, Rosenzweig E, Sinclair LV, Feijoo-Carnero C, Hukelmann JL, Rolf J, Panteleyev AA, Okkenhaug K, Cantrell DA. PDK1 regulation of mTOR and hypoxia-inducible factor 1 integrate metabolism and migration of CD8+ T cells. J Exp Med. 2012;209:2441–53.
29. Mantovani A, Sozzani S, Locati M, Allavena P, Sica A. Macrophage polarization: tumor-associated macrophages as a paradigm for polarized M2 mononuclear phagocytes. Trends Immunol. 2002;23:549–55.
30. Lewis JS, Landers RJ, Underwood JC, Harris AL, Lewis CE. Expression of vascular endothelial growth factor by macrophages is up-regulated in poorly vascularized areas of breast carcinomas. J Pathol. 2000;192:150–8.
31. White JR, Harris RA, Lee SR, Craigon MH, Binley K, Price T, Beard GL, Mundy CR, Naylor S. Genetic amplification of the transcriptional response to hypoxia as a novel means of identifying regulators of angiogenesis. Genomics. 2004;83:1–8.
32. Werno C, Menrad H, Weigert A, Dehne N, Goerdt S, Schledzewski K, Kzhyshkowska J, Brune B. Knockout of HIF-1alpha in tumor-associated macrophages enhances M2 polarization and attenuates their pro-angiogenic responses. Carcinogenesis. 2010;31:1863–72.
33. Doedens AL, Stockmann C, Rubinstein MP, Liao D, Zhang N, DeNardo DG, Coussens LM, Karin M, Goldrath AW, Johnson RS. Macrophage expression of hypoxia-inducible factor-1 alpha suppresses T-cell function and promotes tumor progression. Cancer Res. 2010; 70:7465–75.
34. Burke B, Giannoudis A, Corke KP, Gill D, Wells M, Ziegler-Heitbrock L, Lewis CE. Hypoxia-induced gene expression in human macrophages: implications for ischemic tissues and hypoxia-regulated gene therapy. Am J Pathol. 2003;163:1233–43.
35. Fingleton B, Vargo-Gogola T, Crawford HC, Matrisian LM. Matrilysin [MMP-7] expression selects for cells with reduced sensitivity to apoptosis. Neoplasia. 2001;3:459–68.
36. Gabrilovich DI, Nagaraj S. Myeloid-derived suppressor cells as regulators of the immune system. Nat Rev Immunol. 2009;9:162–74.
37. Gabrilovich D. Mechanisms and functional significance of tumour-induced dendritic-cell defects. Nat Rev Immunol. 2004;4:941–52.

38. Serafini P, Mgebroff S, Noonan K, Borrello I. Myeloid-derived suppressor cells promote cross-tolerance in B-cell lymphoma by expanding regulatory T cells. Cancer Res. 2008;68: 5439–49.
39. Corzo CA, Condamine T, Lu L, Cotter MJ, Youn JI, Cheng P, Cho HI, Celis E, Quiceno DG, Padhya T, McCaffrey TV, McCaffrey JC, Gabrilovich DI. HIF-1alpha regulates function and differentiation of myeloid-derived suppressor cells in the tumor microenvironment. J Exp Med. 2010;207:2439–53.
40. Trinchieri G. Interleukin-12 and the regulation of innate resistance and adaptive immunity. Nat Rev Immunol. 2003;3:133–46.
41. Clambey ET, McNamee EN, Westrich JA, Glover LE, Campbell EL, Jedlicka P, de Zoeten EF, Cambier JC, Stenmark KR, Colgan SP, Eltzschig HK. Hypoxia-inducible factor-1 alpha-dependent induction of FoxP3 drives regulatory T-cell abundance and function during inflammatory hypoxia of the mucosa. Proc Natl Acad Sci U S A. 2012;109:E2784–93.
42. Sitkovsky MV, Kjaergaard J, Lukashev D, Ohta A. Hypoxia-adenosinergic immunosuppression: tumor protection by T regulatory cells and cancerous tissue hypoxia. Clin Cancer Res. 2008;14:5947–52.
43. Bailey C, Negus R, Morris A, Ziprin P, Goldin R, Allavena P, Peck D, Darzi A. Chemokine expression is associated with the accumulation of tumour associated macrophages (TAMs) and progression in human colorectal cancer. Clin Exp Metastasis. 2007;24:121–30.
44. Byrne SN, Knox MC, Halliday GM. TGFbeta is responsible for skin tumour infiltration by macrophages enabling the tumours to escape immune destruction. Immunol Cell Biol. 2008;86:92–7.
45. Yang P, Li QJ, Feng Y, Zhang Y, Markowitz GJ, Ning S, Deng Y, Zhao J, Jiang S, Yuan Y, Wang HY, Cheng SQ, Xie D, Wang XF. TGF-beta-miR-34a-CCL22 signaling-induced Treg cell recruitment promotes venous metastases of HBV-positive hepatocellular carcinoma. Cancer Cell. 2012;22:291–303.
46. Mauge L, Terme M, Tartour E, Helley D. Control of the adaptive immune response by tumor vasculature. Front Oncol. 2014;4:61.
47. Engelhardt JJ, Boldajipour B, Beemiller P, Pandurangi P, Sorensen C, Werb Z, Egeblad M, Krummel MF. Marginating dendritic cells of the tumor microenvironment cross-present tumor antigens and stably engage tumor-specific T cells. Cancer Cell. 2012;21:402–17.
48. Blohm U, Potthoff D, van der Kogel AJ, Pircher H. Solid tumors "melt" from the inside after successful CD8 T cell attack. Eur J Immunol. 2006;36:468–77.
49. Collet G, Lamerant-Fayel N, Tertil M, El Hafny-Rahbi B, Stepniewski J, Guichard A, Foucault-Collet A, Klimkiewicz K, Petoud S, Matejuk A, Grillon C, Jozkowicz A, Dulak J, Kieda C. Hypoxia-regulated overexpression of soluble VEGFR2 controls angiogenesis and inhibits tumor growth. Mol Cancer Ther. 2014;13:165–78.
50. Hamzah J, Jugold M, Kiessling F, Rigby P, Manzur M, Manzur M, Marti HH, Rabie T, Kaden S, Gröne HJ, Hämmerling GJ, Arnold B, Ganss R. Vascular normalization in Rgs5-deficient tumours promotes immune destruction. Nature. 2008;453:410–4.
51. Rolny C, Mazzone M, Tugues S, Laoui D, Johansson I, Coulon C, Squadrito ML, Segura I, Li X, Knevels E, Costa S, Vinckier S, Dresselaer T, Åkerud P, De Mol M, Salomäki H, Phillipson M, Wyns S, Larsson E, Buysschaert I, Botling J, Himmelreich U, Van Ginderachter JA, De Palma M, Dewerchin M, Claesson-Welsh L, Carmeliet P. HRG inhibits tumor growth and metastasis by inducing macrophage polarization and vessel normalization through downregulation of PlGF. Cancer Cell. 2011;19:31–44.
52. Huang Y, Yuan J, Righi E, Kamoun WS, Ancukiewicz M, Nezivar J, Santosuosso M, Martin JD, Martin MR, Vianello F, Leblanc P, Munn LL, Huang P, Duda DG, Fukumura D, Jain RK, Poznansky MC. Vascular normalizing doses of antiangiogenic treatment reprogram the immunosuppressive tumor microenvironment and enhance immunotherapy. Proc Natl Acad Sci U S A. 2012;109:17561–6.
53. Reya T, Morrison SJ, Clarke MF, Weissman IL. Stem cells, cancer, and cancer stem cells. Nature. 2001;414:105–11.

54. Pardal R, Clarke MF, Morrison SJ. Applying the principles of stem-cell biology to cancer. Nat Rev Cancer. 2003;3:895–902.
55. Visvader JE, Lindeman GJ. Cancer stem cells in solid tumours: accumulating evidence and unresolved questions. Nat Rev Cancer. 2008;8:755–68.
56. Jogi A, Ora I, Nilsson H, Lindeheim A, Makino Y, Poellinger L, Axelson H, Pahlman S. Hypoxia alters gene expression in human neuroblastoma cells toward an immature and neural crest-like phenotype. Proc Natl Acad Sci U S A. 2002;99:7021–6.
57. McCord AM, Jamal M, Shankavaram UT, Lang FF, Camphausen K, Tofilon PJ. Physiologic oxygen concentration enhances the stem-like properties of CD133+ human glioblastoma cells in vitro. Mol Cancer Res. 2009;7:489–97.
58. Chen Y, De Marco MA, Graziani I, Gazdar AF, Strack PR, Miele L, Bocchetta M. Oxygen concentration determines the biological effects of NOTCH-1 signaling in adenocarcinoma of the lung. Cancer Res. 2007;67:7954–9.
59. Morrison SJ, Perez SE, Qiao Z, Verdi JM, Hicks C, Weinmaster G, Anderson DJ. Transient Notch activation initiates an irreversible switch from neurogenesis to gliogenesis by neural crest stem cells. Cell. 2000;101:499–510.
60. Wilson A, Radtke F. Multiple functions of Notch signaling in self-renewing organs and cancer. FEBS Lett. 2006;580:2860–8.
61. Li Z, Bao S, Wu Q, Wang H, Eyler C, Sathornsumetee S, Shi Q, Cao Y, Lathia J, McLendon RE, Hjelmeland AB, Rich JN. Hypoxia-inducible factors regulate tumorigenic capacity of glioma stem cells. Cancer Cell. 2009;15:501–13.
62. Pietras A, Gisselsson D, Ora I, Noguera R, Beckman S, Navarro S, Pahlman S. High levels of HIF-2alpha highlight an immature neural crest-like neuroblastoma cell cohort located in a perivascular niche. J Pathol. 2008;214:482–8.
63. Heddleston JM, Li Z, McLendon RE, Hjelmeland AB, Rich JN. The hypoxic microenvironment maintains glioblastoma stem cells and promotes reprogramming towards a cancer stem cell phenotype. Cell Cycle. 2009;8:3274–84.
64. Moreno-Manzano V, Rodriguez-Jimenez FJ, Acena-Bonilla JL, Fustero-Lardies S, Erceg S, Dopazo J, Montaner D, Stojkovic M, Sanchez-Puelles JM. FM19G11, a new hypoxia-inducible factor (HIF) modulator, affects stem cell differentiation status. J Biol Chem. 2010;285:1333–42.
65. Wang Y, Liu Y, Malek SN, Zheng P. Targeting HIF1alpha eliminates cancer stem cells in hematological malignancies. Cell Stem Cell. 2011;8:399–411.
66. Hasmim M, Noman MZ, Lauriol J, Benlalam H, Mallavialle A, Rosselli F, Mami-Chouaib F, Alcaide-Loridan C, Chouaib S. Hypoxia-dependent inhibition of tumor cell susceptibility to CTL-mediated lysis involves NANOG induction in target cells. J Immunol. 2011;187: 4031–9.
67. Noh KH, Kim BW, Song KH, Cho H, Lee YH, Kim JH, Chung JY, Hewitt SM, Seong SY, Mao CP, Wu TC, Kim TW. Nanog signaling in cancer promotes stem-like phenotype and immune evasion. J Clin Invest. 2012;122:4077–93.
68. Dobrila-Dintinjana R. Circulating cancer cells are potential weapon for future generations. Hepatogastroenterology. 2014;61:5–8.
69. Kallergi G, Markomanolaki H, Giannoukaraki V, Papadaki MA, Strati A, Lianidou ES, Georgoulias V, Mavroudis D, Agelaki S. Hypoxia-inducible factor-1alpha and vascular endothelial growth factor expression in circulating tumor cells of breast cancer patients. Breast Cancer Res. 2009;11:R84.
70. Eliane JP, Repollet M, Luker KE, Brown M, Rae JM, Dontu G, Schott AF, Wicha M, Doyle GV, Hayes DF, Luker GD. Monitoring serial changes in circulating human breast cancer cells in murine xenograft models. Cancer Res. 2008;68:5529–32.
71. Steinert G, Scholch S, Niemietz T, Iwata N, Garcia SA, Behrens B, Voigt A, Kloor M, Benner A, Bork U, Rahbari NN, Büchler MW, Stoecklein NH, Weitz J. Immune escape and survival mechanisms in circulating tumor cells of colorectal cancer. Cancer Res. 2014;74:1694–704.
72. Yie SM, Luo B, Ye NY, Xie K, Ye SR. Detection of survivin-expressing circulating cancer cells in the peripheral blood of breast cancer patients by a RT-PCR ELISA. Clin Exp Metastasis. 2006;23:279–89.

73. Hoffmann AC, Warnecke-Eberz U, Luebke T, Prenzel K, Metzger R, Heitmann M, Neiss S, Vallbohmer D, Hoelscher AH, Schneider PM. Survivin mRNA in peripheral blood is frequently detected and significantly decreased following resection of gastrointestinal cancers. J Surg Oncol. 2007;95:51–4.
74. Vegran F, Boidot R. Survivin-3B promotes chemoresistance and immune escape by inhibiting caspase-8 and -6 in cancer cells. Oncoimmunology. 2013;2:e26328.
75. Mani SA, Guo W, Liao MJ, Eaton EN, Ayyanan A, Zhou AY, Brooks M, Reinhard F, Zhang CC, Shipitsin M, Campbell LL, Polyak K, Brisken C, Yang J, Weinberg RA. The epithelial-mesenchymal transition generates cells with properties of stem cells. Cell. 2008;133: 704–15.
76. Tsai JH, Donaher JL, Murphy DA, Chau S, Yang J. Spatiotemporal regulation of epithelial-mesenchymal transition is essential for squamous cell carcinoma metastasis. Cancer Cell. 2012;22:725–36.
77. Kudo-Saito C, Shirako H, Takeuchi T, Kawakami Y. Cancer metastasis is accelerated through immunosuppression during Snail-induced EMT of cancer cells. Cancer Cell. 2009; 15:195–206.
78. Akalay I, Janji B, Hasmim M, Noman MZ, Andre F, De Cremoux P, Bertheau P, Badoual C, Vielh P, Larsen AK, Sabbah M, Tan TZ, Keira JH, Hung NT, Thiery JP, Mami-Chouaib F, Chouaib S. Epithelial-to-mesenchymal transition and autophagy induction in breast carcinoma promote escape from T-cell-mediated lysis. Cancer Res. 2013;73:2418–27.
79. Akalay I, Tan TZ, Kumar P, Janji B, Mami-Chouaib F, Charpy C, Vielh P, Larsen AK, Thiery JP, Sabbah M, Chouaib S. Targeting WNT1-inducible signaling pathway protein 2 alters human breast cancer cell susceptibility to specific lysis through regulation of KLF-4 and miR-7 expression. Oncogene. 2014;0. doi:10.1038/onc.
80. Sullivan R, Graham CH. Hypoxia-driven selection of the metastatic phenotype. Cancer Metastasis Rev. 2007;26:319–31.
81. Volm M, Koomagi R. Hypoxia-inducible factor (HIF-1) and its relationship to apoptosis and proliferation in lung cancer. Anticancer Res. 2000;20:1527–33.
82. Liu L, Cash TP, Jones RG, Keith B, Thompson CB, Simon MC. Hypoxia-induced energy stress regulates mRNA translation and cell growth. Mol Cell. 2006;21:521–31.
83. Fink T, Ebbesen P, Koppelhus U, Zachar V. Natural killer cell-mediated basal and interferon-enhanced cytotoxicity against liver cancer cells is significantly impaired under in vivo oxygen conditions. Scand J Immunol. 2003;58:607–12.
84. Siemens DR, Hu N, Sheikhi AK, Chung E, Frederiksen LJ, Pross H, Graham CH. Hypoxia increases tumor cell shedding of MHC class I chain-related molecule: role of nitric oxide. Cancer Res. 2008;68:4746–53.
85. Noman MZ, Buart S, Van Pelt J, Richon C, Hasmim M, Leleu N, Suchorska WM, Jalil A, Lecluse Y, El Hage F, Giuliani M, Pichon C, Azzarone B, Mazure N, Romero P, Mami-Chouaib F, Chouaib S. The cooperative induction of hypoxia-inducible factor-1 alpha and STAT3 during hypoxia induced an impairment of tumor susceptibility to CTL-mediated cell lysis. J Immunol. 2009;182:3510–21.
86. Bromberg JF, Wrzeszczynska MH, Devgan G, Zhao Y, Pestell RG, Albanese C, Darnell Jr JE. Stat3 as an oncogene. Cell. 1999;98:295–303.
87. Catlett-Falcone R, Landowski TH, Oshiro MM, Turkson J, Levitzki A, Savino R, Ciliberto G, Moscinski L, Fernandez-Luna JL, Nuñez G, Dalton WS, Jove R. Constitutive activation of Stat3 signaling confers resistance to apoptosis in human U266 myeloma cells. Immunity. 1999;10:105–15.
88. Wang T, Niu G, Kortylewski M, Burdelya L, Shain K, Zhang S, Bhattacharya R, Gabrilovich D, Heller R, Coppola D, Dalton W, Jove R, Pardoll D, Yu H. Regulation of the innate and adaptive immune responses by Stat-3 signaling in tumor cells. Nat Med. 2004;10:48–54.
89. Hussain SF, Kong LY, Jordan J, Conrad C, Madden T, Fokt I, Priebe W, Heimberger AB. A novel small molecule inhibitor of signal transducers and activators of transcription 3 reverses immune tolerance in malignant glioma patients. Cancer Res. 2007;67:9630–6.

90. Xin H, Zhang C, Herrmann A, Du Y, Figlin R, Yu H. Sunitinib inhibition of Stat3 induces renal cell carcinoma tumor cell apoptosis and reduces immunosuppressive cells. Cancer Res. 2009;69:2506–13.
91. Ozao-Choy J, Ma G, Kao J, Wang GX, Meseck M, Sung M, Schwartz M, Divino CM, Pan PY, Chen SH. The novel role of tyrosine kinase inhibitor in the reversal of immune suppression and modulation of tumor microenvironment for immune-based cancer therapies. Cancer Res. 2009;69:2514–22.
92. Chouaib S. Integrating the quality of the cytotoxic response and tumor susceptibility into the design of protective vaccines in tumor immunotherapy. J Clin Invest. 2003;111:595–7.
93. Mizushima N. Autophagy: process and function. Genes Dev. 2007;21:2861–73.
94. Yang Z, Klionsky DJ. Eaten alive: a history of macroautophagy. Nat Cell Biol. 2010; 12:814–22.
95. Mathew R, Karantza-Wadsworth V, White E. Role of autophagy in cancer. Nat Rev Cancer. 2007;7:961–7.
96. Corcelle EA, Puustinen P, Jaattela M. Apoptosis and autophagy: Targeting autophagy signalling in cancer cells -'trick or treats'? FEBS J. 2009;276:6084–96.
97. Glick D, Barth S, Macleod KF. Autophagy: cellular and molecular mechanisms. J Pathol. 2010;221:3–12.
98. Yang Z, Klionsky DJ. Mammalian autophagy: core molecular machinery and signaling regulation. Curr Opin Cell Biol. 2010;22:124–31.
99. Mazure NM, Pouyssegur J. Hypoxia-induced autophagy: cell death or cell survival? Curr Opin Cell Biol. 2010;22:177–80.
100. Bellot G, Garcia-Medina R, Gounon P, Chiche J, Roux D, Pouyssegur J, Mazure NM. Hypoxia-induced autophagy is mediated through hypoxia-inducible factor induction of BNIP3 and BNIP3L via their BH3 domains. Mol Cell Biol. 2009;29:2570–81.
101. Rouschop KM, van den Beucken T, Dubois L, Niessen H, Bussink J, Savelkouls K, Keulers T, Mujcic H, Landuyt W, Voncken JW, Lambin P, van der Kogel AJ, Koritzinsky M, Wouters BG. The unfolded protein response protects human tumor cells during hypoxia through regulation of the autophagy genes MAP1LC3B and ATG5. J Clin Invest. 2010;120:127–41.
102. Livesey KM, Tang D, Zeh HJ, Lotze MT. Autophagy inhibition in combination cancer treatment. Curr Opin Investig Drugs. 2009;10:1269–79.
103. Levine B, Mizushima N, Virgin HW. Autophagy in immunity and inflammation. Nature. 2011;469:323–35.
104. Chemali M, Radtke K, Desjardins M, English L. Alternative pathways for MHC class I presentation: a new function for autophagy. Cell Mol Life Sci. 2011;68:1533–41.
105. Crotzer VL, Blum JS. Autophagy and adaptive immunity. Immunology. 2010;131:9–17.
106. Wightman B, Ha I, Ruvkun G. Posttranscriptional regulation of the heterochronic gene lin-14 by lin-4 mediates temporal pattern formation in C. elegans. Cell. 1993;75:855–62.
107. Alvarez-Garcia I, Miska EA. MicroRNA functions in animal development and human disease. Development. 2005;132:4653–62.
108. Kulshreshtha R, Davuluri RV, Calin GA, Ivan M. A microRNA component of the hypoxic response. Cell Death Differ. 2008;15:667–71.
109. Kulshreshtha R, Ferracin M, Wojcik SE, Garzon R, Alder H, Agosto-Perez FJ, Davuluri R, Liu CG, Croce CM, Negrini M, Calin GA, Ivan M. A microRNA signature of hypoxia. Mol Cell Biol. 2007;27:1859–67.
110. Loscalzo J. The cellular response to hypoxia: tuning the system with microRNAs. J Clin Invest. 2010;120:3815–7.
111. Devlin C, Greco S, Martelli F, Ivan M. miR-210. More than a silent player in hypoxia. IUBMB Life. 2011;63:94–100.
112. Huang X, Ding L, Bennewith KL, Tong RT, Welford SM, Ang KK, Story M, Le QT, Giaccia AJ. Hypoxia-inducible mir-210 regulates normoxic gene expression involved in tumor initiation. Mol Cell. 2009;35:856–67.

113. Huang X, Le QT, Giaccia AJ. MiR-210—micromanager of the hypoxia pathway. Trends Mol Med. 2010;16:230–7.
114. Camps C, Buffa FM, Colella S, Moore J, Sotiriou C, Sheldon H, Harris AL, Gleadle JM, Ragoussis J. hsa-miR-210 Is induced by hypoxia and is an independent prognostic factor in breast cancer. Clin Cancer Res. 2008;14:1340–8.
115. Gee HE, Camps C, Buffa FM, Patiar S, Winter SC, Betts G, Homer J, Corbridge R, Cox G, West CM, Ragoussis J, Harris AL. hsa-mir-210 is a marker of tumor hypoxia and a prognostic factor in head and neck cancer. Cancer. 2010;116:2148–58.
116. Pulkkinen K, Malm T, Turunen M, Koistinaho J, Yla-Herttuala S. Hypoxia induces microRNA miR-210 in vitro and in vivo ephrin-A3 and neuronal pentraxin 1 are potentially regulated by miR-210. FEBS Lett. 2008;582:2397–401.
117. Chouaib S, El Hage F, Benlalam H, Mami-Chouaib F. Immunotherapy of cancer: promise and reality. Med Sci (Paris). 2006;22:755–9 (Article in French).
118. Dunn GP, Old LJ, Schreiber RD. The immunobiology of cancer immunosurveillance and immunoediting. Immunity. 2004;21:137–48.
119. Patiar S, Harris AL. Role of hypoxia-inducible factor-1alpha as a cancer therapy target. Endocr Relat Cancer. 2006;13 Suppl 1:S61–75.

Chapter 7
Mechanisms and Modulation of Tumor Microenvironment-Induced Immune Resistance

Tuna Mutis, Niels W.C.J. van de Donk, and Richard W.J. Groen

Abstract In the quest for developing more effective immune therapy strategies for cancer, to date, unraveling and successful modulation of the mechanisms of tumor escape in the microenvironment became an urgent challenge. While immune suppression is considered an important mode of immune escape, this overview will deal with another important mechanism of immune escape in the tumor microenvironment: the microenvironment-regulated resistance of tumor cells toward the cytotoxic machinery of immune effector cells. We have recently studied the impact of the microenvironment to the development of immune resistance in multiple myeloma (MM) and will outline the backgrounds and current knowledge about the mechanisms and modulation of this type of immune escape.

Keywords Cytotoxic T cells • Cancer immunotherapy • Bone marrow • Microenvironment • Apoptosis • Drug resistance • Immune resistance • Multiple myeloma

Abbreviations

BM	Bone marrow
BMSC	Bone marrow mesenchymal stromal cells
CTL	Cytotoxic T cell
MM	Multiple myeloma
MSC	Mesenchymal stromal cells
NK cell	Natural killer cells

No conflict statement: No potential conflicts of interest were disclosed.

T. Mutis (✉) • N.W.C.J. van de Donk • R.W.J. Groen
Department of Hematology, VU University Medical Center,
CCA 4.28 De Boelelaan 1118, 1081 HV Amsterdam, The Netherlands
e-mail: t.mutis@vumc.nl

B. Bonavida, S. Chouaib (eds.), *Resistance of Cancer Cells to CTL-Mediated Immunotherapy*, Resistance to Targeted Anti-Cancer Therapeutics 7,
DOI 10.1007/978-3-319-17807-3_7

7.1 Introduction

Eradication of malignant cells through the cytotoxic machinery of immune cells such as cytotoxic T cells (CTLs) and natural killer (NK) cells is the ultimate aim of cellular immunotherapy of cancer. Starting from the early applications of allogeneic stem cell transplantation, followed by successful donor lymphocyte infusions, clinicians and immunologists have witnessed and appreciated the potential power of cellular immunotherapy in the battle of hematological and non-hematological malignancies [1]. Over the past two decades, the rapid identification of tumor-associated antigens [2, 3], development of new technologies such as T cell receptor (TCR)-gene transfer [4] and recently the remarkable successes of virus-specific T cells [5], tumor infiltrating lymphocytes (TIL) [6] and chimeric antigen receptor (CAR)-engineered T cells [7–9] in the treatment of various hematologic cancers, have elevated cancer immunotherapy to a new level, with high expectations. Nonetheless, despite the optimal activation and infiltration of abundant numbers of tumor-reactive CTLs or NK cells at tumor sites, human cancers, mainly due to genetic heterogeneity as well as micro-environmental influences, display various mechanisms to evade the immune attack [10, 11]. To date, the unraveling and the successful modulation of the mechanisms of tumor escape in the microenvironment became the most urgent challenges to achieve the next level of success in the immunotherapy of cancer [12, 13].

Currently, most scientists consider immune suppression as the main mechanism of immune escape in the tumor microenvironment [14–17]. There is, indeed, a large body of evidence that the tumor microenvironment is a suppressive inflammatory niche [18, 19], with the presence of several immune suppressive soluble factors, such as IDO, Arginase, INOS or TGF-β [20–22], secreted either from tumor cells [23], accessory cells (vascular endothelium, stromal cells, fibroblasts) [24] or from suppressive immune cells such as regulatory T cells [25], tumor associated macrophages [26], and myeloid derived suppressor cells [27, 28], many of which are recruited or induced in the microenvironment through crosstalk with tumor cells and tumor stroma [29]. This immune suppressive milieu also involves the strong upregulation of the immune checkpoint molecules PD1 on T cells and PD-L1/2 on tumor cells [30–35], and in some reported cases through interaction with stroma [36].

This chapter will, however, deal with another, entirely distinct mechanism of immune escape in the tumor microenvironment: the microenvironment-regulated resistance of tumor cells toward the cytotoxic machinery of immune effector cells. This resistance of tumor cells against cytotoxic attack, although extensively documented in the melanoma setting, and may be as important as "immune suppression", has not received sufficient attention yet, probably because it has not been seen as a microenvironment-mediated phenomenon. We have recently studied the impact of the microenvironment to the development of immune resistance in multiple myeloma (MM) and will outline below the backgrounds and current knowledge about the mechanisms and modulation of this type of immune escape.

7.2 MM the Model for Investigating the Role of the Microenvironment in Human Cancers

MM is the malignant disorder of antibody producing clonal plasma cells [37]. It is the second most common hematological malignancy worldwide. Despite four exciting decades of drug development, MM remains incurable by chemotherapy due to the induction of drug resistance [38, 39]. Although experimental and clinical studies indicate the immune competence of MM cells and possibility to treat the disease with cellular immunotherapy [40–42], the overall outcome of allo-SCT, DLI or other experimental immunotherapies in MM is at most moderate, underscoring the ability of MM cells to evade the cellular immune attack.

Traditionally, the biology of MM and its therapy-response is studied preferably in the context of the microenvironment [43–46] because MM, especially in the initial phases of the disease, is entirely dependent on its natural habitat, the bone marrow (BM). Over the past decades, it has been extensively documented that the BM provides MM cells an ideal sanctuary by the production of several survival cytokines such as IL-6 and IL-8, VEGF, SDF-1 and many others, and by interactions of MM cells with extracellular matrix and BM accessory cells, in particular with stromal cells (BMSCs) and vascular endothelial cells (VECs) [47, 48]. In fact, once taken out of this natural niche, primary human MM cells rapidly die, and are very difficult to engraft even in the BM of immune deficient mice [49–51].

7.3 Importance of the Tumor Microenvironment in Drug Resistance

Investigations aiming at understanding the molecular basis of drug resistance of MM have demonstrated that the many soluble factors produced in the BM microenvironment not only provide proliferative and survival signals to MM cells, but also -individually or collectively- contribute to the development of drug resistance [52]. Perhaps, more important is the induction of drug resistance through the (integrin-mediated) adhesion of MM cells to BMSCs and VECs. This type of environmentally, thus epigenetically, regulated drug resistance, which is generally known as “Cell Adhesion-Mediated Drug Resistance” (CAM-DR), has originally been demonstrated for MM cells in the late nineties [53], and has subsequently been described also for several other hematological and non-hematological malignancies [54–58]. While integrins were initially shown to play a key role in this type of drug resistance, another important molecule appears to be NOTCH [59–61]. The relation of this environmentally regulated drug resistance with immune resistance will become obvious upon outlining the molecular nature of both types of resistance mechanisms.

7.4 The Apoptotic Pathways: Immune Resistance Meets Drug Resistance

Studies have shown that the molecular basis of CAM-DR is the cell adhesion-dependent triggering of a complex series of signaling events resulting in the transcriptional or posttranscriptional regulation of intracellular molecules involved in apoptotic signaling for programmed cell death [45, 46]. This ability of the microenvironment to modulate apoptotic pathways was, in fact, for us a major reason to start studying the relation of the microenvironment with immune resistance, because not only drugs, but also cytotoxic immune cells kill the tumor cells via the induction of apoptosis.

In general terms, apoptosis involves a complex cascade of molecular events that can be initiated inside the cell or by external dead signals. Accordingly, two main apoptotic pathways have been described: the intrinsic or mitochondrial pathway and the extrinsic or death receptor pathway [62, 63] (Fig. 7.1). Several pro-apoptotic anticancer drugs are designed for activating either of these pathways [64–71]. While immune cells can trigger the extrinsic death receptor pathway [72], a major mechanism of tumor cell lysis by CTLs and NK cells is the apoptosis induced by the degranulation of granzyme/perforin from the cytotoxic granules upon engagement with the target cells [73]. This specific mechanism has traditionally been defined as a separate pathway, although it is also initiated by external signals. As will be outlined below, more important is the considerable overlap between these pathways. All three signaling pathways eventually converge and mediate the execution phase of apoptosis via the activation of caspase-3. Hence, although immune cells may in some cases kill drug resistant tumor cells, specific drug resistance mechanisms may overlap with immune resistance mechanisms, with potentially important clinical consequences.

7.5 The Modulation of Intrinsic, Extrinsic and Granzyme/Perforin Mediated Pathways of Apoptosis by the Microenvironment

The intrinsic apoptosis pathway, which involves mitochondrial depolarization, is initiated with the activation of pro-apoptotic proteins BAX and BAK, by BIM and BID, respectively [74] (Fig. 7.1). Oligomers or multimers of activated BAX and BAK engage with the mitochondrial membrane [75], induce the formation of mitochondrial pores and cause the release of cytochrome-c and SMAC/Diablo from the mitochondria into the cytosol [76]. By binding to the APAF-1 protein, cytochrome-c generates a large cytoplasmic complex, the apoptosome [77]. This complex binds and activates caspase-9, which in turn can activate several executioner caspases including the caspase-3 [78]. Several members of the BCL-2 family of proteins are important regulators of this pathway. Briefly, the mitochondrial

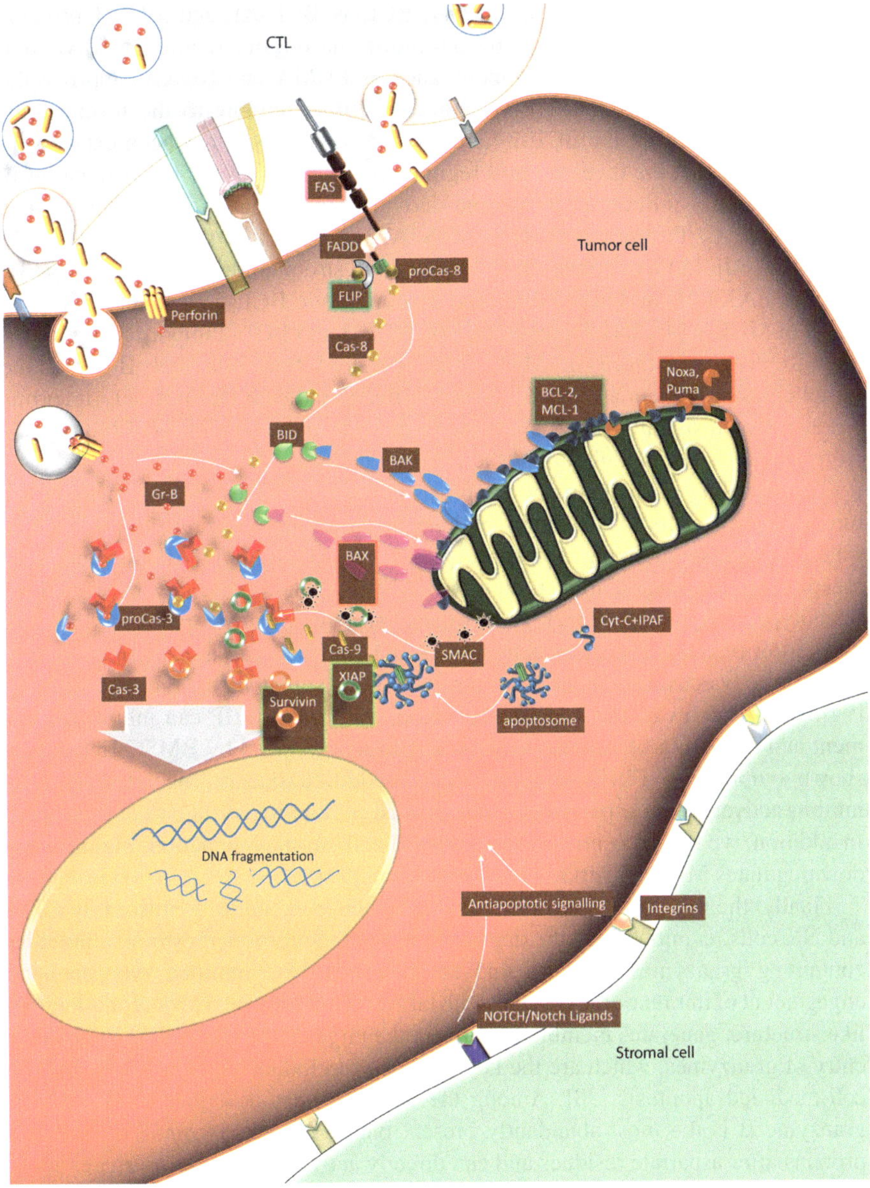

Fig. 7.1 Apoptotic pathways activated by immune effector cells (CTLs/NK cells) and their regulation by the microenvironment. The simplified scheme demonstrates the key molecules and the overlap between the intrinsic, extrinsic and granzyme pathways of apoptosis. Also note the convergence of these pathways at the level of caspase 3 (Cas-3). The molecules that are known to be modulated by the stroma-tumor interactions are indicated with *red* (downregulated) and *green* (upregulated) boxes. *Cas-3* caspase 3, *Cas-8* caspase 8, *Cas-9* caspase 9, *Cyt-C* cytochrome C, *Gr-B* granzyme B

membrane-associated BCL-2, BCL-2A1, BCL-W BCL-XL and MCL-1 proteins protect the cells form apoptosis by inhibiting the oligomerization of BAX and BAK. In contrast, the other members, such as PUMA and NOXA, improve the oligomerization of BAX and BAK via competitive binding to the former anti-apoptotic members of the BCL-2 family of proteins [79]. It has been extensively demonstrated that the mediator and regulatory molecules of the intrinsic pathway are significantly influenced by stroma-derived soluble factors and adhesion. For instance, IL-6, through activation of STAT3 upregulates the transcription of BCL-XL [80], induces adhesion of MM cells to stroma, downregulates BIM [81, 82] and BAX [83] and upregulates the anti-apoptotic BCL-2 proteins [83], especially of MCL-1 [44, 84]. Upregulation of MCL-1 and BCL-2 importantly contributes to drug resistance in MM, acute myeloid leukemia and B-cell acute lymphoblastic leukemia [85, 86]. Several studies indicate that not only integrins but also Notch signaling can have a major impact on the protection of tumor cells from apoptosis via modulation of the intrinsic pathway [59–61].

The signaling of the extrinsic apoptosis pathway involves the triggering of the tumor necrosis factor (TNF) family of death receptors including FAS (CD95), TNF-related apoptosis-inducing ligand-receptor 1 (TRAIL-R1), TRAIL-R2 and TNF receptor apoptosis-mediating protein (TRAMP). CTLs, especially of the CD4+ phenotype, frequently trigger FAS to activate the extrinsic pathway [87–93]. Triggering of death receptors activates FADD and then caspase-8, which in turn either directly activates caspase-3 or cleaves BID to signal via the intrinsic pathway [94]. In this pathway, the FLICE-like inhibitory protein FLIP can inhibit recruitment and activation of caspase-8. Soluble factors produced by BMSCs have been shown to upregulate FLIP expression [95]. In addition, integrin-mediated adhesion inhibits activation of caspase-8 due to increased cellular redistribution of FLIP [96]. In addition, we have recently shown that MM cell-stroma interactions significantly downregulates MM cell surface FAS expression [97].

Finally, the Granzyme/perforin pathway, which is exclusively utilized by CTLs and NK cells, is initiated by the degranulation of the preformed cytotoxic granules containing granzymes, perforin and serglycin into the immune synapse upon engagement of immune effector cells with target cells. Perforin, with its complement-like structure, generates membrane pores in the target cell to enable the cytotosolic entry of granzymes, which are the key molecules to induce signaling for cytotoxic cell-mediated apoptosis [98]. Among the 12 granzymes described until now, the granzyme B is the most abundantly present one in cytotoxic granules. It cleaves proteins after aspartate residues and can directly activate caspase-3 to trigger apoptosis. But, similar to caspase 8, granzyme-B can also trigger the intrinsic pathway of apoptosis through the activation of BID [98]. This clear overlap between the intrinsic pathway and granzyme-mediated lysis may have important consequences: for instance, melanoma cells that have been made resistant to CTL killing display signatures for hyperactivation of the NF-κB pathway, and overexpression of BCL-2, BCL-XL, and MCL-1 [99]. In fact, the efficacy of (CAR) T cell therapy can be significantly upregulated by inhibition of BCL-2 family of proteins [100, 101].

Thus the above described microenvironment-mediated drug resistance mechanisms of intrinsic pathway, may very well influence the outcome of CTL therapy.

In human cells, granzyme B can be inhibited by the proteinase inhibitor-9 (PI-9) [102]. The expression levels of this molecule in pediatric ALL cells correlate with their resistance against immune cell mediated lysis [103]. In the clinical setting, PI-9 expression is an important predictor of disease-free survival in melanoma patients treated with immunotherapy [104]. Interestingly, PI-9 gene expression can be induced by NF-κB signaling [105] as well as by hypoxia [106], which is a typical feature of the bone marrow microenvironment and has been shown to induce resistance against NK mediated lysis of MM cells [107].

Since all major apoptotic pathways converge at the level of caspase-3 activation, the (microenvironment-mediated) signals that regulate the activity of this executioner caspase may contribute to the development of both immune- and drug resistance. A specific group of molecules that regulates the activation of caspases is the IAP family of proteins [108–110]. XIAP, one of the best characterized IAPs, inhibits the activity of caspase-3, -7, and -9. Survivin (BIRC5), another well-known IAP, is frequently expressed in human tumor cells, and inhibits caspase-3 and -7. The activities of these molecules can be controlled, in turn, by the proapoptotic protein SMAC/Diablo, which is released upon mitochondrial depolarization [111, 112]. IAPs are indeed important in mediating both drug and immune resistance: for instance, in a recent study, cis-platinum resistant human ovarian cancer cells were found less susceptible toward NK-cell mediated killing than the parental cells partly due to the upregulation of cIAP-1 and -2 [113], Also survivin-3B, an alternative splice variant of survivin, was recently associated with chemotherapy resistance as well as with resistance to FAS-mediated immune cell toxicity [114]. Taken together, these and some earlier studies [115] demonstrate that drug resistance mechanisms show substantial overlap with the documented mechanisms of immune resistance. Unfortunately, however, the impact of the microenvironment on the induction of immune resistance has not been widely studied, except for MM.

The first indirect evidence for the microenvironment-mediated immune resistance in MM was provided by a study in which BM stroma conferred resistance to Apo2 ligand/TRAIL induced lysis in part by regulating c-FLIP [95]. In this case, soluble factors were found responsible for immune resistance. Using mainly an in vitro co-culture system, which was originally developed to study BMSC-induced drug resistance [44], we and other investigators have recently questioned whether the BM microenvironment can also cause a CAM-DR like immune resistance. Indeed, MM cells were protected against NK cells by co-culture with autologous BMSCs [116]. Subsequently, we have reported in vitro and in vivo evidence that MM cells are protected from CD4+ and CD8+ CTL-mediated lysis upon direct cellular interactions with VECs and BMSCs derived either from MM patients or from healthy individuals [97]. In our study, the protection of MM cells by accessory cells could be observed in the absence of immune suppression; hence, analogous to CAM-DR, we designated this type of cell adhesion-mediated immune resistance as CAM-IR. In further analysis, we discovered that MM cell-stroma interactions significantly downregulated MM cell FAS surface expression, but correction of FAS expression by bortezomib, did not entirely abrogate CAM-IR. By contrast, upregulation of survivin/MCL-1 appeared a central mechanism of CAM-IR, since we could entirely neutralize the immune resistance, in vitro as well as in a recently developed MM model in vivo [51], by combining T cells with the small molecule YM155, a suppressant of survivin and MCL-1 [117, 118]. Although we have not elucidated the entire mechanisms of CAM-IR yet, we have observed that CAM-IR, like CAM-DR, can be inhibited by interfering with integrin binding on intact cells, but unlike CAM-DR, cannot be induced by sole binding of MM cells to fibronectin, vitronectin, or laminin. Signals initiating CAM-IR are therefore most likely triggered by the collective action of integrins with other receptor-ligand systems. A possible candidate is the NOTCH signaling pathway, since we have recently observed that CAM-IR could also be abrogated by inhibition of the NOTCH pathway by gamma secretase inhibitors (GSI) (unpublished observations).

7.6 Towards the Design of Immune-Chemotherapy Strategies to Overcome Microenvironment-Mediated Immune Resistance

Our findings as well as evidence provided from other studies underscore the notion that the interactions between tumor cells and the cells of the microenvironment can induce resistance toward the cytotoxic machinery of immune cells through upregulation of anti-apoptotic molecules such as survivin, BCL-2 and MCL-1. Thus, successful anti-tumor immunotherapy may rely not only on eliminating the immune suppressive factors from the microenvironment, but also on modulation of the mechanisms that induce or mediate immune resistance. Among several theoretically conceivable strategies, specific attention needs to be paid for modulating the target molecules/pathways without compromising T cell function. With this respect, neutralizing survivin/MCL-1 with YM155 is a suitable strategy as we have not observed any T cell compromising effects of YM155. Several other pathways such as the PI3-K/AKT pathway, that are activated by microenvironmental influences play important roles in tumor development, survival, proliferation and drug resistance through induction of anti-apoptotic molecules [119]. The modulation of these pathways may be beneficial but need to be cautiously explored as these pathways may also play essential roles in T cell activation. For instance, the popular MEK inhibitors appear to impair T cell functions and are probably not suitable candidates to combine with immune therapy. On the other hand, selective inhibitors of BRAF were shown to enhance T-cell recognition of melanoma without affecting lymphocyte function [120]. More practical choices may be the general regulators of epigenetic mechanisms, such as histone deacetylase (HDAC) inhibitors as they have been shown to modulate drug resistance as well as to improve CTL-mediated lysis of tumor cells through upregulation of death receptors [121], and downregulating intracellular c-IAP-2 and BCL-XL expressions [122].

Among all these choices, however, the most appealing strategies may be disrupting the tumor-stroma interactions. Since T cells require integrins to generate a proper immune synapse, targeting integrin-mediated adhesion may not be feasible. However, in the BM an effective disruption of stroma-tumor interactions may be achieved using CXCR4 inhibitors, which induce mobilization of stem cells and myeloma cells from the BM. Such a strategy has already been shown to successfully overcome stroma-mediated activation of STAT3 [123] and HGF/MET [124] pathways, and to prevent the drug resistance of myeloma cells induced by BMSCs [125]. Furthermore, disturbing the stroma-tumor interactions may also prevent the upregulation of immune checkpoint molecules [36]. Finally, since NOTCH signaling also seems important in the microenvironment-mediated drug resistance and similarly may induce immune resistance, its modulation can also be explored. Nonetheless, more investigation is required on NOTCH, as there are conflicting reports on its role, especially on the cytotoxic activity of T cells [126–128].

7.7 Concluding Remarks

The appreciation of the role of the microenvironment, not only in the induction of immune suppressive events but also in the protection of tumor cells against cytotoxic T cell attack, will stimulate the research and encourage the scientists and clinicians to combine immunotherapy not only with agents that can modulate immune suppression but also with those that can eliminate the resistance mechanisms induced by the microenvironment. Furthermore, the increasing consciousness that drug resistance may in several cases also cause immune-resistance may stimulate the discussion whether heavily pretreated and multidrug resistant patients are suitable candidates for clinical testing of cellular immunotherapy strategies.

Acknowledgments We thank Prof. Dr. H. Lokhorst and Dr. A. Martens from VUmc Amsterdam, the Netherlands and for Dr. C. Mitsiades from Dana Farber Cancer Institute, Boston US for significant conceptual contributions, inputs with experimental models, critical reading, and stimulating discussions.

References

1. Ringden O. Immunotherapy by allogeneic stem cell transplantation. Adv Cancer Res. 2007; 97:25–60.
2. Wang RF, Rosenberg S. A human tumor antigens for cancer vaccine development. Immunol Rev. 1999;170:85–100.
3. Lewis JD, Reilly BD, Bright RK. Tumor-associated antigens: from discovery to immunity. Int Rev Immunol. 2003;22:81–112.
4. Schumacher TN. T-cell-receptor gene therapy. Nat Rev Immunol. 2002;2:512–9.
5. Bollard CM, Rooney CM, Heslop HE. T-cell therapy in the treatment of post-transplant lymphoproliferative disease. Nat Rev Clin Oncol. 2012;9:510–9.

6. Rosenberg SA, Dudley ME. Adoptive cell therapy for the treatment of patients with metastatic melanoma. Curr Opin Immunol. 2009;21:233–40.
7. Maus MV, Grupp SA, Porter DL, June CH. Antibody-modified T cells: CARs take the front seat for hematologic malignancies. Blood. 2014;123:2625–35.
8. Kochenderfer JN, Rosenberg SA. Treating B-cell cancer with T cells expressing anti-CD19 chimeric antigen receptors. Nat Rev Clin Oncol. 2013;10:267–76.
9. Brentjens RJ, Curran KJ. Novel cellular therapies for leukemia: CAR-modified T cells targeted to the CD19 antigen. Hematology Am Soc Hematol Educ Program. 2012;2012:1 43–51.
10. Gajewski TF, Meng Y, Blank C, Brown I, Kacha A, Kline J, Harlin H. Immune resistance orchestrated by the tumor microenvironment. Immunol Rev. 2006;213:131–45.
11. Runger TM, Klein CE, Becker JC, Brocker EB. The role of genetic instability, adhesion, cell motility, and immune escape mechanisms in melanoma progression. Curr Opin Oncol. 1994;6:188–96.
12. Gajewski TF, Fuertes M, Spaapen R, Zheng Y, Kline J. Molecular profiling to identify relevant immune resistance mechanisms in the tumor microenvironment. Curr Opin Immunol. 2011;23:286–92.
13. Leen AM, Rooney CM, Foster AE. Improving T cell therapy for cancer. Annu Rev Immunol. 2007;25:243–65.
14. Kim R, Emi M, Tanabe K, Arihiro K. Tumor-driven evolution of immunosuppressive networks during malignant progression. Cancer Res. 2006;66:5527–36.
15. Becker JC, Andersen MH, Schrama D, Thor Straten P. Immune-suppressive properties of the tumor microenvironment. Cancer Immunol Immunother. 2013;62:1137–48.
16. Zumsteg A, Christofori G. Corrupt policemen: inflammatory cells promote tumor angiogenesis. Curr Opin Oncol. 2009;21:60–70.
17. Gajewski TF, Meng Y, Harlin H. Immune suppression in the tumor microenvironment. J Immunother. 2006;29:233–40.
18. Mantovani A, Romero P, Palucka AK, Marincola FM. Tumour immunity: effector response to tumour and role of the microenvironment. Lancet. 2008;371:771–83.
19. Yu H, Pardoll D, Jove R. STATs in cancer inflammation and immunity: a leading role for STAT3. Nat Rev Cancer. 2009;9:798–809.
20. Munn DH. Indoleamine 2,3-dioxygenase, tumor-induced tolerance and counter-regulation. Curr Opin Immunol. 2006;18:220–5.
21. Ochoa AC, Zea AH, Hernandez C, Rodriguez PC. Arginase, prostaglandins, and myeloid-derived suppressor cells in renal cell carcinoma. Clin Cancer Res. 2007;13:721s–6s.
22. Wakefield LM, Hill CS. Beyond TGFbeta: roles of other TGFbeta superfamily members in cancer. Nat Rev Cancer. 2013;13:328–41.
23. Rabinovich GA, Gabrilovich D, Sotomayor EM. Immunosuppressive strategies that are mediated by tumor cells. Annu Rev Immunol. 2007;25:267–96.
24. Anderson KC. Targeted therapy of multiple myeloma based upon tumor-microenvironmental interactions. Exp Hematol. 2007;35:155–62.
25. Wang HY, Wang RF. Regulatory T cells and cancer. Curr Opin Immunol. 2007;19:217–23.
26. Pollard JW. Macrophages define the invasive microenvironment in breast cancer. J Leukoc Biol. 2008;84:623–30.
27. Diaz-Montero CM, Finke J, Montero AJ. Myeloid-derived suppressor cells in cancer: therapeutic, predictive, and prognostic implications. Semin Oncol. 2014;41:174–84.
28. Lindau D, Gielen P, Kroesen M, Wesseling P, Adema GJ. The immunosuppressive tumour network: myeloid-derived suppressor cells, regulatory T cells and natural killer T cells. Immunology. 2013;138:105–15.
29. Gabrilovich DI, Ostrand-Rosenberg S, Bronte V. Coordinated regulation of myeloid cells by tumours. Nat Rev Immunol. 2012;12:253–68.
30. Blank C, Brown I, Peterson AC, Spiotto M, Iwai Y, Honjo T, Gajewski TF. PD-L1/B7H-1 inhibits the effector phase of tumor rejection by T cell receptor (TCR) transgenic CD8+ T cells. Cancer Res. 2004;64:1140–5.

31. Myklebust JH, Irish JM, Brody J, Czerwinski DK, Houot R, Kohrt HE, Timmerman J, Said J, Green MR, Delabie J, Kolstad A, Alizadeh AA, Levy R. High PD-1 expression and suppressed cytokine signaling distinguish T cells infiltrating follicular lymphoma tumors from peripheral T cells. Blood. 2013;121:1367–76.
32. Deng L, Liang H, Burnette B, Beckett M, Darga T, Weichselbaum RR, Fu YX. Irradiation and anti-PD-L1 treatment synergistically promote antitumor immunity in mice. J Clin Invest. 2014;124:687–95.
33. Topalian SL, Drake CG, Pardoll DM. Targeting the PD-1/B7-H1(PD-L1) pathway to activate anti-tumor immunity. Curr Opin Immunol. 2012;24:207–12.
34. Thompson RH, Kuntz SM, Leibovich BC, Dong H, Lohse CM, Webster WS, Sengupta S, Frank I, Parker AS, Zincke H, Blute ML, Sebo TJ, Cheville JC, Kwon ED. Tumor B7-H1 is associated with poor prognosis in renal cell carcinoma patients with long-term follow-up. Cancer Res. 2006;66:3381–5.
35. Yang H, Bueso-Ramos C, DiNardo C, Estecio MR, Davanlou M, Geng QR, Fang Z, Nguyen M, Pierce S, Wei Y, Parmar S, Cortes J, Kantarjian H, Garcia-Manero G. Expression of PD-L1, PD-L2, PD-1 and CTLA4 in myelodysplastic syndromes is enhanced by treatment with hypomethylating agents. Leukemia. 2014;28:1280–8.
36. Tamura H, Ishibashi M, Yamashita T, Tanosaki S, Okuyama N, Kondo A, Hyodo H, Shinya E, Takahashi H, Dong H, Tamada K, Chen L, Dan K, Ogata K. Marrow stromal cells induce B7-H1 expression on myeloma cells, generating aggressive characteristics in multiple myeloma. Leukemia. 2013;27:464–72.
37. Raab MS, Podar K, Breitkreutz I, Richardson PG, Anderson KC. Multiple myeloma. Lancet. 2009;374:324–39.
38. Dalton WS. Drug resistance and drug development in multiple myeloma. Semin Oncol. 2002;29:21–5.
39. Kastritis E, Palumbo A, Dimopoulos MA. Treatment of relapsed/refractory multiple myeloma. Semin Hematol. 2009;46:143–57.
40. Kroger N, Badbaran A, Lioznov M, Schwarz S, Zeschke S, Hildebrand Y, Ayuk F, Atanackovic D, Schilling G, Zabelina T, Bacher U, Klyuchnikov E, Shimoni A, Nagler A, Corradini P, Fehse B, Zander A. Post-transplant immunotherapy with donor-lymphocyte infusion and novel agents to upgrade partial into complete and molecular remission in allografted patients with multiple myeloma. Exp Hematol. 2009;37:791–8.
41. van de Donk NW, Kröger N, Hegenbart U, Corradini P, San Miguel JF, Goldschmidt H, Perez-Simon JA, Zijlmans M, Raymakers RA, Montefusco V, Ayuk FA, van Oers MH, Nagler A, Verdonck LF, Lokhorst HM. Prognostic factors for donor lymphocyte infusions following non-myeloablative allogeneic stem cell transplantation in multiple myeloma. Bone Marrow Transplant. 2006;37:1135–41.
42. Lokhorst HM, Schattenberg A, Cornelissen JJ, van Oers MH, Fibbe W, Russell I, Donk NW, Verdonck LF. Donor lymphocyte infusions for relapsed multiple myeloma after allogeneic stem-cell transplantation: predictive factors for response and long-term outcome. J Clin Oncol. 2000;18:3031–7.
43. McMillin DW, Mitsiades CS. High-throughput approaches to discover novel immunomodulatory agents for cancer. Oncoimmunology. 2012;1:1406–8.
44. McMillin DW, Delmore J, Weisberg E, Negri JM, Geer DC, Klippel S, Mitsiades N, Schlossman RL, Munshi NC, Kung AL, Griffin JD, Richardson PG, Anderson KC, Mitsiades CS. Tumor cell-specific bioluminescence platform to identify stroma-induced changes to anticancer drug activity. Nat Med. 2010;16:483–9.
45. Dalton WS. The tumor microenvironment: focus on myeloma. Cancer Treat Rev. 2003;29 Suppl 1:11–9.
46. Mahtouk K, Moreaux J, Hose D, Rème T, Meissner T, Jourdan M, Rossi JF, Pals ST, Goldschmidt H, Klein B. Growth factors in multiple myeloma: a comprehensive analysis of their expression in tumor cells and bone marrow environment using Affymetrix microarrays. BMC Cancer. 2010;10:198.

47. Mitsiades CS, Hayden PJ, Anderson KC, Richardson PG. From the bench to the bedside: emerging new treatments in multiple myeloma. Best Pract Res Clin Haematol. 2007;20: 797–816.
48. Hideshima T, Mitsiades C, Tonon G, Richardson PG, Anderson KC. Understanding multiple myeloma pathogenesis in the bone marrow to identify new therapeutic targets. Nat Rev Cancer. 2007;7:585–98.
49. Tassone P, Neri P, Burger R, Di Martino MT, Leone E, Amodio N, Caraglia M, Tagliaferri P. Mouse models as a translational platform for the development of new therapeutic agents in multiple myeloma. Curr Cancer Drug Targets. 2012;12:814–22.
50. Mitsiades CS, Anderson KC, Carrasco DR. Mouse models of human myeloma. Hematol Oncol Clin North Am. 2007;21:1051–69.
51. Groen RW, Noort WA, Raymakers RA, Prins HJ, Aalders L, Hofhuis FM, Moerer P, van Velzen JF, Bloem AC, van Kessel B, Rozemuller H, van Binsbergen E, Buijs A, Yuan H, de Bruijn JD, de Weers M, Parren PW, Schuringa JJ, Lokhorst HM, Mutis T, Martens AC. Reconstructing the human hematopoietic niche in immunodeficient mice: opportunities for studying primary multiple myeloma. Blood. 2012;120:e9–16.
52. Shain KH, Dalton WS. Environmental-mediated drug resistance: a target for multiple myeloma therapy. Expert Rev Hematol. 2009;2:649–62.
53. Damiano JS, Cress AE, Hazlehurst LA, Shtil AA, Dalton WS. Cell adhesion mediated drug resistance (CAM-DR): role of integrins and resistance to apoptosis in human myeloma cell lines. Blood. 1999;93:1658–67.
54. Nakagawa Y, Nakayama H, Nagata M, Yoshida R, Kawahara K, Hirosue A, Tanaka T, Yuno A, Matsuoka Y, Kojima T, Yoshitake Y, Hiraki A, Shinohara M. Overexpression of fibronectin confers cell adhesion-mediated drug resistance (CAM-DR) against 5-FU in oral squamous cell carcinoma cells. Int J Oncol. 2014;44:1376–84.
55. Mraz M, Zent CS, Church AK, Jelinek DF, Wu X, Pospisilova S, Ansell SM, Novak AJ, Kay NE, Witzig TE, Nowakowski GS. Bone marrow stromal cells protect lymphoma B-cells from rituximab-induced apoptosis and targeting integrin alpha-4-beta-1 (VLA-4) with natalizumab can overcome this resistance. Br J Haematol. 2011;155:53–64.
56. Li ZW, Dalton WS. Tumor microenvironment and drug resistance in hematologic malignancies. Blood Rev. 2006;20:333–42.
57. Damiano JS, Hazlehurst LA, Dalton WS. Cell adhesion-mediated drug resistance (CAM-DR) protects the K562 chronic myelogenous leukemia cell line from apoptosis induced by BCR/ABL inhibition, cytotoxic drugs, and gamma-irradiation. Leukemia. 2001;15:1232–9.
58. Mudry RE, Fortney JE, York T, Hall BM, Gibson LF. Stromal cells regulate survival of B-lineage leukemic cells during chemotherapy. Blood. 2000;96:1926–32.
59. Roodhart JM, He H, Daenen LG, Monvoisin A, Barber CL, van Amersfoort M, Hofmann JJ, Radtke F, Lane TF, Voest EE, Iruela-Arispe ML. Notch1 regulates angio-supportive bone marrow-derived cells in mice: relevance to chemoresistance. Blood. 2013;122:143–53.
60. Nefedova Y, Sullivan DM, Bolick SC, Dalton WS, Gabrilovich DI. Inhibition of Notch signaling induces apoptosis of myeloma cells and enhances sensitivity to chemotherapy. Blood. 2008;111:2220–9.
61. Nefedova Y, Cheng P, Alsina M, Dalton WS, Gabrilovich DI. Involvement of Notch-1 signaling in bone marrow stroma-mediated de novo drug resistance of myeloma and other malignant lymphoid cell lines. Blood. 2004;103:3503–10.
62. Debatin KM. Apoptosis pathways in cancer and cancer therapy. Cancer Immunol Immunother. 2004;53:153–9.
63. Zimmermann KC, Green DR. How cells die: apoptosis pathways. J Allergy Clin Immunol. 2001;108:S99–103.
64. Hu W, Kavanagh JJ. Anticancer therapy targeting the apoptotic pathway. Lancet Oncol. 2003;4:721–9.
65. Cao X, Bennett RL, May WS. c-Myc and caspase-2 are involved in activating Bax during cytotoxic drug-induced apoptosis. J Biol Chem. 2008;283:14490–6.

66. Corazza N, Kassahn D, Jakob S, Badmann A, Brunner T. TRAIL-induced apoptosis: between tumor therapy and immunopathology. Ann N Y Acad Sci. 2009;1171:50–8.
67. Ledgerwood EC, Morison IM. Targeting the apoptosome for cancer therapy. Clin Cancer Res. 2009;15:420–4.
68. Kang MH, Reynolds CP. Bcl-2 inhibitors: targeting mitochondrial apoptotic pathways in cancer therapy. Clin Cancer Res. 2009;15:1126–32.
69. Papenfuss K, Cordier SM, Walczak H. Death receptors as targets for anti-cancer therapy. J Cell Mol Med. 2008;12:2566–85.
70. Akiyama T, Dass CR, Choong PF. Bim-targeted cancer therapy: a link between drug action and underlying molecular changes. Mol Cancer Ther. 2009;8:3173–80.
71. Lessene G, Czabotar PE, Colman PM. BCL-2 family antagonists for cancer therapy. Nat Rev Drug Discov. 2008;7:989–1000.
72. Wajant H. CD95L/FasL and TRAIL in tumour surveillance and cancer therapy. Cancer Treat Res. 2006;130:141–65.
73. Bleackley RC. A molecular view of cytotoxic T lymphocyte induced killing. Biochem Cell Biol. 2005;83:747–51.
74. Sarosiek KA, Chi X, Bachman JA, Sims JJ, Montero J, Patel L, Flanagan A, Andrews DW, Sorger P, Letai A. BID preferentially activates BAK while BIM preferentially activates BAX, affecting chemotherapy response. Mol Cell. 2013;51:751–65.
75. Westphal D, Kluck RM, Dewson G. Building blocks of the apoptotic pore: how Bax and Bak are activated and oligomerize during apoptosis. Cell Death Differ. 2014;21:196–205.
76. Luo X, Budihardjo I, Zou H, Slaughter C, Wang X. Bid, a Bcl2 interacting protein, mediates cytochrome c release from mitochondria in response to activation of cell surface death receptors. Cell. 1998;94:481–90.
77. Rodriguez J, Lazebnik Y. Caspase-9 and APAF-1 form an active holoenzyme. Genes Dev. 1999;13:3179–84.
78. Slee EA, Harte MT, Kluck RM, Wolf BB, Casiano CA, Newmeyer DD, Wang HG, Reed JC, Nicholson DW, Alnemri ES, Green DR, Martin SJ. Ordering the cytochrome c-initiated caspase cascade: hierarchical activation of caspases-2, -3, -6, -7, -8, and -10 in a caspase-9-dependent manner. J Cell Biol. 1999;144:281–92.
79. Kale J, Liu Q, Leber B, Andrews DW. Shedding light on apoptosis at subcellular membranes. Cell. 2012;151:1179–84.
80. Catlett-Falcone R, Landowski TH, Oshiro MM, Turkson J, Levitzki A, Savino R, Ciliberto G, Moscinski L, Fernández-Luna JL, Nuñez G, Dalton WS, Jove R. Constitutive activation of Stat3 signaling confers resistance to apoptosis in human U266 myeloma cells. Immunity. 1999;10:105–15.
81. Reginato MJ, Mills KR, Paulus JK, Lynch DK, Sgroi DC, Debnath J, Muthuswamy SK, Brugge JS. Integrins and EGFR coordinately regulate the pro-apoptotic protein Bim to prevent anoikis. Nat Cell Biol. 2003;5:733–40.
82. Hazlehurst LA, Argilagos RF, Dalton WS. Beta1 integrin mediated adhesion increases Bim protein degradation and contributes to drug resistance in leukaemia cells. Br J Haematol. 2007;136:269–75.
83. de la Fuente MT, Casanova B, Garcia-Gila M, Silva A, Garcia-Pardo A. Fibronectin interaction with alpha4beta1 integrin prevents apoptosis in B cell chronic lymphocytic leukemia: correlation with Bcl-2 and Bax. Leukemia. 1999;13:266–74.
84. Balakrishnan K, Burger JA, Wierda WG, Gandhi V. AT-101 induces apoptosis in CLL B cells and overcomes stromal cell-mediated Mcl-1 induction and drug resistance. Blood. 2009; 113:149–53.
85. Matsunaga T, Takemoto N, Sato T, Takimoto R, Tanaka I, Fujimi A, Akiyama T, Kuroda H, Kawano Y, Kobune M, Kato J, Hirayama Y, Sakamaki S, Kohda K, Miyake K, Niitsu Y. Interaction between leukemic-cell VLA-4 and stromal fibronectin is a decisive factor for minimal residual disease of acute myelogenous leukemia. Nat Med. 2003;9:1158–65.
86. Wang L, Fortney JE, Gibson LF. Stromal cell protection of B-lineage acute lymphoblastic leukemic cells during chemotherapy requires active Akt. Leuk Res. 2004;28:733–42.

87. Paludan C, Bickham K, Nikiforow S, Tsang ML, Goodman K, Hanekom WA, Fonteneau JF, Stevanović S, Münz C. Epstein-Barr nuclear antigen 1-specific CD4(+) Th1 cells kill Burkitt's lymphoma cells. J Immunol. 2002;169:1593–603.
88. Silva CL, Lowrie DB. Identification and characterization of murine cytotoxic T cells that kill Mycobacterium tuberculosis. Infect Immun. 2000;68:3269–74.
89. Wilson AD, Redchenko I, Williams NA, Morgan AJ. CD4+ T cells inhibit growth of Epstein-Barr virus-transformed B cells through CD95–CD95 ligand-mediated apoptosis. Int Immunol. 1998;10:1149–57.
90. Yi S, Feng X, Wang Y, Kay TW, Wang Y, O'Connell PJ. CD4+ cells play a major role in xenogeneic human anti-pig cytotoxicity through the Fas/Fas ligand lytic pathway. Transplantation. 1999;67:435–43.
91. Doherty PC, Topham DJ, Tripp RA, Cardin RD, Brooks JW, Stevenson PG. Effector CD4+ and CD8+ T-cell mechanisms in the control of respiratory virus infections. Immunol Rev. 1997;159:105–17.
92. Komada Y, Zhou YW, Zhang XL, Chen TX, Tanaka S, Azuma E, Sakurai M. Fas/APO-1 (CD95)-mediated cytotoxicity is responsible for the apoptotic cell death of leukaemic cells induced by interleukin-2-activated T cells. Br J Haematol. 1997;96:147–57.
93. Hahn S, Gehri R, Erb P. Mechanism and biological significance of CD4-mediated cytotoxicity. Immunol Rev. 1995;146:57–79.
94. Shelton SN, Shawgo ME, Robertson JD. Cleavage of Bid by executioner caspases mediates feed forward amplification of mitochondrial outer membrane permeabilization during genotoxic stress-induced apoptosis in Jurkat cells. J Biol Chem. 2009;284:11247–55.
95. Perez LE, Parquet N, Shain K, Nimmanapalli R, Alsina M, Anasetti C, Dalton W. Bone marrow stroma confers resistance to Apo2 ligand/TRAIL in multiple myeloma in part by regulating c-FLIP. J Immunol. 2008;180:1545–55.
96. Shain KH, Landowski TH, Dalton WS. Adhesion-mediated intracellular redistribution of c-Fas-associated death domain-like IL-1-converting enzyme-like inhibitory protein-long confers resistance to CD95-induced apoptosis in hematopoietic cancer cell lines. J Immunol. 2002;168:2544–53.
97. de Haart SJ, van de Donk NW, Minnema MC, Huang JH, Aarts-Riemens T, Bovenschen N, Yuan H, Groen RW, McMillin DW, Jakubikova J, Lokhorst HM, Martens AC, Mitsiades CS, Mutis T. Accessory cells of the microenvironment protect multiple myeloma from T-cell cytotoxicity through cell adhesion-mediated immune resistance. Clin Cancer Res. 2013; 19:5591–601.
98. Barry M, Bleackley RC. Cytotoxic T lymphocytes: all roads lead to death. Nat Rev Immunol. 2002;2:401–9.
99. Jazirehi AR, Baritaki S, Koya RC, Bonavida B, Economou JS. Molecular mechanism of MART-1+/A*0201+ human melanoma resistance to specific CTL-killing despite functional tumor-CTL interaction. Cancer Res. 2011;71:1406–17.
100. Karlsson H, Lindqvist AC, Fransson M, Paul-Wetterberg G, Nilsson B, Essand M, Nilsson K, Frisk P, Jernberg-Wiklund H, Loskog A. CAR T cells and the Bcl-2 family apoptosis inhibitor ABT-737 for treating B-cell malignancy. Cancer Gene Ther. 2013;20:386–93.
101. Thakur A, Lum LG, Schalk D, Azmi A, Banerjee S, Sarkar FH, Mohommad R. Pan-Bcl-2 inhibitor AT-101 enhances tumor cell killing by EGFR targeted T cells. PLoS One. 2012; 7:e47520.
102. Medema JP, de Jong J, Peltenburg LT, Verdegaal EM, Gorter A, Bres SA, Franken KL, Hahne M, Albar JP, Melief CJ, Offringa R. Blockade of the granzyme B/perforin pathway through overexpression of the serine protease inhibitor PI-9/SPI-6 constitutes a mechanism for immune escape by tumors. Proc Natl Acad Sci U S A. 2001;98:11515–20.
103. Classen CF, Ushmorov A, Bird P, Debatin KM. The granzyme B inhibitor PI-9 is differentially expressed in all main subtypes of pediatric acute lymphoblastic leukemias. Haematologica. 2004;89:1314–21.
104. van Houdt IS, Oudejans JJ, van den Eertwegh AJ, Baars A, Vos W, Bladergroen BA, Rimoldi D, Muris JJ, Hooijberg E, Gundy CM, Meijer CJ, Kummer JA. Expression of the apoptosis

inhibitor protease inhibitor 9 predicts clinical outcome in vaccinated patients with stage III and IV melanoma. Clin Cancer Res. 2005;11:6400–7.
105. Kannan-Thulasiraman P, Shapiro DJ. Modulators of inflammation use nuclear factor-kappa B and activator protein-1 sites to induce the caspase-1 and granzyme B inhibitor, proteinase inhibitor 9. J Biol Chem. 2002;277:41230–9.
106. Holmquist-Mengelbier L, Fredlund E, Löfstedt T, Noguera R, Navarro S, Nilsson H, Pietras A, Vallon-Christersson J, Borg A, Gradin K, Poellinger L, Påhlman S. Recruitment of HIF-1alpha and HIF-2alpha to common target genes is differentially regulated in neuroblastoma: HIF-2alpha promotes an aggressive phenotype. Cancer Cell. 2006;10:413–23.
107. Sarkar S, Germeraad WT, Rouschop KM, Steeghs EM, van Gelder M, Bos GM, Wieten L. Hypoxia induced impairment of NK cell cytotoxicity against multiple myeloma can be overcome by IL-2 activation of the NK cells. PLoS One. 2013;8:e64835.
108. Roy N, Deveraux QL, Takahashi R, Salvesen GS, Reed JC. The c-IAP-1 and c-IAP-2 proteins are direct inhibitors of specific caspases. EMBO J. 1997;16:6914–25.
109. Deveraux QL, Roy N, Stennicke HR, Van Arsdale T, Zhou Q, Srinivasula SM, Alnemri ES, Salvesen GS, Reed JC. IAPs block apoptotic events induced by caspase-8 and cytochrome c by direct inhibition of distinct caspases. EMBO J. 1998;17:2215–23.
110. Liston P, Roy N, Tamai K, Lefebvre C, Baird S, Cherton-Horvat G, Farahani R, McLean M, Ikeda JE, MacKenzie A, Korneluk RG. Suppression of apoptosis in mammalian cells by NAIP and a related family of IAP genes. Nature. 1996;379:349–53.
111. Du C, Fang M, Li Y, Li L, Wang X. Smac, a mitochondrial protein that promotes cytochrome c-dependent caspase activation by eliminating IAP inhibition. Cell. 2000;102:33–42.
112. Verhagen AM, Ekert PG, Pakusch M, Silke J, Connolly LM, Reid GE, Moritz RL, Simpson RJ, Vaux DL. Identification of DIABLO, a mammalian protein that promotes apoptosis by binding to and antagonizing IAP proteins. Cell. 2000;102:43–53.
113. Hahne JC, Meyer SR, Gambaryan S, Walter U, Dietl J, Engel JB, Honig A. Immune escape of AKT overexpressing ovarian cancer cells. Int J Oncol. 2013;42:1630–5.
114. Vegran F, Mary R, Gibeaud A, Mirjolet C, Collin B, Oudot A, Charon-Barra C, Arnould L, Lizard-Nacol S, Boidot R. Survivin-3B potentiates immune escape in cancer but also inhibits the toxicity of cancer chemotherapy. Cancer Res. 2013;73:5391–401.
115. Classen CF, Fulda S, Friesen C, Debatin KM. Decreased sensitivity of drug-resistant cells towards T cell cytotoxicity. Leukemia. 1999;13:410–8.
116. McMillin DW, Delmore J, Negri JM, Vanneman M, Koyama S, Schlossman RL, Munshi NC, Laubach J, Richardson PG, Dranoff G, Anderson KC, Mitsiades CS. Compartment-specific bioluminescence imaging platform for the high-throughput evaluation of antitumor immune function. Blood. 2012;119:e131–8.
117. Nakahara T, Kita A, Yamanaka K, Mori M, Amino N, Takeuchi M, Tominaga F, Hatakeyama S, Kinoyama I, Matsuhisa A, Kudoh M, Sasamata M. YM155, a novel small-molecule survivin suppressant, induces regression of established human hormone-refractory prostate tumor xenografts. Cancer Res. 2007;67:8014–21.
118. Tang H, Shao H, Yu C, Hou J. Mcl-1 downregulation by YM155 contributes to its synergistic anti-tumor activities with ABT-263. Biochem Pharmacol. 2011;82:1066–72.
119. Datta SR, Dudek H, Tao X, Masters S, Fu H, Gotoh Y, Greenberg ME. Akt phosphorylation of BAD couples survival signals to the cell-intrinsic death machinery. Cell. 1997;91:231–41.
120. Boni A, Cogdill AP, Dang P, Udayakumar D, Njauw CN, Sloss CM, Ferrone CR, Flaherty KT, Lawrence DP, Fisher DE, Tsao H, Wargo JA. Selective BRAFV600E inhibition enhances T-cell recognition of melanoma without affecting lymphocyte function. Cancer Res. 2010;70:5213–9.
121. Jazirehi AR, Kurdistani SK, Economou JS. Histone deacetylase inhibitor sensitizes apoptosis-resistant melanomas to cytotoxic human T lymphocytes through regulation of TRAIL/DR5 pathway. J Immunol. 2014;192:3981–9.
122. Hodge JW, Garnett CT, Farsaci B, Palena C, Tsang KY, Ferrone S, Gameiro SR. Chemotherapy-induced immunogenic modulation of tumor cells enhances killing by cytotoxic T lymphocytes and is distinct from immunogenic cell death. Int J Cancer. 2013;133:624–36.

123. Li J, Favata M, Kelley JA, Caulder E, Thomas B, Wen X, Sparks RB, Arvanitis A, Rogers JD, Combs AP, Vaddi K, Solomon KA, Scherle PA, Newton R, Fridman JS. INCB16562, a JAK1/2 selective inhibitor, is efficacious against multiple myeloma cells and reverses the protective effects of cytokine and stromal cell support. Neoplasia. 2010;12:28–38.
124. Straussman R, Morikawa T, Shee K, Barzily-Rokni M, Qian ZR, Du J, Davis A, Mongare MM, Gould J, Frederick DT, Cooper ZA, Chapman PB, Solit DB, Ribas A, Lo RS, Flaherty KT, Ogino S, Wargo JA, Golub TR. Tumour micro-environment elicits innate resistance to RAF inhibitors through HGF secretion. Nature. 2012;487:500–4.
125. Azab AK, Runnels JM, Pitsillides C, Moreau AS, Azab F, Leleu X, Jia X, Wright R, Ospina B, Carlson AL, Alt C, Burwick N, Roccaro AM, Ngo HT, Farag M, Melhem MR, Sacco A, Munshi NC, Hideshima T, Rollins BJ, Anderson KC, Kung AL, Lin CP, Ghobrial IM. CXCR4 inhibitor AMD3100 disrupts the interaction of multiple myeloma cells with the bone marrow microenvironment and enhances their sensitivity to therapy. Blood. 2009;113:4341–51.
126. Gogoi D, Dar AA, Chiplunkar SV. Involvement of Notch in activation and effector functions of gammadelta T cells. J Immunol. 2014;192:2054–62.
127. Sandy AR, Chung J, Toubai T, Shan GT, Tran IT, Friedman A, Blackwell TS, Reddy P, King PD, Maillard I. T cell-specific notch inhibition blocks graft-versus-host disease by inducing a hyporesponsive program in alloreactive CD4+ and CD8+ T cells. J Immunol. 2013; 190:5818–28.
128. Zhang Y, Sandy AR, Wang J, Radojcic V, Shan GT, Tran IT, Friedman A, Kato K, He S, Cui S, Hexner E, Frank DM, Emerson SG, Pear WS, Maillard I. Notch signaling is a critical regulator of allogeneic CD4+ T-cell responses mediating graft-versus-host disease. Blood. 2011; 117:299–308.

Chapter 8
Evasion of Cytotoxic Lymphocyte and Pulmonary Macrophage-Mediated Immune Responses in Lung Cancer

Sandra Hodge and Greg Hodge

Abstract Lung cancer is responsible for more cancer-related deaths than colon, breast and prostate cancers combined. Survival rates for lung cancer are generally lower than those for most cancers, with an overall 5-year survival rate for lung cancer of about 16 % compared to 65 % for colon cancer, 89 % for breast cancer, and over 99 % for prostate cancer. Lung cancer comprises several types with varying response to therapy and survival rates; although they can be broadly grouped into small cell lung carcinoma (SCLC) and non-small cell lung carcinoma (NSCLC). NSCLC includes squamous cell carcinoma, adenocarcinoma, and large cell carcinoma. SCLC accounts for approximately 20 % of all primary lung cancers and in general and tends to be more aggressive; some studies suggest that 60–70 % of patients with small cell lung cancer have evidence of distant spread at the time of initial diagnosis; treatment usually is limited to chemotherapy and/or radiation therapy. By contrast, surgical resection for NSLC may be an option.

COPD/emphysema is a highly prevalent airways disease that arises as a result of noxious injury to the lungs. Cigarette smoke plays a significant role in the aetiology of both COPD and lung cancer. Both smokers and COPD patients have an increased risk of developing lung cancer; however, there is an increased risk of developing lung cancer in smokers with COPD far above that of smokers without COPD. The carcinogenic effects of tobacco smoke have been well-described with over 80 % of lung cancer cases occurring in smokers or ex-smokers. The burden of COPD and the associated prevalence of COPD-associated lung cancer are

---

The authors have no potential conflicts of interest to disclose.

S. Hodge (✉) • G. Hodge
Department of Lung Research, Hanson Institute; Thoracic Medicine, Royal Adelaide Hospital, and Medicine, University of Adelaide, Adelaide, South Australia
e-mail: Sandra.hodge@health.sa.gov.au

B. Bonavida, S. Chouaib (eds.), *Resistance of Cancer Cells to CTL-Mediated Immunotherapy*, Resistance to Targeted Anti-Cancer Therapeutics 7,
DOI 10.1007/978-3-319-17807-3_8

projected to increase in the coming decades due to continued exposure to COPD risk factors and the changing age structure of the world's population. Despite these alarming statistics, it is unknown why many lung cancers are relatively resistant to conventional therapies.

Keywords Lung cancer • Immune evasion • Cytotoxic T-cell • CD8 T-cell • NK cells • NKT-like cells • Tregs • Granzyme B • PI-9 • Macrophage phagocytosis

Abbreviations

AA	Arachidonic acid
COPD	Chronic obstructive pulmonary disease
COX	Cyclooxygenase-2
CTL	Cytotoxic T-cells
EP1–4	E-prostanoid 2 receptor 1–4
IFN	Interferon
IL-	Interleukin
LC-ESI-MSMS	High performance liquid chromatography—electrospray tandem mass spectrometry
NK cells	Natural killer cells
NSCLC	Non small cell lung cancer
PGE2	Eicosanoid prostaglandin E2
PI-9	Proteinase inhibitor 9
SCLC	Small cell lung cancer
TGF	Transforming growth factor
TNF	Tumour necrosis factor
Tregs	Regulatory T lymphocytes

8.1 Introduction

8.1.1 Lung Cancer

Lung cancer is responsible for more cancer-related deaths than colon, breast and prostate cancers combined [1]. For small cell lung cancer (SCLC), many patients have evidence of distant spread at the time of initial diagnosis thus management is usually limited to chemotherapy and/or radiation therapy. For non-small cell lung cancer (NSLC), surgical resection for NSLC may be an option [2–4]. Both cigarette smokers and patients with chronic obstructive pulmonary disease (COPD) have an increased risk of developing lung cancer [5, 6]. It is currently unclear why many lung cancers are relatively resistant to conventional therapies.

8.1.2 Elimination of Tumour Cells by Natural Killer (NK) and Cytotoxic T-cells (CTL)

CTLs are important barriers against virally infected cells and tumour cells. Elimination of tumour cells by NK and CTL's is induced through two major cytolytic pathways; the death receptor pathway (mediated by the TNF/Fas family) and the calcium-dependent granule exocytosis pathway [7, 8]. The latter pathway involves removal of the target cell by the process of apoptosis mediated by the release of pore-forming perforin and enzymes that are stored in the cytoplasmic granules of CTL's. These enzymes comprise granzymes, perforin and granulysin [9–11]. After a cytotoxic/target cell junction, perforin is released by exocytosis before forming pores upon the target cell membrane. Granzyme B and granulysin are passively conducted through the target cell membrane, followed by caspase cleavage and induction of DNA fragmentation. Although widely considered to be essential for the entrance of these mediators into the target cell, accumulating evidence suggests that perforin is not absolutely necessary for this function, although it is required for granzyme B-induced cytolysis (cleaving several intracellular proteins, including caspase-3, and inducing DNA fragmentation). Granulysin, in contrast, has a structural similarity to the saposin family and it has been suggested that its lytic activity occurs due to cell membrane damage as a result of interactions between granulysin and negative charges from target cell mitochondrial membrane lipids, although this is augmented by the presence of perforin.

8.2 Resistance of Tumour Cells to CTL-Induced Apoptosis

It is becoming increasingly documented, however, that many tumour cells have the ability to resist CTL-induced apoptosis. Of particular importance to the survival and proliferation of lung cancer cells may be resistance to granzyme B-mediated attack. One means of this resistance may be the expression of specific proteins that inhibit tumour cell death induced by the granzyme pathway. The only known specific inhibitor of granzyme B is the intracellular serine protease inhibitor PI-9 [12–14]. PI-9 is a serpin that inactivates granzyme B, thereby inhibiting progression of the apoptotic pathway. PI-9 is normally found in lymphoid tissue, immune-privileged sites and CTL's. PI-9 is normally present in the cytoplasm and nucleus. When present in the cytoplasm of CTL's PI-9 is thought to protect the cells from destruction by their own granzyme B [14, 15]. Secreted PI-9 has also been found, although the study did not ascertain whether the PI-9 was actually released from the cells or released as a result of cellular necrosis [12].

Interestingly, the expression of PI-9 has been reported in various cancer cells, where it is likely to act by preventing granzyme B/perforin-mediated apoptosis of the cancer cell [15–19]. This potential evasion mechanism was highlighted in a study of anaplastic large cell lymphoma where a relationship between high numbers of cancer cells expressing PI-9 and poor outcome was shown [17]. In B cell non-Hodgkins lymphoma, high PI-9 expression was shown to be associated with high grade malignancy [15]. PI-9 is also thought to directly inhibit the caspase (caspase-1 and potentially caspases-8 and -10) and Fas/FasL pathways of apoptosis induction [20]. The anti-apoptotic protein cellular FLICE inhibitory protein (cFLIP) is a further anti-apoptotic protein that may bind via two death effector domains and functions as an inactive caspase-8 surrogate [21–23]. Increased expression of cFLIP has been reported in colonic carcinoma where it may act to inhibit apoptosis induced by the CTL mediators [24].

8.3 PI-9 in Lung Cancer

Increased granzyme B in CTL's associated with increased cell death in BAL and blood from COPD patients has been reported [25]. However, based on the findings described above, it is likely that lung tumour-associated CTLs will exhibit reduced expression of granzyme B even in the presence of COPD, and this could result from increased production of the granzyme B inhibitor PI-9 by the lung cancer cells. Consistent with the presence of PI-9 in other cancer types discussed above, high expression of PI-9 has been shown in some NSCLC cell lines and tumour cells from lung cancer resection [18]. The PI-9 was shown to form a complex with granzyme B and inhibit granzyme B-mediated cytotoxicity. Soriano et al. applied both flow cytometry and immunohistochemistry to show that reduced granzyme B expression by CD8+ T-cells in curative lung cancer tissue resected from lung cancer patients and increased PI-9 expression by the lung cancer cells (Fig. 8.1) [26]. The authors compared PI-9 expression between bronchial brushing-derived primary large airway epithelial cells and disaggregated epithelial cells from non-cancer areas of resected lung tissue, validating the use of these cells as controls.

Soriano et al. further investigated whether soluble mediators secreted by the various lung cancer cell lines could inhibit granzyme B by CD8+ T-cells [26]. All cancer cell lines with the exception of H1466 significantly reduced expression of this cytotoxic mediator. Cytotoxicity was also assessed in CD8+ T-cells positively

Fig. 8.1 (**a**) PI-9 expression by A. primary large airway epithelial cells collected by bronchial brushing at flexible bronchoscopy from 16 healthy controls ('Large airway EC') B. epithelial cells obtained from non-cancer areas of resected lung tissue ('Non-cancer tissue') and C. cancer cells from cancer areas of lung tissue ('Cancer tissue') from a cohort of 17 cancer patients. PI-9 expression determined using flow cytometry. *Reproduced with permission from Soriano et al. Lung Cancer* 2012;77(1):38–45. (**b**) Immunohistochemical analysis of PI-9 expression in cancer and non-cancer lung tissue. PI-9 expression as measured by a scoring index in epithelial cells from non-cancer and cancer tissue from lung cancer tissue from patients with no COPD ('Non-cancer Tissue; No COPD' and 'Cancer Tissue; No COPD'), epithelial cells from non-cancer and cancer lung tissue from subjects with Cancer + COPD ('Non-cancer Tissue; + COPD' and 'Cancer Tissue; + COPD'). (A) Positive PI-9 expression in primary lung cancer tissue (*brown staining*). (B) Negative staining with serum only. (C) Low staining for PI-9 in epithelial cells from non-cancer tissue. Original magnification 200× (A) and 400× (B) and (C). (D) Data summarized in histogram (mean ± SEM). *Reproduced with permission from Soriano et al. Lung Cancer* 2012;77(1):38–45

a

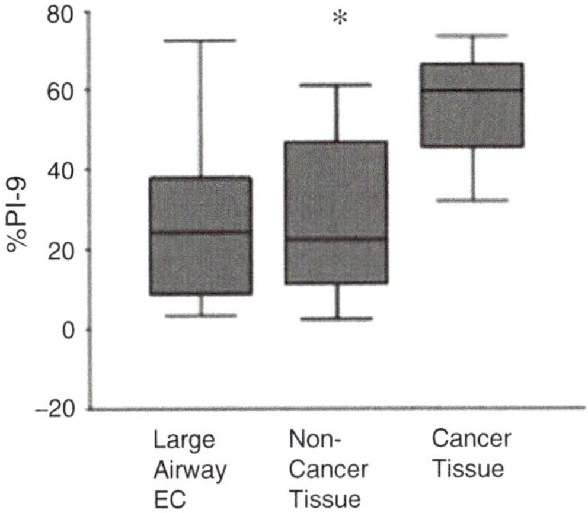
80
60
40
20
0
–20
%PI-9
*
Large Airway EC
Non-Cancer Tissue
Cancer Tissue

b

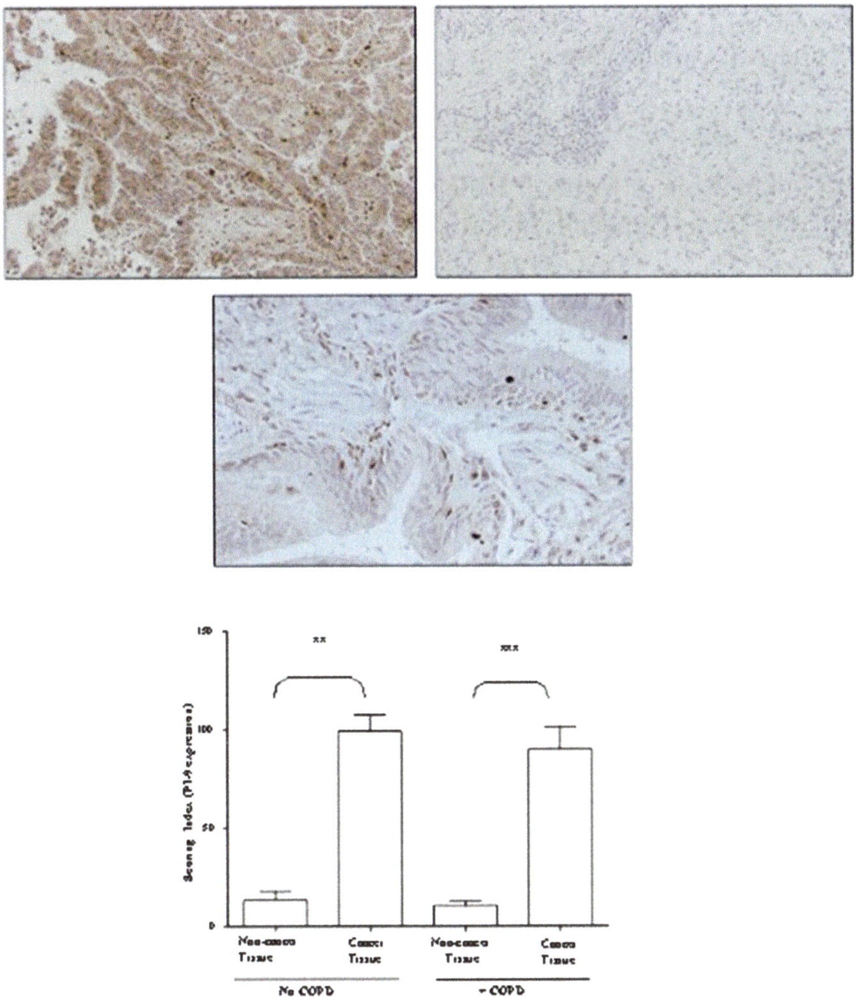
**
***

selected from PBMC and stimulated with a Dynabeads CD3/CD28 T cell expander [26]. After removal of beads, CD8+ T-cells were resuspended in cancer cell supernatants. Cytotoxicity using K562 human myeloid leukemia cells was analysed by a modified flow-cytometric method described by Kim et al. [27].

Again, soluble mediators secreted by the various lung cancer cell lines induced a reduction in the cytotoxic potential of the CD8+ T-cells. Interestingly, H1466 cells with relatively low expression of PI-9 also had a relatively low effect on cytotoxicity and granzyme B production by CD8+ T-cells. Thus, available evidence suggests that PI-9 over-expression by lung cancer cells and a resultant down-regulation of granzyme B expression by lung cancer-associated CD8+ T-cells may provide an immune evasion mechanism against granzyme B-mediated cytotoxicity in lung cancer. Whether the levels of perforin and granulysin follow the same pattern of expression as granzyme B remains to be determined; it is also possible that levels of one or all of these mediators are decreased in T-cells from the tumour vs the normal tissue environment contributing to reduced apoptosis and tumour evasion. Treatment strategies that inhibit expression of these mediators within cancer cells will enhance the cell's sensitivity to granzyme B/perforin-mediated apoptosis and/or apoptosis induced by other agents.

8.4 The Role of Natural Killer (NK) and NKT-Like Cells in Lung Cancer Evasion

The preceding section described the ability of cytotoxic cells including CD8+ T-cells to mount immune responses to cancer via the release of cytolytic enzymes including granzyme B and perforin. Hodge et al. showed that NK and NKT-like cells are also potent producers of these cytotoxic and proinflammatory mediators, suggesting a strong role for these cell types in the elimination of tumour cells [28]. The gating strategy applied to identify NK and NKT-like cells is shown in Fig. 8.2.

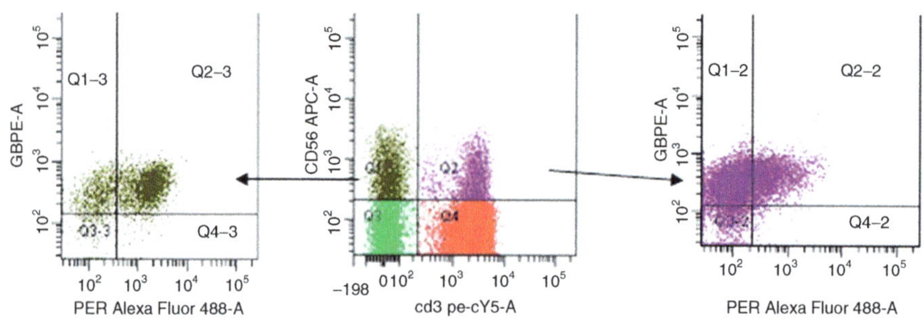

Fig. 8.2 Flow cytometry gating strategy to identify perforin and granzyme B positive NK (CD56+CD3–) cells and NKT-like (CD56+CD3+) cells. The *central panel* shows staining with CD3-PE-Cy5 vs CD56 APC. The *left panel* shown staining for perforin (FITC) vs. granzyme B (PE) on NK cells gated on the basis of negative staining for CD3 and positive staining for CD56. The *right panel* shows staining for perforin (FITC) vs. granzyme B (PE) on NKT-like cells gated on the basis of positive staining for both CD3 and CD56

Resistance to attack by NK and NKT-like cells is, therefore, essential for the survival and proliferation of lung cancer cells, although until recently it was unknown whether their production of cytotoxic mediators was changed in the pro-tumour environment. Resistance to attack by NK and NKT-like cells is therefore essential for the survival and proliferation of lung cancer cells, although until recently, it was unknown whether their production of cytotoxic mediators was changed in the pro-tumour environment. Recently, Hodge et al. further described the relative expression of NK and NKT-like cells in lung cancer vs non-cancer lung tissue, and their relative production of granzyme B, perforin and pro-inflammatory cytokines [29]. They investigated lung cancer and normal tissue (from lung resection surgery for management of lung cancer), identified by experienced pathologists. Tissue was dissaggregated into single cells. Following adherence and removal of macrophages, pro-inflammatory **c**ytokines and expression of the cytotoxic mediators granzyme B and perforin were measured in CD4 and CD8+ T, NKT-like cells and NK cells by flow cytometry. They found a significant decrease in the percentage of T, NKT-like subsets and NK cells expressing perforin and IFN-γ compared with normal tissue. There was also a decrease in the percentages of CD8+ T cells and CD8+ NKT-like cells expressing granzyme B compared with normal tissue (Fig. 8.3a). Thus, lung cancer is associated with decreased expression of perforin (Fig. 8.3b), granzyme B and IFN-γ (Fig. 8.3c) by infiltrating T cells, NKT-like and NK cells and may be an important immune evasion mechanism.

Hodge et al. then investigated whether the cancer cells secrete soluble mediators that exert a suppressive effect on the production of pro-inflammatory cytokines by NK and NKT-like cells.

Treatment of lung cancer supernatants with a Cox-2 inhibitor, indomethacin, significantly negated the suppressive effect of lung cancer supernatants on IFNγ and TNFα production by CD4 and CD8 T and NKT-like and NK cells [29] (Fig. 8.4).

8.5 Decreased Pulmonary Macrophage Function in Lung Cancer as a Potential Immune Evasion Mechanism

Dehle et al. continued the theme of immune surveillance, again utilizing well-characterized lung tissue samples obtained at lobectomy for the management of lung cancer [30]. They focused on the lung macrophage as this cell has been extensively shown to have a significant defect in the ability to phagocytose apoptotic cells (efferocytosis) with resultant airway inflammation [31–34]. The potential relevance of effective macrophage phagocytic ability in cancer was shown in patients treated with rituximab, a drug which acts, in part, by opsonizing cells and increasing phagocytosis. The treatment had a positive prognostic value despite the high number of tumour-associated macrophages [31].

Un-cleared apoptotic material is likely to be important in the progression of lung cancer as this material can then undergo secondary necrosis and perpetuate the inflammatory response [35–37]. Importantly, uncleared apoptotic material induces

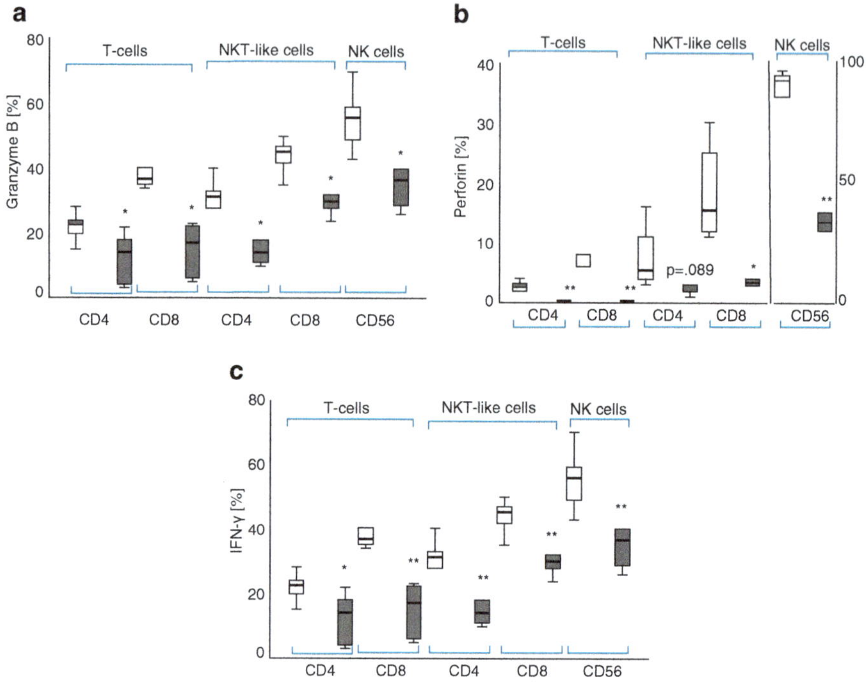

Fig. 8.3 (**a**) Intracellular granzyme B expression in CD4+ and CD8+ T cell and NKT-like subsets and NK cells from normal (*clear bars*) and cancer tissue (*grey bars*). There was a significant decrease in the percentage of CD8+ T cells expressing granzyme B from cancer tissue compared with normal tissue. There was also an decrease in the percentage of CD8+ NKT-like cells and NK cells expressing granzyme B compared with normal tissue (*$p<0.05$). *Reproduced from Hodge et al. Clinical and Experimental Immunology 2014 in press.* (**b**) Perforin expression in CD4+ and CD8+ T cell and NKT-like subsets and NK cells from normal (*clear bars*) and cancer tissue (*grey bars*). There was a decrease in the percentage of CD4+ and CD8+ T cells expressing perforin from cancer tissue compared with normal tissue. There was also a decrease in the percentage of CD8+ NKT-like cells and NK cells expressing perforin compared with normal tissue (*$p<0.05$; **$p<0.01$). *Reproduced from Hodge et al. Clinical and Experimental Immunology 2014 in press.* (**c**) IFN-γ production in CD4+ and CD8+ T cell and NKT-like subsets and NK cells from normal (*clear bars*) and cancer tissue (*grey bars*). There was a decrease in the percentage of CD4+ and CD8+ T cells, CD4+ and CD8+ NKT-like cells and NK cells producing IFN-γ from cancer tissue compared with normal tissue (*$p<0.05$; **$p<0.01$). *Reproduced from Hodge et al. Clinical and Experimental Immunology 2014 in press*

anti-DNA antibodies to self antigens, that results in a "pseudo-autoimmune status" leading to an influx of immature dendritic cells and the induction of regulatory T lymphocytes (Tregs) [38, 39]. Tregs are endogenous regulators of the immune response that are capable of attenuating immune responses to self and non-self antigens. There is abundant evidence for the role of these cells in cancer development [40]. One study showed that the inhibition of Tregs in a mouse model of cancer induced an increase in intra-tumoural CTL numbers and reduced tumour burden [41]. Jarnicki et al. reported in a cancer model that tumour growth facilitated

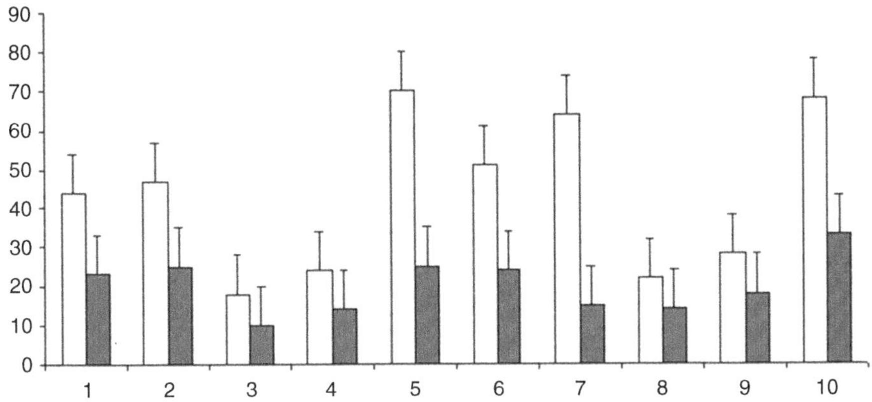

Fig. 8.4 The percentage inhibition of IFN-γ and TNFα by CD4 and CD8 T and NKT-like and CD56+ NK cells in the presence of lung cancer supernatant (*clear bars*). Inhibition of pro-inflammatory cytokines in the presence of lung cancer supernatants was significantly negated in the presence of indomethacin in most lymphocyte subsets (*grey bars*). *Reproduced from Hodge et al. Clinical and Experimental Immunology 2014 in press*

the induction or recruitment of CD4 Tregs that secreted IL-10 and TGF-β and suppressed the effector CD8 T cell responses [42]. Chen et al. further reported that Tregs derived from mice with hepatocellular carcinoma down-regulated the expression of costimulatory molecules CD80/CD86 and inhibited the production of TNF-α and IL-12 by dendritic cells, further supporting the essential role for Tregs in the establishment and persistence of tumor immune suppression [43].

The role of Tregs in the increased susceptibility of COPD patients to lung cancer has not been fully assessed. One study showed a lower frequency of Tregs, Foxp3 and IL-10 in the blood of patients with moderate and severe COPD [44]. Interestingly, the study also reported that increased ratios of Th17 to Tregs were negatively correlated with the values of forced vital capacity (FVC), forced expiratory volume in 1 s (FEV1) and FEV1/FVC, suggesting that an imbalance of circulating Th17 cells and Tregs is associated with the deterioration of pulmonary function in COPD [44]. The same authors found that mice with chronic cigarette smoke exposure showed significant increase in lung Th17 prevalence and Th17-related cytokines (IL-17A, IL-6 and IL-23) accompanied by a decrease in the prevalence of Tregs, Forkhead box (Fox) p3 mRNA and the Treg-related regulatory cytokine IL-10, as compared to mice that underwent sub-acute CS exposure and air-exposure [45]. A similar trend was also found for the Th17/Treg ratios in peripheral blood. A further study showed that Tregs from COPD patients suppressed lipoprotein P6-specific T cell proliferation to a greater extent than Tregs from healthy subjects. Plasma levels of Treg-generated regulatory cytokines and both IL-10 and TGF-β were elevated. Taken together these data suggest that functionally suppressive Tregs may contribute to effector T cell dysfunction and the development and perpetuation of inflammation in COPD [46]. However, the mechanisms by which the chronic airway inflammation

COPD is associated with an enhanced risk for lung cancer, and the role of Tregs in the progression to lung cancer are not well-defined. In one study that applied a mouse model of lung cancer, using an oncogenic form of K-ras (K-ras(G12D)) that is frequently found in human lung cancer, an increased presence of Th17 and Tregs in the lung cancer tissues was shown [47]. A further study applied a doxycycline-treated IKTA (IKKβ trans-activated) mouse model that developed chronic airway inflammation and markedly increased numbers of lung tumours in response to urethane. The lungs of these mice were shown to have a substantial increase in functional Tregs. Importantly, Treg depletion using repetitive injections of anti-CD25 antibodies limited excessive tumour formation in the mice, while at 6 weeks following urethane injection, antibody-mediated Treg depletion in the IKTA mice reduced the number of premalignant lesions in the lungs. Thus, persistent inflammatory signalling in the airway may facilitate tumourigenesis by effects on the immune/inflammatory environment in the lungs. There is, however, still a need for more comprehensive studies to define the differential expression of Tregs in blood, BAL and lung/tumour tissues from subjects with COPD with/without lung cancer. Whether there is differential expression of Tregs in the various compartments and whether these are related to a higher risk of developing lung cancer remain to be explored.

To investigate whether the macrophage phagocytic defect was present in cancer (no COPD), Dehle et al. investigated efferocytosis in both alveolar and lung tissue macrophages and found that decreased efferocytosis was noted in all cancer/COPD groups in both compartments (presented in Fig. 8.5) [30]. Others have also

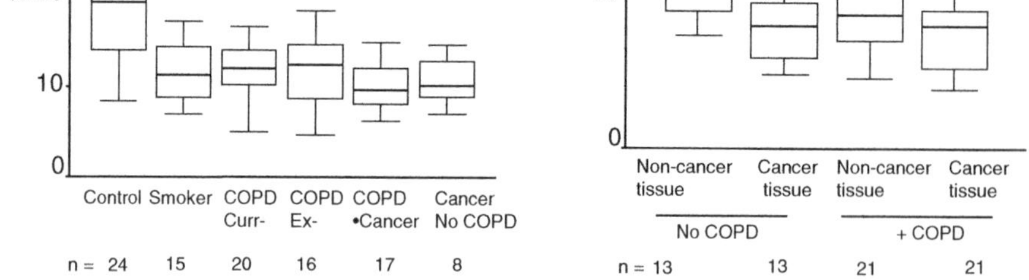

Fig. 8.5 Efferocytosis ability of (**a**) alveolar and (**b**) lung tissue macrophages. (**a**) Controls ('C'), smokers, current- and ex- smokers with COPD ('COPD Cur' and 'COPD Ex'), COPD subjects with lung cancer ('COPD Cancer') and patients with lung cancer and no COPD ('Cancer'); (**b**) Tissue from Controls ('C Non-Tumor') (non-cancer area from patients with cancer/no COPD), 'COPD Non-Tumor' (non-cancer area from patients with cancer+COPD), 'COPD Tumor' (cancer site from patients with cancer+COPD) and 'Control Tumor' (cancer site from patients with cancer/no COPD). *significantly ($p<0.05$) lower expression vs. controls *Reproduced with permission from Dehle et al. PLoS One April 26 2013* http://dx.plos.org/10.1371/journal.pone.0061573

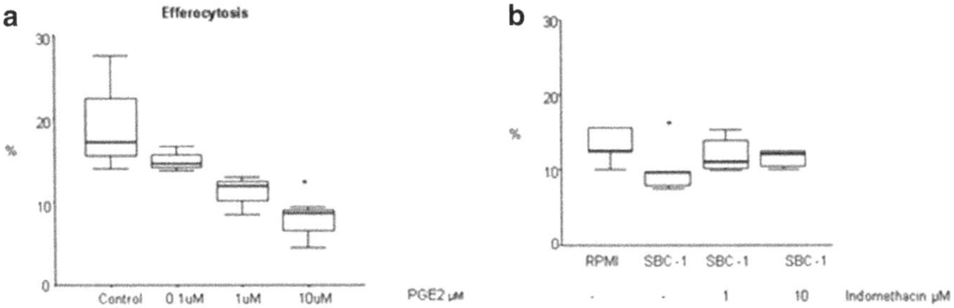

Fig. 8.6 (**a**) Prostaglandins inhibit efferocytosis and partially mediate the inhibitory effect of cancer cell line supernatants on the phagocytosis of apoptotic bronchial epithelial cells by U937 cells. U937 cells were incubated with varying concentrations of PGE2 for 18 h and efferocytosis assessed. (**b**) Prostaglandin inhibition of efferocytosis involves COX-2 U937 cells were incubated in normal RPMI media or SBC-1 supernatant that had been treated with indomethacin. Values are presented as percentage of macrophages ingesting apoptotic cells *, $p<0.05$ compared with control (RPMI media treatment). Reproduced with permission from *Dehle et al. PLoS One April 26 2013*

found evidence for defective macrophage phagocytic function in lung cancer [48]. The investigators showed that phagocytosis of fluorescent beads and surface expression of mannose receptor (required for effective phagocytosis) on alveolar macrophages from patients with lung cancer was reduced. However, the study did not investigate the link between COPD and cancer and it is currently unknown whether there is variability in the ability of macrophages to phagocytose various lung cancer cells or whether COPD subjects with lung cancer demonstrate further reduced ability to phagocytose the tumour cells.

Further in vitro experiments confirmed that the presence of supernatant from the lung cancer cells decreased the ability of alveolar macrophages to phagocytose apoptotic cells (Fig. 8.6a). To identify the mediators responsible for these effects, Arachidonic Acid (AA) metabolites in cancer cells were qualitatively identified by LC-ESI-MSMS, and the effects of COX inhibition (using indomethacin) on efferocytosis were assessed. All three lung cancer cell lines tested (A549, H2009, SBC-1) showed detectable levels of PGE2, PGD2, PGF2α, TXN2 and 6ketoPGF1. 11-HETE, TxB2; 12- and 5- HETE; EPA, DHA, 8-HODE, LTB4, 12(5)TETE, PGB2 and 13(5)HODE were not identified. The eicosanoid prostaglandin E2 (PGE2) is present to some degree in nearly all cell types including cancer cells, and exerts it effects by interacting with four different receptors termed E-prostanoid 2 receptor (EP1–EP4). PGE2 release is mediated by phospholipase A2 followed by metabolism by cyclooxygenase-2 (COX-2). Based on the presence of PGE2, the investigators assessed the effects of the COX inhibitor, indomethacin, on efferocytosis (Fig. 8.6b). It was shown that the phagocytic defect is at least partially a result of inhibition by soluble mediators produced by cancer cells that include PGE2. These data are consistent with another study of NSCLC cell lines A549 and H1299 [49]. PGE2 was also shown to have a suppressive effect on phagocytosis of bacteria [50]. In mesothelioma cancer cells co-cultured with macrophages induced a decrease in phagocytosis but an increase in the PGE-2 release [51]. Taken together, this data describe the new and exciting findings that decreased efferocytosis in airway and lung tissues in lung cancer and the inhibition of efferocytosis via release of soluble prostaglandins by lung cancer cells may be a potential immune evasion mechanism in lung cancer.

8.6 The Effect of Cancer Stage on Mediators of Immune Evasion

Soriano et al. found that PI-9 expression positively correlated with cancer stage among the patients with NSCLC [26]. Others also reported that PI-9 expression is associated with poor prognosis or clinical outcome in anaplastic large B-cell lymphoma, or in vaccinated patients with stage III and IV melanoma [16]. There remains, however, a need for further investigations of large numbers of lung cancer cases over a 5 year period to allow for the important investigation of the correlation of PI-9 with long-term patient outcomes in lung cancer. As curative lobectomy is not routinely applied for the management of SCLC, assessing the association between SCLC stage and PI-9 expression in cells obtained from lung tissue is more difficult. Consistent with the concept that the more aggressive SCLC would exhibit increased expression of PI-9, one study reported that SBC1 and SBC3 expressed more PI-9 than NSCLC lines [26]. In contrast, Rousalova et al. reported higher expression of PI-9 in NSCLC cell lines compared to SCLC cell lines [18]. The varying data may have resulted from the two studies using different cell lines. The wide variability in the expression of PI-9 in NSCLC cell lines may have also contributed [26], and further larger studies are warranted. Also required are investigations of the association between PI-9 levels and survival rates. Preliminary studies in our laboratory using cell lines have found a significant negative correlation between levels of PI-9 in the lung cancer cells and the reported 5 year survival rate for the various cancer types and stages (unpublished).

Interestingly, and consistent with the PI-9 data from Soriano et al. [26], Dehle reported that the most significant suppressive effects of cancer cell supernatant on macrophage function were noted using the SCLC cell line, SBC-1 [30]. It is tempting to speculate that this is representative of the more aggressive nature of this lung cancer type. Another study of primary NSCLC demonstrated the highest levels of both mRNA and protein COX-2 expression in adenocarcinoma cells compared with large cell and squamous cell carcinoma [38] (Fig. 8.7). They did not, however, investigate SCLC.

In a subsequent publication, Hodge et al. retrospectively performed a correlation of cancer stage and CD8+ production of granzyme B for 21 patients with NSCLC that had been recruited for previous studies [29]. Cancer stage ranged from 1A to 3A. They showed a significant negative correlation between granzyme expression by CD8+ T-cells and cancer stage (correlation coefficient −0.508, $p=0.019$) [30].

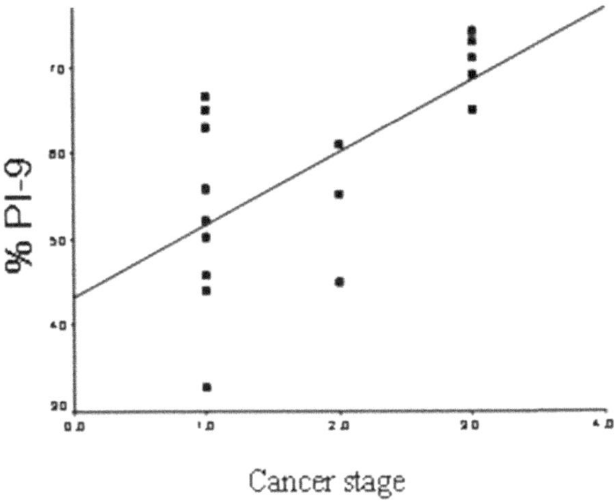

Fig. 8.7 Significant correlation (Spearman correlation 654; p=0.004) between % PI-9 expression in cancer cells from cancer areas of lung tissue and cancer stage. Adapted with permission from *Soriano et al. Lung Cancer* 2012;77(1):38–45

8.7 Conclusion

Further understanding the mechanisms for the evasion of cytotoxic lymphocyte and macrophage-mediated immune responses in lung cancer will have direct significance in providing new therapeutic strategies with high potential for clinical translation. Treatment strategies for lung cancer that target immune suppressive factors (e.g. PI-9) represent a potentially effective approach to improving treatment efficacy or as cancer preventatives in COPD. Moreover, their combination with current and new chemotherapeutic agents may revolutionize lung cancer treatment.

Acknowledgements The authors acknowledge the expert contributions by Jessica Ahern, Geoffrey Matthews, Cyd Soriano, Frances Dehle, Paul N Reynolds, Hubertus Jersmann and Mark Holmes.

References

1. The global burden of disease: Updated projections. In. Geneva: Health statistics and informatics Department, World Health Organisation 2004.
2. Alberg AJ, Samet JM. Epidemiology of lung cancer. Chest. 2003;123(1 Suppl):21S–49.
3. Herbst RS, Heymach JV, Lippman SM. Lung cancer. N Engl J Med. 2008;35:1367–80.
4. Ries LAG, Young YJ, Keel GE, Eisner MP, Lin YD, Horner MJ. National Cancer Institute SP: SEER Survival Monograph: Cancer Survival among Adults: U.S. SEER Program, 1988-2001, Patient and Tumor Characteristics. Bethesda 2007.

5. Mannino DM, Aguayo SM, Petty TL, Redd SC. Low lung function and incident lung cancer in the United States: data From the First National Health and Nutrition Examination Survey follow-up. Arch Intern Med. 2003;163:1475–80.
6. Brody JS, Spira A. State of the art. Chronic obstructive pulmonary disease, inflammation, and lung cancer. Proc Am Thorac Soc. 2006;3:535–7.
7. Krysko DV, Vanden Berghe T, D'Herde K, Vandenabeele P. Apoptosis and necrosis: detection, discrimination and phagocytosis. Methods. 2008;44:205–21.
8. Lieberman J. The ABCs of granule-mediated cytotoxicity: new weapons in the arsenal. Nat Rev Immunol. 2003;3:361–70.
9. Chávez-Galán L, Arenas-Del Angel MC, Zenteno E, Chávez R, Lascurain R. Cell death mechanisms induced by cytotoxic lymphocytes. Cell Mol Immunol. 2009;6:15–25.
10. Kroemer G, Reed JC. Mitochondrial control of cell death. Nat Med. 2000;6:513–9.
11. Heusel JW, Wesselschmidt RL, Shresta S, Russell JH, Ley TJ. Cytotoxic lymphocytes require granzyme B for the rapid induction of DNA fragmentation and apoptosis in allogeneic target cells. Cell. 1994;76:977–87.
12. Bladergroen BA, Strik MCM, Wolbink AM, Wouters D, Broekhuizen R, Kummer JA, Hack CE. The granzyme B inhibitor proteinase inhibitor (PI9) is expressed by human mast cells. Eur J Immunol. 2005;35:1175–83.
13. Buzza MS, Hirst CE, Bird CH, Hosking P, McKendrick J, Bird PI. The granzyme B inhibitor, PI-9, is present in endothelial and mesothelial cells, suggesting that it protects bystander cells during immune responses. Cell Immunol. 2010;2001:21–9.
14. Medema JP, de Jong J, Peltenburg LT, Verdegaal EM, Gorter A, Bres SA, Franken KL, Hahne M, Albar JP, Melief CJ, et al. Blockade of the granzyme B/perforin pathway through overexpression of the serine protease inhibitor PI-9/SPI-6 constitutes a mechanism for immune escape by tumors. Proc Natl Acad Sci U S A. 2001;98:11515–20.
15. Bladergroen BA, Meijer CJ, ten Berge RL, Hack CE, Muris JJ, Dukers DF, Chott A, Kazama Y, Oudejans JJ, van Berkum O, et al. Expression of the granzyme B inhibitor, protease inhibitor 9, by tumor cells in patients with non-Hodgkin and Hodgkin lymphoma: a novel protective mechanism for tumor cells to circumvent the immune system? Blood. 2002;99:232–7.
16. van Houdt IS, Oudejans JJ, van den Eertwegh AJ, Baars A, Vos W, Bladergroen BA, Rimoldi D, Muris JJ, Hooijberg E, Gundy CM, et al. Expression of the apoptosis inhibitor protease inhibitor 9 predicts clinical outcome in vaccinated patients with stage III and IV melanoma. Clin Cancer Res. 2005;11:6400–7.
17. ten Berge RL, Meijer CJ, Dukers DF, Kummer JA, Bladergroen BA, Vos W, Hack CE, Ossenkoppele GJ, Oudejans JJ. Expression levels of apoptosis-related proteins predict clinical outcome in anaplastic large cell lymphoma. Blood. 2002;99:4540–6.
18. Rousalova I, Krepela E, Prochazka J, Cermak J, Benkova K. Expression of proteinase inhibitor-9/serpinB9 in non-small cell lung carcinoma cells and tissues. Int J Oncol. 2010;36:275–83.
19. Bossard C, Belhadj K, Reyes F, Martin-Garcia N, Berger F, Kummer JA, Brière J, Baglin AC, Cheze S, Bosq J, Ribrag V, Gisselbrecht C, Mounier N, Gaulard P. Expression of the granzyme B inhibitor PI9 predicts outcome in nasal NK/T-cell lymphoma: results of a Western series of 48 patients treated with first-line polychemotherapy within the Groupe d'Etude des Lymphomes de l'Adulte (GELA) trials. Blood. 2007;109:2183–9.
20. Cunningham TD, Jiang X, Shapiro DJ. Expression of high levels of human proteinase inhibitor 9 blocks both perforin/granzyme and Fas/Fas ligand-mediated cytotoxicity. Cell Immunol. 2007;245:32–41.
21. Milano F, Jorritsma T, Rygiel AM, Bergman JJ, Sondermeijer C, Ten Brinke A, van Ham SM, Krishnadath KK. Expression pattern of immune suppressive cytokines and growth factors in oesophageal adenocarcinoma reveal a tumour immune escape-promoting microenvironment. Scand J Immunol. 2008;68:616–23.
22. Okano H, Shiraki K, Inoue H, Kawakita T, Yamanaka T, Deguchi M, Sugimoto K, Sakai T, Ohmori S, Fujikawa K, Murata K, Nakano T. Cellular FLICE/caspase-8-inhibitory protein as a principal regulator of cell death and survival in human hepatocellular carcinoma. Lab Invest. 2003;83:1033–43.

23. Thome M, Schneider P, Hofmann K, Fickenscher H, Meinl E, Neipel F, Mattmann C, Burns K, Bodmer JL, Schröter M, Scaffidi C, Krammer PH, Peter ME, Tschopp J. Viral FLICE-inhibitory proteins (FLIPs) prevent apoptosis induced by death receptors. Nature. 1997;386:517–21.
24. Ryu BK, Lee MG, Chi SG, Kim YW, Park JH. Increased expression of cFLIP(L) in colonic adenocarcinoma. J Pathol. 2001;194:15–9.
25. Hodge S, Hodge G, Nairn J, et al. Increased airway granzyme b and perforin in current and ex-smoking COPD subjects. COPD. 2006;3:179–87.
26. Soriano C, Mukaro V, Hodge G, Ahern J, Holmes M, Jersmann H, Moffat D, Meredith D, Jurisevic C, Reynolds P, Hodge S. Increased proteinase inhibitor-9 (PI-9) and reduced granzyme B in lung cancer: mechanism for immune evasion? Lung Cancer. 2012;77:38–45.
27. Kim GG, Donnenberg VS, Donnenberg AD, Gooding W, Whiteside TL. A novel multiparametric flow cytometry-based cytotoxicity assay simultaneously immunophenotypes effector cells: comparisons to a 4 h 51Cr-release assay. J Immunol Methods. 2007;325:51–66.
28. Hodge GL, Hodge S, Liew CL, Reynolds PN, Holmes M. Increased NKT-like cells are a major source of pro-inflammatory cytokines and granzymes in lung transplant patients. Respirology. 2012;17:155–63.
29. Hodge G, Barnawi J, Jurisevic C, Moffat D, Holmes M, Reynolds PN, Jersmann H, Hodge S. Lung cancer is associated with decreased expression of perforin, granzyme B and IFNγ by infiltrating lung tissue T cells, NKT-like and NK cells. Clin Exp Immunol. 2014;178(1): 79–85.
30. Dehle F, Mukaro V, Jurisevic C, Moffat D, Meredith D, Holmes M, Hodge G, Jersmann H, Reynolds PN, Hodge S. Defective efferocytosis in patients with lung cancer with or without COPD- mediated by PGE2 produced by lung cancer cells? PLoS One. 2013;26:0061573.
31. Hodge S, Hodge G, Flower R, et al. Alveolar macrophages from subjects with COPD are deficient in their ability to phagocytose apoptotic airway epithelial cells. Immunol Cell Biol. 2003;81:289–96.
32. Hodge S, Hodge G, Ahern J, et al. Azithromycin improves macrophage phagocytic function and expression of mannose receptor in COPD. Am J Respir Crit Care Med. 2008;178:139–48.
33. Hodge S, Hodge G, Ahern J, et al. Smoking alters alveolar macrophage recognition and phagocytic ability: implications in chronic obstructive pulmonary disease. Am J Respir Cell Mol Biol. 2007;37:748–55.
34. Taskinen M, Karjalainen-Lindsberg ML, Nyman H, Eerola LM, Leppa S. A high tumor-associated macrophage content predicts favorable outcome in follicular lymphoma patients treated with rituximab and cyclophosphamidedoxorubicin-vincristine-prednisone. Clin Cancer Res. 2007;13:5784–9.
35. Canioni D, Salles G, Mournier N, et al. High numbers of tumor-associated macrophages have an adverse prognostic value that can be circumvented by rituximab in patients with follicular lymphoma enrolled onto the GELA-GOELAMS FL-2000 trial. J Clin Oncol. 2008;26:440–6.
36. Hodge S, Hodge G, Holmes M, et al. Increased apoptosis in the airways in COPD persists after smoking cessation. Eur Respir J. 2005;25:447–54.
37. Vandivier RW, Henson PM, Douglas IS. Burying the dead: the impact of failed apoptotic cell removal (efferocytosis) on chronic inflammatory lung disease. Chest. 2006;129:1673–82.
38. Kim R, Emi M, Tanabe K. Cancer immunosuppression and autoimmune disease: beyond immunosuppressive networks for tumour immunity. Immunology. 2006;119:254–64.
39. Tuve S, Chen BM, Liu Y, Cheng TL, Toure P, Sow PS, Feng Q, Kiviat N, Strauss R, Ni S, et al. Combination of tumor site-located CTL-associated antigen-4 blockade and systemic regulatory T-cell depletion induces tumor destructive immune responses. Cancer Res. 2007;67:5929–39.
40. Quezada SA, Peggs KS, Curran MA, Allison JP. CTLA4 blockade and GM-CSF combination immunotherapy alters the intratumor balance of effector and regulatory T cells. J Clin Invest. 2006;116:1935–45.
41. Zhou Q, Bucher C, Munger ME, Highfill SL, Tolar J, Munn DH, Levine BL, Riddle M, June CH, Vallera DA, Weigel BJ, Blazar BR. Depletion of endogenous tumor-associated regulatory T cells improves the efficacy of adoptive cytotoxic T-cell immunotherapy in murine acute myeloid leukemia. Blood. 2009;114:3793–802.

42. Jarnicki AG, Lysaght J, Todryk S, Mills KH. Suppression of antitumor immunity by IL-10 and TGF-beta-producing T cells infiltrating the growing tumor: influence of tumor environment on the induction of CD4 and CD8 regulatory T cells. J Immunol. 2006;177:896–904.
43. Chen X, Du Y, Huang Z. CD4+CD25+ Treg derived from hepatocellular carcinoma mice inhibits tumor immunity. Immunol Lett. 2012;148:83–9.
44. Wang H, Ying H, Wang S, Gu X, Weng Y, Peng W, Xia D, Yu W. Imbalance of peripheral blood Th17 and Treg responses in patients with chronic obstructive pulmonary disease. Clin Respir J. 2014. doi:10.1111/crj.12147 [Epub ahead of print].
45. Wang H, Peng W, Weng Y, Ying H, Li H, Xia D, Yu W. Imbalance of Th17/Treg cells in mice with chronic cigarette smoke exposure. Int Immunopharmacol. 2012;14:504–12.
46. Kalathil SG, Lugade AA, Pradhan V, Miller A, Parameswaran GI, Sethi S, Thanavala Y. T regulatory cells and PD-1+ T cells contribute to effector T cell dysfunction in COPD patients. Am J Respir Crit Care Med. 2014;190:40–50.
47. Chang SH, Mirabolfathinejad SG, Katta H, Cumpian AM, Gong L, Caetano MS, Moghaddam SJ, Dong C. T helper 17 cells play a critical pathogenic role in lung cancer. Proc Natl Acad Sci U S A. 2014;111:5664–9.
48. Pouniotis DS, Plebanski M, Apostolopoulos V, et al. Alveolar macrophage function is altered in patients with lung cancer. Clin Exp Immunol. 2006;143:363–72.
49. Watkins DN, Peroni DJ, Lenzo JC, Knight DA, Garlepp MJ, Thompson PJ. Expression and localization of COX-2 in human airways and cultured airway epithelial cells. Eur Respir J. 1999;13:999–1007.
50. Aronoff DM, Canetti C, Peters-Golden M. Prostaglandin E2 inhibits alveolar macrophage phagocytosis through an E-prostanoid 2 receptor-mediated increase in intracellular cyclic AMP. J Immunol. 2004;173:559–65.
51. Izzi V, Chiurchiu V, D'Aquilio F, Palumbo C, Tresoldi I, Modesti A, Baldini PM. Differential effects of malignant mesothelioma cells on THP-1 monocytes and macrophages. Int J Oncol. 2009;34:543–50.

Part III
Resistance to Death Ligands-Mediated Apoptosis and Sensitization

Chapter 9
Sensitization of Immune-Resistant Tumor Cells to CTL-Mediated Apoptosis via Interference at the Dysregulated NF-κB/Snail/YY1/PI3K/RKIP/PTEN Resistant Loop

Benjamin Bonavida

Abstract Cancer cells respond initially to various cytotoxic therapies (chemotherapy, radiation, immunotherapy), however, a subset of cancer cells is unresponsive or develops resistance as a consequence of the therapy. Immunotherapy has gained a significant momentum recently by the positive clinical response rates achieved with either anti-tumor cytotoxic T lymphocytes (CTL) or anti-tumor monoclonal antibodies-based therapies that are more specific and less toxic than chemotherapy. A prerequisite of CTL-mediated successful immunotherapy is that the tumor cells, following recognition by the CTL, have to be sensitive to CTL-mediated cell death. This prerequisite is not being encountered in many cancers and is a major factor for the clinical failure of immunotherapy. Tumor cells develop several mechanisms to escape cell death, hence, for successful immunotherapy, one must interfere with these resistance mechanisms in an effort to sensitize the tumor cells to CTL-mediated cell death. This review discusses one mechanism by which tumor cells developed resistance to CTLs, namely, via a dysregulated NF-κB/Snail/YY1/RKIP/PTEN loop. This loop has been shown to regulate tumor cell resistance to cytotoxic agents, including CTLs. Various examples are provided to discuss the roles each of the gene products in this loop and, also, examples of various agents that have been shown to interfere with expression of factors of this loop and resulting in the reversal resistance when used in combination with CTL/death ligands. It is proposed that the combination of agents that target the resistant gene product that regulates resistance in this loop in tumors with anti-tumor CTL death ligands should result in a more successful response to immunotherapy.

Keywords Apoptosis • CTL • NF-κB • PI3K • Resistance • RKIP • Snail • TRAIL • YY1

Conflict of interest: No potential conflicts of interest were disclosed

B. Bonavida (✉)
Department of Microbiology, Immunology and Molecular Genetics, David Geffen School of Medicine, Jonsson Comprehensive Cancer Center, University of California, Los Angeles, CA 90095, USA
e-mail: bbonavida@mednet.ucla.edu

B. Bonavida, S. Chouaib (eds.), *Resistance of Cancer Cells to CTL-Mediated Immunotherapy*, Resistance to Targeted Anti-Cancer Therapeutics 7,
DOI 10.1007/978-3-319-17807-3_9

Abbreviations

Akt	Protein kinase B
CTL	Cytotoxic T lymphocytes
DcR1	Decoy receptor 1
DcR2	Decoy receptor 2
DETANONOate	(*Z*)-1-[2-(2-aminoethyl)-*N*-(2-ammonioethyl)amino]diazen-1-ium-1,2-diolate
DR4	Death receptor 4
DR5	Death receptor 5
Fas	Fas receptor
Fas-L	Fas ligand
MHC	Major histocompatibility complex
NF-κB	Nuclear factor-kappaB
NK	Natural killer
NPI-0052	Salinosporamide A; marizomib
PI3K	Phosphoinositide 3-kinase
PTEN	Phosphatase and tensin homolog
RKIP	Raf kinase inhibitor protein
YY1	Yin Yang 1

9.1 Introduction

The innate immune system is a primary defense system that has been conserved throughout evolution in plants, fungi, insects and vertebrates [1]. In mammals, the innate immune system consists of effector cells and circulating factors that defend the host immediately after infection or newly-arised transformed or neoplastic cells. The initial response is transient [2] and furthered by the adaptive immune system. The innate immune system effector cells constitute natural killers (NK), mast cells, eosinophils, basophils and phagocytic cells (macrophages and dendritic cells) [3]. The innate immune system is pivotal for the activation of the adaptive immune system [4, 5]. The adaptive primary immune system is endowed with the exquisite capacity to recognize a large number of "non-self" antigens and that is followed by immunological memory. It is mediated by cellular (T-lymphocytes) and humoral (B antibody-producing lymphocytes) responses. Antigen presentation, an innate immune response mediated by APC, stimulates T cells to become helper (CD4+) or cytotoxic (CD8). CTLs are a subset of CD8+ lymphocytes that induce cell death following recognition and interaction with targets expressing the appropriate MHC peptide complex recognized by the specific T cell receptor.

Tumor resistance to conventional therapies, such as chemotherapy, hormonal therapy and radiation, has rejuvenated cancer immunotherapy. Tumor-specific CTLs have been identified and, thus, several strategies were developed to generate tumor-specific CTLs for the therapy of drug-resistant tumors [6–9]. These strategies assumed that the successful generation of tumor-specific CTLs may be sufficient to overcome the acquired resistance in cancer cells to conventional treatments and that such tumors would be sensitive to CTL-mediated killing. However, this assumption was not compatible with reports of patients' failure to respond to CTL anti-tumor killing. Failure of current therapies in cancer patients may result from one or more mechanisms, including the low frequency of tumor-specific CTLs, tumor-mediated immunosuppression, downregulation of MHC expression on tumor surfaces and activation-induced CTL cell death by the tumor [10, 11]. Further, one mechanism of killing by CTL is through the perforin/granzyme-inducing necrosis in tumor cells, and this may be effective in some tumors. However, other mechanisms of apoptosis will not be effective by CTL, since most conventional therapies, including drugs and radiation, mediate their killing through apoptosis. Therefore, cross-resistance to apoptosis is achieved in drug/radiation-resistant tumors and such resistant tumor cells will not be killed by CTLs [12, 13].

To induce sensitivity of tumor cells to apoptosis induced by immunotherapy, several strategies have been devised, including cancer vaccines, monoclonal antibodies, recombinant cytokines, adaptive cellular administration, gene therapy, etc. [14].

9.2 Mechanisms of Killing by CTL

Cytotoxic NK and T lymphocytes mediate their killing by granule exocytosis and death ligands. Granules contain both granzymes and perforin [15–18]. The granules delivered through the exocytotoxic pathway become activated through target cell recognition by the cytotoxic lymphocytes. De-granulation takes place whereby the microtubules are mobilized, leading the pre-formed granules into the lysosomes toward the point of contact with the target cell and, thus, releasing the cytotoxic molecules [19, 20]. Perforin has an amino-terminal domain with lytic activity [21]. It also has an alpha-helix amphipathic domain that regulates its transmembrane insertion and allows the formation of pores on the cell membrane [22]. Once it is released, the anchored perforin polymerizes in the presence of calcium to form cylindrical pores of a diameter of 5–20 nm [23]. Granzymes are soluble proteins of a globular structure and belong to the same proteases family. Granzymes A and B are the most abundant in the lytic granules. Granzymes are released as multi-molecular complexes and can induce apoptosis by both caspase-dependent and independent mechanisms [24, 25]. Granzyme A induces caspase-independent apoptosis. It cleaves single-stranded DNA and hydrolyzes proteins containing basic amino acids such as arginine and lysine [26, 27]. Granzyme B cleaves protein substrates at the carboxyl side of the amino acids, such as aspartic acid. It induces apoptosis through (1) activation of caspase 3 directly [28] and (2) promotes the permeability of the mitochondrial membrane and cleaves Bid [28] and Bid induces cytochrome C release and other apoptotic molecules such as HtrA2/Omni, endoG and AIF into the cytoplasm and leading to the activation of caspases and inducing apoptosis.

In addition to perforin and granzyme killing, CTL can also be triggered by activation of death ligands such as TNF-α, Fas-L and TRAIL by corresponding death receptors on the target cells [29]. Death receptors consist of TNF-R1/R2, Fas, and DR4 and DR5 [30].

Apoptotic cell death is manifested by two main pathways, namely, the type I and type II pathways. These are mediated by a family of caspases (cysteine proteases) with aspartic acid specificity. These caspases are present in living cells as inactive zymogens (pro-caspases) and their activation results in an auto-catalytic processing of caspase cascades. They are divided into two categories: initiators (examples caspases 8–10) and effector/executioners (examples caspases 3, 6 and 7) [31]. In the type I apoptotic pathway, a caspase cascade is triggered following the oligomerization of surface death receptors (Fas, DR4, DR5, TNF-αR1) and undergoes activation of caspase 8 that activates caspase 3, resulting in the activation of PARP and DNA cleavage. In the type II pathway, it involves the mitochondrion and its damage results in its permeabilization and release of cytochrome C and Smac/DIABLO and resulting in the activation of caspases 9 and 3, PARP and DNA cleavages. The released cytochrome C binds to an adaptor module, Apaf-1, which recruits precaspase 9 and forms the apoptotic complex (cytochrome C/Apaf-1/pro-caspase 9) and results in the activation of caspases 9, 7 and 3. Hence, the activation of caspase 3 by type I and type II is their merging point [32–35].

TRAIL binds to four receptors, two death receptors (DR4 and DR5) and two decoy receptors (DcR1 and DcR2). The decoy receptors lack the functional cytoplasmic domain that is needed for apoptotic signaling. Like TNF-α and Fas-L, TRAIL initiates the apoptotic signal upon binding to its cognate receptors, DR4 and DR5, all in trimeric forms, resulting in the formation of the death-inducing signaling complex (DISC). This complex recruits pro-caspase 8 by means of the death domain interaction with the adaptive molecule FADD [36, 37]. This leads to activation of pro-caspase 8 into caspase 8, which, in turn, leads to a caspase activation cascade involving caspase 3. In type II, TRAIL activates caspase 8 and generates a truncated BID, and, in turn, it triggers the mitochondria to release cytochrome C, leading to activation of caspases 9 and 3 and resulting in apoptosis [38].

9.3 Mechanisms of Resistance to CTL Killing

Cancer cells exhibit hyperactivated and constitutively activated survival/anti-apoptotic pathways, including the PI3K/Akt, p38 MAPK, Raf/MEK/ERK, and NF-κB pathways, etc. [39, 40]. These pathways regulate the resistance mechanisms endowed in tumor cells. Several mechanisms have been postulated for tumor cell resistance to CTL-mediated killing and have been reviewed elsewhere [41–44] (Fig. 9.1). Below, additional mechanisms of resistance of tumors to CTL are briefly discussed.

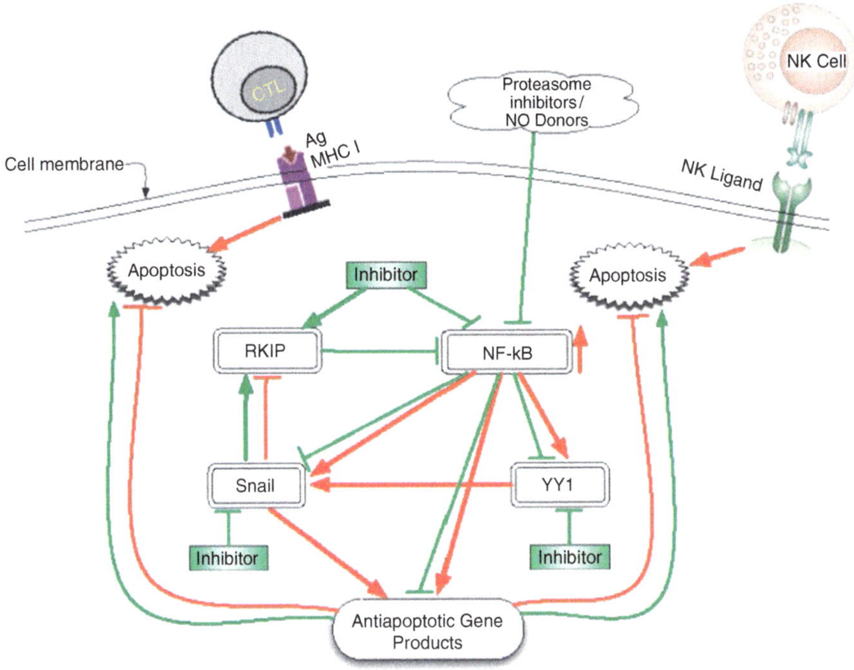

Fig. 9.1 Targeting the NF-κB/Snail/RKIP loop to reverse resistance of tumor or infected cells to apoptosis mediated by CTLs or NK cells. NF-κB hyperactivation in tumor cells or after a viral infection results in overexpression of gene products known to confer tumor cell resistance to apoptotic stimuli such as Snail, YY1, and several anti-apoptotic proteins that are directly involved in the suppression of the intrinsic apoptotic pathway. Targeting of NF-κB by conventional and novel anti-tumor agents, such as nitric oxide donors or proteasome inhibitors, results in downstream inhibition of Snail and YY1 and up-regulation of RKIP and death receptor expression such as DR5 and Fas, respectively. RKIP induction leads to further inhibition of NF-κB and NF-κB targets, while death receptor overexpression confers higher tumor cell susceptibility to cell killing induced by death ligands such as TRAIL or FasL. All of the above demonstrate that the tight regulation of the NF-κB-Snail-RKIP loop could serve as a key modulator of tumor and virus-infected cell response to apoptosis by CTLs or NK cells. (Permission for reproduction by publisher [45])

9.3.1 The Dysregulated NF-κB/Snail/YY1/RKIP/PTEN Resistant Loop in Tumors Resistant to CTL

We have established a dysregulated NF-κB/Snail/YY1/RKIP/PTEN loop in cancer cells. This loop was established by the findings that NF-κB is hyper-activated in most cancers, and it regulates, downstream, several target genes, among which are the metastatic-inducer transcription factor Snail [46, 47] and the immune resistance transcription factor YY1. Overexpression of Snail, in turn, suppresses the metastatic suppressor RKIP, which, when overexpressed, inhibits both the Raf/MEK/ERK and

NF-κB pathways [48, 49]. In addition, YY1 regulates positively Snail [50] and negatively PTEN. Thus, in cancer cells the expressions and activities of NF-κB, Snail and YY1 are upregulated, leading to downregulation of both RKIP and PTEN expressions and activities (Fig. 9.1). This loop, hence, is interconnected by the various gene products, and each individual gene product will, invariably, modify the other gene products in the loop. NF-κB has been shown to regulate cell survival and resistance to apoptosis and, hence, its overexpression and downstream overexpression of Snail and YY1 will also regulate tumor cell resistance. Likewise, overexpression of RKIP and PTEN will, in turn, regulates sensitivity to apoptosis [45].

Below, the role of each of the loop factors in the regulation of tumor cell resistance to immunotherapy is briefly described.

9.3.1.1 NF-κB

NF-κB is a transcription factor that regulates many genes associated with inflammation and apoptosis [51]. It is activated by many factors [52]. NF-κB and Rel proteins constitute a family of structurally-related eukaryotic transcription factors that are involved in the control of a large number of normal cellular processes [53]. Generally, NF-κB is present as a latent, inactive IκB-based complex in the cytoplasm. It is activated by extracellular factors. The activation of NF-κB facilitates tumor cells' escape from immune surveillance [54]. NF-κB regulates death signaling pathways through the overexpression of c-FLIP, Bcl-$_{XL}$ and IAPs, which are inhibitors of apoptosis by death ligands [53].

Several mouse models showed an association between NF-κB activation and tumor promotion, progression and metastasis [55]. The NF-κB-mediated inhibition of programmed cell death involves an alteration of the c-Jun-N-terminal kinase (JNK) cascade mediated through the induction of the expression of a JNK inhibitor [56] or induction of selected downstream targets such as the caspase inhibitor XIAP, the zinc-finger protein A20, the inhibition of the MKK/JNKCC2 kinases, GADD45β/MYD118 [57].

The NF-κB signaling pathway, in part, regulates innate and adaptive immune responses [58] and, clearly, plays a role in cancer development and progression. NF-κB is involved in the bridge of inflammation and cancer and particularly, cancer immune surveillance by killer lymphocytes. Most tumor cells exhibit hyper-activated NF-κB and downstream upregulation of anti-apoptotic target gene products that result in tumor cell resistance to apoptotic stimuli including cytotoxic lymphocytes [59–62]. Inhibition of NF-κB sensitizes tumor cells to cytotoxicity by chemo and immuno drugs and CTL [63, 64] (Fig. 9.2).

9.3.1.2 Snail

Snail is a member of the Snail superfamily of zinc-finger transcription factors and plays a pivotal role in embryonic development and cell survival [66, 67]. Snail is intrinsically involved in the regulation of epithelial mesenchymal transition (EMT)

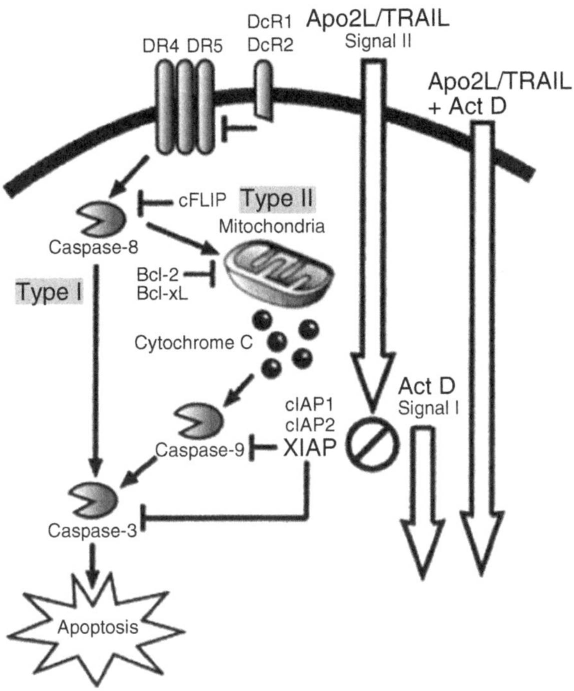

Fig. 9.2 NPI-0052 sensitizes tumor cells to apoptosis via activation of the intrinsic apoptotic pathway and inhibition of Bcl-xL expression. Schematic diagram representing the role of the NF-κB-Snail-RKIP circuitry in the regulation of tumor cell sensitivity to TRAIL- and CDDP-induced apoptosis by NPI-0052. The constitutively active NF-κB pathway induces high levels of Snail and antiapoptotic gene products and represses RKIP expression, thus conferring to tumor chemoimmunoresistance. NPI-0052 regulates cell survival and apoptosis via inhibition of phosphorylated IκBα degradation and consequently NF-κB inactivation. NPI-0052-mediated NF-κB inhibition leads to the induction of RKIP through downregulation of its transcriptional repressor Snail. NPI-0052-induced RKIP upregulation potentiates further NF-κB inhibition and suppression of NF-κB-regulated antiapoptotic gene targets, thus leading to tumor chemoimmunosensitization. (Permission for reproduction by publisher [65])

during metastasis by inhibiting the expression of the metastatic suppressor genes E-cadherin and RKIP [3, 68], downregulation of tight functional components (occludin and claudin) and induces the expression of metalloproteinases [69, 70]. In addition to Snail regulation by NF-κB, it is also self-regulated by binding to its own promoter [71]. Also, YY1 is an activator of Snail [50].

Inhibition of NF-κB results in the inhibition of Snail and YY1 and induction of RKIP. Likewise, overexpression of RKIP inhibits NF-κB, Snail and YY1 (Figs. 9.1 and 9.2). The role of Snail in the regulation of resistance to TRAIL was demonstrated by treatment of cells with Snail siRNA, and such treated cells were sensitized to TRAIL apoptosis. These treated cells expressed high RKIP, low NF-κB and Snail and upregulation of DR5 [45, 72–74].

9.3.1.3 YY1

YY1 is a ubiquitously expressed zinc-finger transcription factor that is involved in several cellular functions and in both tumor establishment and progression [75]. YY1 is overexpressed in many tumors and correlates with prostate tumor progression [76, 77]. NF-κB has been reported to regulate YY1 transcription and expression [78]. YY1 has been shown to regulate resistance of tumor cells to Fas-L-induced apoptosis [79] and TRAIL-induced apoptosis [80]. YY1 was found to regulate tumor cell resistance to TRAIL via its binding to one binding site on the DR5 promoter [80]. Inhibition of NF-κB or direct inhibition of YY1 by siRNA sensitized tumor cells to TRAIL apoptosis concurrently with upregulation of DR5 [63, 80]. The inhibition of YY1 by siRNA and sensitization to TRAIL may be due to an indirect mechanism in which the inhibition of YY1 would result in the inhibition of Snail and leading to de-repression of RKIP. Upregulation of RKIP in tumor cells, in turn, would inhibit both NF-κB and Raf/MEK/ERK and downstream anti-apoptotic gene products (Fig. 9.2). Alternatively, YY1 may have a direct effect independent of Snail and NF-κB and this mechanism has not yet been explored.

Most tumor cells are resistant to TRAIL. Zhang and Fang [81] reviewed several resistance mechanisms. Genotoxic drugs such as ADR, VP16 and CDDP sensitize tumor cells to TRAIL apoptosis concomitantly with upregulation of DR5 expression [82–85] (Fig. 9.3). We have also reported that rituximab sensitized cells to Fas-L apoptosis via upregulation of Fas as a consequence of the inhibition of DR5 repressor YY1 [87, 88] (Fig. 9.4). Hence, we hypothesized that drug-induced sensitization to TRAIL may also involve the inhibition of YY1 and upregulation of DR5. We have identified a putative binding site for YY1 on the DR5 promoter [89]. The findings revealed that treatment of tumor cells with chemotherapeutic drugs sensitized tumor cells to TRAIL concomitantly with inhibition of YY1 and upregulation of DR5. Synergy was achieved by the combination treatment in apoptosis. The role of YY1 in the negative transcriptional regulation of DR5 was corroborated by us using a reporter system whereby the putative YY1 binding site was deleted or mutated [90]. The inhibition of YY1 may be the result of drug-induced inhibition of NF-κB, as inhibitors of NF-κB also inhibited YY1 [91]. Furthermore, treatment of cells with siRNA YY1 mimicked drug-induced sensitization of tumor cells to TRAIL apoptosis.

9.3.1.4 RKIP

We discussed above in Sec. 9.3.1.1 the role of NF-κB in the regulation of resistance and, downstream, its target the transcription factor YY1 in the regulation of resistance to both Fas-L and TRAIL. Inhibition of NF-κB reversed the resistance and sensitized the cells to Fas-L and TRAIL apoptosis. Clearly, the intrinsic inhibitors of NF-κB may mimic chemical inhibitors and would also sensitize tumor cells to Fas-L and TRAIL apoptosis. Hence, Yeung et al. [48, 49] have reported the cloning of a new gene product, Raf kinase inhibitor protein (RKIP) that was shown to inhibit

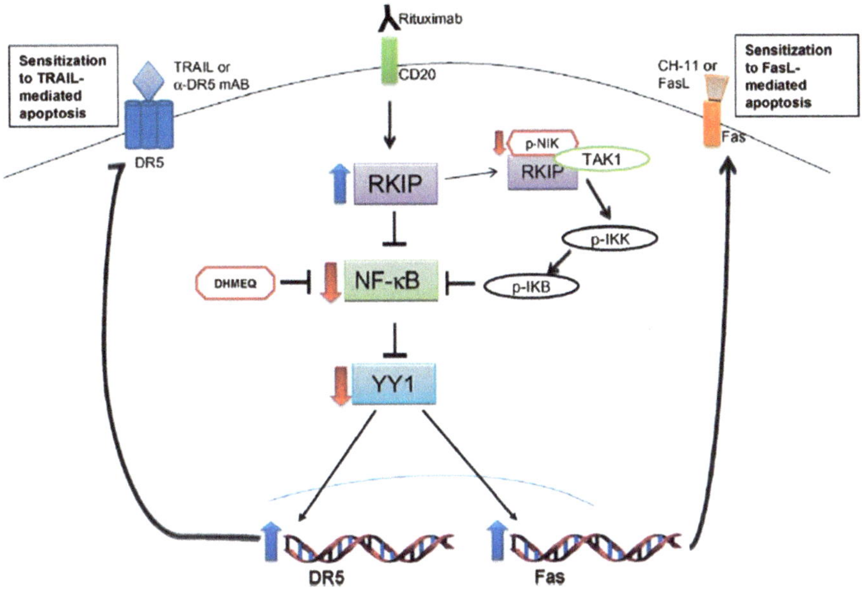

Fig. 9.3 Schematic diagram representing the role of the proteasome inhibitor NPI-0052 in the regulation of tumor cells sensitivity to TRAIL-induced apoptosis. Treatment with NPI-0052 results in the modification of several genes regulating the apoptotic pathways. NPI-0052 inhibits the NF-κB pathway via inhibition of Iκβα and p65 phosphorylation. NF-κB inhibition by NPI-0052 leads to the down-regulation of Bcl-xL and the induction of Bax contributing to the mitochondrial membrane depolarization. Furthermore, NPI-0052 inhibits the transcription repressor YY1, leading to up-regulation of DR5. Thus, the combination of NPI-0052 and TRAIL results in the activation of the mitochondrial apoptotic pathway, inhibition of antiapoptotic gene products, activation of procaspases-9 and -7, formation of the apoptosome, and altogether downstream activation of the effector caspase-3 resulting in apoptosis. (Permission for reproduction by publisher [86])

both the Raf/MEK/ERK and NF-κB pathways. The expression of RKIP is low in many cancers and absent in metastatic cancer [45]. The induction of RKIP was reported to inhibit metastatic prostate cancer in a murine model and where it has been coined a "metastatic suppressor" [92]. RKIP depletion resulted in a decrease of the mitotic index, a short time for the metaphase to anaphase transition and also a defect in the spindle checkpoint [93]. Altogether, the above findings suggested that RKIP expression is involved in tumor cell arrest, apoptosis and the regulation of metastasis. Further, the fact that RKIP inhibits the NF-κB and Raf/MEK/ERK pathways is concordant with above effects and its expression shifts the balance from proliferation toward cytostasis and apoptosis. Several agents that result in the induction of RKIP resulted in the reversal of resistance and sensitization to Fas-L and TRAIL apoptosis [63, 86, 90, 94, 95]. Baritaki et al. reported that RKIP induction resulted in the inhibition of NF-κB and YY1 and sensization to TRAIL apoptosis concomitantly with upregulation of DR5. Treatment of tumor cells with RKIP siRNA reversed tumor cell sensitization to TRAIL [63]. The findings with RKIP

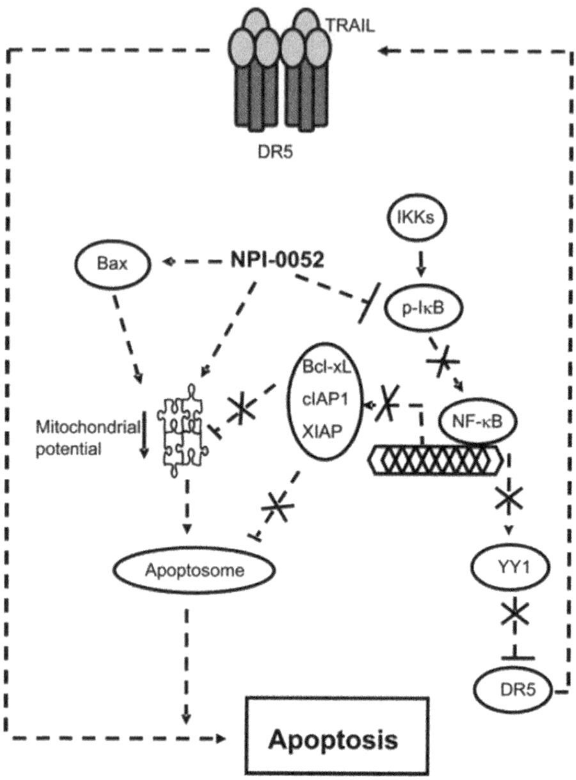

Fig. 9.4 DHMEQ-induced immunosensitization in resistant tumor cells. The schematic diagram illustrates tumor cells that constitutively express the activated NF-κB pathway. Activation of the NF-κB pathway results in the upregulation of the transcription repressor YY1. YY1 has been shown to negatively regulate the transcription and expression of the death receptors Fas and DR5 and thus regulates tumor cell resistance to Fas-L or TRAIL-induced apoptosis. Inhibition of NF-κB by DHMEQ results in inhibition of YY1, upregulation of Fas and DR5 and sensitization to Fas-L-mediated apoptosis and TRAIL-mediated apoptosis, respectively. In addition, the diagram illustrates an example of Rituximab-mediated inhibition of the NF-κB pathway via the induction of RKIP, thus inhibiting YY1 like DHMEQ and resulting in tumor cell sensitization to immunotherapy. (Permission for reproduction by publisher [64])

induction on TRAIL sensitization is also likely to be involved in sensitization to Fas-L, since both ligands are regulated by YY1. The findings on the role of RKIP in the sensitization to Fas-L and TRAIL are consistent with its role as an "immunosurveillance gene" in addition to its role as a "metastatic suppressor gene."

9.3.1.5 PTEN

It has been reported that metastatic melanoma cells are resistant to CTL [96]. In comparison with primary melanoma cells that are susceptible to CTL, in contrast, the metastatic cells are resistant and shown to express less ICAM-1. Treatment of metastatic cells with interferon-gamma increased the expression of ICAM-1 and susceptibility to CTL-killing. Further, there was an inverse correlation between the expressions of ICAM-1 and PTEN. ICAM-1-knockdown was shown to increase PTEN and inhibit PI3K/Akt signaling. These findings implicate the role of PTEN in the regulation of tumor cell sensitivity to CTL.

Reddy et al. [97] have reported that the metastasis-associated protein 1 (MTA1) is overexpressed in many human cancers and contributes to metastasis. MTA1 represses PTEN by recruiting HDAC4 with YY1 on the PTEN promoter. Upregulation of MTA1 decreases PTEN expression and stimulates the PI3K/Akt pathway. Hence, the upregulation of YY1 in cancer cells is accompanied by the inhibition of PTEN, the activation of PI3K/Akt and NF-κB pathways and the downstream expression of anti-apoptotic gene products; all of these affects the resistance to apoptosis by CTL and cytotoxic drugs.

Gao et al. [98] have stably expressed PTEN in a squamous carcinoma cell line and resulted in the induction of apoptosis via the negative regulation of the PI3K/Akt pathway and inhibition of anti-apoptotic gene products. New findings also implicate the sensitivity of CTL to apoptosis. Nguyen et al. [99] have reported the study on engineered ePTEN whereby its expression in tumor cells with a suppressed PTEN resulted in a decrease in PIP3 levels, inhibition of the phosphorylation of the PI3K pathway, inhibition of both the proliferation and migration, and reversal of resistance. Kim et al. [100] have examined the resistance of cancer stem cells (CSCs) to apoptotic stimuli and the roles of the PTEN/PI3K/Akt/NF-κB pathway in CSCs and the regulation of ABCG2. Knock-out of PTEN increased stem-like properties of CSCs in prostate cancer cells (sphere formation, number of stem cells, EMT, and ABCG2 expression). The loss of PTEN in prostate cancer cells resulted in the development of CSCs and resistance.

Wang et al. [101] have established TRAIL-resistant breast cancer cell lines for investigation. These cell lines exhibited the EMT phenotype, invasiveness and downregulation of PTEN. Silencing miR-221 resulted in the upregulation of PTEN and the inhibition of both EMT and invasion. Likewise, knock-out miR-221 sensitized the cells to TRAIL apoptosis by targeting PTEN. The resistance to TRAIL correlated with the inhibition of PTEN.

Hao et al. [102] have examined the role Twist and Snail transcription. The PI3K/Akt pathway has been shown to regulate the twist and Snail transcription. Since Snail has been reported by us in the inhibition of TRAIL apoptosis [45] its inhibition by PTEN, via mediated-inhibition of PI3K/Akt, resulted in sensitization to TRAIL apoptosis. Thus, PTEN plays a role indirectly in the regulation of CTL-mediated killing.

Fang et al. [103] have examined the differential expression of microRNAs between chemo-sensitive and chemo-resistant colorectal cancer (CRC) cell lines and found an increased expression of miR-17-5p in the resistant cell line as well as in the metastatic CRC from patients. Higher levels of miR-17-5p correlated with poor survival. PTEN was a target of miR17-5p in colon cancer and the repression of PTEN correlated with chemo-resistance. This finding suggested indirectly the cross-resistance and, most likely, resistance to CTL. Zhang et al. [104] have reported that PTEN is a target gene of miR-205. MiR-205 inhibited PTEN, resulting in the activation of the PI3K/Akt pathway and resistance to apoptosis.

9.4 Reversal of Tumor Resistance to CTL Apoptosis

9.4.1 The NF-κB Inhibitor DHMEQ

DHMEQ is an inhibitor that prevents the translocation of NF-κB into the nucleus [105] DHMEQ exerts anti-tumor effects in vivo in various experimental model systems [64, 106]. It has also been shown that DHMEQ can act as an immunosensitizing agent. Treatment of B-NHL cells with DHMEQ sensitized the cells to Fas-L apoptosis via inhibition of NF-κB [107]. Both rituximab-sensitive and resistant B-NHL cell lines were sensitized to TRAIL by DHMEQ treatment via inhibition of NF-κB [95] (Fig. 9.4).

9.4.2 Proteasome Inhibitors

NPI-0052 (marizomib) is a non-peptide murine-derived proteasome inhibitor reported to inhibit, irreversibly, all three enzymatic activities (CT-L, trypsin-like and caspase-like) of the 26S proteasome core [108, 109]. NPI-0052 was reported to have an anti-tumor activity in in vivo xenograft tumor models [110]. Treatment of tumor cells with proteasome inhibitors sensitized the cells to TRAIL apoptosis, concomitantly with DR5 upregulation [111–114] (Fig. 9.3). The mechanism by which proteasome inhibitors upregulate DR5 was not known and was examined by Baritaki et al. [86]. The findings demonstrated that NPI-0052 inhibited the DR5 repressor YY1 and resulted in the upregulation of DR5 and sensitization to TRAIL apoptosis. The inhibition of YY1 by NPI-0052 was the result, in part, of the inhibition of NF-κB transcription activity [78]. NPI-0052 treatment in combination with TRAIL activated the mitochondrial type II apoptotic pathway and synergy was achieved in apoptosis. There was inhibition of the anti-apoptotic gene products XIAP, IAPs and Bcl-$_{XL}$ along with the induction of Bax. The role of DR5 upregulation in sensitization was corroborated by findings demonstrating that treatment of cells with siRNA DR5 attenuated significantly TRAIL-induced apoptosis [115]. These findings above demonstrated for the first time that proteasome inhibitors-induced upregulation of DR5 was due in large part to the inhibition of YY1, a repressor of DR5 transcription [63]. Both NF-κB inhibitors such as DHMEQ and/or siRNA YY1 treatment sensitized tumor cells to TRAIL apoptosis with the upregulation of DR5 and, thus, mimicked proteasome inhibitors.

We have reported previously that induction of RKIP sensitized tumor cells to TRAIL via inhibition of NF-κB and YY1 and upregulation of DR5. Beach and colleagues [3] have reported that Snail, a target of NF-κB, represses RKIP transcription and expression. Snail is a member of the Snail superfamily of zinc-finger transcription factors with a pivotal role in embryonic development and cell survival [66]. Snail is regulated, in part, by NF-κB [46, 47] and, in part, by itself [71]. Thus, we hypothesized that since NPI-0052-mediated sensitization to TRAIL resulted from the inhibition of NF-κB and its target YY1, it was likely that NPI-0052-mediated inhibition of NF-κB would also result in the inhibition of Snail and de-repression of RKIP transcription, and this modification may be involved in TRAIL sensitization. Hence, the NF-κB/Snail/YY1/RKIP dysregulated loop will be modified by NPI-0052, and each modulated gene product will be involved in sensitization. Treatment with specific NF-κB inhibitors, such as DHMEQ, mimicked NPI-0052 in the inhibition of NF-κB and Snail, along with upregulation of RKIP and sensitization to TRAIL [65] (Fig. 9.4). In addition, RKIP overexpression mimicked treatment with Snail siRNA or NPI-0052 in sensitization of cells to TRAIL apoptosis, concomitant with a decrease of Bcl-$_{XL}$. In contrast, treatment with RKIP siRNA reversed the sensitization to TRAIL. Collectively, the findings above established the NF-κB/Snail/YY1/RKIP circuitry in tumor cells that regulates tumor cell sensitivity to TRAIL apoptosis (Figs. 9.2 and 9.3).

Several immunotherapeutic strategies have been developed and applied in the treatment of cancer patients. These include cancer vaccines, immunotherapy (ex vivo activated dendritic cells, IL2, adoptive T cell therapy, antibodies, genetically engineered T and B cells). In patients with melanoma, the above various approaches have resulted in clinical responses initially, though the majority of patients experiences relapses and no longer responds to further treatments [116]. T cells genetically engineered expressing anti-tumor T cell receptors were developed and showed significant anti-tumor response in animal model systems [117, 118] and were reported the outgrowth of immune-resistant tumor variants in patients treated with immunotherapy. Noteworthy, the Rosenberg group genetically engineered peripheral blood T cells to express high affinity TCR for melanoma MART-1 and called F5 MART-1 TCR cells and achieved a partial complete response in patients [119]. The low clinical response in patients by F5 suggested that either the CTL are not recognizing the tumor targets or reaching the targets or, alternatively, the tumor cells were resistant to CTL-killing. These possibilities were examined by Jazirehi et al. [120]. The approach used was to generate F5 CTL-resistant tumor clones and examine their mechanism of resistance. The resistant clones expressed the same levels of MART-1 and HLA-1 complexes, though they proliferated faster than the parental cells. Further, the resistant clones exhibited more hyper-activated NF-κB activity and, downstream, higher expression of anti-apoptotic gene products as compared to parental cells. In the absence of killing of the clones by F5 CTL, however, the F5 CTL still recognized the targets via binding and conjugate formation and also were triggered to release interferon γ and IL2 comparable to the sensitive tumor cells. The hyper-activated NF-κB activity in the clones suggested it may be regulating the resistance to CTL as it has been reported to confer immune resistance [121], and its inhibition reverses resistance. We treated the resistant clones with bortezomib and resulted in the sensitization of those cells to F5 CTL. Protective factors regulated by NF-κB (Bcl-2, Bcl-$_{XL}$ and Mcl-1) were also shown to reverse resistance following their inhibition using various inhibitors or siRNA. The above findings implied that, in vivo, in patients treated with immunotherapy and have circulating CTL that the failure of response may be due to the acquisition of resistance of the tumor cells. Hence, interventions are needed to target the tumor cells' resistance and to be used in combination with immunotherapy to result in an effective clinical response.

9.4.3 NO

Many cancers exhibit constitutively activated NF-κB and it was reported that NF-κB regulates tumor cell sensitivity to TRAIL apoptosis in hepatoma cells [122]. Downstream targets of NF-κB include the Bcl2 family and the Bcl2-related gene ($Bcl\text{-}_{XL}$), and those were reported to regulate tumor cell sensitivity to drug-mediated apoptosis [123]. The roles each of NF-κB and $Bcl\text{-}_{XL}$ in the regulation of TRAIL apoptosis were examined [91]. NO donors such as DETANONOate were reported to sensitize tumor cells to Fas-L and TRAIL-induced apoptosis [37, 124–126]. The mechanism by which NO sensitizes tumor cells to TRAIL apoptosis was examined. The findings demonstrated that NO inactivates NF-κB activity by S-nitrosylation of NF-κB p50 and downstream $Bcl\text{-}_{XL}$ expression. Inhibition of either NF-κB or $Bcl\text{-}_{XL}$ sensitized tumor cells to TRAIL apoptosis. The synergy achieved by the combination treatment with DETANONOate and TRAIL resulted in the activation of type II apoptotic pathway and resulted in apoptosis. While each treatment resulted in the activation of the mitochondria, associated with membrane depolarization and release of cytochrome C and Smac/DIABLO, however, neither achieved subsequent activation of caspases 9 and 3. In contrast, the combination treatment resulted in complementary activities and activated caspases 9 and 3, leading to apoptosis. Using prostate cancer cell lines as a model, DETANONOate sensitized both androgen-dependent and androgen-independent lines to TRAIL apoptosis (Fig. 9.5). While treatment with ActD or VP16 sensitized tumor cells to TRAIL via inhibition of XIAP [127], DETANONOate treatment did not affect XIAP, but primarily inhibited $Bcl\text{-}_{XL}$ (Fig. 9.6). These studies suggest that tumor cells' resistance to TRAIL is mediated by several mechanisms that can be altered by different agents. The mechanism by which NO perturbs the mitochondria has been reported by several investigators. Poderoso et al. [128] have reported that NO binds to cytochrome C oxidase (Complex IV) in the mitochondria electron transfer chain and resulting in the

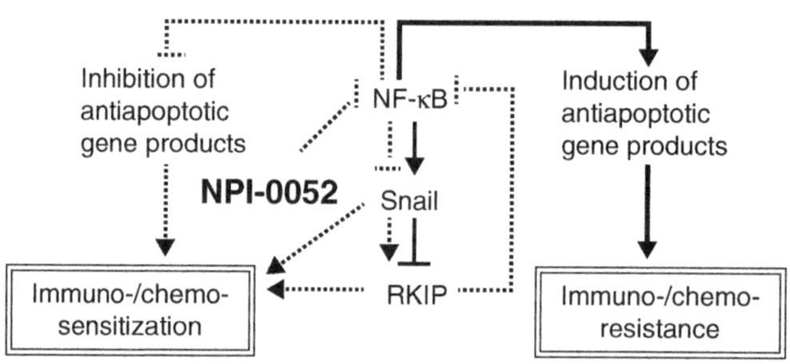

Fig. 9.5 Schematic diagram of the role of YY1 in the negative regulation of DR5 transcription and resistance to TRAIL-induced apoptosis. The tumor cells constitutively express activated NF-κB and YY1 activities and express low levels of DR5. These cells are resistant to TRAIL-induced apoptosis. Treatment of the tumor cells with DETANONOate inhibits NF-κB and YY1 and results in the inhibition of YY1 repressor activity. These lead to the upregulation of DR5 and sensitization to TRAIL-induced apoptosis. (Permission for reproduction by publisher [80])

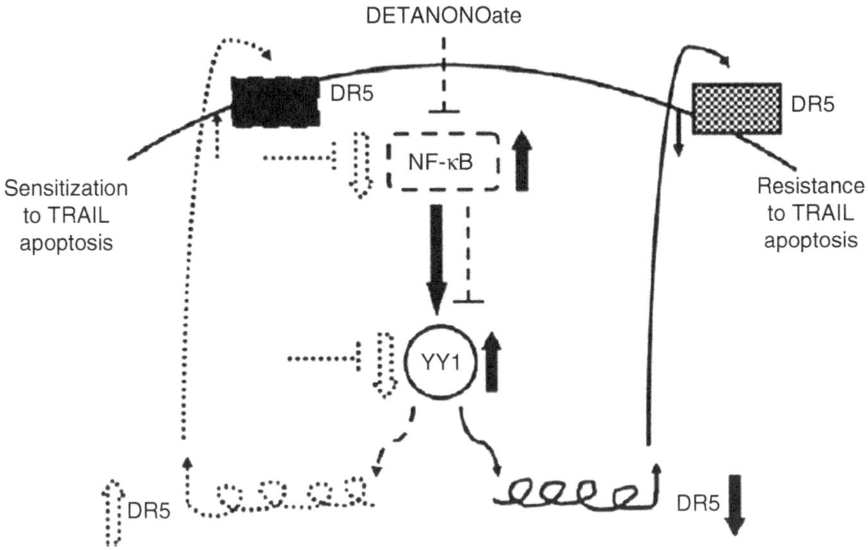

Fig. 9.6 Proposed model of actinomycin D (Act D)-sensitized tumor necrosis factor-related apoptosis-inducing ligand (Apo2L/TRAIL)-mediated apoptosis. Apo2L/TRAIL initiates apoptosis by trimerization of its cognate receptors DR4 and DR5, followed by activation of the initiator caspase-8. Active caspase-8 can directly activate caspase-3 or indirectly activate caspase-9 by means of the mitochondrial pathway. The direct pathway that activates caspase-3 after caspase-8 activation is known as the type I pathway; the indirect activation of caspase-3 by means of the activation of caspase-9 is termed the type II pathway. In the type II pathway, caspase-9 is activated when cytochrome C is released from the mitochondria, which is triggered by active caspase-8. The activation of caspase-3 leads to the final apoptotic phenotypes such as DNA fragmentation and chromosomal condensation. Various anti-apoptotic proteins inhibit each signaling event throughout the pathway. c-FLIP inhibits the activation of caspase- 8. Bcl-2-related family proteins guard against mitochondrial release of cytochrome C. IAP family proteins directly inhibit the activation of caspase-9 and-3. Apo2L/TRAIL could induce cytochrome C but did not activate caspase-9 (Signal II). The blockade of signal I is potentially mediated primarily through XIAP (stop sign). Pretreatment with Act D suppresses the expression of XIAP, thus, removing the block (Signal I). The combination treatment of Apo2L/TRAIL and Act D then leads to completion of the apoptotic pathway. (Permission for reproduction by publisher [127])

generation of superoxide. Superoxide interacts with NO to form peroxinitrite, which induces mitochondrial dysfunction and the release of cytochrome C.

NO donors inhibit NF-κB DNA-binding activity and downstream targets, including anti-apoptotic gene products. In addition, NO inhibits p50 and p65 through nitrosylation. We have reported that treatment of tumor cells with DETANONOate sensitizes cells to TRAIL apoptosis [91]. Sensitization of tumor cells by NO involved the inhibition of NF-κB and downstream, the DR5 repressor YY1, leading to upregulation of DR5. Hence, we hypothesized that DETA treatment will inhibit YY1 and sensitize the cells to TRAIL apoptosis. YY1 was identified as a resistant factor and regulates resistance to both chemotherapy and irradiation. For TRAIL, YY1 represses DR5 and is responsible, in part, for TRAIL resistance, and, thus, its inhibition by NO will reverse resistance. The DR5 promoter has a consensus binding site for YY1 and was corroborated by its interaction, directly, by ChIP analysis and, indirectly, by deletion or mutation of the YY1 consensus binding site on the DR5 promoter. The in vitro findings were corroborated in vivo in mice bearing human tumor xenografts and in which the treatment with DETANONOate was shown to result in the inhibition of YY1 and upregulation of DR5 as assessed ex vivo in tumors derived from the DETANONOate-treated mice.

The direct role of DR5 upregulation in TRAIL sensitization has been reported [129]. However, with DETANONOate, many other factors are involved, such as the inhibition of anti-apoptotic gene products. In addition to YY1 repression of DR5, Yoshida et al. [7], using a reporter system for human DR5, identified two SP-1 sites, respectively, for the basal transcriptional activity of the DR5 gene promoter. Nakata et al. [130] reported that HDAC inhibitors upregulate DR5 expression and sensitize the cells to TRAIL apoptosis. Other inducers of DR5 have also been reported. For example, p53 transactivates DR5 gene expression [131, 132]. Genotoxic agents (doxorubicin, VP16, gamma irradiation) induced DR5 in a p53-dependent or independent manners [129, 133]. Dexamethasone and interferon gamma induce apoptosis by DR5 expression in a p53-independent manner [134]. Sulindac sulfite [134] and 2-methoxy-estradiol [135] induced DR5 through mechanisms that are not yet known.

9.4.4 Rituximab and Galiximab

9.4.4.1 Rituximab

The standard treatment of B-NHL is the combination of rituximab and chemotherapy (R-CHOP) [136]. We have reported that rituximab treatment of B-NHL cell lines sensitized the cells to drug-induced apoptosis [137–140]. Rituximab treatment inhibited the constitutively activated survival pathways, such as NF-κB and MEK/ERK1/2 [138] and the p38 MAPK [73]. Based on the findings of rituximab-mediated sensitization to drugs, we sought to investigate whether it would also sensitize the cells to Fas-L apoptosis. The hypothesis put forth was that inhibition of NF-κB in ovarian cancer cells by interferon γ sensitized the cells to Fas-L via inhibition of NF-κB and its target YY1. Inhibition of YY1 was accompanied by the induction of Fas, as well as the inhibition of YY1 sensitized the cells to Fas-L apoptosis [79]. Therefore, the possible inhibition of YY1 by rituximab via inhibition of NF-κB may sensitize the B-NHL cells to Fas-L apoptosis. The findings established synergy in apoptosis in B-NHL cells treated with a combination of rituximab and Fas-L. The synergy was the result, in part, of inhibition of the Fas-repressor YY1 and other anti-apoptotic gene products regulated by NF-κB. Chemical inhibitors established the roles of p38 MAPK, NF-κB and YY1 in the regulation of resistance. The observed synergy in apoptosis was the result of the activation of type II mitochondrial apoptotic pathway.

We speculated that in an in vivo setting, rituximab may exert a new mechanism of cytotoxicity by sensitizing tumor cells to Fas-L expressing cells, such as T and NK lymphocytes and contributes to its in vivo anti-tumor activities [88].

We have reported that rituximab treatment of TRAIL-resistant B-NHL cell lines are sensitized to TRAIL apoptosis. Hence, we postulated that the treatment of tumor cells with rituximab will also sensitize them to CTL circulating in vivo alone or in combination with adoptive immunotherapy and/or other approaches to generate anti-tumor CTL. Vega et al. [141] have examined the above hypothesis in vitro. In previous studies, we reported that rituximab sensitizes Fas-resistant B-NHL to Fas-L apoptosis [87, 88]. In other studies, by us and others, rituximab also sensitized tumor cells to TRAIL apoptosis [142–144]. The in vitro studies were validated in vivo, in which administration of rituximab and TRAIL inhibited B-NHL tumor xenografts growth [143]. The mechanism by which rituximab sensitized tumor cells to TRAIL was predicated on the finding that inhibition of NF-κB reverses resistance to TRAIL via inhibition, downstream, of the DR5 repressor YY1 [90]. We have previously reported that rituximab inhibits NF-κB activity in B-NHL cell lines [95] delineating the mechanism of rituximab resistance. The above findings on rituximab-mediated sensitization to Fas-L and TRAIL add a novel mechanism to be involved in vivo (Fig. 9.7) in which rituximab activates lymphocyte-mediated cytotoxicity of tumor cells in vivo in addition to the postulated mechanisms of ADCC and CDC. The patients' effector cells, CTL and NK, express the death ligands that can trigger corresponding receptor on the B-NHL tumors, and their interaction mediate tumor cell apoptosis. These findings strongly suggested that patients with B-NHL may respond to a combination of rituximab and CTL-mediated immunotherapy. However, not all cells are sensitive, and that may explain one mechanism of failures of patients to respond to rituximab treatment.

9.4.4.2 Galiximab

The anti-CD80 mAb galiximab has been tested for its signal mediating effects on CD80-positive B-NHL cell lines. Galiximab is a high affinity primitized anti-CD80 (IgG-1λ) that contains variable regions of primate cynolmogous macaque origin and constant regions of human origin [145]. It has been considered for clinical treatment. The studies undertaken were reminiscent of prior studies discussed above with the anti-CD20 mAb rituximab. The CD80 membrane bound co-stimulatory molecule has been reported in its activity in the regulation of T cells and is a member of the B7 co-stimulatory molecules [146]. CD80 expression is found at the surface of B cells, APCs and T cells [147] and on the surface of a variety of lymphoid malignancies [148] Anti-CD80 antibody inhibits cell proliferation and induces ADCC in vivo against B-NHL xenografts [149] and in vitro cytotoxicity [150]. Galiximab also exerted anti-tumor effects in vivo in mice bearing human lymphoma xenografts [151].

Cell signaling in B-NHL by galiximab was reported by Martinez-Paniagna et al. [152]. The findings revealed that galiximab exerts anti-proliferative effects and

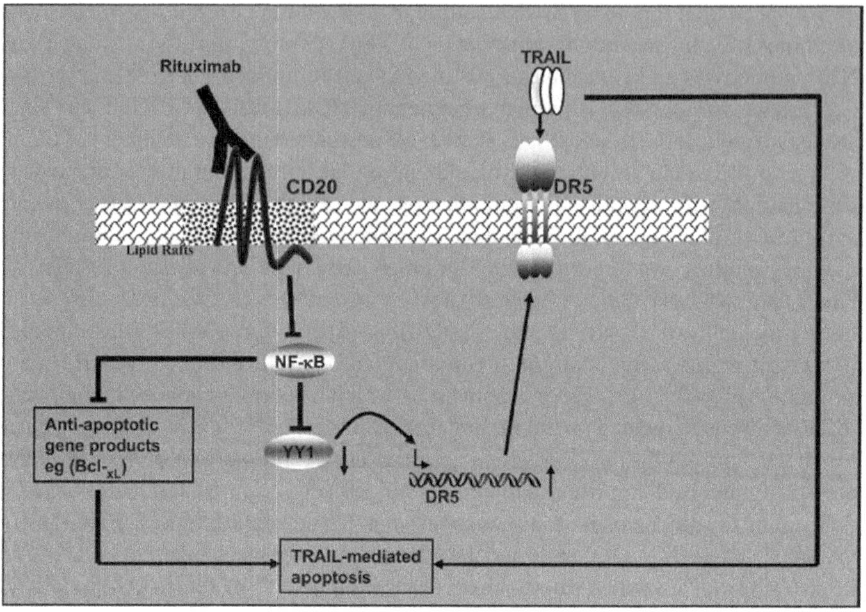

Fig. 9.7 Schematic diagram of the mechanism by which rituximab sensitizes B-NHL cells to TRAIL-induced apoptosis. B-NHL cells maintain their resistance to TRAIL-induced apoptosis through constitutively active NF-κB and YY1, which negatively regulate DR5 expression. Cell treatment with rituximab inhibits NF-κB and YY1 leading to the inhibition of YY1 repressor activity on the DR5 promoter and up-regulation of DR5 expression. In parallel, rituximab-mediated NF-κB inhibition downstream inhibits the expression of anti-apoptotic gene products, such as Bcl-XL and Mcl-1. The combination of rituximab and TRAIL results in the cleavage of caspases 9, 8, and 3 and PARP, all of which lead to apoptosis. (Permission for reproduction by publisher [141])

sensitized the B-NHL cells to apoptosis by both chemotherapy and immunotherapy. Galiximab signals the cells via the CD80 receptor, resulting in the inhibition of the activation of the NF-κB pathway and also inhibited the Akt pathway and downstream targets YY1 and Snail and Bcl-$_{XL}$. Individually, each of these gene products inhibited by galiximab sensitizes cells to TRAIL apoptosis. Thus, galiximab interferes with the dysregulated NF-κB/Snail/YY1/RKIP loop to reverse drug and immune resistance. Overall, treatment of tumor cells with galiximab inhibited both NF-κB and Akt and resulted in the sensitization to TRAIL, Fas-L and chemotherapy.

9.4.5 Chemotherapeutic Drugs

Lymphokine activated killer cells (LAK) and tumor-infiltrating lymphocytes (TIL) are promising immunotherapeutic anti-cancer strategies [153–155]. LAK and TIL kill autologous and allogeneic tumor cells via the perforin/granzyme pathway and

TNF family of apoptosis-inducing ligand [155–158]. The TIL in tumors are not effective and not cytolytic and may become anergic [159]. Alternatively, TIL may be functional, but the surviving tumor cells may be resistant to killing. The study by Frost et al. [160] demonstrated that patients-derived TIL kill tumor cell lines if the tumor cells are pre-treated with low concentrations of chemotherapeutic drugs such as CDDP and VP16. The above studies point to the findings that tumor cells develop resistance to CTL, LAK and TIL in vivo, and it should be considered that in addition to the generation of anti-tumor CTL response, one has to consider resistance of tumor cells to killing and the tumor cells must be treated to reverse their resistance so that the combination treatment will be effective.

TRAIL is a member of the TNF superfamily that has been reported to kill sensitive tumor cells selectively and not killing normal cells; hence, it has been considered a potential therapeutic target. Both in vitro and in vivo studies reported TRAIL-mediated anti-tumor activities [83, 161–163]. Noteworthy, while both Fas-L and TNF-α exert in vivo toxicities, in contrast, TRAIL is not toxic [164].

Tumor cell resistance to TRAIL apoptosis can be sensitized by sub-toxic concentrations of chemotherapeutic drugs [83, 163–168]. The findings that actinomycin D (ActD) sensitized AIDS-Kaposi sarcoma cells to TRAIL apoptosis [166], we examined the sensitizing activity of ActD in TRAIL-resistant prostate cancer cell lines [127]. Indeed, ActD sensitized several human prostate carcinoma cell lines to TRAIL apoptosis. The combination treatment resulted in caspase activation following activation of the type II mitochondrial apoptotic pathway. The combination treatment activated caspases 8 and 9, but no activation with single agent alone. Earlier times following treatment revealed upregulation of Bcl-$_{XL}$ and downregulation of XIAP. The upregulation of Bcl-$_{XL}$ did not allow the cytochrome C release. The direct role of XIAP inhibition in sensitization was corroborated by overexpression of Smac/DIABLO that mimicked ActD in tumor sensitization to TRAIL apoptosis. Of interest, treatment with TRAIL activated the mitochondria (membrane depolarization) and release of cytochrome C in the absence of downstream activation. Hence, the overexpression of XIAP protein prevented cytochrome C activation of caspase 9. The IAP family members exert their anti-apoptotic function downstream of cytochrome C by directly binding to caspases and preventing the activation of effector caspases (9 and 3) [169]. XIAP is the most potent anti-apoptotic protein among the IAP family. ActD treatment suppresses XIAP very early after treatment and there was little effect on other anti-apoptotic proteins. Smac/DIABLO is an inactivator of IAP family proteins [170] (Fig. 9.6). Resistance to TRAIL involves loss of agonist receptors (DR4 and DR5) and overexpression of decoy receptors [168, 171, 172].

Several mechanisms have been postulated to delineate how ActD inhibits XIAP. Two signal models were proposed for the sensitization of cells by ActD to TRAIL apoptosis. This model explains the synergy achieved by ActD and TRAIL as complementary pro-apoptotic effects. TRAIL initiates the necessary type II apoptotic signal and perturbing the mitochondrial and cytochrome C but was not sufficient to activate caspases (Signal II). Signal I was required to inhibit the anti-apoptotic gene product XIAP and other resistant factors. The combination resulted in the activation of caspases and resulted in apoptosis [85]. Like TRAIL, ActD also sensitized to Fas-L apoptosis [173]. Hence, ActD is a good example of the reversal of tumor cell resistance to CTL apoptosis (Fig. 9.6).

The overexpression of Smac/DIABLO inhibits XIAP, which is overexpressed in resistant tumor cells and was shown to be responsible, in part, for resistance to TRAIL apoptosis [85, 127]. The inability to induce apoptosis by translocation of cytochrome C and endogenous Smac/DIABLO by TRAIL highlights the importance of the inhibitors downstream of the apoptotic events in tumor resistance. The overexpression of XIAP protein is associated with poor response to apoptosis-inducing therapies. In leukemia patients, high level of XIAP in tumor cells correlated with poor survival [174]. XIAP was also found to be highly expressed in resistant ovarian cancers to chemotherapy and radiation, and treatment with antisense XIAP reversed resistance [175, 176].

The effect of TRAIL treatment on representative tumor MM cell lines, 8226 and ADR-resistant variant 8226/dox40, were used to determine the relative effects of TRAIL on both ADR-sensitive (8226) and ADR-resistant (8226/dox40) cell lines. The findings revealed that 8226/dox40 was more resistant to TRAIL than 8226. Further, treatment of 8226/dox40 with ADR sensitized the cells to ADR apoptosis [139]. These findings suggested that ADR may exert a different signaling than a cytotoxic killing since the 8226/dox40 was resistant to ADR-induced cell death and that such signaling by ADR must have altered the anti-apoptotic pathways and resulted in sensitization to TRAIL apoptosis. The 8226/dox40 resistance to TRAIL was not the result of poor or absent expression of DR4 or DR5. The synergy achieved by ADR and also by VP16 in combination with TRAIL and apoptosis of 8226/dox40 is consistent with previous findings of drug-induced sensitization to TRAIL [168, 176–179]. Lower concentrations of ADR were used for sensitization than the concentrations used for cytotoxicity in the sensitization of tumor cells. Of interest, the low concentration of ADR activity was active in the MDR-expressing 8226/dox variant [180].

The mechanism of ADR-induced sensitization of 8226/dox40 to TRAIL apoptosis was examined. There was some modest upregulation of DR5 by ADR. There was little change in any of the pro- or anti-apoptotic gene products by ADR, though there was upregulation of both caspase 9 and Apaf-1. The combination treatment resulted in depolarization of the mitochondrial membrane. These findings demonstrated that ADR sensitizes TRAIL-resistant MDR-positive tumor cells to TRAIL apoptosis as a result of the activation of the type II apoptotic pathway. The sensitization was independent of the MDR phenotype by a drug that is resistant to MDR. Since CTL mediates its cytotoxic activity, in part, by TRAIL, thus, treatment of tumor cells with low concentrations of drugs (example ADR and VP16) would sensitize tumor cells to CTL-apoptosis. Similar findings were also reported for sensitization of Fas-L resistant tumor cells by drugs and their sensitivity to CTL-mediated apoptosis [165].

9.4.6 Gene Modification (siRNA/Overexpression): RKIP as a Model

The development of tumor cell resistance to CTL-mediated cytotoxic mechanisms underlies the search for molecular targets that govern resistance and their possible consideration as potential therapeutic targets. TRAIL and agonist DR4/DR5 mAbs are currently being explored in the clinic for treatment of various cancers [181, 182]. We and others have reported on possible mechanisms that regulate resistance to TRAIL and their reversal by sensitizing agents [63, 82–84].

Chatterjee et al. [94] have reported that drug resistance of tumor cells can be sensitized to drug apoptosis by overexpression of RKIP. RKIP is a member of the phosphatidyl-ethanolamine-binding protein family and it inhibits both the NF-κB and the Raf/MEK/ERK pathways [48, 49]. The finding that constitutively activated NF-κB and Raf/MEK/ERK survival anti-apoptotic pathways mediated resistance, their inhibition by RKIP may reverse resistance and render the cells sensitive to apoptotic stimuli. For instance, inhibition of NF-κB resulted in downstream inhibition of the Fas and DR5 repressor factor YY1 and resulting in deregulation of Fas and DR5 expression, leading to sensitization to Fas-L and TRAIL apoptosis, respectively [12, 79, 87, 88]. The findings reported by Baritaki et al. [90] demonstrated overexpression of RKIP in tumor cell lines sensitizes cells to TRAIL apoptosis and, in contrast, inhibition of RKIP reversed the sensitization to TRAIL. The induction of RKIP correlated with inhibition of YY1 and upregulation of DR5. The combination of TRAIL and overexpression of RKIP resulted in activation of both type I and type II apoptotic pathways. Similar to the inhibition of NF-κB and YY1 and the upregulation of DR5 that sensitized the cells to TRAIL, therefore, RKIP expression was shown to mimic these inhibitions.

RKIP acts upstream of the kinase complex that regulates NF-κB activity [49]. These findings suggested that RKIP induction inhibits NF-κB and YY1 and augments DR5 expression underlying the mechanism of RKIP-induced sensitization to TRAIL. However, RKIP-induced inhibition of the Raf/MEK/ERK pathway may also be involved in sensitization, since this pathway was reported to override the apoptotic signaling by death receptors, including TRAIL [183]. We have suggested that since YY1 is involved in the regulation of both Fas-L and TRAIL resistance, therefore, RKIP overexpression may also sensitize the cells to Fas-L apoptosis by inhibiting YY1 and inducing Fas.

Overexpression of RKIP is manifested in the cells by depolarization of the mitochondrial membrane potential, activation of caspases and also, downregulation of anti-apoptotic gene products such as XIAP and Bcl-$_{XL}$. Treatment of cells overexpressing RKIP potentiated the type II apoptotic pathway (Fig. 9.3). The findings above suggest strongly that RKIP regulates the immune response by CTL and NK cells and it is a new role, in addition to its metastatic suppressor role previously identified.

Since the levels of RKIP are low in most tumors, thus, it may be a critical determinant in cancer progression through modulation of the anti-tumor immune response. Hence, RKIP is a target whereby its induction may inhibit metastasis and sensitize the cells to both drugs and the immune response.

9.5 Clinical Applications

The resistance of tumor cells to cytotoxic lymphocytes leads to disease progression in the host. The resistance to killing by CTL is not restricted to the lymphocytes as mechanisms governing anti-apoptotic outcomes in cancer cells are also governed for various agents-mediated apoptosis (chemotherapy, hormonal, irradiation, antibody, chemical inhibitors, etc.). The identification of the mechanism of a gene(s) product that regulates killing by CTL and cytotoxic agents have been represented by various manipulations discussed herein. For example, the dysregulated NF-κB/Snail/YY1/RKIP/PI3K/PTEN loop offers novel intervention approaches to modulate its role in resistance and shift the balance from anti- to pro-apoptotic activities [45].

9.6 Conclusions and Future Directions

In this review, the resistance of model cancer tumor cells to CTL/ligands-mediated cytotoxicity was analyzed via one mechanism, among many other mechanisms discussed elsewhere, that tumor cells use to inhibit CTL-mediated cytotoxicity. The dysregulated NF-κB/Snail/RKIP/YY1/PTEN was shown to regulate resistance to apoptotic stimuli induced by CTL ligands (examples Fas-L, TRAIL, TNF-α) and how its interference, by various selective agents that disrupted this loop, resulted in the sensitization of tumor cells to CTL-induced apoptosis. The various findings that have been discussed in in vitro model systems must be confirmed and validated in clinical trials. In addition, since the interference by specific agents directed against each one of the various factors in the loop was sufficient to sensitize the tumor cells to CTL, it suggests that one must be able to develop novel agents that target specifically any of these factors and possibly achieving the same results. In addition to the reversal of resistance to CTL-mediated apoptosis via modulation of the loop, that same loop has been shown to also regulate the resistance to chemotherapeutic drugs, on one hand, as well as in the regulation of EMT and metastasis. Therefore, the agents that will interfere and sensitize the cells to CTL-mediated apoptosis will also be able to override the cross-resistance between chemotherapy and immunotherapy, as well as inhibit EMT and metastasis. Such an approach has unique attributes and functions that is not achieved by agents that are more selective and more confined.

Acknowledgments The authors acknowledge the laboratory personnel at UCLA and collaborators outside of UCLA whose reported research investigations in the YY1 field have been referenced and used in the preparation of this review. These investigators are doctors: Baritaki S (UCLA), Berenson J (Institute for Myeloma and Bone Marrow Cancer Research, Hollywood, CA), Chatterjee D (Brown University), Garban H (UCLA), Huerta-Yepez S (UCLA and Hospital Infantil de Mexico, Mexico City), Jazirehi AR (UCLA), Katsman A (UCLA), Palladino M (Nereus Pharmaceuticals, San Diego), Rapozzi V (University of Udine, Italy), Spandidos D (University of Crete, Greece), Vega MI (UCLA and Hospital de Infectologia CMN La Raza, Mexico City), Wu K (UCLA) and Yeung KC (Medical College of Ohio).

The authors also acknowledge the research supports that were funded throughout the YY1 investigations for the reported and include: the Jonsson Comprehensive Cancer Center at UCLA; the University of California Gene Medicine Program; the UCLA AIDS Institute; the UCLA Fogarty International Center Fellowship (D43. TW0013-14); the UCLA SPORE in Prostate Cancer; the Department of Defense (DOD/U.S. ARMY, DAMD, 17-02-1-0023,) UC-MEXUS-CONACYT; Bodasaki Foundation (Greece); NCI-RO1-CA133479; NCICA107023-02S1; NCICA05715213S1; NIHR21149938.

The assistance of Kathy Nguyen is also acknowledged in the preparation of this manuscript.

References

1. Cooper EL, Kauschke E, Cossarizza A. Digging for innate immunity since Darwin and Metchnikoff. Bioessays. 2002;24:319–33.
2. Uthaisangsook S, Day NK, Bahna SL, Good RA, Haraguchi S. Innate immunity and its role against infections. Ann Allergy Asthma Immunol. 2002;88:253–64.
3. Beach S, Tang H, Park S, Dhillon AS, Keller ET, Kolch W, Yeung KC. Snail is a repressor of RKIP transcription in metastatic prostate cancer cells. Oncogene. 2008;27:2243–8.
4. Guermonprez P, Valladeau J, Zitvogel L, Thery C, Amigorena S. Antigen presentation and T cell stimulation by dendritic cells. Annu Rev Immunol. 2002;20:621–67.
5. Janeway Jr CA, Medzhitov R. Innate immune recognition. Annu Rev Immunol. 2002;20: 197–216.
6. Rosenberg SA, Spiess P, Lafreniere R. A new approach to the adoptive immunotherapy of cancer with tumor-infiltrating lymphocytes. Science. 1986;233:1318–21.
7. Yoshida S, Tanaka R, Takai N, Ono K. Local administration of autologous lymphokine-activated killer cells and recombinant interleukin 2 to patients with malignant brain tumors. Cancer Res. 1988;48:5011–6.
8. Kimoto Y, Taguchi T. Adoptive immunotherapy of malignant diseases with IL-2-activated lymphocytes. Biken J. 1987;30:29–38.
9. Rizzo S, Silvotti MG, Martano F, Santamaria AB, Pontiggia P. Long-term primary human tumor cell cultures and mixed autologous tumor-lymphocyte cultures for adoptive specific anti-tumoral immunotherapy. Anticancer Res. 1998;18:41–4.
10. Frost PJ, Belldegrun A, Bonavida B. Sensitization of immunoresistant prostate carcinoma cell lines to Fas/Fas ligand-mediated killing by cytotoxic lymphocytes: independence of de novo protein synthesis. Prostate. 1999;41:20–30.
11. Bonavida B, Safrit J, Morimoto H, Mizutani Y, Uslu R, Borsellino N, Frost P, Berek J, Belldegrun A, Zighelboim J, Ng CP, Mori S. Cross-resistance of tumor cells to chemotherapy and immunotherapy: approaches to reverse resistance and implications in gene therapy. Oncol Rep. 1997;4:201–5.
12. Thompson CB. Apoptosis in the pathogenesis and treatment of disease. Science. 1995;267: 1456–62.
13. Landowski TH, Gleason-Guzman MC, Dalton WS. Selection for drug resistance results in resistance to Fas-mediated apoptosis. Blood. 1997;89:1854–61.
14. Hodi FS, Dranoff G. Combinatorial cancer immunotherapy. Adv Immunol. 2006;90: 341–68.
15. Trambas CM, Griffiths GM. Delivering the kiss of death. Nat Immunol. 2003;4:399–403.
16. Metkar SS, Wang B, Ebbs ML, Kim JH, Lee YJ, Raja SM, Froelich CJ. Granzyme B activates procaspase-3 which signals a mitochondrial amplification loop for maximal apoptosis. J Cell Biol. 2003;160:875–85.
17. Lieberman J. Anatomy of a murder: how cytotoxic T cells and NK cells are activated, develop, and eliminate their targets. Immunol Rev. 2010;23:5–9.

18. Bonavida B. NK cell phenotypic and functional heterogeneities and molecular mechanisms of cytotoxicity. Crit Rev Oncog. 2014;19:21–45.
19. Shen DT, Ma JS, Mather J, Vukmanovic S, Radoja S. Activation of primary T lymphocytes results in lysosome development and polarized granule exocytosis in CD4+ and CD8+ subsets, whereas expression of lytic molecules confers cytotoxicity to CD8+ T cells. J Leukoc Biol. 2006;80:827–37.
20. Ma JS. Protein kinase Cdelta regulates antigen receptor-induced lytic granule polarization in mouse CD8+ CTL. J Immunol. 2007;178:7814–21.
21. Natarajan K, Cowan JA. Solution structure of a synthetic lytic peptide: the perforin amino terminus. Chem Biol. 1998;5:147–54.
22. Voskoboinik I, Thia MC, Fletcher J, Ciccone A, Browne K, Smyth MJ, Trapani JA. Calcium-dependent plasma membrane binding and cell lysis by perforin are mediated through its C2 domain: a critical role for aspartate residues 429, 435, 483, and 485 but not 491. J Biol Chem. 2005;280:8426–34.
23. Liu CC, Walsh CM, Young JD. Perforin: structure and function. Immunol Today. 1995;16: 194–201.
24. Waterhouse NJ, Sedelies KA, Sutton VR, Pinkoski MJ, Thia KY, Johnstone R, Bird PI, Green DR, Trapani JA. Functional dissociation of DeltaPsim and cytochrome c release defines the contribution of mitochondria upstream of caspase activation during granzyme B-induced apoptosis. Cell Death Differ. 2006;13:607–18.
25. Waterhouse NJ, Sedelies KA, Trapani JA. Role of Bid-induced mitochondrial outer membrane permeabilization in granzyme B-induced apoptosis. Immunol Cell Biol. 2006;84: 72–8.
26. Fan Z, Beresford PJ, Oh DY, Zhang D, Lieberman J. Tumor suppressor NM23-H1 is a granzyme A-activated DNase during CTL-mediated apoptosis, and the nucleosome assembly protein SET is its inhibitor. Cell. 2003;112:659–72.
27. Zhang D, Beresford PJ, Greenberg AH, Lieberman J. Granzymes A and B directly cleave lamins and disrupt the nuclear lamina during granule-mediated cytolysis. Proc Natl Acad Sci U S A. 2001;98:5746–51.
28. Pinkoski MJ, Waterhouse NJ, Heibein JA, Wolf BB, Kuwana T, Goldstein JC, Newmeyer DD, Bleackley RC, Green DR. Granzyme B-mediated apoptosis proceeds predominantly through a Bcl-2-inhibitable mitochondrial pathway. J Biol Chem. 2001;276:12060–7.
29. Jin Z, El-Deiry WS. Overview of cell death signaling pathways. Cancer Biol Ther. 2005;4: 139–63.
30. Wilson NS, Dixit V, Ashkenazi A. Death receptor signal transducers: nodes of coordination in immune signaling networks. Nat Immunol. 2009;10:348–55.
31. Scaffidi C, Fluda S, Srinivasan A, Friesen C, Li F, Tomaselli KJ, Debatin KM, Krammer PH, Peter ME. Two CD95(APO-1/Fas) signaling pathways. EMBO J. 1998;17:1675–87.
32. Finucane DM, Bossy-Wetzel E, Waterhouse NJ, Cotter TG, Green DR. Bax-induced caspase activation and apoptosis via cytochrome c release from mitochondria is inhibitable by Bcl-XL. J Biol Chem. 1999;274:2225–33.
33. Bossy-Wetzel E, Green DR. Caspases induce cytochrome c release from mitochondria by activating cytosolic factors. J Biol Chem. 1999;274:17484–90.
34. Wolf BB, Schuler M, Echeverri F, Green DR. Caspase 3 is the primary activator of apoptotic DNA fragmentation via DNA fragmentation factor-45/inhibitor of caspase-activated DNase inactivation. J Biol Chem. 1999;274:30651–6.
35. Perkins CL, Fang G, Kim CN, Bhalla KN. The role of Apaf-1, caspase 9 and Bid proteins in etoposide or paclitaxel-induced mitochondrial events during apoptosis. Cancer Res. 2000;60:1645–53.
36. Sprick MR, Weigand MA, Rieser E, Rauch CT, Juo P, Blenis J, Krammer PH, Walczak H. FADD/MORT1 and caspase-8 are recruited to TRAIL receptors 1 and 2 and are essential for apoptosis mediated by TRAIL receptor 2. Immunity. 2000;12:599–609.
37. Kischkel FC, Lawrence DA, Chuntharapai A, Schow P, Kim KJ, Ashkenazi A. Apo2L/TRAIL-dependent recruitment of endogenous FADD and caspase-8 to death receptors 4 and 5. Immunity. 2000;12:611–20.

38. Zou H, Li Y, Liu X, Wang X. An APAF-1.cytochrome c multimeric complex is a functional apoptosome that activates procaspase-9. J Biol Chem. 1999;274:11549–56.
39. Faivre S, Djelloul S, Raymond E. New paradigms in anticancer therapy: targeting multiple signaling pathways with kinase inhibitors. Semin Oncol. 2006;4:407–20.
40. Shukla S, Maclennan GT, Marengo SR, Resnick MI, Gupta S. Constitutive activation of P I3 K-Akt and NF-kappaB during prostate cancer progression in autochthonous transgenic mouse model. Prostate. 2005;64:224–39.
41. Classen CF, Falk CS, Friesen C, Fulda S, Herr I, Debatin KM. Natural killer resistance of a drugresistant leukemia cell line, mediated by up-regulation of HLA class I expression. Haematologica. 2003;88:509–21.
42. Huang Y, Obholzer N, Fayad R, Qiao L. Turning on/off tumor-specific CTL response during progressive tumor growth. J Immunol. 2005;175:3110–6.
43. Ferris RL, Whiteside TL, Ferrone S. Immune escape associated with functional defects in antigen-processing machinery in head and neck cancer. Clin Cancer Res. 2006;12:3890–5.
44. Frey AB, Monu N. Signaling defects in anti-tumor T cells. Immunol Rev. 2008;222: 192–205.
45. Baritaki S, Bonavida B. Viral infection and cancer: the NF-κB/Snail/RKIP loop regulates target cell sensitivity to apoptosis by cytotoxic lymphocytes. Crit Rev Immunol. 2010;30: 31–46.
46. Barbera MJ, Puig I, Dominguez D, Julien-Grille S, Guaita-Esteruelas S, Peiro S, Baulida J, Franci C, Dedhar S, Larue L, Garcia de Herreros A. Regulation of Snail transcription during epithelial to mesenchymal transition of tumor cells. Oncogene. 2004;23:7345–54.
47. Julien S, Puig I, Caretti E, Bonaventure J, Nelles L, van Roy F, Dargemont C, de Herreros AG, Bellacosa A, Larue L. Activation of NF-kappaB by Akt upregulates Snail expression and induces epithelium mesenchyme transition. Oncogene. 2007;26:7445–56.
48. Yeung K, Seitz T, Li S, Janosch P, McFerran B, Kaiser C, Fee F, Katsanakis KD, Rose DW, Mischak H, Sedivy JM, Kolch W. Suppression of Raf-1 kinase activity and MAP kinase signalling by RKIP. Nature. 1999;401:173–7.
49. Yeung KC, Rose DW, Dhillon AS, Yaros D, Gustafsson M, Chatterjee D, McFerran B, Wyche J, Kolch W, Sedivy JM. Raf kinase inhibitor protein interacts with NF-kappaB-inducing kinase and TAK1 and inhibits NF-kappaB activation. Mol Cell Biol. 2001;21:7207–17.
50. Palmer MB, Majumder P, Cooper JC, Yoon H, Wade PA, Boss JM. Yin yang 1 regulates the expression of snail through a distal enhancer. Mol Cancer Res. 2009;7(2):221–9.
51. Karin M. Nuclear factor-κB in cancer development and progression. Nature. 2006;441: 431–6.
52. Luo JL, Kamata H, Karin M. IKK/NF-kappaB signaling: balancing life and death—a new approach to cancer therapy. J Clin Invest. 2005;115:2625–32.
53. Ravi R, Bedi A. NF-κB in cancer—a friend turned foe. Drug Resist Updat. 2004;7:53–67.
54. Ghosh S, May MJ, Kopp EB. NF-kappa B and Rel proteins: evolutionarily conserved mediators of immune responses. Annu Rev Immunol. 1998;16:225–60.
55. Hoesel B, Schmid JA. The complexity of NF-κB signaling in inflammation and cancer. Mol Cancer. 2013;12:86.
56. Tang G, Minemoto Y, Dibling B, et al. Inhibition of JNK activation through NF-kappaB target genes. Nature. 2001;414:313–7.
57. Lerebours F, Vacher S, Andrieu C, Espie M, Marty M, Lidereau R, Bieche I. NF-kappa B genes have a major role in inflammatory breast cancer. BMC Cancer. 2008;8:41.
58. Hayden MS, West AP, Ghosh S. NF-kappaB and the immune response. Oncogene. 2006;25:6758–80.
59. Bours V, Bentires-Alj M, Hellin AC, Viatour P, Robe P, Delhalle S, Benoit V, Merville MP. Nuclear factorkappa B, cancer, and apoptosis. Biochem Pharmacol. 2000;60:1085–9.
60. Bubici C, Papa S, Pham CG, Zazzeroni F, Franzoso G. The NF-kappaB-mediated control of ROS and JNK signaling. Histol Histopathol. 2006;21:69–80.
61. Arlt A, Schafer H. NFkappaB-dependent chemoresistance in solid tumors. Int J Clin Pharmacol Ther. 2002;40:336–47.

62. Lu T, Stark GR. Cytokine overexpression and constitutive NFkappaB in cancer. Cell Cycle. 2004;3:1114–7.
63. Baritaki S, Huerta-Yepez S, Sakai T, Spandidos DA, Bonavida B. Chemotherapeutic drugs sensitize cancer cells to TRAIL-mediated apoptosis: up-regulation of DR5 and inhibition of Yin Yang 1. Mol Cancer Ther. 2007;6:1387–99.
64. Katsman A, Umezawa K, Bonavida B. Reversal of resistance to cytotoxic cancer therapies: DHMEQ as a chemo-sensitizing and immune-sensitizing agent. Drug Resist Updat. 2007; 10:1–12.
65. Baritaki S, Yeung K, Palladino M, Berenson J, Bonavida B. Pivotal roles of snail inhibition and RKIP induction by the proteasome inhibitor NPI-0052 in tumor cell chemoimmunosensitization. Cancer Res. 2009;69:8376–85.
66. Nieto MA. The snail superfamily of zinc-finger transcription factors. Nat Rev Mol Cell Biol. 2002;3:155–66.
67. Kaufhold S, Bonavida B. Central role of Snail1 in the regulation of EMT and resistance in cancer: a target for therapeutic intervention. J Exp Clin Cancer Res. 2014;33:62.
68. Peinado H, Portillo F, Cano A. Transcriptional regulation of cadherins during development and carcinogenesis. Int J Dev Biol. 2004;48:365–75.
69. Miyoshi A, Kitajima Y, Kido S, Shimonishi T, Matsuyama S, Kitahara K, Miyazaki K. Snail accelerates cancer invasion by upregulating MMP expression and is associated with poor prognosis of hepatocellular carcinoma. Br J Cancer. 2005;92:252–8.
70. Zha YH, He JF, Mei YW, Yin T, Mao L. Zinc-finger transcription factor snail accelerates survival, migration and expression of matrix metalloproteinase-2 in human bone mesenchymal stem cells. Cell Biol Int. 2007;31:1089–96.
71. Peiro S, Escriva M, Puig I, Barbera MJ, Dave N, Herranz N, Larriba MJ, Takkunen M, Franci C, Munoz A, Virtanen I, Baulida J, Garcia de Herreros A. Snail1 transcriptional repressor binds to its own promoter and controls its expression. Nucleic Acids Res. 2006;34:2077–84.
72. Kajita M, McClinic KN, Wade PA. Aberrant expression of the transcription factors snail and slug alters the response to genotoxic stress. Mol Cell Biol. 2004;24:7559–66.
73. Vega MI, Huerta-Yepaz S, Garban H, Jazirehi A, Emmanouilides C, Bonavida B. Rituximab inhibits p38 MAPK activity in 2F7 B NHL and decreases IL-10 transcription: pivotal role of p38 MAPK in drug resistance. Oncogene. 2004;23:3530–40.
74. Zhuo W, Wang Y, Zhuo X, Zhang Y, Ao X, Chen Z. Knockdown of Snail, a novel zinc finger transcription factor, via RNA interference increases A549 cell sensitivity to cisplatin via JNK/mitochondrial pathway. Lung Cancer. 2008;62:8–14.
75. Gordon S, Akopyan G, Garban H, Bonavida B. Transcription factor YY1: structure, function, and therapeutic implications in cancer biology. Oncogene. 2006;25:1125–42.
76. Seligson DB, Hongo F, Huerta-Yepez S, Mizutani Y, Miki T, Yu H, Horvath S, Chia D, Goodglick L, Bonavida B. Expression of X-linked inhibitor of apoptosis protein is a strong predictor of human prostate cancer recurrence. Clin Cancer Res. 2007;13:6056–63.
77. Castellano G, Torrisi E, Ligresti G, Malaponte G, Militello L, Russo AE, McCubrey JA, Canevari S, Libra M. The involvement of the transcription factor Yin Yang 1 in cancer development and progression. Cell Cycle. 2009;8:1367–72.
78. Wang H, Hertlein E, Bakkar N, Sun H, Acharyya S, Wang J, Carathers M, Davuluri R, Guttridge DC. NFkappaB regulation of YY1 inhibits skeletal myogenesis through transcriptional silencing of myofibrillar genes. Mol Cell Biol. 2007;27:4374–87.
79. Garban HJ, Bonavida B. Nitric oxide inhibits the transcription repressor Yin-Yang 1 binding activity at the silencer region of the Fas promoter: a pivotal role for nitric oxide in the up-regulation of Fas gene expression in human tumor cells. J Immunol. 2001;167:75–81.
80. Huerta-Yepez S, Vega M, Escoto-Chavez SE, Murdock B, Sakai T, Baritaki S, Bonavida B. Nitric oxide sensitizes tumor cells to TRAIL-induced apoptosis via inhibition of the DR5 transcription repressor Yin Yang 1. Nitric Oxide. 2009;20:39–52.
81. Zhang L, Fang B. Mechanisms of resistance to TRAIL-induced apoptosis in cancer. Cancer Gene Ther. 2005;12:228–37.

82. Sheikh MS, Burns TF, Huang Y, Wu GS, Amundson S, Brooks KS, Fornace Jr AJ, el-Deiry WS. p53-dependent and -independent regulation of the death receptor KILLER/DR5 gene expression in response to genotoxic stress and tumor necrosis factor α. Cancer Res. 1998; 58:1593–8.
83. Nagane M, Pan G, Weddle JJ, Dixit VM, Cavenee WK, Huang HJ. Increased death receptor 5 expression by chemotherapeutic agents in human gliomas causes synergistic cytotoxicity with tumor necrosis factor-related apoptosis-inducing ligand in vitro and in vivo. Cancer Res. 2000;60:847–53.
84. Shankar S, Chen XTR, Srivastava RK. Effects of sequential treatments with chemotherapeutic drugs followed by TRAIL on prostate cancer in vitro and in vivo. Prostate. 2005; 62:165–86.
85. Ng CP, Bonavida B. X-linked inhibitor of apoptosis (XIAP) blocks Apo2 ligand/tumor necrosis factor-related apoptosis-inducing ligand-mediated apoptosis of prostate cancer cells in the presence of mitochondrial activation: sensitization by overexpression of second mitochondria-derived activator of caspase/direct IAP-binding protein with low pl (Smac/DIABLO). Mol Cancer Ther. 2002;1:1051–8.
86. Baritaki S, Suzuki E, Umezawa K, Spandidos DA, Berenson J, Daniels TR, Penichet ML, Jazirehi AR, Palladino M, Bonavida B. Inhibition of Yin Yang 1-dependent repressor activity of DR5 transcription and expression by the novel proteasome inhibitor NPI-0052 contributes to its TRAIL-enhanced apoptosis in cancer cells. J Immunol. 2008;180:6199–210.
87. Vega MI, Jazirehi AR, Huerta-Yepez S, Bonavida B. Rituximab-induced inhibition of YY1 and Bcl-x_L expression in Ramos non-Hodgkin's lymphoma cell line via inhibition of NF-κB activity: role of YY1 and Bcl-x_L in Fas resistance and chemoresistance, respectively. J Immunol. 2005;175:2174–83.
88. Vega MI, Huerta-Yepez S, Jazirehi A, Garban H, Bonavida B. Rituximab (chimeric anti-CD20) sensitizes B-NHL cell lines to Fas-induced apoptosis. Oncogene. 2005;24:8114–27.
89. Yoshida T, Maeda A, Tani N, Sakai T. Promoter structure and transcription initiation sites of the human death receptor 5/TRAIL-R2 gene. FEBS Lett. 2001;507:381–5.
90. Baritaki S, Katsman A, Chatterjee D, Yeung KC, Spandidos DA, Bonavida B. Regulation of tumor cell sensitivity to TRAIL-induced apoptosis by the metastatic suppressor Raf kinase inhibitor protein via Yin Yang 1 inhibition and death receptor 5 up-regulation. J Immunol. 2007;179:5441–53.
91. Huerta-Yepez S, Vega M, Jazirehi A, Garban H, Hongo F, Cheng G, Bonavida B. Nitric oxide sensitizes prostate carcinoma cell lines to TRAIL-mediated apoptosis via inactivation of NF-kappa B and inhibition of Bcl-xl expression. Oncogene. 2004;23:4993–5003.
92. Fu Z, Smith PC, Zhang L, Rubin MA, Dunn RL, Yao Z, Keller ET. Effects of raf kinase inhibitor protein expression on suppression of prostate cancer metastasis. J Natl Cancer Inst. 2003;95:878–89.
93. Eves EM, Shapiro P, Naik K, Klein UR, Trakul N, Rosner MR. Raf kinase inhibitory protein regulates aurora B kinase and the spindle checkpoint. Mol Cell. 2006;23:561–74.
94. Chatterjee D, Bai Y, Wang Z, Beach S, Mott S, Roy R, Braastad C, Sun Y, Mukhopadhyay A, Aggarwal BB, Darnowski J, Pantazis P, Wyche J, Fu Z, Kitagwa Y, Keller ET, Sedivy JM, Yeung KC. RKIP sensitizes prostate and breast cancer cells to drug-induced apoptosis. J Biol Chem. 2004;279:17515–23.
95. Jazirehi A, Bonavida B. Cellular and molecular signal transduction pathways modulated by rituximab (rituxan, anti-CD20 mAb) in non-Hodgkin's lymphoma: implications in chemosensitization and therapeutic intervention. Oncogene. 2005;24:2121–43.
96. Hamaï A, Meslin F, Benlalam H, Jalil A, Mehrpour M, Faure F, Lecluse Y, Vielh P, Avril MF, Robert C, Chouaib S. ICAM-1 has a critical role in the regulation of metastatic melanoma tumor susceptibility to CTL lysis by interfering with PI3K/AKT pathway. Cancer Res. 2008;68:9854–64.
97. Reddy SD, Pakala SB, Molli PR, Sahni N, Karanam NK, Mudvari P, Kumar R. Metastasis-associated protein 1/histone deacetylase 4-nucleosome remodeling and deacetylase complex

regulates phosphatase and tensin homolog gene expression and function. J Biol Chem. 2012;287:27843–50.
98. Gao Q, Zhang L, Zhang B, Wang QY, Sun CF, Dong XT, Ying J. Phosphatase and tensin homolog overexpression decreases proliferation and invasion and increases apoptosis in oral squamous cell carcinoma cells. Oncol Lett. 2014;8:1058–64.
99. Nguyen HN, Yang JM, Afkari Y, Park BH, Sesaki H, Devreotes PN, Iijima M. Engineering ePTEN, an enhanced PTEN with increased tumor suppressor activities. Proc Natl Acad Sci U S A. 2014;111:E2684–93.
100. Kim RJ, Bae E, Hong YK, Hong JY, Kim NK, Ahn HJ, Oh JJ, Park DS. PTEN loss-mediated Akt activation increases the properties of cancer stem-like cell populations in prostate cancer. Oncology. 2014;87:270–9.
101. Wang H, Xu C, Kong X, Li X, Kong X, Wang Y, Ding X, Yang Q. Trail resistance induces epithelial-mesenchymal transition and enhances invasiveness by suppressing PTEN via miR-221 in breast cancer. PLoS One. 2014;9:e99067.
102. Hao L, Ha JR, Kuzel P, Garcia E, Persad S. Cadherin switch from E- to N-cadherin in melanoma progression is regulated by the PI3K/PTEN pathway through Twist and Snail. Br J Dermatol. 2012;166:1184–97.
103. Fang L, Li H, Wang L, Hu J, Jin T, Wang J, Yang BB. MicroRNA-17-5p promotes chemotherapeutic drug resistance and tumour metastasis of colorectal cancer by repressing PTEN expression. Oncotarget. 2014;5:2974–87.
104. Zhang G, Hou X, Li Y, Zhao M. MiR-205 inhibits cell apoptosis by targeting phosphatase and tensin homolog deleted on chromosome ten in endometrial cancer Ishikawa cells. BMC Cancer. 2014;14:440.
105. Ariga A, Namekawa J, Matsumoto N, Inoue J, Umezawa K. Inhibition of TNF-induced nuclear translocation and activation of NF-κB by dehydroxymethyl-epoxyquinomicin. J Biol Chem. 2002;277:24625–30.
106. Umezawa K. Inhibition of tumor growth by NF-κB inhibitors. Cancer Sci. 2006;97:990–5.
107. Bonavida B, Vega MI. Rituximab-mediated chemosensitization of AIDS and non-AIDS non-Hodgkin's lymphoma. Drug Resist. 2005;8:27–41.
108. Feling RH, Buchanan GO, Mincer TJ, Kauffman CA, Jensen PR, Fenical W. Salinosporamide A: a highly cytotoxic proteasome inhibitor from a novel microbial source, a marine bacterium of the new genus Salinospora. Angew Chem Int Ed Engl. 2003;42:355–7.
109. Macherla VR, Mitchell SS, Manam RR, Reed KA, Chao TH, Nicholson B, Deyanat-Yazdi G, Mai B, Jensen PR, Fenical WF, Neuteboom ST, Lam KS, Palladino MA, Potts BC. Structure-activity relationship studies of salinosporamide A (NPI-0052), a novel marine derived proteasome inhibitor. J Med Chem. 2005;48:3684–7.
110. Cusack Jr JC, Liu R, Xia L, Chao TH, Pien C, Niu W, Palombella VJ, Neuteboom ST, Palladino MA. NPI-0052 enhances tumoricidal response to conventional cancer therapy in a colon cancer model. Clin Cancer Res. 2006;12:6758–64.
111. An J, Sun YP, Adams J, Fisher M, Belldegrun A, Rettig MB. Drug interactions between the proteasome inhibitor bortezomib and cytotoxic chemotherapy, tumor necrosis factor (TNF) α, and TNF-related apoptosis-inducing ligand in prostate cancer. Clin Cancer Res. 2003;9:4537–45.
112. He Q, Huang Y, Sheikh MS. Proteasome inhibitor MG132 upregulates death receptor 5 and cooperates with Apo2L/TRAIL to induce apoptosis in Bax-proficient and -deficient cells. Oncogene. 2004;23:2554–8.
113. Sayers TJ, Brooks AD, Koh CY, Ma W, Seki N, Raziuddin A, Blazar BR, Zhang X, Elliott PJ, Murphy WJ. The proteasome inhibitor PS-341 sensitizes neoplastic cells to TRAIL-mediated apoptosis by reducing levels of c-FLIP. Blood. 2003;102:303–10.
114. La Ferla-Brühl K, Westhoff MA, Karl S, Kasperczyk H, Zwacka RM, Debatin KM, Fulda S. NF-κB-independent sensitization of glioblastoma cells for TRAIL-induced apoptosis by proteasome inhibition. Oncogene. 2007;26:571–82.
115. Liu X, Yue P, Chen S, Hu L, Lonial S, Khuri FR, Sun SY. The proteasome inhibitor PS-341 (bortezomib) up-regulates DR5 expression leading to induction of apoptosis and enhancement

of TRAIL-induced apoptosis despite up-regulation of c-FLIP and survivin expression in human NSCLC cells. Cancer Res. 2007;67:4981–8.

116. Rosenberg SA, Restifo NP, Yang JC, Morgan RA, Dudley ME. Adoptive cell transfer: a clinical path to effective cancer immunotherapy. Nat Rev Cancer. 2008;8:299–308.
117. Kessels HW, Wolkers MC, Van Den Boom MD, Van Der Valk MA, Schumacher TN. Immunotherapy through TCR gene transfer. Nat Immunol. 2001;2:957–61.
118. Morgan RA, Dudley ME, Yu YY, Zheng Z, Robbins PF, Theoret MR, et al. High efficiency TCR gene transfer into primary human lymphocytes affords avid recognition of melanoma tumor antigen glycoprotein 100 and does not alter the recognition of autologous melanoma antigens. J Immunol. 2003;171:3287–95.
119. Morgan RA, Dudley ME, Wunderlich JR, Hughes MS, Yang JC, Sherry RM, et al. Cancer regression in patients after transfer of genetically engineered lymphocytes. Science. 2006;314:126–9.
120. Jazirehi AR, Baritaki S, Koya RC, Bonavida B, Economou JS. Molecular mechanism of MART-1^+/A*0201^+ human melanoma resistance to specific CTL-killing despite functional tumor-CTL interaction. Cancer Res. 2011;71:1406–17.
121. Vallabhapurapu S, Karin M. Regulation and function of NF-kappaB transcription factors in the immune system. Annu Rev Immunol. 2009;27:693–733.
122. Shigero M, Nakao K, Ichikawa T, Suzuki K, Kawakami A, Abiru S, Miyazoe S, Akagawa Y, Ishikawa H, Hamasaki K, Nakata K, Ishii N, Eguchi K. Oncogene. 2003;22:1653–62.
123. Raffo AJ, Perlman H, Chen MW, Day ML, Streitman JS, Bttyan R. Cancer Res. 1995;55:4438–45.
124. Huerta-Yepez S, Vega M, Garban H and Bonavida B. 94th Annual Meeting of American Association for Cancer Research, Vol. 44, p. 918, 2003. Abstract #4012.
125. Lee YJ, Lee KH, Kim HR, Jessup JM, Seol DW, Kim TH, Billiar T, Song YK. Oncogene. 2001;20:1476–85.
126. Secchiero P, Gonelli A, Celeghini C, Mirandola P, Guidotti L, Visani G, Capitani S, Zauli G. Blood. 2001;98:2220–8.
127. Ng CP, Zisman A, Bonavida B. Synergy is achieved by complementation with Apo2L/TRAIL and actinomycin D in Apo2L/TRAIL-mediated apoptosis of prostate cancer cells: role of XIAP in resistance. Prostate. 2002;53:286–99.
128. Poderoso JJ, Carreras MC, Lisdero C, Riobo N, Schopfer F, Boveris A. Arch Biochem Biophys. 1996;328:85–92.
129. Kuang AA, Diehl GE, Zhang J, Winoto A. FADD is required for DR4- and DR5-mediated apoptosis: lack of trail-induced apoptosis in FADD-deficient mouse embryonic fibroblasts. J Biol Chem. 2000;275:25065–8.
130. Nakata S, Yoshida T, Horinaka M, Shiraishi T, Wakada M, Sakai T. Histone deacetylase inhibitors upregulate death receptor 5/TRAIL-R2 and sensitize apoptosis induced by TRAIL/APO2-L in human malignant tumor cells. Oncogene. 2004;23:6261–71.
131. Wu GS, Burns TF, McDonald 3rd ER, Meng RD, Kao G, Muschel R, Yen T, El-Deiry WS. Induction of the TRAIL receptor KILLER/DR5 in p53-dependent apoptosis but not growth arrest. Oncogene. 1999;18:6411–8.
132. Takimoto R, El-Deiry WS. Wild-type p53 transactivates the KILLER/DR5 gene through an intronic sequence-specific DNA-binding site. Oncogene. 2000;19:1735–43.
133. Wen J, Ramadevi N, Nguyen D, Perkins C, Worthington E, Bhalla K. Antileukemic drugs increase death receptor 5 levels and enhance Apo-2L-induced apoptosis of human acute leukemia cells. Blood. 2000;96:3900–6.
134. Meng RD, El-Deiry WS. p53-independent upregulation of KILLER/DR5 TRAIL receptor expression by glucocorticoids and interferon-gamma. Exp Cell Res. 2001;262:154–69.
135. LaVallee TM, Zhan XH, Johnson MS, Herbstritt CJ, Swartz G, Williams MS, Hembrough WA, Green SJ, Pribluda VS. 2-Methoxyestradiol up-regulates death receptor 5 and induces apoptosis through activation of the extrinsic pathway. Cancer Res. 2003;63:468–75.
136. Emmanouilides C, Territo M, Menco H, Patel R, Rosen P. Mitoxantrone-cyclophosphamide-rituximab: an effective and safe combination for indolent NHL. Hematol Oncol. 2003;21: 99–108.

137. Jazirehi AR, Gan XH, De Vos S, Emmanouilides C, Bonavida B. Rituximab (anti-CD20) selectively modifies Bcl-xL and apoptosis protease activating factor-1 (Apaf-1) expression and sensitizes human non-Hodgkin's lymphoma B cell lines to paclitaxel-induced apoptosis. Mol Cancer Ther. 2003;2:1183–93.
138. Jazirehi AR, Huerta-Yepez S, Cheng G, Bonavida B. Rituximab (chimeric anti-CD20 monoclonal antibody) inhibits the constitutive nuclear factor-{kappa}B signaling pathway in non-Hodgkin's lymphoma B-cell lines: role in sensitization to chemotherapeutic drug-induced apoptosis. Cancer Res. 2005;65:264–76.
139. Jazirehi AR, Ng CP, Gan XH, Schiller G, Bonavida B. Adriamycin sensitizes the adriamycin-resistant 8226/Dox40 human multiple myeloma cells to Apo2L/tumor necrosis factor-related apoptosis-inducing ligand-mediated (TRAIL) apoptosis. Clin Cancer Res. 2001;7:3874–83.
140. Jazirehi AR, Vega MI, Chatterjee D, Goodglick L, Bonavida B. Inhibition of the Raf-MEK1/2-ERK1/2 signaling pathway, Bcl-xL down-regulation, and chemosensitization of non-Hodgkin's lymphoma B cells by Rituximab. Cancer Res. 2007;64:7117–26.
141. Vega MI, Baritaki S, Huerta-Yepez S, Martinez-Paniagua MA, Bonavida B. A potential mechanism of rituximab-induced inhibition of tumor growth through its sensitization to tumor necrosis factor-related apoptosis-inducing ligand-expressing host cytotoxic cells. Leuk Lymphoma. 2011;52:108–21.
142. Vega MI, Huerta-Yepez S, Baritaki S, Martinez-Paniagua MA, Gonzalez-Bonilla CR, Bonavida B. Rituximab sensitizes TRAIL-resistant B-NHL lines to apoptosis by both TRAIL and fully humanized antibodies targeting TRAIL-R1 (mapatumumab) and TRAIL-R2 (lexatumumab). Blood. 2007;110(Suppl 1):Abstract 2350.
143. Daniel D, Yang B, Lawrence DA, et al. Cooperation of the proapoptotic receptor agonist rhApo2L/TRAIL with the CD20 antibody rituximab against non-Hodgkin lymphoma xenografts. Blood. 2007;110:4037–46.
144. Sancilio S, Grill V, Di Pietro R. A combined approach with rituximab plus anti-TRAIL-R agonistic antibodies for the treatment of haematological malignancies. Curr Pharm Des. 2008;14:2085–99.
145. Newman R, Alberts J, Anderson D, Carner K, Heard C, Norton F, et al. "Primatization" of recombinant antibodies for immunotherapy of human diseases: a macaque/human chimeric antibody against human CD4. Biotechnology (NY). 1992;10:1455–60.
146. Schultze J, Nadler LM, Gribben JG. B7-mediated costimulation and the immune response. Blood Rev. 1996;10:111–27.
147. Vyth-Dreese FA, Dellemijn TA, Majoor D, de Jong D. Localization in situ of the co-stimulatory molecules B7.1, B7.2, CD40 and their ligands in normal human lymphoid tissue. Eur J Immunol. 1995;25:3023–9.
148. Munro JM, Freedman AS, Aster JC, Gribben JG, Lee NC, Rhynhart KK, et al. In vivo expression of the B7 costimulatory molecule by subsets of antigen-presenting cells and the malignant cells of Hodgkin's disease. Blood. 1994;83:793–8.
149. Plumas J, Chaperot L, Jacob MC, Molens JP, Giroux C, Sotto JJ, et al. Malignant B lymphocytes from non-Hodgkin's lymphoma induce allogeneic proliferative and cytotoxic T cell responses in primary mixed lymphocyte cultures: an important role of co-stimulatory molecules CD80 (B7-1) and CD86 (B7-2) in stimulation by tumor cells. Eur J Immunol. 1995;25:3332–41.
150. Bolognesi A, Polito L, Tazzari PL, Lemoli RM, Lubelli C, Fogli M, et al. In vitro anti-tumour activity of anti-CD80 and anti-CD86 immunotoxins containing type 1 ribosome-inactivating proteins. Br J Haematol. 2000;110:351–61.
151. Hariharan K, Anderson D, Leigh B. Therapeutic activity of IDEC-114 (anti-CD80) and rituximab (Rituxan) in B-cell lymphoma. Blood. 2001;98:608a.
152. Martinez-Paniagua MA, Vega MI, Huerta-Yepez S, Baritaki S, Vega GG, Hariharan K, Bonavida B. Galiximab signals B-NHL cells and inhibits the activities of NF-κB-induced YY1- and snail-resistant factors: mechanism of sensitization to apoptosis by chemoimmunotherapeutic drugs. Mol Cancer Ther. 2012;11:572–81.

153. Rosenberg SA, Packard BS, Aebersold PM, Solomon D, Topalian SL, Toy ST, Simon P, Lotze MT, Yang JC, Seipp CA, Simpson C, Carter C, Bock S, Schwartzentruber D, Wei JP, White DE. Use of tumor-infiltrating lymphocytes and interleukin-2 in the immunotherapy of patients with metastatic melanoma. N Engl J Med. 1988;319:1676–80.
154. Topalian SL, Solomon D, Rosenberg SA. Tumor-specific cytolysis by lymphocytes infiltrating human melanomas. J Immunol. 1989;142:3714–25.
155. Lee RK, Spielman J, Zhao DY, Olsen KJ, Podack ER. Perforin, Fas ligand, and tumor necrosis factor are the major cytotoxic molecules used by lymphokine-activated killer cells. J Immunol. 1996;157:1919–25.
156. Frost P, Ng CP, Belldegrun A, Bonavida B. Immunosensitization of prostate carcinoma cell lines for lymphocytes (CTL, TIL, LAK)-mediated apoptosis via the Fas-Fas-ligand pathway of cytotoxicity. Cell Immunol. 1997;180:70–83.
157. Kagi D, Vignaux F, Ledermann B, Burki K, Depraetere V, Nagata S, Hengartner H, Golstein P. Fas and perforin pathways as major mechanisms of T cell-mediated cytotoxicity. Science. 1994;265:528–30.
158. Hishii M, Kurnick JT, Ramirez-Montagut T, Pandolfi F. Studies of the mechanisms of cytolysis by tumour-infiltrating lymphocytes. Clin Exp Immunol. 1999;116:388–94.
159. Mulder WM, Stukart MJ, Roos M, van Lier RA, Wagstaff J, Scheper RJ, Bloemena E. Culture of tumour-infiltrating lymphocytes from melanoma and colon carcinoma: removal of tumour cells does not affect tumour-specificity. Cancer Immunol Immunother. 1995;41:293–301.
160. Frost P, Caliliw R, Belldegrun A, Bonavida B. Immunosensitization of resistant human tumor cells to cytotoxicity by tumor infiltrating lymphocytes. Int J Oncol. 2003;22:431–7.
161. Ashkenazi A, Pai RC, Fong S, Leung S, Lawrence DA, Marsters SA, Blackie C, Chang L, McMurtrey AE, Hebert A, DeForge L, Koumenis IL, Lewis D, Harris L, Bussiere J, Koeppen H, Shahrokh Z, Schwall RH. Safety and antitumor activity of recombinant soluble Apo2 ligand. J Clin Invest. 1999;104:155–62.
162. Walczak H, Miller RE, Ariail K, Gliniak B, Griffith TS, Kubin M, Chin W, Jones J, Woodward A, Le T, Smith C, Smolak P, Goodwin RG, Rauch CT, Schuh JC, Lynch DH. Tumoricidal activity of tumor necrosis factor-related apoptosis-inducing ligand in vivo. Nat Med. 1999; 5:157–63.
163. Gliniak B, Le T. Tumor necrosis factor-related apoptosis-inducing ligand's antitumor activity in vivo is enhanced by the chemotherapeutic agent CPT-11. Cancer Res. 1999;59:6153–8.
164. Bonavida B, Ng CP, Jazirehi A, Schiller G, Mizutani Y. Selectivity of TRAIL-mediated apoptosis of cancer cells and synergy with drugs: the trail to non-toxic cancer therapeutics [review]. Int J Oncol. 1999;15:793–802.
165. Mizutani Y, Yoshida O, Miki T, Bonavida B. Synergistic cytotoxicity and apoptosis by Apo-2 ligand and adriamycin against bladder cancer cells. Clin Cancer Res. 1999;5:2605–12.
166. Mori S, Murakami-Mori K, Nakamura S, Ashkenazi A, Bonavida B. Sensitization of AIDS-Kaposi's sarcoma cells to Apo-2 ligand-induced apoptosis by actinomycin D. J Immunol. 1999;162:5616–23.
167. Gibson SB, Oyer R, Spalding AC, Anderson SM, Johnson GL. Increased expression of death receptors 4 and 5 synergizes the apoptosis response to combined treatment with etoposide and TRAIL. Mol Cell Biol. 2000;20:205–12.
168. Keane MM, Ettenberg SA, Nau MM, Russell EK, Lipkowitz S. Chemotherapy augments TRAIL-induced apoptosis in breast cell lines. Cancer Res. 1999;59:734–41.
169. Deveraux QL, Roy N, Stennicke HR, Van Arsdale T, Zhou Q, Srinivasula SM, Alnemri ES, Salvesen GS, Reed JC. IAPs block apoptotic events induced by caspase-8 and cytochrome c by direct inhibition of distinct caspases. EMBO J. 1998;17:2215–23.
170. Verhagen AM, Ekert PG, Pakusch M, Silke J, Connolly LM, Reid GE, Moritz RL, Simpson RJ, Vaux DL. Identification of DIABLO, a mammalian protein that promotes apoptosis by binding to and antagonizing IAP proteins. Cell. 2000;102:43–53.
171. Leverkus M, Neumann M, Mengling T, Rauch CT, Brocker EB, Krammer PH, Walczak H. Regulation of tumor necrosis factor-related apoptosis-inducing ligand sensitivity in primary and transformed human keratinocytes. Cancer Res. 2000;60:553–9.

172. Sheikh MS, Huang Y, Fernandez-Salas EA, El-Deiry WS, Friess H, Amundson S, Yin J, Meltzer SJ, Holbrook NJ, Fornace Jr AJ. The antiapoptotic decoy receptor TRID/TRAIL-R3 is a p53-regulated DNA damage-inducible gene that is overexpressed in primary tumors of the gastrointestinal tract. Oncogene. 1999;18:4153–9.
173. Zisman A, Ng C-P, Pantuck AJ, Bonavida B, Belldegrun AS. Actinomycin D and gemcitabine synergistically sensitize androgen-independent prostate cancer cells to Apo2L/TRAIL-mediated apoptosis. J Immunother. 2001;24:459–71.
174. Tamm I, Kornblau SM, Segall H, Krajewski S, Welsh K, Kitada S, Scudiero DA, Tudor G, Qui YH, Monks A, Andreeff M, Reed JC. Expression and prognostic significance of IAP-family genes in human cancers and myeloid leukemias. Clin Cancer Res. 2000;6:1796–803.
175. Sasaki H, Sheng Y, Kotsuji F, Tsang BK. Down-regulation of X-linked inhibitor of apoptosis protein induces apoptosis in chemoresistant human ovarian cancer cells. Cancer Res. 2000;60:5659–66.
176. Holcik M, Yeh C, Korneluk RG, Chow T. Translational upregulation of X-linked inhibitor of apoptosis (XIAP) increases resistance to radiation induced cell death. Oncogene. 2000;19:4174–7.
177. Shiraishi T, Yoshida T, Nakata S, Horinaka M, Wakada M, Mizutani Y, Miki T, Sakai T. Tunicamycin enhances tumor necrosis factor-related apoptosis-inducing ligand-induced apoptosis in human prostate cancer cells. Cancer Res. 2005;65:6364–70.
178. Kim R, Fisher MJ, Xu SQ, El-Deiry WS. Molecular determinants of response to TRAIL in killing of normal and cancer cells. Clin Cancer Res. 2000;6:335–46.
179. Doroshow JH. Anthracyclines and anthracenediones. In: Chabner BA, Longo DL, editors. Cancer chemotherapy and biotherapy. 2nd ed. Philadelphia: Lippincott-Raven; 1996. p. 409–34.
180. Abbaszadegan MR, Foley NE, Gleason-Guzman MC, Dalton WS. Resistance to the chemosensitizer verapamil in a multidrug-resistant (MDR) human multiple myeloma cell line. Int J Cancer. 1996;66:506–14.
181. Shankar S, Srivastava RK. Enhancement of therapeutic potential of TRAIL by cancer chemotherapy and irradiation: mechanisms and clinical implications. Drug Resist Updat. 2004;7:139–56.
182. Holland PM. Death receptor agonist therapies for cancer, which is the right TRAIL? Cytokine Growth Factor Rev. 2014;25:185–93.
183. Soderstrom TS, Poukkula M, Holmstrom TH, Heiskanen KM, Eriksson JE. Mitogen-activated protein kinase/extracellular signal-regulated kinase signaling in activated T cells abrogates TRAIL-induced apoptosis upstream of the mitochondrial amplification loop and caspase-8. J Immunol. 2002;169:2851–60.

Chapter 10
Overcoming Cancer Cell Resistance to Death Receptor Targeted Therapies

Julianne D. Twomey, William Hallett, and Baolin Zhang

Abstract Death receptors (DRs) are promising targets for cancer therapies because of their ability to induce apoptosis in cancer cells. These receptors are characterized by an intracellular death domain, which transmits a death signal from their cognate ligands, including TNF-related apoptosis inducing ligand (TRAIL). Currently, multiple clinical trials are underway to evaluate the antitumor activity of recombinant human TRAIL and agonistic antibodies to its receptors DR4 and DR5. Although the products have shown a tolerated safety profile in the completed phase 1 studies, a large number of cancer cell lines are found to be resistant to these agents, raising a concern about their clinical efficacy. This review provides an update of recent advances in understanding the molecular mechanisms involved in cancer cell resistance to DR4/DR5 targeted therapies. This information will be further discussed with respect to combinational strategies to overcome or bypass resistance mechanisms towards a better treatment outcome.

Keywords Death receptors • Apoptosis • Targeted therapies • Drug resistance • Predictive biomarkers • Combinational therapies

Abbreviations

5-dAzaC	5-Aza-2′-deoxycytidine
5-FU	5-Fluorouracil
AE	Adverse effects

No Conflict of Interest/Disclaimer: The comments and discussions in this paper are based on our experimental data and a survey of the related scientific publications. They do not necessarily reflect the official views of the US Food and Drug Administration with respect to the development of the death receptor targeted therapies. The use of product names is for product identification purpose only and does not imply endorsement.

J.D. Twomey • W. Hallett • B. Zhang (✉)
Office of Biotechnology Products, Center for Drug Evaluation and Research, Food and Drug Administration, Bethesda, MD 20892, USA
e-mail: Baolin.Zhang@fda.hhs.gov

B. Bonavida, S. Chouaib (eds.), *Resistance of Cancer Cells to CTL-Mediated Immunotherapy*, Resistance to Targeted Anti-Cancer Therapeutics 7,
DOI 10.1007/978-3-319-17807-3_10

BH	Bcl-2 homology
c-FLIP	Cellular FADD-like IL-1 beta-converting enzyme inhibitor protein
DISC	Death inducing signaling complex
DLT	Dose limiting toxicities
DR	Death receptors
EGFR	Epidermal growth factor receptor
FADD	Fas-associated death domain
FOLFIRI	Fololinic acid, fluorouracil, and irinotecan
FOLFOX	Fololinic acid, fluorouracil, and oxiplatin
HER	Human epidermal receptor
IAP	Inhibitor of apoptosis proteins
IFN	Interferon
IGFR	Insulin-like growth factor receptor
MOA	Mechanism of action
NSCLC	Non-small cell lung cancer
PNET	Primitive neuroectodermal
rhTRAIL	Recombinant human TRAIL
SCLC	Small cell lung cancer
siRNA	Small interfering RNA
SMAC/DIABLO	Second mitochondrial activator of caspases/direct inhibitor of apoptosis-binding protein with low pI
tBid	Truncated Bid
TNFR	Tumor necrosis factor
TRAIL	TNF-related apoptosis inducing ligand
XIAP	x Chromosome-linked inhibitor of apoptosis

10.1 Introduction

The cell surface death receptors are promising targets for cancer therapy due to their ability to induce apoptosis in cancer cells. To date, six human death receptors (DRs) have been identified, including Tumor Necrosis Factor Receptor (TNFR) 1, Fas (CD95), DR3, DR4 (TRAIL-R1), DR5 (TRAIL-R2) and DR6. These receptors are characterized by an intracellular death domain that transmits a death signal from their respective cognate ligands including TNFα, FasL, and TNF-related apoptosis inducing ligand (TRAIL/Apo2L). Despite the ability of TNFα and FasL to induce apoptosis in cancer cells, severe toxicities to normal cells leading to hypertension and hepatotoxicity preclude their use in systemic cancer therapy [1, 2]. In contrast, recombinant human TRAIL (rhTRAIL) preferentially induces apoptosis in a variety of tumor cell lines without harming many normal cell types [3, 4]. Moreover, administration of rhTRAIL into mice bearing human tumor xenografts induces significant tumor regression without systemic toxicity. These promising results have led to multiple clinical trials of rhTRAIL and agonistic antibodies to DR4 or DR5 as potential anticancer therapies (Table 10.1). These products have shown a

Table 10.1 Phase I and II clinical trials involving rhTRAIL and DR4/5 agonistic antibody therapies[a]

	Drug name	Clinical trial arms	Phase	Tumor type	Patients
Apo2L/rhTRAIL	Dulanermin [7]	*Single Agent: Dose Escalation*	I	Advanced Cancer	71
	Dulanermin [65]	Arm 1: FOLFOX + Bevacizumab + Dulanermin	Ib	Metastatic Colorectal Cancer	23
	Dulanermin	Arm 1: Cetuximab + Irinotecan + Dulanermin Arm 2: Bevacizumab + FOLFIRI + Dulanermin	Ib	Colorectal Cancer	42
	Dulanermin	Arm 1: Rituximab + Dulanermin Arm 2: Rituximab	II	Non-Hodgkin's Lymphoma	72
	AMG 951	Arm 1: Carboplatin + Paclitaxel + Bevacizumab Arm 2: Carboplatin + Paclitaxel + Bevacizumab + AMG 951 Arm 3: Carboplatin + Paclitaxel Arm 4: Carboplatin + Bevacizumab + AMG 951	II	NSCLC[b]	213
Anti-DR4	Mapatumumab [8]	Arm 1: Paclitaxel + Carboplatin + Mapatumumab	I	Advanced Solid Tumors	27
	Mapatumumab [54]	*Single Agent: Dose Escalation*	I	Advanced Solid Tumors	41
	Mapatumumab [75]	Arm 1: Gemcitabine + Cisplatin + Mapatumumab	I	Advanced Solid Tumors	49
	Mapatumumab [52]	*Single Agent*	I	Advanced Solid Tumors	49
	Mapatumumab	Arm 1: Paclitaxel + Carboplatin Arm 2: Carboplatin + Mapatumumab Arm 3: Paclitaxel + Carboplatin + Mapatumumab	Ib/II	Cervical Cancer	9
	Mapatumumab	Arm 1: Mapatumumab + Sorafenib Arm 2: Placebo + Sorafenib	II	Hepatocellular Carcinoma	101
	Mapatumumab	Arm 1: Mapatumumab + Cisplatin + Radiotherapy	II	Multiple Myeloma	105
	Mapatumumab [56]	*Single Agent*	II	NSCLC	32
	Mapatumumab [55]	*Single Agent*	II	Refractory Colorectal Cancer	38
	Mapatumumab	Arm 1: Paclitaxel + Carboplatin Arm 2: Paclitaxel + Carboplatin + Mapatumumab (low dose) Arm 3: Paclitaxel + Carboplatin + Mapatumumab (high dose)	II	NSCLC	111
	Mapatumumab [53]	*Single Agent*	II	Relapsed/Refractory Non-Hodgkin's Lymphoma	40

(continued)

Table 10.1 (continued)

	Drug name	Clinical trial arms	Phase	Tumor type	Patients
Anti-DR5	Conatumumab	Arm 1: Conatumumab + Birinapant	I	Relapsed Ovarian Cancer	40
	Conatumumab [61]	*Single Agent: Dose Escalation*	I	Advanced Solid Tumors	37
	Conatumumab	Arm 1: Conatumumab (low dose) + mFOLFOX6 + Bevacizumab Arm 2: Conatumumab (high dose) + mFOLFOX6 + Bevacizumab Arm 3: Placebo + mFOLFOX6 + Bevacizumab	Ib/II	Metastatic Colon Cancer	202
	Conatumumab	Arm 1: Conatumumab (low dose) + AMG 479 Arm 2: Conatumumab (moderate dose) + AMG 479 Arm 3: Conatumumab (high dose) + AMG 470	Ib/II	Advanced/Refractory Solid Tumors	89
	Conatumumab [78]	Arm 1: Conatumumab (2 mg/kg) + mFOLFOX Arm 2: Conatumumab (10 mg/kg) + mFOLFOX Arm 3: Placebo + mFOLFOX	Ib/2	Metastatic Colorectal Cancer	190
	Conatumumab [62]	Arm 1: Paclitaxel + Carboplatin + Conatumumab (low dose) Arm 1: Paclitaxel + Carboplatin + Conatumumab (high dose) Arm 1: Paclitaxel + Carboplatin + Placebo	Ib/II	NSCLC	172
	Conatumumab	Arm 1: Conatumumab + Panitumumab	Ib/II	Metastatic Colorectal Cancer	53
	Conatumumab [64]	Arm 1: Conatumumab + Doxorubicin Arm 2: Placebo + Doxorubicin	I/II	Metastatic/Unresectable soft tissue sarcoma	134
	Conatumumab	Arm 1: Conatumumab + FOLFOX6 + Bevacizumab + AMG 479 Arm 2: Conatumumab Arm 3: AMG479	II	Advanced Cancer	12
	Conatumumab [81]	Arm 1: FOLFIRI + Conatumumab Arm 2: FOLFIRI + Ganitumab Arm 3: FOLFIFI + Placebo	II	Metastatic Colorectal Cancer	155
	Conatumumab [63]	Arm 1: Ganitumab + Gemcitabine Arm 2: Conatumumab + Gemcitabine Arm 3: Placebo + Gemcitabine	II	Metastatic Pancreatic Cancer	125

	Conatumumab	Arm 1: Conatumumab (intermediate dose) + Vorinostat Arm 2: Conatumumab (low dose) + Vortezomib Arm 3: Conatumumab (low dose) + Vorinostat Arm 4: Conatumumab (high dose) + Bortezomib Arm 5: Conatumumab (high dose) + Vorinostat Arm 6: Conatumumab (TBD dose) + Bortezomib Arm 7: Conatumumab (intermediate dose) + Bortezomib	II	Lymphoma	33
	Lexatumumab [57]	*Single Agent: Dose Escalation*	I	Advanced Solid Tumors	24
	Lexatumumab [59]	*Single Agent: Dose Escalation*	I	Advanced Solid Tumors	37
	Lexatumumab [58]	*Single Agent: Dose Escalation*	I	Advanced Solid Tumors	31
	Drozitumab [6]	*Single Agent*	I	Advanced Solid Tumors or Non-Hodgkin's Lymphoma	50
	Drozitumab [77]	Arm 1: Drozitumab + FOLFOX + Bevacizumab	Ib	Metastatic Colorectal Cancer	9
	Drozitumab	Arm 1: Cetuximab + Irinotecan + Drozitumab Arm 2: Bevacizumab + FOLFIRI + Drozitumab	Ib	Metastatic Colorectal Cancer	20
	Drozitumab	Arm 1: Bevacizumab + Carboplatin + Paclitaxel + Drozitumab Arm 2: Bevacizumab + Carboplatin + Paclitaxel + Placebo	II	NSCLC	128
	Drozitumab	Arm 1: Drozitumab + Rituximab	II	Non-Hodgkin's Lymphoma	49
	Tigatuzumab [60]	*Single Agent*	I	Relapsed/Refractory Carcinomas or Lymphomas	17
	Tigatuzumab	Arm 1 Tigatuzumab (dose escalation + low dose maintenance) + Sorafenib Arm 2: Tigatuzumab (dose escalation + high dose maintenance) + Sorafenib Arm 3: Sorafenib	I	Advanced Liver Cancer	160
	Tigatuzumab	Arm 1: Tigatuzumab + Abraxane Arm 2: Abraxane	I	Metastatic TNBC[c]	66
	Tigatuzumab	*Single Agent: Dose Escalation*	I	Lymphoma	40
	Tigatuzumab	Arm 1: Tigatuzumab + FOLFIRI	I	Metastatic Colorectal Cancer	21

(continued)

Table 10.1 (continued)

	Drug name	Clinical trial arms	Phase	Tumor type	Patients
	Tigatuzumab	Arm 1: Tigatuzumab + Irinotecan Arm 2: Irinotecan	II	Metastatic Colorectal Carcinoma	8
	Tigatuzumab	Arm 1: Tigatuzumab + Paclitaxel + Carboplatin	II	Metastatic Ovarian	24
	Tigatuzumab	Arm 1: Tigatuzumab + Carboplatin + Paclitaxel Arm 2: Placebo + Carboplatin + Paclitaxel	II	NSCLC	109
	Tigatuzumab [74]	Arm 1: Gemcitabine + Tigatuzumab	II	Unresectable/Metastatic Pancreatic Cancer	62
	Tigatuzumab [71]	Arm 1: Tigatuzumab + Carboplatin + Paclitaxel Arm 2: Placebo + Carboplatin + Paclitaxel	II	Unresectable/Metastatic NSCLC	97

[a] Additional information obtained from https://clinicaltrials.gov
[b] Non-small cell lung cancer
[c] Triple Negative Breast Cancer

well-tolerated safety profile in the completed Phase I studies [5–9]. However, a significant portion of tumor cell lines as well as primary human tumor cells are found to be resistant to these therapies due to intrinsic or acquired mechanisms [10–14]. Undoubtedly, non-responsive patients will not benefit from the treatments but may still suffer from the potential side effects. An in-depth analysis of resistance mechanisms could facilitate the identification of biomarkers for predicting tumor response to the DR-targeted therapies and aiding in the development of combinational therapies to overcome resistance towards a better clinical outcome of cancer treatment.

10.2 Apoptosis Signaling Through Death Receptors

Like other TNF ligands, native TRAIL exists as a homotrimer that cross-links its death receptors (DRs) 4 and/or 5 on the surface membrane of target cells (Fig. 10.1). The agonistic antibodies act in a similar mode. Activation of DR4 and/or DR5 results in the recruitment of the adaptor molecule Fas-associated death domain (FADD) and the procaspase-8 or -10 into a death-inducing signaling complex (DISC). Within the DISC, caspase-8 or -10 is activated by self-processing that subsequently activates the downstream effector caspases such as caspase-3, -6, and -7 in a mitochondrial-independent or -dependent manner. The latter process is linked by caspase-8 mediated truncation of Bid (tBid) [15–17]. The activated caspases propagate apoptotic programming by cleaving a wide range of structural and signaling proteins, ultimately leading to apoptosis of the target cell. TRAIL resistance has been associated with defects in the relevant apoptosis signaling components or regulatory proteins. These factors will be discussed with respect to their functional relevance in cancer resistance: (1) functionality of receptors, (2) availability of caspases, and (3) status of regulatory proteins.

10.2.1 Deficiency of Surface Death Receptors

Initiation of a death-signaling cascade relies on the surface expression of DR4 and DR5 for TRAIL or antibody ligation. Deficiency of these receptors on the cell membrane is enough to render cancer cells resistant to TRAIL-induced apoptosis, regardless of the expression status of other signaling proteins. This lack of surface expression is seen in a variety of cancer lines and primary tumor cells, including those derived from breast [14] and oral squamous carcinoma [18]. The absence of death receptors on the surface membrane of the cell does not correlate with receptor total protein levels [14], indicating these receptors are trapped within the cell. Many mechanisms have been implicated in this mislocalization of the death receptors, such as unsuccessful trafficking to the plasma membrane [19–22], increased endocytosis [13, 14, 23–25], and autophagosome localization [26]. Studies have shown

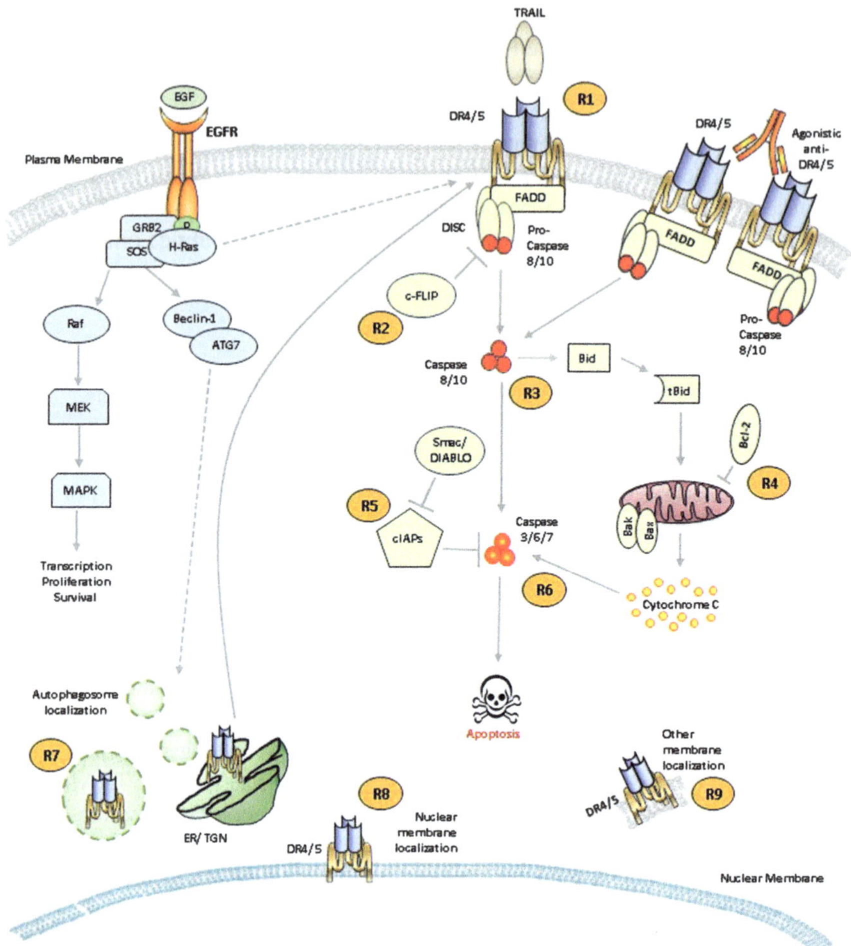

Fig. 10.1 Checkpoints of TRAIL-induced apoptosis signaling pathway. The TRAIL apoptotic signaling pathway is initiated through ligation of TRAIL or agonistic antibodies targeting DR4/5. This ligation induces assembly of a DISC composed of FADD and pro-caspase 8/10. Caspase 8 is activated and released to initiate caspase 3/7 to induce apoptosis. Caspase 8 can also cause the cleavage of Bid to truncated Bid (tBid), linking to the mitochondrial-dependent caspase activation. The key resistance mechanisms include surface deficiency of DR4/5 (R1), upregulated c-FLIP (R2), caspase 8 deficiency (R3), Bcl2 protein family over-expression (R4), inhibitor of apoptosis proteins (R5), caspase 3 deficiency (R6), and mislocalization of the DRs to autophagosomes (R7), the nuclear membrane (R8) or other membrane localization (R9) within the cytoplasm. To achieve better cancer treatment outcomes, combinational therapies can be used to circumvent the specific resistance mechanisms in cancer cells

in cells with deficient surface expression, the DRs are mainly found in the cytoplasm and the nucleus [19–22, 27, 28]. Our work has shown that both DR4 and DR5 undergo constitutive or ligand-induced internalization in some breast cancer cell lines [12–14]. Constitutive endocytosis may occur through faulty dileucine-based sorting signals, such as EAQC337LL within DR4. DR4/DR5 endocytosis is just beginning to be understood, but may be a mechanism to terminate apoptosis signaling through TRAIL receptors [13].

Autophagy and Ras-dependent events have also been implicated in the surface deficiency of the death receptors. Our work has shown that TRAIL-resistant breast cancer cells have higher levels of basal autophagosomes, with DR4 and DR5 located within LC3-II labeled autophagosomes [26]. This autophagosomal localization may confer TRAIL resistance to the cell, preventing receptor trafficking to the membrane. This resistance due to autophagy has been reported in pancreatic cancer cell lines [29]. Implications of Ras small GTPase in DR-mediated apoptosis come from a study of oral squamous cell carcinomas, which found that TRAIL sensitivity correlated with expression of endogenous Ras [18]. In fact, constitutive expression of active Ras with mutant RasV12 selectively upregulated surface expression of DR5 and restored TRAIL-sensitivity in resistant cell lines. Similar findings were observed in colon cancers where overexpression of H-Ras increased death receptors through a MEK-dependent pathway [30]. Conversely, K-Ras mutations confer resistance to pancreatic and lung cancer cell lines [31]. Our laboratory has recently shown that wild-type H-Ras is upregulated in some cancer cells where it renders cancer resistance to TRAIL and is closely correlated with a deficiency of surface DR4 and DR5 [18]. Mutations in the Ras family are commonly found in tumors and, therefore, further studies on Ras' effect on TRAIL sensitivity are warranted to better understand the pleiotropic effects Ras family members have on tumor resistance.

DR5 was thought to be the primary receptor for TRAIL leading to apoptosis in various types of cancer cells. At least six anti-DR5 antibodies, which compares with only one anti-DR4 antibody, are currently under development (Table 10.1). Indeed, our studies have shown that DR4 is deficient at a much higher frequency than DR5 [14]. This observation suggests that targeting DR5 would be more beneficial in cancer treatment in several types of cancer lines. Our studies also show that TRAIL requires both DR4 and DR5 for a maximal killing in breast cancer cells. The two death receptors may act synergistically by forming hetero-receptor complexes [14]. The surface deficiency in either receptor would lower the sensitivity of target cells to TRAIL. Paradoxically, other studies show that TRAIL induces apoptosis exclusively through DR4 in cancer cell lines from skin [32], ovary [33], and leukocytes [34] as well as primary cells from chronic lymphocytic leukemia and mantle cell lymphoma [35]. The molecular basis for this preference of TRAIL is not clear but may be due to differences in the functional status of death receptors in a specific tumor.

10.2.2 Deficiency of Caspase 8 and 10

Inhibition of initiator caspases is another mechanism of preventing death receptor-mediated apoptosis. Cells that lack expression of critical initiator caspases-8 and -10 are found to be resistant to TRAIL-induced apoptosis [36].

For instance, some colon cancer cell lines resist TRAIL-mediated apoptosis by reducing basal procaspase-8 and by increasing active caspase-8 degradation after TRAIL exposure [37]. Alteration of the genetic code, deletion of genetic material, and aberrant gene methylation are also common pathways leading to loss of gene function in human cancers. Many human tumors reduce expression of caspase-8 through hyper-methylation, as was observed in glioma cells with stem cell features [38] in primitive neuroectodermal (PNET) brain tumors [39], small cell lung cancers (SCLC) [40] and in neuroblastomas [41]. The study with PNET tumors found that caspase-8 mRNA and protein expression of caspase-8 could be restored with the DNA methylation inhibitor 5-aza-2′-deoxycytidine [39]. Other studies have demonstrated that interferon (IFN)-γ is capable of restoring caspase-8 expression that is silenced by methylation [40]. The identification of new strategies to overcome methylation of caspase-8 is critical to the promotion of DR-mediated therapies.

10.2.3 Upregulation of Anti-Apoptosis Proteins

DR-mediated caspase activation is also regulated by intracellular proteins such as c-FLIP, IAPs and Bcl2 family members. Cellular FLICE (FADD-like IL-1-beta-converting enzyme) inhibitory protein (c-FLIP) is a master anti-apoptotic regulator and resistance factor that suppresses death receptors including TNF-α, Fas, and TRAIL. c-FLIP is a family of alternatively spliced variants that primarily consist of long (c-FLIP(L)) and short (c-FLIP(S)) splice variants, and both forms can protect cells from apoptosis [42]. c-FLIP competes with the initiator caspases for binding to FADD due to the high sequence homology to the caspase death domains [43]. The binding of c-FLIP to the death domain of the death receptors prevents DISC formation and subsequent activation of the caspase cascade.

Another mechanism utilized by cancer cells to resist TRAIL-induced apoptosis is upregulation of the inhibitor of apoptosis proteins (IAP). IAP family members are characterized by the presence of a ~70 amino acid motif referred to as the baculovirus IAP Repeat (BIR) domain [44]. These BIR domains mediate IAP binding and caspases inhibition. The most potent IAP is the X chromosome-linked inhibitor of apoptosis (XIAP), which inhibits the function of effector caspases including Caspase-3, -7, and -9 [45]. The inhibitory activity of XIAP is overcome by a protein called second mitochondrial activator of caspases/direct inhibitor of apoptosis-binding protein with low pI (Smac/DIABLO). Smac/DIABLO is released from mitochondria during apoptosis and antagonizes XIAP, promoting apoptosis in a positive feedback loop [46].

Apoptosis is also prevented by upregulation of Bcl-2 family members, which include at least 20 proteins, all of which contain one or more conserved Bcl-2 homology (BH) domains. Bcl-2, Bcl-xL, Bcl-w, and Mcl-1 are members of the Bcl-2 family that inhibit apoptosis in response to many cytotoxic agents. Bcl-2 overexpression protects neuroblastoma, glioblastoma, and breast cancer cells from TRAIL-mediated apoptosis by blocking caspase-3, -7, and -9 cleavage as well as cleavage of XIAP [47, 48]. Resistance to TRAIL mediated by Bcl-xL was demonstrated in pancreatic cancer cell lines [49]. These studies demonstrated that TRAIL treated BCL-xL expressing cells resulted in normal caspase-8 cleavage, but suppression of caspase-3 activity and apoptosis, which was abrogated by the administration of antisense oligonucleotides to BCL-xL mRNA [49]. Bcl-2 was also seen to be highly expressed in TRAIL-resistant tissues [50]. The upregulation of anti-apoptotic proteins will aid in cancer survival to TRAIL receptor agonists.

10.3 Ongoing Clinical Trials Evaluating DR-Targeted Therapies

Multiple clinical trials are underway to evaluate recombinant human TRAIL and agonistic antibodies against DR4 or DR5. Dulanermin (Apo2L/TRAIL/AMG951; Amgen/Genentech) is presently the only recombinant form of human TRAIL in clinical trials. Monoclonal antibodies against DR4 such as mapatumumab (human IgG1; GSK) or DR5 which include lexatumumab (human IgG1; GSK), drozitumab (human IgG1; Genentech/Roche), tigatuzumab (humanized IgG1; Daiichi-Sankyo), conatumumab (human IgG1; Amgen), and LBY135 (chimeric mouse/human IgG1; Novartis) are being developed to in phase I/II clinical studies. Another possible solution is a recombinant adenovirus encoding TRAIL, Ad-TRAIL, is in early development for cancer therapy [51]. A summary of the clinical trials that involved these therapies is found in Table 10.1. Understanding the resistance mechanisms to these drugs will advance the development of combinational therapies to overcome cancer death evasion.

10.3.1 Major Safety Findings from Phase 1 Studies

Clinical trials have shown death receptor targeting therapeutics do not have substantial toxicity, with the majority of side effects being fatigue and nausea. Dulanermin was given to 71 patients in a Phase 1 trial to patients with advanced cancer [7]. The adverse events (AE) associated with treatment were mostly mild, though two patients with sarcoma (synovial and undifferentiated) experienced serious AEs associated with rapid tumor necrosis. Agonistic anti-DR4 therapy, mapatumumab, was also well tolerated in Phase 1 studies, with no drug-related hepatic or dose-limiting toxicities (DLT) [52, 53]. Mapatumumab was given to 41 patients with advanced cancer and the majority of adverse events were grade 1 (mild) or 2 (moderate) on a 5 point scale [54]. Clinical studies which passed into phase II did not demonstrate an ability to shrink tumors within refractory colon cancer [55] or non-SCLC (NSCLC) [56]. Agonistic antibodies targeting DR5 have also shown tolerance in clinical studies across a variety of tumor types with minor

DLT [57, 58]. In one study, lexatumumab was given to 37 patients, resulting in DLTs including asymptomatic elevations of serum amylase, transaminases, and bilirubin [59]. Similar observations were seen for drozitumab [6], tigatuzumab [60], and conatumumab [61].

10.3.2 Current Combinational Therapies

Survival mechanisms for cancer cells result from multiple pathways, suggesting a combination of therapeutics could potentially work well together to target TRAIL-resistance. In anticipation of tumor resistance to TRAIL signaling pathway targets, the ongoing Phase 2 studies are focused on evaluation of the DR-targeted therapies in combination with classical chemotherapies or other targeted therapies. These include paclitaxel and carboplatin used for NSCLC [62], gemcitabine for advanced pancreatic cancer [63], doxorubicin in unresectable soft tissue sarcomas [64] and FOLFOX for colorectal cancer [65].

The primary mechanisms of action (MOA) for Paclitaxel is inhibition of mitosis by stabilizing microtubules during cell division, while the MOA for platinum compounds like carboplatin is binding DNA, forming crosslinks that affect DNA replication. These compounds may combine well with DR-targeting therapies. Paclitaxel, and other taxanes such as docetaxel, increase the surface expression of DR4/DR5 [66, 67] and decrease AKT activity [68]. Additionally, the platinum family of compounds, such as carboplatin, cisplatin, and oxaliplatin, increase DR4/DR5 [65, 66] and decrease levels of c-FLIP [69]. Current trials have combined Dulanermin with paclitaxel, carboplatin, and bevacizumab in NSCLC and were well tolerated with 58 % progression free survival [70] but in studies combining carboplatin/paclitaxel with tigatuzumab there was no improvement over the efficacy of the chemotherapeutics [71]. Fully understanding the mechanisms through which chemotherapies can enhance DR-induced apoptosis is needed.

Gemcitabine is the standard treatment for patients with advanced pancreatic cancer. Gemcitabine is a nucleoside analog of cytidine but with fluorine atoms replacing the hydrogen atoms on the secondary carbon, resulting in inhibited DNA replication. There is evidence to suggest that gemcitabine may also combine well with DR-targeted therapies. Pyrimidine chemotherapies such as gemcitabine and 5-Fluorouracil reduce the levels of c-FLIP [42] and increase caspase-8 activity [72, 73], both of which are common mechanisms of resistance against DR-induced apoptosis. When gemcitabine was combined with tigatuzumab, 45 % of patients with metastatic pancreatic cancer within a phase II trial showed disease stability [74]. Gemcitabine was also tested in combination with cisplatin and mapatumumab, showing toleration and stable disease progression for a median of 6 months in 25 out of 49 patients [75].

Additionally, there are a series of chemotherapy regimens used for the treatment of colorectal cancer with names such as FOLFOX or FOLFIRI. Combining *FOLol*inic acid, *F*luorouracil, and *OX*aliplatin is known as FOLFOX, while replacing oxaliplatin with *IRI*notecan is known as FOLFIRI. Fluorouracil, in particular 5-fluorouracil (5-FU), is a pyrimidine analog that inhibits thymidylate synthase. Folinic acid (leucovorin) augments the function of 5-FU. Oxaliplatin, similar to carboplatin, cross-links DNA preventing replication and transcription. Irinotecan is a topoisomerase inhibitor. The dosage regimens of FOLFOX can be modified and the resulting treatments include names like FOLFOX6 and modified FOLFOX6 (reviewed in [76]). The 5-fluorouracil and oxaliplatin components of FOLFOX are known to sensitize tumors to DR-targeted therapies. Drozitumab combined with both mFOLFOX6 and Bevacizumab resulted in stable disease for three out of eight patients treated [77]. FOLFOX combined with Conatumumab has also been explored in metastatic pancreatic cancer [78].

When treating the apoptotic signaling pathway, combinational therapies can expand to incorporate alternate signaling pathways. Current work is focusing on combining targets against the insulin-like growth factor receptor (IGFR) pathway [79] and the epidermal growth factor receptor (EGFR) pathway [80] with anti-DR5. IGFR agonistic antibody ganitumab with conatumumab showed tumor shrinkage and 36 % stable disease across patients with NSCLC, colorectal cancer, sarcoma, pancreatic cancer, and ovarian cancer [79]. Ganitumab was also combined with conatumumab and FOLFIRI, but resulted in patients with the FOLFIRI and conatumumab demonstrating progression-free survival [81]. Combining conatumumab and soluble TRAIL has shown increased DR clustering, resulting in increased DISC creation [82, 83]. Further studies combining different DR-agonists could yield interesting results for apoptosis induction.

10.3.3 Alternate Combination Strategies

Studies aim to improve the antitumor activity of DR4/DR5 by rationally designing mixtures that would overcome or bypass the resistance mechanisms within cancer cells. These include combinations with classical chemotherapies such as the ones discussed earlier. To further improve synergistic therapies, the main resistance mechanisms within the cell described earlier should be targeted, such as surface deficiency of DR4 and DR5, increased c-FLIP expression, decreased caspase-8 activity, and overexpression of anti-apoptotic proteins, such as XIAP.

Receptor deficiency on the cell surface is sufficient to render cancer cells resistant to TRAIL-induced apoptosis. Chemotherapies such as cisplatin and carboplatin can be used in combination with DR targeting therapeutics due to their ability to increase the surface expression of DR5 [66]. The proteasome inhibitor bortezomib [84, 85], the anti-melanoma drug ADI-PEG20 [86], p53 activating agents [87], anti-angiogenic therapies such as 3TSR [88], and histone deacetylase inhibitors [89, 90] have shown increases in surface DR expression, sensitizing cells to TRAIL. Therapies which increase DR expression can act synergistically with rhTRAIL or antibodies, dependent on a functional caspase signaling cascade.

c-FLIP is an important target for cancer therapy. Small interfering RNAs (siRNAs) that inhibited the expression of c-FLIP(L) in human cancer cell lines augmented TRAIL-induced DISC recruitment, activation, processing, and release of caspase-8 [91, 92]. The siRNA knockdown of c-FLIP is also postulated to target the tumor initiating cells within breast cancer lines [93]. Additionally, bortezomib is known to reduce c-FLIP expression [94] and sensitize cells to recombinant or immune-mediated TRAIL killing [95]. Small molecule-mediated inhibition of c-FLIP may have a strong therapeutic outlook [96].

Hyper-methylation of caspase-8 is a well-studied mechanism of caspase-8 silencing [38, 40]. Demethylating agents, such as 5-Aza-2′-deoxycytidine (5-dAzaC), are capable of restoring caspase-8 expression caused by hyper-methylation [38, 97]. In fact, treatment of neuroblastoma with a combination of low concentrations of 5-dAzaC and IFN-γ restored caspase-8 expression and sensitized tumors to TRAIL-mediated apoptosis [98]. Overexpression of IFN-γ combined with XIAP inhibitors increased caspase-8 activity in pancreatic cell lines sensitized cancer cells to TRAIL [99].

XIAP inhibitors also present a promising approach to augmenting TRAIL-mediated apoptosis. Small molecule inhibitors of XIAP cooperate with TRAIL to induce apoptosis in childhood acute leukemia cells via enhanced TRAIL-induced activation of caspases, loss of mitochondrial membrane potential, and cytochrome c release in a caspase-dependent manner [100]. Another potential method of reducing XIAP levels is through the sub-toxic doses of roscovitine, a specific inhibitor of Cdc2 and Cdk2 [101]. Roscovitine treated TRAIL-resistant glioma cells reduced their expression of XIAP and survivin, two major inhibitors of caspases, and sensitized the cells to TRAIL-mediated apoptosis. Treatment of selumetinib (therapeutic targeting the MEK pathway) [102] or Dacarbazine [103] both downregulated IAPs and sensitized the cells to TRAIL. Modulation of the pro-apoptotic and anti-apoptotic signaling pathways through chemotherapy and alternative targeted therapeutics will combine well with DR-targeted therapies to induce cancer cell death.

10.3.4 Predictive Biomarkers for Cancer Response

Successful application of combinational therapies relies on predictive biomarkers of patient response. Biomarkers are currently being evaluated to improve therapeutics targeting the apoptosis signaling pathway [104]. The first indicator of potential responsiveness to DR targeted therapies is expression of DR4 or DR5. However, many studies have demonstrated that sensitivity cannot be predicted based on DR4 or DR5 surface expression alone [18, 27, 105, 106]. Studies from our laboratory have pursued this research topic.

We have identified a gene signature of over 71 over-expressed genes that were predictive of TRAIL sensitivity by examining the genome-wide mRNA expression profiles of 95 human cancer cell lines [11]. The over-expressed genes were dominated by two functionally related gene families: interferon-induced genes and major histocompatibility genes. These data a[...]t with the findings that treatment of cancers with interferon sensitizes the[...] TRAIL-related therapies [98]. Another study approached the identificatio[...]arkers for TRAIL via mRNA expression and had very interesting results. T[...] expression profiles of pancreatic, NSCLC, and melanoma cell lines show[...] to 30 % of these tumors had increased expression of GALNT14, a pept[...]lycosyltransferase. The investigators were able to increase or decrease TR[...]sitivity by selectively overexpressing or silencing GALNT14 [27].

Another possibility for identifying biomarkers that ind[...]poptosis sensitivity is to look at autophagy. Autophagy and apoptosis have a [...]lex relationship, either being triggered together or developing through mutually [...]sive processes. Our studies indicate one role for autophagy is to protect tumor ce[...]rom TRAIL-mediated apoptosis. During autophagy, cellular components, includ[...] membrane components containing DR4 and DR5, are invaginated into autopha[...] vesicles (autophagosomes). These autophagosomes fuse with lysosomes to form a[...]lysosomes wherein autophagic cargos are degraded. Our studies indicate that this process also provides tumors with resistance to death receptor-mediated therapies [26]. Breast cancer cell lines with high levels of basal autophagic function in nutrient rich conditions have a high level of TRAIL resistance. Similar levels of basal autophagy were found in pancreatic [107], melanoma [108], and NSCLC [109]. The basal autophagic activity sequesters death receptors into intracellular compartments where they are not exposed to TRAIL and thus are resistant. Our studies indicate that the death receptors were housed in LC3-II labeled autophagosomes, and disruption of the autophagosomes restored surface expression of death receptors and increased sensitivity to TRAIL. Analysis of tumors for LC3-II may provide predictive markers of tumor resistance to TRAIL-related therapies.

Oncogenic proteins, such as Ras GTPases, may also provide unique opportunities to identify biomarkers for TRAIL sensitivity. Many cancer types upregulate the Ras signaling pathway due to gain of function mutations in *ras* genes themselves or alterations in the proteins that regulate Ras [110–112]. Ras is also shown to promote activation of cell death pathways, in contrast to its best known function of promoting growth [113]. Ras interacts with various downstream effector targets such as MEK, PI3K, and Rho GTPases [114, 115]. Recent evidence suggests that Ras regulates the expression of death receptors and increases TRAIL sensitivity [30, 116, 117]. In fact, transfection of oral squamous cell carcinomas with H-RasV12, a constitutively active H-Ras mutant, increased surface expression of DR5 and sensitivity to either TRAIL or anti-DR5 [18]. These findings support the idea of using Ras as a biomarker for predicting DR sensitivity.

The involvement of Ras in TRAIL sensitivity of tumors is pertinent because of the expansion of growth factor inhibitors currently used to treat cancer. The human epidermal receptor (HER) family of growth factor receptors, including members EGFR and HER2, are important regulators of tumor cell proliferation, survival, angiogenesis, and metastasis [118]. Engagement of an HER by its cognate ligand initiates the Ras signaling pathway. EGFR and HER2 are frequently aberrantly overexpressed or mutated in a wide range of tumors; therefore, these receptors represent attractive targets for treatment. This has resulted in the development of multiple anti-HER therapeutics, including mAbs trastuzumab (anti-HER2), cetuximab (anti-EGFR), and multiple small molecule tyrosine kinases inhibitors targeting EGFR (e.g. gefitinib, erlotnib) and HER2 (e.g. CP-724, 714, M578440).

It has been reported that TRAIL activates the EGRF pathway, and that the cetuximab-mediated sensitization to TRAIL is due to the inhibition of TRAIL-mediated EGFR activation in colorectal cancers [119]. Additionally, the combination of cetuximab and TRAIL resulted in increased clustering of DR4 and FADD into lipid rafts, which is known to enhance the function of death receptors [121]. Breast and ovarian cancers treated with trastuzumab are also sensitized to DR-mediated apoptosis. Trastuzumab treatment decreases Akt kinase activation but not mitogen-activated protein kinase activation and sensitizes cell lines to TRAIL [122]. These studies indicate that anti-HER therapeutics, in addition to their direct suppression of tumor growth, also provide favorable conditions for TRAIL-triggered apoptosis.

10.4 Perspectives

There is great potential in TRAIL-based therapies, yet the limitations of TRAIL receptor agonists as a single agent need to be overcome. The benefits of TRAIL as a targeted therapeutic with mild toxicity are outweighed by the lack of efficacy in clinical trials due to the protein's short half-life and the cancer cell's TRAIL resistance mechanisms. Thus, a renewed effort into combinational therapies that counter these resistances allowing DR targeted therapies to initiate apoptosis is needed.

The most effective combinational therapies will overcome DR surface deficiency, loss of the initiator caspases-8 and -10, and overexpression of anti-apoptotic molecules such as c-FLIP and XIAP. Many current combinations use chemotherapies to upregulate DR expression or inhibit anti-apoptotic proteins. The clinical use of combination therapy promotes investigation of molecular interactions of combination components, as not all chemotherapies will improve the efficacy of agonistic antibodies. The effectiveness of DR-targeted therapies will be maximized by optimizing therapies based on the resistances of different cancer types and for individual patients.

The next generation of combination therapies that exploit cellular machinery to augment DR therapies is another exciting realm of future discoveries. The combination of DR-targeted therapies with EGFR inhibitors, such as cetuximab and trastuzumab, offer new potential avenues for cancer treatment now that scientists have a growing understanding of the influence that the EGFR-Ras pathway has on DR-mediated apoptosis. Our recent work demonstrating the high basal level of autophagy causing surface deficiencies of DRs recommend combinational therapies that target the Ras/EGFR pathway in combination with the DR pathway. Chemotherapeutics that inhibit autophagy offer promise by reducing the trafficking of DR4 and DR5 from the surface into autophagosomes. In fact, treatment of cells with hydroxychloroquine, an inhibitor of autophagy, increased caspase-3 activation and DR-mediated apoptosis [123, 124]. Future studies that directly inhibit autophagy with DR targeted therapies are needed to examine the enhancement of apoptotic signaling.

Recent studies analyzing the synergistic effects of combining DR targeted therapeutics that overcome DR signaling pathway deficiencies such as insufficient receptor clustering and DISC formation are clinically relevant [82, 83]. Combining DR-specific therapeutics provides an alternative to chemotherapeutic administration, taking advantage of the benefits of targeted therapeutic and cancer-specific toxicity. This could potentially further the use of rhTRAIL in cancer patients.

Additionally, there is an unmet need for biomarkers that predict tumor sensitivities to TRAIL receptor targeted therapies. Much of the basic science needed to identify biomarkers is available; we are well aware of inducers and inhibitors of apoptosis that generally indicate TRAIL resistance, such as lack of surface DR4/5. However, the apoptotic machinery is redundant, and multiple lines of attack are needed to overcome resistances. Therefore, these biomarkers need additional sophistication than simply surface expression of DR5 or lack of caspase-8. When well designed, combinational drugs could lead to improved outcomes of cancer treatment by circumventing the specific resistance mechanisms in cancer cells.

Acknowledgment This work was partly supported by funding from the FDA/CDER Critical Path initiatives.

References

1. Lenk H, Tanneberger S, Muller U, Ebert J, Shiga T. Phase II clinical trial of high-dose recombinant human tumor necrosis factor. Cancer Chemother Pharmacol. 1989;24:391–2.
2. Creaven PJ, Plager JE, Dupere S, Huben RP, Takita H, Mittelman A, Proefrock A. Phase I clinical trial of recombinant human tumor necrosis factor. Cancer Chemother Pharmacol. 1987;20:137–44.
3. Ashkenazi A, Pai RC, Fong S, Leung S, Lawrence DA, Marsters SA, Blackie C, Chang L, McMurtrey AE, Hebert A, DeForge L, Koumenis IL, Lewis D, Harris L, Bussiere J, Koeppen H, Shahrokh Z, Schwall RH. Safety and antitumor activity of recombinant soluble Apo2 ligand. J Clin Invest. 1999;104:155–62.
4. Lawrence D, Shahrokh Z, Marsters S, Achilles K, Shih D, Mounho B, Hillan K, Totpal K, DeForge L, Schow P, Hooley J, Sherwood S, Pai R, Leung S, Khan L, Gliniak B, Bussiere J, Smith CA, Strom SS, Kelley S, Fox JA, Thomas D, Ashkenazi A. Differential hepatocyte toxicity of recombinant Apo2L/TRAIL versions. Nat Med. 2001;7:383–5.
5. Daniel D, Wilson NS. Tumor necrosis factor: renaissance as a cancer therapeutic? Curr Cancer Drug Targets. 2008;8:124–31.
6. Camidge DR, Herbst RS, Gordon MS, Eckhardt SG, Kurzrock R, Durbin B, Ing J, Tohnya TM, Sager J, Ashkenazi A, Bray G, Mendelson D. A phase I safety and pharmacokinetic study of the death receptor 5 agonistic antibody PRO95780 in patients with advanced malignancies. Clin Cancer Res. 2010;16:1256–63.
7. Herbst RS, Eckhardt SG, Kurzrock R, Ebbinghaus S, O'Dwyer PJ, Gordon MS, Novotny W, Goldwasser MA, Tohnya TM, Lum BL, Ashkenazi A, Jubb AM, Mendelson DS. Phase I

dose-escalation study of recombinant human Apo2L/TRAIL, a dual proapoptotic receptor agonist, in patients with advanced cancer. J Clin Oncol. 2010;28:2839–46.

8. Leong S, Cohen RB, Gustafson DL, Langer CJ, Camidge DR, Padavic K, Gore L, Smith M, Chow LQ, von Mehren M, O'Bryant C, Hariharan S, Diab S, Fox NL, Miceli R, Eckhardt SG. Mapatumumab, an antibody targeting TRAIL-R1, in combination with paclitaxel and carboplatin in patients with advanced solid malignancies: results of a phase I and pharmacokinetic study. J Clin Oncol. 2009;27:4413–21.
9. Roberts NJ, Zhou S, Diaz Jr LA, Holdhoff M. Systemic use of tumor necrosis factor alpha as an anticancer agent. Oncotarget. 2011;2:739–51.
10. Walczak H. Death receptor-ligand systems in cancer, cell death, and inflammation. Cold Spring Harb Perspect Biol. 2013;5:a008698.
11. Chen JJ, Knudsen S, Mazin W, Dahlgaard J, Zhang B. A 71-gene signature of TRAIL sensitivity in cancer cells. Mol Cancer Ther. 2012;11:34–44.
12. Yoshida T, Zhang Y, Rivera Rosado LA, Zhang B. Repeated treatment with subtoxic doses of TRAIL induces resistance to apoptosis through its death receptors in MDA-MB-231 breast cancer cells. Mol Cancer Res. 2009;7:1835–44.
13. Zhang Y, Yoshida T, Zhang B. TRAIL induces endocytosis of its death receptors in MDA-MB-231 breast cancer cells. Cancer Biol Ther. 2009;8:917–22.
14. Zhang Y, Zhang B. TRAIL resistance of breast cancer cells is associated with constitutive endocytosis of death receptors 4 and 5. Mol Cancer Res. 2008;6:1861–71.
15. Deng Y, Lin Y, Wu X. TRAIL-induced apoptosis requires Bax-dependent mitochondrial release of Smac/DIABLO. Genes Dev. 2002;16:33–45.
16. Suliman A, Lam A, Datta R, Srivastava RK. Intracellular mechanisms of TRAIL: apoptosis through mitochondrial-dependent and -independent pathways. Oncogene. 2001;20: 2122–33.
17. Yin XM. Signal transduction mediated by Bid, a pro-death Bcl-2 family proteins, connects the death receptor and mitochondria apoptosis pathways. Cell Res. 2000;10:161–7.
18. Chen JJ, Mikelis CM, Zhang Y, Gutkind JS, Zhang B. TRAIL induces apoptosis in oral squamous carcinoma cells—a crosstalk with oncogenic Ras regulated cell surface expression of death receptor 5. Oncotarget. 2013;4:206–17.
19. Liu GC, Zhang J, Liu SG, Gao R, Long ZF, Tao K, Ma YF. Detachment of esophageal carcinoma cells from extracellular matrix causes relocalization of death receptor 5 and apoptosis. World J Gastroenterol. 2009;15:836–44.
20. Leithner K, Stacher E, Wurm R, Ploner F, Quehenberger F, Wohlkoenig C, Balint Z, Polachova J, Olschewski A, Samonigg H, Popper HH, Olschewski H. Nuclear and cytoplasmic death receptor 5 as prognostic factors in patients with non-small cell lung cancer treated with chemotherapy. Lung Cancer. 2009;65:98–104.
21. Kojima Y, Nakayama M, Nishina T, Nakano H, Koyanagi M, Takeda K, Okumura K, Yagita H. Importin beta1 protein-mediated nuclear localization of death receptor 5 (DR5) limits DR5/tumor necrosis factor (TNF)-related apoptosis-inducing ligand (TRAIL)-induced cell death of human tumor cells. J Biol Chem. 2011;286:43383–93.
22. Jin Z, McDonald III ER, Dicker DT, El-Deiry WS. Deficient tumor necrosis factor-related apoptosis-inducing ligand (TRAIL) death receptor transport to the cell surface in human colon cancer cells selected for resistance to TRAIL-induced apoptosis. J Biol Chem. 2004;279:35829–39.
23. Kohlhaas SL, Craxton A, Sun XM, Pinkoski MJ, Cohen GM. Receptor-mediated endocytosis is not required for tumor necrosis factor-related apoptosis-inducing ligand (TRAIL)-induced apoptosis. J Biol Chem. 2007;282:12831–41.
24. Austin CD, Lawrence DA, Peden AA, Varfolomeev EE, Totpal K, De Maziere AM, Klumperman J, Arnott D, Pham V, Scheller RH, Ashkenazi A. Death-receptor activation halts clathrin-dependent endocytosis. Proc Natl Acad Sci U S A. 2006;103:10283–8.
25. Chen JJ, Shen HC, Rivera Rosado LA, Zhang Y, Di X, Zhang B. Mislocalization of death receptors correlates with cellular resistance to their cognate ligands in human breast cancer cells. Oncotarget. 2012;3:833–42.

26. Di X, Zhang G, Zhang Y, Takeda K, Rivera Rosado LA, Zhang B. Accumulation of autophagosomes in breast cancer cells induces TRAIL resistance through downregulation of surface expression of death receptors 4 and 5. Oncotarget. 2013;4:1349–64.
27. Wagner KW, Punnoose EA, Januario T, Lawrence DA, Pitti RM, Lancaster K, Lee D, von Goetz M, Yee SF, Totpal K, Huw L, Katta V, Cavet G, Hymowitz SG, Amler L, Ashkenazi A. Death-receptor O-glycosylation controls tumor-cell sensitivity to the proapoptotic ligand Apo2L/TRAIL. Nat Med. 2007;13:1070–7.
28. Haselmann V, Kurz A, Bertsch U, Hubner S, Olempska-Muller M, Fritsch J, Hasler R, Pickl A, Fritsche H, Annewanter F, Engler C, Fleig B, Bernt A, Roder C, Schmidt H, Gelhaus C, Hauser C, Egberts JH, Heneweer C, Rohde AM, Boger C, Knippschild U, Rocken C, Adam D, Walczak H, Schutze S, Janssen O, Wulczyn FG, Wajant H, Kalthoff H, Trauzold A. Nuclear death receptor TRAIL-R2 inhibits maturation of let-7 and promotes proliferation of pancreatic and other tumor cells. Gastroenterology. 2014;146:278–90.
29. Monma H, Harashima N, Inao T, Okano S, Tajima Y, Harada M. The HSP70 and autophagy inhibitor pifithrin-mu enhances the antitumor effects of TRAIL on human pancreatic cancer. Mol Cancer Ther. 2013;12:341–51.
30. Drosopoulos KG, Roberts ML, Cermak L, Sasazuki T, Shirasawa S, Andera L, Pintzas A. Transformation by oncogenic RAS sensitizes human colon cells to TRAIL-induced apoptosis by up-regulating death receptor 4 and death receptor 5 through a MEK-dependent pathway. J Biol Chem. 2005;280:22856–67.
31. Sahu RP, Batra S, Kandala PK, Brown TL, Srivastava SK. The role of K-ras gene mutation in TRAIL-induced apoptosis in pancreatic and lung cancer cell lines. Cancer Chemother Pharmacol. 2011;67:481–7.
32. Leverkus M, Sprick MR, Wachter T, Denk A, Brocker EB, Walczak H, Neumann M. TRAIL-induced apoptosis and gene induction in HaCaT keratinocytes: differential contribution of TRAIL receptors 1 and 2. J Invest Dermatol. 2003;121:149–55.
33. Horak P, Pils D, Haller G, Pribill I, Roessler M, Tomek S, Horvat R, Zeillinger R, Zielinski C, Krainer M. Contribution of epigenetic silencing of tumor necrosis factor-related apoptosis inducing ligand receptor 1 (DR4) to TRAIL resistance and ovarian cancer. Mol Cancer Res. 2005;3:335–43.
34. Cheng J, Hylander BL, Baer MR, Chen X, Repasky EA. Multiple mechanisms underlie resistance of leukemia cells to Apo2 ligand/TRAIL. Mol Cancer Ther. 2006;5:1844–53.
35. MacFarlane M, Kohlhaas SL, Sutcliffe MJ, Dyer MJ, Cohen GM. TRAIL receptor-selective mutants signal to apoptosis via TRAIL-R1 in primary lymphoid malignancies. Cancer Res. 2005;65:11265–70.
36. Crowder RN, El-Deiry WS. Caspase-8 regulation of TRAIL-mediated cell death. Exp Oncol. 2012;34:160–4.
37. van Geelen CM, Pennarun B, Ek WB, Le PT, Spierings DC, de Vries EG, de Jong S. Downregulation of active caspase 8 as a mechanism of acquired TRAIL resistance in mismatch repair-proficient colon carcinoma cell lines. Int J Oncol. 2010;37:1031–41.
38. Capper D, Gaiser T, Hartmann C, Habel A, Mueller W, Herold-Mende C, von Deimling A, Siegelin MD. Stem-cell-like glioma cells are resistant to TRAIL/Apo2L and exhibit downregulation of caspase-8 by promoter methylation. Acta Neuropathol. 2009;117:445–56.
39. Grotzer MA, Eggert A, Zuzak TJ, Janss AJ, Marwaha S, Wiewrodt BR, Ikegaki N, Brodeur GM, Phillips PC. Resistance to TRAIL-induced apoptosis in primitive neuroectodermal brain tumor cells correlates with a loss of caspase-8 expression. Oncogene. 2000;19:4604–10.
40. Hopkins-Donaldson S, Ziegler A, Kurtz S, Bigosch C, Kandioler D, Ludwig C, Zangemeister-Wittke U, Stahel R. Silencing of death receptor and caspase-8 expression in small cell lung carcinoma cell lines and tumors by DNA methylation. Cell Death Differ. 2003;10:356–64.
41. Rebbaa A, Chou PM, Emran M, Mirkin BL. Doxorubicin-induced apoptosis in caspase-8-deficient neuroblastoma cells is mediated through direct action on mitochondria. Cancer Chemother Pharmacol. 2001;48:423–8.
42. Haag C, Stadel D, Zhou S, Bachem MG, Moller P, Debatin KM, Fulda S. Identification of c-FLIP(L) and c-FLIP(S) as critical regulators of death receptor-induced apoptosis in pancreatic cancer cells. Gut. 2011;60:225–37.

43. Safa AR, Day TW, Wu CH. Cellular FLICE-like inhibitory protein (C-FLIP): a novel target for cancer therapy. Curr Cancer Drug Targets. 2008;8:37–46.
44. Finlay D, Vamos M, Gonzalez-Lopez M, Ardecky RJ, Ganji SR, Yuan H, Su Y, Cooley TR, Hauser CT, Welsh K, Reed JC, Cosford ND, Vuori K. Small-molecule IAP antagonists sensitize cancer cells to TRAIL-induced apoptosis: roles of XIAP and cIAPs. Mol Cancer Ther. 2014;13:5–15.
45. Cummins JM, Kohli M, Rago C, Kinzler KW, Vogelstein B, Bunz F. X-linked inhibitor of apoptosis protein (XIAP) is a nonredundant modulator of tumor necrosis factor-related apoptosis-inducing ligand (TRAIL)-mediated apoptosis in human cancer cells. Cancer Res. 2004;64:3006–8.
46. Maas C, Verbrugge I, de Vries E, Savich G, van de Kooij LW, Tait SW, Borst J. Smac/DIABLO release from mitochondria and XIAP inhibition are essential to limit clonogenicity of Type I tumor cells after TRAIL receptor stimulation. Cell Death Differ. 2010;17:1613–23.
47. Fulda S, Meyer E, Debatin KM. Inhibition of TRAIL-induced apoptosis by Bcl-2 overexpression. Oncogene. 2002;21:2283–94.
48. Zhang L, Fang B. Mechanisms of resistance to TRAIL-induced apoptosis in cancer. Cancer Gene Ther. 2005;12:228–37.
49. Hinz S, Trauzold A, Boenicke L, Sandberg C, Beckmann S, Bayer E, Walczak H, Kalthoff H, Ungefroren H. Bcl-XL protects pancreatic adenocarcinoma cells against. Oncogene. 2000; 19:5477–86.
50. Subbiah V, Brown RE, Buryanek J, Trent J, Ashkenazi A, Herbst R, Kurzrock R. Targeting the apoptotic pathway in chondrosarcoma using recombinant human Apo2L/TRAIL (dulanermin), a dual proapoptotic receptor (DR4/DR5) agonist. Mol Cancer Ther. 2012; 11:2541–6.
51. Vanoosten RL, Earel Jr JK, Griffith TS. Enhancement of Ad5-TRAIL cytotoxicity against renal cell carcinoma with histone deacetylase inhibitors. Cancer Gene Ther. 2006;13: 628–32.
52. Tolcher AW, Mita M, Meropol NJ, von Mehren M, Patnaik A, Padavic K, Hill M, Mays T, McCoy T, Fox NL, Halpern W, Corey A, Cohen RB. Phase I pharmacokinetic and biologic correlative study of mapatumumab, a fully human monoclonal antibody with agonist activity to tumor necrosis factor-related apoptosis-inducing ligand receptor-1. J Clin Oncol. 2007;25:1390–5.
53. Younes A, Vose JM, Zelenetz AD, Smith MR, Burris HA, Ansell SM, Klein J, Halpern W, Miceli R, Kumm E, Fox NL, Czuczman MS. A phase 1b/2 trial of mapatumumab in patients with relapsed/refractory non-Hodgkin's lymphoma. Br J Cancer. 2010;103:1783–7.
54. Hotte SJ, Hirte HW, Chen EX, Siu LL, Le LH, Corey A, Iacobucci A, MacLean M, Lo L, Fox NL, Oza AM. A phase 1 study of mapatumumab (fully human monoclonal antibody to TRAIL-R1) in patients with advanced solid malignancies. Clin Cancer Res. 2008;14: 3450–5.
55. Trarbach T, Moehler M, Heinemann V, Kohne CH, Przyborek M, Schulz C, Sneller V, Gallant G, Kanzler S. Phase II trial of mapatumumab, a fully human agonistic monoclonal antibody that targets and activates the tumour necrosis factor apoptosis-inducing ligand receptor-1 (TRAIL-R1), in patients with refractory colorectal cancer. Br J Cancer. 2010;102:506–12.
56. Greco FA, Bonomi P, Crawford J, Kelly K, Oh Y, Halpern W, Lo L, Gallant G, Klein J. Phase 2 study of mapatumumab, a fully human agonistic monoclonal antibody which targets and activates the TRAIL receptor-1, in patients with advanced non-small cell lung cancer. Lung Cancer. 2008;61:82–90.
57. Merchant MS, Geller JI, Baird K, Chou AJ, Galli S, Charles A, Amaoko M, Rhee EH, Price A, Wexler LH, Meyers PA, Widemann BC, Tsokos M, Mackall CL. Phase I trial and pharmacokinetic study of lexatumumab in pediatric patients with solid tumors. J Clin Oncol. 2012;30:4141–7.

58. Wakelee HA, Patnaik A, Sikic BI, Mita M, Fox NL, Miceli R, Ullrich SJ, Fisher GA, Tolcher AW. Phase I and pharmacokinetic study of lexatumumab (HGS-ETR2) given every 2 weeks in patients with advanced solid tumors. Ann Oncol. 2010;21:376–81.
59. Plummer R, Attard G, Pacey S, Li L, Razak A, Perrett R, Barrett M, Judson I, Kaye S, Fox NL, Halpern W, Corey A, Calvert H, de Bono J. Phase 1 and pharmacokinetic study of lexatumumab in patients with advanced cancers. Clin Cancer Res. 2007;13:6187–94.
60. Forero-Torres A, Shah J, Wood T, Posey J, Carlisle R, Copigneaux C, Luo FR, Wojtowicz-Praga S, Percent I, Saleh M. Phase I trial of weekly tigatuzumab, an agonistic humanized monoclonal antibody targeting death receptor 5 (DR5). Cancer Biother Radiopharm. 2010;25:13–9.
61. Herbst RS, Kurzrock R, Hong DS, Valdivieso M, Hsu CP, Goyal L, Juan G, Hwang YC, Wong S, Hill JS, Friberg G, LoRusso PM. A first-in-human study of conatumumab in adult patients with advanced solid tumors. Clin Cancer Res. 2010;16:5883–91.
62. Paz-Ares L, Balint B, de Boer RH, van Meerbeeck JP, Wierzbicki R, De SP, Galimi F, Haddad V, Sabin T, Hei YJ, Pan Y, Cottrell S, Hsu CP, RamLau R. A randomized phase 2 study of paclitaxel and carboplatin with or without conatumumab for first-line treatment of advanced non-small-cell lung cancer. J Thorac Oncol. 2013;8:329–37.
63. Kindler HL, Richards DA, Garbo LE, Garon EB, Stephenson Jr JJ, Rocha-Lima CM, Safran H, Chan D, Kocs DM, Galimi F, McGreivy J, Bray SL, Hei Y, Feigal EG, Loh E, Fuchs CS. A randomized, placebo-controlled phase 2 study of ganitumab (AMG 479) or conatumumab (AMG 655) in combination with gemcitabine in patients with metastatic pancreatic cancer. Ann Oncol. 2012;23:2834–42.
64. Demetri GD, Le CA, Chawla SP, Brodowicz T, Maki RG, Bach BA, Smethurst DP, Bray S, Hei YJ, Blay JY. First-line treatment of metastatic or locally advanced unresectable soft tissue sarcomas with conatumumab in combination with doxorubicin or doxorubicin alone: a phase I/II open-label and double-blind study. Eur J Cancer. 2012;48:547–63.
65. Wainberg ZA, Messersmith WA, Peddi PF, Kapp AV, Ashkenazi A, Royer-Joo S, Portera CC, Kozloff MF. A phase 1B study of dulanermin in combination with modified FOLFOX6 plus bevacizumab in patients with metastatic colorectal cancer. Clin Colorectal Cancer. 2013; 12:248–54.
66. El-Gazzar A, Perco P, Eckelhart E, Anees M, Sexl V, Mayer B, Liu Y, Mikulits W, Horvat R, Pangerl T, Zheng D, Krainer M. Natural immunity enhances the activity of a DR5 agonistic antibody and carboplatin in the treatment of ovarian cancer. Mol Cancer Ther. 2010; 9:1007–18.
67. Nimmanapalli R, Perkins CL, Orlando M, O'Bryan E, Nguyen D, Bhalla KN. Pretreatment with paclitaxel enhances apo-2 ligand/tumor necrosis factor-related apoptosis-inducing ligand-induced apoptosis of prostate cancer cells by inducing death receptors 4 and 5 protein levels. Cancer Res. 2001;61:759–63.
68. Asakuma J, Sumitomo M, Asano T, Asano T, Hayakawa M. Selective Akt inactivation and tumor necrosis actor-related apoptosis-inducing ligand sensitization of renal cancer cells by low concentrations of paclitaxel. Cancer Res. 2003;63:1365–70.
69. Ding L, Yuan C, Wei F, Wang G, Zhang J, Bellail AC, Zhang Z, Olson JJ, Hao C. Cisplatin restores TRAIL apoptotic pathway in glioblastoma-derived stem cells through up-regulation of DR5 and down-regulation of c-FLIP. Cancer Invest. 2011;29:511–20.
70. Soria JC, Smit E, Khayat D, Besse B, Yang X, Hsu CP, Reese D, Wiezorek J, Blackhall F. Phase 1b study of dulanermin (recombinant human Apo2L/TRAIL) in combination with paclitaxel, carboplatin, and bevacizumab in patients with advanced non-squamous non-small-cell lung cancer. J Clin Oncol. 2010;28:1527–33.
71. Reck M, Krzakowski M, Chmielowska E, Sebastian M, Hadler D, Fox T, Wang Q, Greenberg J, Beckman RA, von Pawel J. A randomized, double-blind, placebo-controlled phase 2 study of tigatuzumab (CS-1008) in combination with carboplatin/paclitaxel in patients with chemotherapy-naive metastatic/unresectable non-small cell lung cancer. Lung Cancer. 2013;82:441–8.

72. Yi TB, Yang LY. Caspase-8 in apoptosis of hepatoma cell induced by 5-fluorouracil. Hepatobiliary Pancreat Dis Int. 2003;2:98–101.
73. Yang L, Wu D, Luo K, Wu S, Wu P. Andrographolide enhances 5-fluorouracil-induced apoptosis via caspase-8-dependent mitochondrial pathway involving p53 participation in hepatocellular carcinoma (SMMC-7721) cells. Cancer Lett. 2009;276:180–8.
74. Forero-Torres A, Infante JR, Waterhouse D, Wong L, Vickers S, Arrowsmith E, He AR, Hart L, Trent D, Wade J, Jin X, Wang Q, Austin T, Rosen M, Beckman R, von Roemeling R, Greenberg J, Saleh M. Phase 2, multicenter, open-label study of tigatuzumab (CS-1008), a humanized monoclonal antibody targeting death receptor 5, in combination with gemcitabine in chemotherapy-naive patients with unresectable or metastatic pancreatic cancer. Cancer Med. 2013;2:925–32.
75. Mom CH, Verweij J, Oldenhuis CN, Gietema JA, Fox NL, Miceli R, Eskens FA, Loos WJ, de Vries EG, Sleijfer S. Mapatumumab, a fully human agonistic monoclonal antibody that targets TRAIL-R1, in combination with gemcitabine and cisplatin: a phase I study. Clin Cancer Res. 2009;15:5584–90.
76. Pasetto LM, Jirillo A, Iadicicco G, Rossi E, Paris MK, Monfardini S. FOLFOX versus FOLFIRI: a comparison of regimens in the treatment of colorectal cancer metastases. Anticancer Res. 2005;25:563–76.
77. Rocha Lima CM, Bayraktar S, Flores AM, MacIntyre J, Montero A, Baranda JC, Wallmark J, Portera C, Raja R, Stern H, Royer-Joo S, Amler LC. Phase Ib study of drozitumab combined with first-line mFOLFOX6 plus bevacizumab in patients with metastatic colorectal cancer. Cancer Invest. 2012;30:727–31.
78. Fuchs CS, Fakih M, Schwartzberg L, Cohn AL, Yee L, Dreisbach L, Kozloff MF, Hei YJ, Galimi F, Pan Y, Haddad V, Hsu CP, Sabin A, Saltz L. TRAIL receptor agonist conatumumab with modified FOLFOX6 plus bevacizumab for first-line treatment of metastatic colorectal cancer: a randomized phase 1b/2 trial. Cancer. 2013;119:4290–8.
79. Tabernero J, Chawla SP, Kindler H, Reckamp K, Chiorean EG, Azad NS, Lockhart AC, Hsu CP, Baker NF, Galimi F, Beltran P, Baselga J. Anticancer activity of the type I insulin-like growth factor receptor antagonist, ganitumab, in combination with the death receptor 5 agonist, conatumumab. Oncol: Target; 2014.
80. Dolloff NG, Mayes PA, Hart LS, Dicker DT, Humphreys R, El-Deiry WS. Off-target lapatinib activity sensitizes colon cancer cells through TRAIL death receptor up-regulation. Sci Transl Med. 2011;3:86ra50.
81. Cohn AL, Tabernero J, Maurel J, Nowara E, Sastre J, Chuah BY, Kopp MV, Sakaeva DD, Mitchell EP, Dubey S, Suzuki S, Hei YJ, Galimi F, McCaffery I, Pan Y, Loberg R, Cottrell S, Choo SP. A randomized, placebo-controlled phase 2 study of ganitumab or conatumumab in combination with FOLFIRI for second-line treatment of mutant KRAS metastatic colorectal cancer. Ann Oncol. 2013;24:1777–85.
82. Tuthill MH, Montinaro A, Zinngrebe J, Prieske K, Draber P, Prieske S, Newsom-Davis T, von Karstedt S, Graves J, Walczak H. TRAIL-R2-specific antibodies and recombinant TRAIL can synergise to kill cancer cells. Oncogene. 2015;34:2138–44.
83. Graves JD, Kordich JJ, Huang TH, Piasecki J, Bush TL, Sullivan T, Foltz IN, Chang W, Douangpanya H, Dang T, O'Neill JW, Mallari R, Zhao X, Branstetter DG, Rossi JM, Long AM, Huang X, Holland PM. Apo2L/TRAIL and the death receptor 5 agonist antibody AMG 655 cooperate to promote receptor clustering and antitumor activity. Cancer Cell. 2014; 26:177–89.
84. Lundqvist A, Abrams SI, Schrump DS, Alvarez G, Suffredini D, Berg M, Childs R. Bortezomib and depsipeptide sensitize tumors to tumor necrosis factor-related apoptosis-inducing ligand: a novel method to potentiate natural killer cell tumor cytotoxicity. Cancer Res. 2006;66:7317–25.
85. Ames E, Hallett WH, Murphy WJ. Sensitization of human breast cancer cells to natural killer cell-mediated cytotoxicity by proteasome inhibition. Clin Exp Immunol. 2009;155: 504–13.

86. You M, Savaraj N, Wangpaichitr M, Wu C, Kuo MT, Varona-Santos J, Nguyen DM, Feun L. The combination of ADI-PEG20 and TRAIL effectively increases cell death in melanoma cell lines. Biochem Biophys Res Commun. 2010;394:760–6.
87. Pishas KI, Neuhaus SJ, Clayer MT, Adwal A, Brown MP, Evdokiou A, Callen DF, Neilsen PM. Pre-activation of the p53 pathway through Nutlin-3a sensitises sarcomas to drozitumab therapy. Oncol Rep. 2013;30:471–7.
88. Ren B, Song K, Parangi S, Jin T, Ye M, Humphreys R, Duquette M, Zhang X, Benhaga N, Lawler J, Khosravi-Far R. A double hit to kill tumor and endothelial cells by TRAIL and antiangiogenic 3TSR. Cancer Res. 2009;69:3856–65.
89. Jazirehi AR, Kurdistani SK, Economou JS. Histone deacetylase inhibitor sensitizes apoptosis-resistant melanomas to cytotoxic human T lymphocytes through regulation of TRAIL/DR5 pathway. J Immunol. 2014;192:3981–9.
90. Earel Jr JK, Vanoosten RL, Griffith TS. Histone deacetylase inhibitors modulate the sensitivity of tumor necrosis factor-related apoptosis-inducing ligand-resistant bladder tumor cells. Cancer Res. 2006;66:499–507.
91. Sharp DA, Lawrence DA, Ashkenazi A. Selective knockdown of the long variant of cellular FLICE inhibitory protein augments death receptor-mediated caspase-8 activation and apoptosis. J Biol Chem. 2005;280:19401–9.
92. Bijangi-Vishehsaraei K, Saadatzadeh MR, Huang S, Murphy MP, Safa AR. 4-(4-Chloro-2-methylphenoxy)-N-hydroxybutanamide (CMH) targets mRNA of the c-FLIP variants and induces apoptosis in MCF-7 human breast cancer cells. Mol Cell Biochem. 2010;342: 133–42.
93. Piggott L, Omidvar N, Marti PS, Eberl M, Clarkson RW. Suppression of apoptosis inhibitor c-FLIP selectively eliminates breast cancer stem cell activity in response to the anti-cancer agent, TRAIL. Breast Cancer Res. 2011;13:R88.
94. Sayers TJ, Brooks AD, Koh CY, Ma W, Seki N, Raziuddin A, Blazar BR, Zhang X, Elliott PJ, Murphy WJ. The proteasome inhibitor PS-341 sensitizes neoplastic cells to TRAIL-mediated apoptosis by reducing levels of c-FLIP. Blood. 2003;102:303–10.
95. Hallett WH, Ames E, Motarjemi M, Barao I, Shanker A, Tamang DL, Sayers TJ, Hudig D, Murphy WJ. Sensitization of tumor cells to NK cell-mediated killing by proteasome inhibition. J Immunol. 2008;180:163–70.
96. Schimmer AD, Thomas MP, Hurren R, Gronda M, Pellecchia M, Pond GR, Konopleva M, Gurfinkel D, Mawji IA, Brown E, Reed JC. Identification of small molecules that sensitize resistant tumor cells to tumor necrosis factor-family death receptors. Cancer Res. 2006; 66:2367–75.
97. Hopkins-Donaldson S, Bodmer JL, Bourloud KB, Brognara CB, Tschopp J, Gross N. Loss of caspase-8 expression in neuroblastoma is related to malignancy and resistance to TRAIL-induced apoptosis. Med Pediatr Oncol. 2000;35:608–11.
98. Fulda S, Debatin KM. 5-Aza-2′-deoxycytidine and IFN-gamma cooperate to sensitize for TRAIL-induced apoptosis by upregulating caspase-8. Oncogene. 2006;25:5125–33.
99. Buneker CK, Yu R, Deedigan L, Mohr A, Zwacka RM. IFN-gamma combined with targeting of XIAP leads to increased apoptosis-sensitisation of TRAIL resistant pancreatic carcinoma cells. Cancer Lett. 2012;316:168–77.
100. Fakler M, Loeder S, Vogler M, Schneider K, Jeremias I, Debatin KM, Fulda S. Small molecule XIAP inhibitors cooperate with TRAIL to induce apoptosis in childhood acute leukemia cells and overcome Bcl-2-mediated resistance. Blood. 2009;113:1710–22.
101. Kim EH, Kim SU, Shin DY, Choi KS. Roscovitine sensitizes glioma cells to TRAIL-mediated apoptosis by downregulation of survivin and XIAP. Oncogene. 2004;23:446–56.
102. Grazia G, Vegetti C, Benigni F, Penna I, Perotti V, Tassi E, Bersani I, Nicolini G, Canevari S, Carlo-Stella C, Gianni AM, Mortarini R, Anichini A. Synergistic anti-tumor activity and inhibition of angiogenesis by cotargeting of oncogenic and death receptor pathways in human melanoma. Cell Death Dis. 2014;5:e1434.

103. Engesaeter B, Engebraaten O, Florenes VA, Maelandsmo GM. Dacarbazine and the agonistic TRAIL receptor-2 antibody lexatumumab induce synergistic anticancer effects in melanoma. PLoS One. 2012;7:e45492.
104. Zoog SJ, Ma CY, Kaplan-Lefko PJ, Hawkins JM, Moriguchi J, Zhou L, Pan Y, Hsu CP, Friberg G, Herbst R, Hill J, Juan G. Measurement of conatumumab-induced apoptotic activity in tumors by fine needle aspirate sampling. Cytometry A. 2010;77:849–60.
105. Clodi K, Wimmer D, Li Y, Goodwin R, Jaeger U, Mann G, Gadner H, Younes A. Expression of tumour necrosis factor (TNF)-related apoptosis-inducing ligand (TRAIL) receptors and sensitivity to TRAIL-induced apoptosis in primary B-cell acute lymphoblastic leukaemia cells. Br J Haematol. 2000;111:580–6.
106. Kontny HU, Hammerle K, Klein R, Shayan P, Mackall CL, Niemeyer CM. Sensitivity of Ewing's sarcoma to TRAIL-induced apoptosis. Cell Death Differ. 2001;8:506–14.
107. Yang S, Wang X, Contino G, Liesa M, Sahin E, Ying H, Bause A, Li Y, Stommel JM, Dell'antonio G, Mautner J, Tonon G, Haigis M, Shirihai OS, Doglioni C, Bardeesy N, Kimmelman AC. Pancreatic cancers require autophagy for tumor growth. Genes Dev. 2011;25:717–29.
108. Lazova R, Klump V, Pawelek J. Autophagy in cutaneous malignant melanoma. J Cutan Pathol. 2010;37:256–68.
109. Kaminskyy VO, Piskunova T, Zborovskaya IB, Tchevkina EM, Zhivotovsky B. Suppression of basal autophagy reduces lung cancer cell proliferation and enhances caspase-dependent and -independent apoptosis by stimulating ROS formation. Autophagy. 2012;8:1032–44.
110. Sogabe Y, Suzuki H, Toyota M, Ogi K, Imai T, Nojima M, Sasaki Y, Hiratsuka H, Tokino T. Epigenetic inactivation of SFRP genes in oral squamous cell carcinoma. Int J Oncol. 2008;32:1253–61.
111. Kuo MY, Jeng JH, Chiang CP, Hahn LJ. Mutations of Ki-ras oncogene codon 12 in betel quid chewing-related human oral squamous cell carcinoma in Taiwan. J Oral Pathol Med. 1994;23:70–4.
112. Schubbert S, Shannon K, Bollag G. Hyperactive Ras in developmental disorders and cancer. Nat Rev Cancer. 2007;7:295–308.
113. Overmeyer JH, Maltese WA. Death pathways triggered by activated Ras in cancer cells. Front Biosci (Landmark Ed). 2011;16:1693–713.
114. Chin L, Tam A, Pomerantz J, Wong M, Holash J, Bardeesy N, Shen Q, O'Hagan R, Pantginis J, Zhou H, Horner JW, Cordon-Cardo C, Yancopoulos GD, DePinho RA. Essential role for oncogenic Ras in tumour maintenance. Nature. 1999;400:468–72.
115. Li W, Zhu T, Guan KL. Transformation potential of Ras isoforms correlates with activation of phosphatidylinositol 3-kinase but not ERK. J Biol Chem. 2004;279:37398–406.
116. Nesterov A, Nikrad M, Johnson T, Kraft AS. Oncogenic Ras sensitizes normal human cells to tumor necrosis factor-alpha-related apoptosis-inducing ligand-induced apoptosis. Cancer Res. 2004;64:3922–7.
117. Wang Y, Quon KC, Knee DA, Nesterov A, Kraft AS. RAS, MYC, and sensitivity to tumor necrosis factor-alpha-related apoptosis-inducing ligand-induced apoptosis. Cancer Res. 2005;65:1615–6.
118. Ocana A, Pandiella A. Targeting HER receptors in cancer. Curr Pharm Des. 2013;19: 808–17.
119. Van SS, Kelly DM, Kyula J, Stokesberry S, Fennell DA, Johnston PG, Longley DB. Src and ADAM-17-mediated shedding of transforming growth factor-alpha is a mechanism of acute resistance to TRAIL. Cancer Res. 2008;68:8312–21.
120. Xu L, Hu X, Qu X, Hou K, Zheng H, Liu Y. Cetuximab enhances TRAIL-induced gastric cancer cell apoptosis by promoting DISC formation in lipid rafts. Biochem Biophys Res Commun. 2013;439:285–90.
121. Ouyang W, Yang C, Liu Y, Xiong J, Zhang J, Zhong Y, Zhang G, Zhou F, Zhou Y, Xie C. Redistribution of DR4 and DR5 in lipid rafts accounts for the sensitivity to TRAIL in NSCLC cells. Int J Oncol. 2011;39:1577–86.

122. Cuello M, Ettenberg SA, Clark AS, Keane MM, Posner RH, Nau MM, Dennis PA, Lipkowitz S. Down-regulation of the erbB-2 receptor by trastuzumab (herceptin) enhances tumor necrosis factor-related apoptosis-inducing ligand-mediated apoptosis in breast and ovarian cancer cell lines that overexpress erbB-2. Cancer Res. 2001;61:4892–900.
123. Kim WU, Yoo SA, Min SY, Park SH, Koh HS, Song SW, Cho CS. Hydroxychloroquine potentiates Fas-mediated apoptosis of rheumatoid synoviocytes. Clin Exp Immunol. 2006; 144:503–11.
124. Singh K, Sharma A, Mir MC, Drazba JA, Heston WD, Magi-Galluzzi C, Hansel D, Rubin BP, Klein EA, Almasan A. Autophagic flux determines cell death and survival in response to Apo2L/TRAIL (dulanermin). Mol Cancer. 2014;13:70.

Chapter 11
Pancreatic Cancer Resistance to TRAIL Therapy: Regulators of the Death Inducing Signaling Complex

Yabing Chen, Kaiyu Yuan, and Jay McDonald

Abstract Pancreatic cancer is the fourth leading cause of cancer deaths in the United States. It is generally a fatal cancer with poor prognosis. Once pancreatic cancer becomes metastatic, it is uniformly fatal with an overall average survival of typically 6 months. The only potentially curative therapy for pancreatic cancer is surgical resection. Unfortunately, the majority of pancreatic cancer patients have advanced and inoperable disease at the time of diagnosis. Studies from our group and others have supported that modulating tumor necrosis factor-related apoptosis-inducing ligand (TRAIL)-mediated apoptosis provides potential novel avenues for cancer therapy. However, resistance of pancreatic cancer to TRAIL therapy remains a large clinical hurdle. Thus, better understanding of the molecular events regulating pancreatic cancer cell apoptosis would facilitate the development of novel strategies to enhance the efficacy of TRAIL therapy.

Dysregulation of apoptosis of tumor cells plays an important role in the pancreatic cancer pathogenesis and their resistance to therapies. We and others have demonstrated that the formation of death receptor-activated death-inducing signaling complex (DISC) and the recruitment of DISC components determine both the downstream apoptotic and survival signaling pathways. We have identified several components in the death receptor-activated DISC that mediate death receptor-induced survival pathways, including FLIP and three new DISC components,

No conflict statement: "No potential conflicts of interest were disclosed."

Y. Chen (✉) • J. McDonald
Department of Pathology, University of Alabama at Birmingham, 614 Shelby Biomedical Research Bldg., 1825 University Blvd., Birmingham, AL 35294, USA

The Birmingham Veterans Affairs Medical Center, Birmingham, AL 35294, USA
e-mail: ybchen@uab.edu

K. Yuan
Department of Pathology, University of Alabama at Birmingham, 614 Shelby Biomedical Research Bldg., 1825 University Blvd., Birmingham, AL 35294, USA

B. Bonavida, S. Chouaib (eds.), *Resistance of Cancer Cells to CTL-Mediated Immunotherapy*, Resistance to Targeted Anti-Cancer Therapeutics 7,
DOI 10.1007/978-3-319-17807-3_11

calmodulin (CaM), Src and poly(ADP-ribose) polymerase (PARP-1), which contribute to the resistance of cancer cells to death receptor-activated apoptosis. This review discusses the roles of TRAIL death receptors and the molecular regulators in the DISC that contribute to the resistance to TRAIL-induced apoptosis. The specific apoptotic regulators as potential therapeutic targets for TRAIL-resistant pancreatic cancers are emphasized, including death receptor 5 (DR5), FLIP, CaM, Src and PARP-1.

Keywords Pancreatic cancer • TRAIL • Resistance • Apoptosis • Death receptor • Death-inducing signaling complex

Abbreviations

AKT	Protein kinase B
Bak	Bcl-2 homologous antagonist/killer
Bax	Bcl-2-associated X protein
Bcl-2	B-cell lymphoma 2
Bcl-X_L	B-cell lymphoma-extra large
BID	BH3 interacting-domain death agonist
CaM	Calmodulin
DcR	Decoy receptor
DD	Death domain
DED	Death effector domain
DISC	Death-inducing signaling complex
DNA-PK	DNA protein kinase
DR4	Death receptor 4
DR5	Death receptor 5
DRs	Death receptors
FADD	FAS-associated death-domain
FLIP	FLICE (FADD-like IL-1β-converting enzyme)-inhibitory protein
GALNT14	Polypeptide N-acetylgalactosaminyltransferase 14
GALNT3	Polypeptide N-acetylgalactosaminyltransferase 3
HDAC	Histone deacetylase
IAP	Inhibitors of Apoptosis
Mcl-1	Myeloid cell leukemia-1 protein
NF-κB	Nuclear factor kappa-light-chain-enhancer of activated B cells
PARP	Poly (ADP-ribose) polymerase
SH2	Src homology 2
TFP	Trifluoperazine
TMX	Tamoxifen
TNF	Tumor necrosis factor
TNF-R	Tumor necrosis factor receptor
TRADD	TNFR-associated death-domain
TRAIL	TNF-related apoptosis-inducing ligand

TRAIL-R	TNF-related apoptosis-inducing ligand receptor
XIAP	X-linked inhibitor of apoptosis protein.

11.1 Introduction

Pancreatic cancer is the fourth leading cause of cancer deaths in the USA, causing an estimated 227,000 deaths per year worldwide [1]. The American Cancer Society estimated 43,920 new cases and 37,390 deaths from pancreatic cancer in 2012 in the USA. It is the most lethal type of digestive cancer. Since 1975, the 5-year survival rate has only improved from 2 to 6 %. Only 7 % of cases are diagnosed at an early stage, and even with disease localized to the pancreas, the 5-year survival rate is only 22 % (American Cancer Society) [2, 3]. Once pancreatic cancer becomes metastatic, it is uniformly fatal with an overall average survival of typically 6 months. The etiology of pancreatic cancer remains unclear, although smoking, family history of chronic pancreatitis, advancing age, male sex, diabetes mellitus, obesity, non-O blood group, occupational exposures (e.g., to chlorinated hydrocarbon solvents and nickel), African-American ethnic group, high fat diet and diets low in vegetable and folate have all been considered to be risk factors [4–7]. The only potentially curative therapy for pancreatic cancer is surgical resection. Unfortunately, only 20 % of patients are resectable at the time of diagnosis. Even among those patients who undergo resection for pancreatic cancer and have tumor-free margins, the 5-year survival rate after resection is 10–25 % [7]. Gemcitabine or 5-fluorouracil chemotherapy coupled with radiotherapy may improve the quality of life of patients, but their survival benefit is very limited [5, 8]. Despite improved knowledge in our understanding of cancer development, resistance of pancreatic cancer to current therapies remains a large clinical hurdle. Therefore, a better understanding of the pathogenesis of pancreatic cancer and its molecular mediators is essential for developing novel strategies and therapeutic targets to prevent, diagnose and cure this highly fatal tumor.

Dysregulation of apoptosis of tumor cells plays an important role in the pancreatic cancer pathogenesis and their resistance to therapies. Our group has a long-term interest in molecular mechanisms underlying cancer cell resistance to death receptor-activated apoptosis, and we have been seeking effective reagents that overcome the resistance of cancer cells to therapies targeting death receptors. Studies from our group and others have demonstrated that modulating the components in the Death-Inducing Signaling Complex (DISC) determines the downstream survival and apoptosis signals conveyed by the death receptors. We have identified several DISC components that mediate death receptor-activated survival pathways, including FLIP and three new DISC components, calmodulin (CaM), Src and poly(ADP-ribose) polymerase (PARP-1) [9–17]. This review focuses on the roles of death receptors and molecular regulators in the DISC that contribute to the resistance to tumor necrosis factor-related apoptosis-inducing ligand (TRAIL), a promising therapy for pancreatic cancer. The specific apoptotic regulators, including DR5, FLIP, CaM, Src and PARP-1, as potential therapeutic targets for TRAIL-resistant pancreatic cancers are emphasized.

11.2 Apoptosis and Cancer

Apoptosis is a major mechanism of programmed cell death that plays a pivotal role during development and in the control of tissue homeostasis during adult life. Apoptosis is used by multicellular organisms to eliminate unnecessary or irreparably damaged cells. The ability of tumor cell populations to expand in number is determined by increased cell proliferation, resistance to apoptotic cell death, or the combination of both. Altered expression of pro- and/or anti-apoptotic proteins may render cells resistant to apoptosis, a hallmark of many types of cancer, thus resulting in abnormal accumulation of neoplastic cells [18]. At the cellular level, there are two main apoptotic pathways, the extrinsic and intrinsic pathways [19]. The intrinsic pathway, also called the mitochondrial pathway, mediates apoptosis initiated by internal signals, such as growth factor deprivation, exposure to cytotoxic drugs or radiation that cause DNA damage and are mostly engaged by conventional chemotherapeutic drugs [20]. On the other hand, the extrinsic pathway is initiated by activation of death receptors (DRs) present on the cell surface, such as the Fas death receptor (CD95), the tumor necrosis factor receptor (TNF-R) and TRAIL receptors [21]. Since some DRs are selectively increased only in cancer cells, inducing DR-activated apoptosis is a promising venue for cancer therapy, compared to other anticancer drugs, including inhibitors of protein kinases or growth receptors. Additionally, combination therapies of death receptor agonists with chemotherapy or radiotherapy to trigger both extrinsic and intrinsic pathways may reduce excessive systemic toxicity toward normal cells and tumor resistance after recurrent treatments [22].

11.3 DRs-Activated Apoptosis

The DRs belong to a subgroup of the TNF superfamily, including the well-known TNF-R, Fas, TRAIL receptors (TRAIL R1/DR4 and TRAIL R2/DR5) and other DRs such as DR3, DR6 and actodysplasin A receptor and nerve growth factor receptors [19, 21]. These DRs share a ‘death domain’, a conserved 80-amino-acid sequence in the cytoplasmic tail that is necessary for the direct activation of the apoptotic signaling pathways by the DRs [19, 21]. There are two distinct cell surface-expressed TNF-Rs: TNF-R1 and TNF-R2. TNF-R1 mediates TNF-induced apoptotic signaling [23], whereas TNF-R2 does not transmit apoptotic signals due to its lack of death domain [24, 25] TNF-induced apoptosis is mediated by the recruitment of the adaptor proteins TNFR-associated death-domain protein, Fas-associated death-domain protein (FADD) and caspase-8 to the cytoplasmic death domain of the TNF-R1 [25, 26]. Fas is the best characterized among DRs. It is a type I transmembrane receptor expressed in activated lymphocytes and tumor cells [27], which plays a crucial role in regulation of the immune system by triggering autocrine or paracrine cell death [28]. Five TRAIL receptors encoded by separate genes have been identified in humans [29]. TRAIL R1 (DR4, TNFRSF10a) and TRAILR2 (DR5, TNFRSF10b) contain two cysteine-rich extracellular ligand-binding domains and an intracellular DD, which is required for the activation of the extrinsic apoptotic pathway. DR4 and DR5 have been shown to form homomeric and heteromeric complexes [30], Two membrane-bound decoy receptors (DcRs) that lack a functional DD, TRAIL R3 (DcR1, TNFRSF10c) and TRAIL R4 (DcR2, TNFRSF10d), however, block TRAIL-induced apoptosis by competing for ligand binding with DR4 and DR5 or by forming complexes with the signaling receptors to produce non-functional receptor heterocomplexes [31]. Osteoprotogerin (TNFRSF11b), a soluble protein that also binds to TRAIL, may function extracellularly to inhibit TRAIL-binding to the functional death receptors. Among the five receptors, DR5 has the highest binding affinity to TRAIL while osteoprotogerin has the lowest affinity [29, 32].

The molecular events that mediate death receptor-activated signals are similar for Fas and TRAIL receptors. Binding of trimerized Fas ligand and TRAIL to their functional receptors triggers the assembly of the DISC, which recruits FADD that leads to recruitment and activation of the initiating caspases at the DISC, including caspase-8 and -10 [33, 34]. Activation of the initial caspase-8 or 10 in turn activates downstream effector caspases, such as caspase-3, 6 and -7, leading to apoptosis. In type I cells, a high level of caspase-8 activation at the DISC can directly activate the effector caspases that trigger apoptosis [35]. In type II cells, a low level of caspase-8 activation in the DISC is enhanced via the mitochondrial amplification mechanisms, which is initiated by the cleavage of the BH-3-only protein, Bid that induces the accumulation of Bax in the mitochondria and the subsequent release of mitochondrial cytochrome C to the cytoplasm that activates caspase-9 [36]. Therefore, activation of caspase-8 in the DISC is a pivotal trigger for death receptor-mediated apoptotic signals [21]. The death receptor-activated DISC may also recruit the FLICE-like inhibitor protein (FLIP), an enzymatically inactive homologue of caspase-8 [37, 38]. Increased recruitment of FLIP into the DISC may inhibit caspase-8 recruitment and, thus, transmits primarily survival signals through the DISC [37, 38]. Therefore, recruitment of different components in the DISC determines the downstream survival and apoptosis signals conveyed by the death receptors, which play important roles in cancer cell resistance to death receptor-activated apoptosis [10–13, 15–17, 39].

11.4 Trail in Cancer Therapy

The possibility of targeting TNF-R and Fas for tumor-specific killing has been limited due to systemic toxicity and lack of selectivity on tumors over normal tissues [22, 40]. TNF treatment induced severe adverse events including hepatotoxicity and hypotension [41], while Fas ligand was also found to be highly cytotoxic on primary hepatocytes, non-transformed cells and liver in rodents [42, 43]. Recently, local administration of a novel hexameric Fas ligand APO010 [44], a chimera of collagen domain of adiponectin edng to the Fas ligand extracellular domain, was shown to be effective on xenograft tumors in preclinical studies [45–48]. However, its safety and tolerability in human are unknown, which is currently being tested in a phase I study in patients with solid tumors (NCT00437736). In sharp contrast, the selective tumor-killing effects of recombinant human TRAIL has been demonstrated in numerous preclinical studies in a variety of tumor cells without affecting normal cells [49–54].

In mice and non-human primates, soluble TRAIL inhibits growth of TRAIL-sensitive human tumor xenografts, with no apparent systemic toxicity [54, 55]. In addition, monoclonal antibodies for DR4 and DR5 also exhibit potent therapeutic efficacy in mouse xenograft models of several human tumors [56–60]. The antibodies specifically targeting DR4 and DR5 may not only overcome DcRs-mediated resistance to TRAIL but also have benefited from a significantly longer plasma half-life [61]. Many recombinant TRAIL or anti-human DR4 or DR5 monoclonal antibodies have been tested in phase I-III clinical trials for their anti-tumor efficacy, including dulanermin (TRAIL agonist) [62], mapatumumab (for DR4) [61, 63–65], conatumumab (AMG 655, for DR5) [66, 67], CS-1008 (TRA-8, humanized monoclonal antibody for DR5) [68], lexatumumab (for DR5) [68, 69] and PRO95780 (fully human monoclonal antibody DR5 agonist) [70, 71]. Among the antibodies for DR4 or DR5, conatumumab (AMG655, antibody for DR5) [72] and tigatuzumab (CS-1008, TRA-8, monoclonal antibodies for DR5) [73] have been tested for pancreatic tumors (Clinicaltrials.gov). In general, these agents have been well-tolerated, showing low toxicity in patients in several clinical trials [74–76]. However, clinical trials with the TRAIL and DR4/5 agonist antibodies to date have shown limited anti-tumor efficacy. For instance, antitumor activity of dulanermin [62] or PRO95780 [70] was evidenced in few patients. Mapatumumab affected only specific group of lymphomas patients [63], while conatumumab [66] and lexatumumab [69, 77] showed effectiveness only in advanced solid tumors. Moreover, therapies combining the TRAIL, DR4 or DR5 antibodies with other anticancer therapy, such as cytotoxic agents like gemcitabine or doxorubicin and target agents like antibodies for growth factors found minimal or no improvement in response rate or progression-free survival [62, 71, 72, 78–84]. The resistance of tumor cells to TRAIL-induced apoptosis and lack of ability for the other anticancer agents to sensitize TRAIL-induced apoptosis apparently contribute to the limited efficacy of the current TRAIL therapies. Experimental studies have shown that substantial numbers of cancer cells are resistant to TRAIL-induced apoptosis, especially some highly malignant tumors such as pancreatic cancer [85]. Accordingly, resistance to TRAIL-induced apoptosis in cancer cells remains a clinical challenge. Better knowledge of the molecular and cellular mechanisms of TRAIL resistance is critical for the successful application of TRAIL and DR4 or DR5 agonist antibodies in cancer therapy.

11.5 Trail Resistance

TRAIL has been shown to induce both extrinsic and intrinsic apoptotic pathways in human pancreatic cancer cell lines [86, 87] and pancreatic tumors in patients [88]. However, both apoptotic pathways are inhibited in the majority of the human pancreatic cancer cell lines [86, 89] and tumors [88]. Experimental studies have postulated multiple mechanisms that are responsible for TRAIL resistance, including low expression or mutations of the death-inducing receptors DR4 and DR5, high expression of the decoy receptor DcR1 or DcR2, and increased expression of anti-apoptotic molecular such as FLIP [76]. Additionally, recent studies have shown that a secondary signaling complex may be formed subsequent to the assembly of the primary TRAIL-activated DISC that leads to activation of TRAIL-induced non-canonical kinase pathways, which contribute to the TRAIL resistance in normal cells as well as the resistant tumor cells [90].

Despite recent progress, the expression of apoptosis-inducing receptors or the components of the TRAIL-induced apoptosis/survival pathways has not been a consistent predictor of TRAIL sensitivity of pancreatic cancer cells [76, 85, 91]. Therefore, understanding the regulation of basic mechanisms of TRAIL-activated signaling pathways may not only provide molecular insights into the non-toxic effect of TRAIL in normal tissues, but also identify novel molecular targets and strategies to enhance the efficacy of TRAIL therapy in resistant tumors. As TRAIL-activated DISC formation and recruitments determine the downstream apoptotic and survival signaling pathways, the key components of TRAIL-activated DISC that mediate TRAIL-induced apoptosis and their modulation in cancer cells leading to TRAIL resistance are the focuses of this review.

11.6 The TRAIL Receptors

The apoptosis-inducing TRAIL DRs, DR4 or DR5, are selectively expressed in transformed cells while the apoptosis-inhibiting DcRs are generally expressed in normal cells [33, 34], which support the selective tumor-killing effects of TRAIL. However, the expression of the TRAIL apoptosis-inducing death receptors may not predict TRAIL resistance of pancreatic cancer cells [76]. Increased expression of the apoptosis-inhibiting DcRs and altered expression of apoptosis-inducing DRs have been linked to resistance of several cancer cells to TRAIL-induced apoptosis. In many studies, reagents that enhance expression of the apoptosis-inducing DR4 or DR5 are found to sensitize a variety of cancers to TRAIL therapy.

11.6.1 Decoy Receptors

The DcRs are expressed in some primary tumors such as gastrointestinal, prostate, lung and acute myeloid leukemia cancer cells [92–95], but not in other tumors including neuroblastomas, primary breast and lung cancers [96, 97]. In some TRAIL resistant tumor cells, including human pancreatic cancer cells, breast cancer cells and lung cancer cells, TRAIL DcR2 is highly expressed and the relative ratio of DRs to DcRs predicted the sensitivity of these cancer cells to TRAIL-mediated apoptosis [98, 99]. Consistently, knockdown or blocking DcR2 increased TRAIL sensitivity in human prostate cancer cells and lung cancer cells [93, 94]. Additionally, shedding of DcR1 from the cell surface restores TRAIL sensitivity in Hela cells [100]. On the other hand, overexpression of DcR1 or DcR2 in TRAIL sensitive cancer cells rendered them resistance to TRAIL-induced apoptosis [31, 101–104]. Therefore, it was postulated that the expression of DcRs may not only protect normal cells but also render resistance of some cancer cells to TRAIL-induced apoptosis. However, another study found no correlation between the expression of DcRs and TRAIL resistance in a panel of human melanoma cells [105]. For instance, the TRAIL-resistant melanoma cell line WM3211 express DR5, but not DcR1 and DcR2 [106], whereas DcR1, DcR2 or both are expressed in the TRAIL-sensitive melanoma cell lines, WM9, WM793 and WM1205 [106]. Accordingly, high expression of DcR1 and DcR2 may not solely predict TRAIL resistance of cancer cells. As the DcRs inhibit TRAIL-inducing apoptosis signals by blocking TRAIL binding to its functional DRs, selective agonists with higher binding affinity to the DRs than the DcRs may improve therapeutic efficacy on TRAIL-resistant tumors due to high DcRs.

11.6.2 Death Receptors 4 and 5

Among the five TRAIL receptors identified in humans [29], DR4 and DR5 are the only ones that contain both extracellular ligand-binding domains and intracellular DD that mediate TRAIL-induced activation of the extrinsic apoptotic pathway. The expression levels of DR4 and DR5 are much higher in cancer cells compared with those in normal cells [107]. However, a consistent correlation between the expression of DR4 or DR5 and TRAIL sensitivity of cancer cells has not been determined [76, 103, 108–113]. With five pancreatic cancer cell lines, we have recently demonstrated that the expression of DR5 is correlated with the sensitivity of pancreatic cancer cells to DR5-mediated apoptosis [108]. As mutations and post-translational modification on the DR4 and DR5 have been reported in several cancer cells, including pancreatic cancers, it is likely that such modulations on the DRs may interfere with their ligand binding, clustering and lipid raft localization, which are critical initial events for the formation of TRAIL-induced DISC that leads to activation of downstream apoptosis signals.

Mutations on DR4 and DR5

The genes for DR4 and DR5 are located at chromosome 8p21-22 [114], a segment identified by genome-wide searches to be one of the most common sites of loss heterozygosity due to allelic deletions in several cancers including hepatocellular carcinoma and pancreatic cancer [115]. Among many DR4 polymorphisms, the most extensively studied polymorphisms are rs2230229 (A1322G), rs20575 (C626G) and rs20576 (A683C) [116]. Missense mutations on the DR4 gene has been found in human ovarian, bladder, lung, head and neck squamous cell and gastric adenocarcinoma cancer cells [112, 117]. Mutations of the DR5 gene have also been identified in a variety of human cancers, including head and neck [118], non-small-cell lung [119], breast [120], non-Hodgkin's lymphoma [121], hepatocellular carcinoma [122] and gastric cancers [123]. A 2-bp insertion in the DD domain of the DR5 results in a premature stop codon and a truncated DR5A in primary head and neck cancer [118]. Mutations in the death domain region of DR5 was identified in non-small-cell lung cancer specimens [119], human hepatocellular carcinoma [122], non-Hodgkin's lymphoma [121], but not in normal tissues. These mutations resulted in missensed or truncated DR5.

The DR4 and DR5 mutations have been linked to tumor growth and metastasis. The Glu228Ala (A683C, rs20576) mutation in the ligand binding domain of DR4 is associated with increased risk for prostate cancer metastases [124] and higher risk for ovarian cancer in carriers of BRCA1 mutations [125]. In breast cancer, mutations in DR4 at Asn373Asp, Pro376Leu, and Ala402Val are associated with the metastasized cancer [120], suggesting their function during the progression of breast cancer into metastatic stages. Similarly, DR5 mutations within or flanking the DD domain at Gly426Glu, Gln416Arg, and Gly426Arg have been identified in metastasized breast cancer, but no DR5 mutations were detected in non-metastatic breast cancer [120]. The mechanisms and mode of action of these DR4 and DR5 mutations on tumor growth and metastasis have not been fully understood. Overexpression of the above breast cancer metastasis-associated DR4 and DR5 mutants in 293 cells led to suppression of TRAIL-induced apoptosis [120]. Consistently, over-expression of the DR4 A1322G mutant rendered several cancer cells resistant to TRAIL-induced apoptosis, including human ovarian cancer, bladder and colon cancer cells [112]. The DR5 mutations, such as L334F, E326K, E338K and K386N, failed to form a functional DISC to induce apoptosis, and inhibited the function of wild-type DR4 receptor in lymphoma cells [126]. Therefore, it is likely that mutated DR4 and DR5 may impair TRAIL-binding or interact with themselves or normal DR4 or DR5 proteins to form a structurally abnormal DR trimers on the tumor cell surface, which may function as a "dominant negative" regulator to impair the normal function of DR4 or DR5 to activate downstream apoptosis signaling pathways. As a result, DR4 or DR5 mutations may increase TRAIL-resistance of tumor cells, so as to escape immuosurveillance during tumor growth and metastasis as well as TRAIL therapy.

Modification on DR4 and DR5

Post-translational modifications on DR4 and DR5, such as O-glycosylation of DR4 and DR5 [127] or palmitoylation of DR4 [128], have been suggested to affect their trimerization and thus regulate TRAIL resistance in some cancer cells. Palmitoylation modification on DR4 was found to increase its lipid raft localization and oligomerization, which facilitates TRAIL-activated downstream death signaling in breast and leukemia cancer cell lines [128]. In pancreatic cancer cells and some other cancers, the expression of a peptidyl O-glycosyltransferase, GALNT14, is correlated with TRAIL-sensitivity [127]. In myeloma cells, another peptidyl O-glycosyltransferase, GALNT3, regulates TRAIL sensitivity [129]. It is believed that O-glycosylation of DR4 or DR5 promotes ligand-stimulated clustering of these apoptosis-inducing death receptors, thus leading to TRAIL-triggered DISC recruitment and activation of caspase-8. This notion is supported by the observations that inhibition of GALNY14 led to decreased sensitivity of pancreatic cancer and colon cancer cell lines to TRAIL-induced apoptosis [127], while increased expression of GALNT3 enhanced DISC formation and caspase-8 activation [129]. Accordingly, altered post-translational modification on DR4 and DR5, such as O-glycosylation and palmitoylation, may affect DRs trimerization that is an important initial event for TRAIL-induced apoptotic signaling. Therefore, altered post-translational modification on DR4 or DR5 may explain the resistance of some cancer cells to TRAIL-induced apoptosis, despite their expression of high levels of DR4 or DR5.

Upregulation of DR4 and DR5

Although the correlation between the expression levels of DR4 or DR5 and the sensitivity of tumor cells to TRAIL-induced apoptosis has not been demonstrated, pharmacological drugs that upregulate the expression of DR4 and/or DR5 appear to exclusively enhance TRAIL-induced apoptosis. Chemotherapeutic agents such as doxorubin and etoposide increase the expression DR4 and DR5, and enhance sensitivity of cancer cells to TRAIL-induced apoptosis [130, 131]. Nature product derivatives, including quercetin, Gossypol, gamma-T3 and nimbolide, have been shown to upregulate the expression of DR5 and/or DR4, and thus sensitizing TRAIL-induced apoptosis in a verity of cancer cells, including human pancreatic, kidney, leukemia and colon cancer cells [132–135]. In addition, epigenetic modification by histone deacetylase inhibitors [136] and post-translational regulation by the proteasome inhibitor, bortezomib [107] are also found to upregulate the expression of DR4 and DR5 and sensitize the cells to TRAIL-induced apoptosis. Although the selective cytotoxity of these reagents towards cancer cells but not normal cells have not been determined, it supports the concept that safe pharmacological agents that upregulate DR4 and DR5 expression may represent a unique approach to sensitize TRAIL therapy for resistant cancer cells.

11.7 TRAIL-Activated Apoptosis Signals

Engagement of DR4 or DR5 with TRAIL induces extrinsic apoptotic signaling pathways via recruiting several cytosolic proteins to form the TRAIL-activated DISC [30, 137]. Activation of caspase-8 in the DISC is a pivotal trigger for TRAIL-induced apoptotic signals [21], which in turn cleaves and activates downstream effector caspases to execute cell killing. As the TRAIL-activated DISC may also recruit FLIP, the enzymatically inactive homologue of caspase-8 that mediates primarily survival signals through the DISC [37, 38], the relative levels of FLIP and caspase-8 affects the recruitment and activation of caspases-8 in the DISC, and thus determines the activation of downstream apoptosis signals. Additionally, since low levels of caspase-8 activation in the DISC may be enhanced in the mitochondria, the regulators in the mitochondrial, such as the members of the Bcl-2 family, also contribute to the sensitivity of cancer cell to TRAIL-induced apoptosis.

11.7.1 Caspase-8

Caspase-8 is a cysteine protease that has 480 amino acids and contains two death effector domains and a catalytic protease domain [138]. Two major caspase-8 isoforms have been observed, a 55 kDa caspase-8/a and a 53 kDa caspase-8/b [139]. Caspase-8 is expressed as an inactive zymogen, which can be activated by multiple steps that include oligomerization and proteolysis cleavage [140]. The first cleavage of caspase-8 generates p43/41 intermediate fragments, which are further cleaved into p26/24, p18 and p10 fragments [140]. Active caspase-8 consists of a tetramer with two large and small subunits.

Mutations on caspase-8 have been reported in a variety of malignancies and lead to reduced death receptor-mediated cell death [141–144]. A point mutation that altered the stop codon and increased the size of the encoded caspase-8 protein has been identified in human squamous cell carcinoma [141], which render the cells less sensitive to apoptosis [141]. Several other point mutations or missense mutations have also been identified in gastric, hepatocellular and colorectal cancer [142–144]. Cancer cells with these mutations are resistant to DR5-induced apoptosis [142–144], while overexpression of the caspase-8 G1238A, C1237T or 1381 insertion mutant in 293 T cells reduced DR5-induced apoptosis [144]. In addition, decreased expression of caspase-8 has also been demonstrated in TRAIL resistant cancer cells, such as head and neck carcinoma [145], childhood neuroblastomas and medulloblastomas [146–149]. Inhibition of DNA methylation was found to increase caspase-8 expression and thus enhance TRAIL-induced apoptosis in resistant neuroblastoma cells [147, 149]. In contrast, DNA methylation and histone hypoacetylation inhibit caspase-8 and increase TRAIL-induced apoptosis in small cell lung carcinoma [150, 151]. Furthermore, decreased caspase-8 stability and accelerated degradation was determined in TRAIL resistant colon cancer cells, while over expression of caspase-8 protein restore their sensitive to TRAIL-induced apoptosis [152]. TRAIL increased caspase-8 ubiquitination in TRAIL-sensitive lung cancer cells [153], whereas inhibition of caspase-8 ubiquitination was associated with decreased caspase-8 activity and inhibited TRAIL-mediated apoptosis [153], suggesting ubiquitination of caspase-8 is required for TRAIL sensitivity. Therefore, altered expression of caspase-8, by mutation, DNA methylation/acetylation and ubiquitination contribute to reduced caspase-8 activation in TRAIL resistant tumors, and thus inhibiting TRAIL-induced apoptosis.

11.7.2 Inhibitors of Caspase-8 Activation

11.7.2.1 FLICE Like Inhibitory Proteins (FLIP)

Suppression of apoptosis by intracellular survival factors is important in the development of chemoresistance. As the enzymatically inactive homologue of caspase-8, the relative levels of FLIP and caspase-8 determine which of these two proteins is dominant when recruited to the death receptor, thus regulating the survival or death of the cells. Two major FLIP isoforms have been identified, a short FLIP, $FLIP_S$, and a long FLIP, $FLIP_L$ [154]. Both $FLIP_L$ and $FLIP_S$ can be recruited into the TRAIL-activated DISC by binding to FADD [154], however, they affect TRAIL-activated downstream signaling in distinct ways [154]. $FLIP_S$ contains two DEDs that allows its binding to FADD, and thus blocks the recruitment and activation of caspase-8 by FADD [154]. In addition to two DEDs, $FLIP_L$ also contains a caspase-like domain that allows it to form a dimer with pro-caspase 8 and 10 in the DISC. Despite of its lack of an essential cysteine residue for catalytic activity, the $FLIP_L$ and caspase-8 heterodimer results in a lower degree of activation, favoring proliferation and differentiation pathways rather than apoptosis pathways [155]. As the expression of caspase-8 is quite stable, modest changes in expression of FLIP appear to determine whether a cell proliferates or dies in response to upstream stimuli [156]. In hepatocellular carcinoma and melanoma, the ratio of FLIP/caspase-8 has been reported to be correlated with TRAIL resistance [157, 158]. Elevation of FLIP expression has been identified in pancreatic carcinoma [109] and many other tumor cells [106, 109, 112, 159–163], which contributes to their resistance to TRAIL-induced apoptosis. Inhibition of FLIP in the pancreatic cancer or other cancer cells decreases the TRAIL resistance [106, 109, 112, 159–165]. The molecular signals that are linked to FLIP upregulation in cancer cells include activation of AKT, which induces FLIP expression that regulates the resistance of leukemia [166] and gastric cancer cells [160] to TRAIL-induced apoptosis. Inhibition of AKT decreases FLIP expression and sensitizes the gastric cancer cells to TRAIL-mediated apoptosis [160]. Furthermore, a recent study identified a FLIP antisense oligonucleotide that sensitized cancer cells but not a normal lung cell line to TRAIL-induced apoptosis [167], indicating the possibility to specifically target FLIP in cancer cells to enhance TRAIL therapy.

11.7.2.2 BCL-2 Family Proteins

The mitochondrial pathway is important for TRAIL-induced apoptosis. In type II cells, low level of caspase-8 is activated in the DISC. Activation of caspase-8 in the DISC can cleave Bid, which in turn translocates to the mitochondria. Pro- and anti-apoptotic Bcl-2 family members can form hetero- and homo-dimers on the mitochondrial membrane, regulating the release of cytochrome *c* into and subsequential activation of caspase-9 and then downstream effector caspases. Several members of the Bcl-2 family proteins, including the anti-apoptotic protein, Bcl-2, Bcl-X_L and myeloid cell leukemia-1 protein (Mcl-1), and pro-apoptotic proteins, Bid, Bax, and Bak, are involved in the crosstalk between cytosolic and mitochondrial signaling. Therefore, the relative levels of the pro-apoptotic and anti-apoptotic Bcl-2 family members modulate caspase-8 activation and the sensitivity of cancer cells to TRAIL-induced apoptosis [168].

The contribution of the pro-apoptotic members, Bax and Bak, to TRAIL-induced apoptosis has been demonstrated in normal cells as well as cancer cells. In mouse embryonic fibroblasts, TRAIL-induced apoptosis was inhibited when Bak and Bax are deleted [169]; whereas deletion of Bax was sufficient to block TRAIL-induced apoptosis in human colon cancer cell lines [170–172]. The anti-apoptosis effects of Bcl-2 and Bcl-X_L in TRAIL-mediated apoptosis have been well studied. Overexpression of Bcl-2 was found to inhibit TRAIL-induced caspase-8 cleavage, thus inhibiting TRAIL-induced apoptosis in many cancer cells, such as neuroblastoma, glioblastoma, breast cancer and colon cancer cells [173, 174]. Similarly, the expression of Bcl-X_L was highly correlate with sensitivity to TRAIL-induced apoptosis in several pancreatic adenocarcinoma cells [85]. Overexpression of Bcl-X_L in the TRAIL-sensitive Colo357 cells, which express low levels of Bcl-X_L, rendered the cells resistant to TRAIL-induced apoptosis [85]. In contrast, inhibition of Bcl-XL sensitized TRAIL-resistant pancreatic cancer PANC-1 cells to TRAIL-induced cell death [85]. Mcl-1 can inhibit pro-apoptotic Bcl-2 family proteins such as Bid and thus inhibit TRAIL-induced apoptosis [175–177]. High expression of Mcl-1, but not Bcl-2, was demonstrated in invasive cholangiocarcinoma and cultured human cholangiocarcinoma cell lines [176]. Consistently, overexpression of Mcl-1, but not Bcl-2, mediates the resistance of cancer cells to TRAIL-induced apoptosis; while down regulation of Mcl-1 sensitized the cells to TRAIL-mediated apoptosis [175]. Taken together, these studies support the important roles of the anti-apoptotic Bcl-2 family proteins in regulating caspase-8 activation via the mitochondria pathway, and thus mediating resistance of cancer cells to TRAIL-induced apoptosis.

11.7.2.3 Inhibitor of Apoptosis Proteins (IAP)

The IAP proteins mostly execute their inhibitory effects on death receptor-induced apoptosis by directly interacting with the active sites of the effector caspases, such as caspase-3, 6 and -7, or caspase-9, thus inhibiting the catalytic activity of these caspases [178]. Among the eight IAPs were identified in humans, the X-linked IAP (XIAP) is the most potent inhibitor of caspase activity involved in both intrinsic and extrinsic apoptosis pathways [179, 180]. High expression of XIAP mediates the resistance of a variety of cancer cells to TRAIL-induced apoptosis [181–185], while inhibition of XIAP enhances the sensitivity of cancer cells to TRAIL-induced apoptosis [186–188]. A few studies have identified the inhibitory effects of IAPs on DISC assembly and caspase-8 activation in breast cancer and ovarian cancer cells [189]. Nonetheless, the majority of studies have demonstrated the effects of IAPs on death receptor-induced apoptosis downstream of DISC and caspase-8 activation via blocking caspase-9 and caspase-3. Therefore, cancer cells with high expression of

IAPs may be resistant to a variety of apoptosis-inducing agents, including TRAIL, thus targeting IAPs should effectively sensitize such resistant cancer cells to TRAIL-induced apoptosis.

11.8 TRAIL-Induced Survival Regulators in the DISC

In addition to FLIP, we have reported several DISC components that mediate the death receptor-mediated survival pathways, including CaM, Src, and PARP-1 [9–17, 108]. Consistently, we demonstrated that pharmacological inhibition of FLIP, CaM, Src or PARP-1 enhances death receptor-mediated apoptosis in cholangiocarcinoma and pancreatic cancers [11, 15–17, 108]. The roles of death receptor activated-DISC recruitment of CaM, Src and PARP-1 in regulating TRAIL resistance are discussed below.

11.8.1 Calmodulin (CaM)

Previous studies from our group have demonstrated that two potent calmodulin antagonists, tamoxifen (TMX) and trifluoperazine (TFP) induce apoptosis in cholangiocarcinoma and pancreatic cancer cells and decrease tumor cell growth in mouse xenograft models [17, 190, 191]. We have demonstrated that TMX, a known estrogenic inhibitor, is an effective CaM antagonist, being as potent as TFP [192]. CaM is a small intracellular protein that mainly functions as an intracellular mediator of Ca^{2+} signals [193]. The role of Ca^{2+}/CaM in cancer pathogenesis remains unclear and somewhat paradoxical, because Ca^{2+} is critical for both cell division and cell death. Elevated levels of Ca^{2+}-bound CaM are associated with cancer [194]. Antagonists of CaM inhibit tumor cell invasion in vitro and metastasis in vivo [195], suggesting that CaM antagonists are promising chemotherapeutic agents for cancer. Consistently, we have shown that CaM antagonists induce apoptosis in cholangiocarcinoma cells, through caspase-dependent apoptosis pathways and a caspase-independent pathway by inducing depolarization of the mitochondrial membrane [190]. In addition, we found that TMX inhibits phosphorylation of AKT [15]. The expression and activation of other molecules downstream of CaM activation may also play important roles in determining cell responses to apoptotic stimuli. The Ca^{2+}/CaM-dependent kinase II (CaMKII) upregulates the expression of FLIP in astrocytes and glioma cells [196, 197], suggesting CaM may inhibit apoptosis via activating its downstream enzymes. We have identified a Ca^{2+}-dependent interaction between CaM and Fas death receptor in Jurkat cells and osteoclasts that is regulated during Fas and CaM antagonists-induced apoptosis [198, 199]. Recruitment of CaM into the Fas-mediated DISC has been identified in cholangiocarcinoma and pancreatic cancer cells [11, 17]. CaM was found to interact directly and in a Ca^{2+}-dependent manner with FLIP in the DISC, but not FADD and caspase-8 [16]. Furthermore, a direct interaction of CaM and Src has demonstrated in pancreatic cancer cells [17].

The CaM antagonist, TFP, decreased CaM binding to Src and inhibited Fas-induced recruitment of Src into the DISC and Src activation [17]. Similarly, we found that CaM was recruited into DR5-activated DISC. CaM antagonists blocked DISC-recruitment of Src, sensitized DR5-induced apoptosis in vitro and enhanced efficacy of DR5 therapy in pancreatic cancer xenograft model (unpublished data). The recruitment and direct interaction of CaM with survival signals Src and FLIP in the DISC support its role in regulating death receptor-activated signaling in the DISC. This novel regulatory role of CaM in the DISC may present a unique opportunity for the use of the readily available and well tolerated CaM antagonists, such as TMX and TFP, to enhance the efficacy for TRAIL therapy. Further elucidation of the fundamental function of CaM in the TRAIL-DISC may reveal novel molecular insights into the basic mechanisms of TRAIL-induced apoptosis, which will be useful for the development of new specific agents to overcome TRAIL resistance.

11.8.2 Src Kinase

The Src kinase has also been linked to TRAIL resistance that contributes to breast cancer metastasis [200]. In TRAIL resistant hepatic carcinoma cells, inhibition of Src activity sensitized the cancer cells to TRAIL-induced apoptosis [201]. The molecular mechanisms underlying Src-mediated TRAIL resistance remain unclear. TRAIL was shown to active Src kinase that leads to AKT activation and thus resistant of prostate cancer cells [202]. Consistently, inhibition of Src sensitized the prostate cancer cells to TRAIL-induced apoptosis [202]. In addition, TRAIL-activated Src family kinase was also found to active epidermal growth factor receptor and human epidermal receptor 2-mediated survival signaling in colorectal cancer cells, which led to resistance of the cells to TRAIL-induced apoptosis [203]. Src activation has also been demonstrated to inhibit caspase-8 activation in Hela cells, via phosphorylating caspase-8 at Tyrosine 380 that inhibits caspase-8 cleavage [204]. In contrast, increased caspase-8 cleavage was associated with Src inhibition, which contributes to increased apoptosis in TRAIL resistant hepatic carcinoma cells [201]. In pancreatic cancer cells, we have reported that activation of Src kinase by the death receptor Fas promotes survival of the pancreatic cancer cells [17]. Importantly, we have demonstrated that Src is recruited into the Fas-activated DISC via interaction with CaM at amino acids 204–214 that overlaps the Src homology 2 (SH2) domain. The CaM antagonist, TFP, decreased CaM binding to Src, which inhibited Fas-induced recruitment of Src into the DISC and Src phosphorylation at tyrosine 416 that are key to its activation [17]. We also found that Src was recruited into the DR5-activated DISC in pancreatic cancer cells (unpublished data). Accordingly, recruitment of Src, via CaM, into the death receptor-activated DISC may provide the proximity for Src to phosphorylate caspase-8, which inhibits caspase-8 cleavage and activation as seen in Hela cells. Further investigations are warranted to characterize the molecular mechanisms underlying death receptor signaling-induced DISC-recruitment and activation of Src kinase, and its action on DISC proteins, including caspase-8, that lead to TRAIL resistance.

11.8.3 Poly (ADP-Ribose) Polymerase 1

We have recently characterized several lines of human pancreatic cancer cells, and demonstrated that the expression levels of DR5 and anti-apoptotic protein FLIP was not correlated to their resistance to TRA-8 (DR5 agonist antibody)-induced apoptosis [108]. In contrast, we have identified a novel function of poly(ADP-ribose) polymerase-1 (PARP-1) in regulating the resistance of pancreatic cancer cells to TRA-8-induced apoptosis in vitro and in vivo [205].

The PARP proteins are highly abundant nuclear proteins that are activated when DNA is damaged [206]. PARP enzymes modify proteins by adding chains of ADP ribose units (pADPr). To date, 17 members of the PARP family have been identified on the basis of sequence homology. PARP-1 is the prominent member of the family of PARPs and accounts for 75–90 % of cellular pADPr formation and modification [207]. PARP-1 plays an important role in repairing single-strand DNA breaks by modifying proteins associated with DNA repair [208], so as to maintain genomic integrity and cell survival in response to genotoxic insults [209–212]. In many tumors, the expression of PARP-1 is elevated and is associated with a poor prognosis [213–219]. Accordingly, PARP-1 antagonists, used as a mono-therapy for tumors with DNA repair deficiencies or in combination with DNA damage-inducing agents, may increase accumulation of irreparable damaged DNA that triggers intrinsic apoptotic pathways signaling pathway in cancer therapy [208, 220–223]. For example, PARP-1 inhibition has been used to treat cancers with DNA repair deficiencies, such as BRCA-deficient breast and ovarian cancer [224] and BRCA2-associated pancreatic cancer [221]. Combined use of PARP inhibitors with DNA damaging reagents or radiation sensitizes glioma, ovarian and pancreatic cancers to therapy [220, 222, 223]. Currently, several PARP inhibitors in combination with DNA-damaging agents such as platins, cyclophosphamide, ionizing radiation, and gemcitabine are in Phase I and Phase II trials [206]. Importantly, all of these investigations are based on the known function of PARP-1 in regulating DNA repair, and targeting the intrinsic apoptosis pathways.

The function of PARP-1 in the death receptor-activated extrinsic apoptosis pathways have not been studied previously. Our recent studies have identified a novel function of PARP-1 in the DR5-associated DISC, where it regulates the resistance of pancreatic cancer cells to TRA-8-induced apoptosis [108]. We determined a correlation between PARP-1 expression and the resistance of pancreatic cancer cells to TRA-8. Inhibition PARP-1 in resistant pancreatic cell lines, PANC-1 and Suit-2 cells, sensitizes the cells to TRA-8-induced apoptosis. We found that inhibition of PARP-1 alone does not induce apoptosis of pancreatic cancer cells, suggesting that PARP-1 regulates TRA-8-induced extrinsic apoptosis via a mechanism independent of its function in DNA repair. As a novel component of the DR5-activated DISC, PARP-1 contributes to TRAIL resistance of pancreatic cancer cells by inhibiting caspase-8 activation in the DISC [108]. We found that PARP-1 does not modify DR5 under basal conditions, but regulates the pADPr modification of the DR5-associated DISC complex, and thus modulates downstream apoptotic signaling. PARP-1 was found to directly regulate pADPr modification of caspase-8 and thereby inhibiting its activation. The mechanisms underlying PARP-1-mediated pADPr modification of caspase-8 is not clear. It is plausible that the presence of PARP-1 in the DR5-associated complex provides the proximity for PARP-1 to modify (pro)caspase-8 in the DISC. PARP-1 targets aspartate residues [208], and the aspartate residues at 216, 374 and 384 are cleavage of caspase-8 into its active forms [225, 226]. Therefore, pADPr modification on these caspase-8 aspartate residues by PARP-1 may lead to blockage of caspase-8 cleavage and thus inhibiting caspases-8 activation. Consistently, inhibition of PARP-1 blocks pADRr modification of caspase-8, which facilitates DR5-mediated activation of caspase-8 in the DISC and sensitizes tumor cells to TRA-8-induced apoptosis. This novel function of PARP-1 in the DR5-activated apoptotic signaling machinery suggest the use of cytoplasmic PARP-1 expression as a potential diagnostic marker to identify sensitivity of cancer to TRA-8 therapy, and further support interventions combining PARP-1 inhibitors with death receptor agonists to treat resistant pancreatic cancers.

11.9 Conclusion

Pancreatic cancer remains a highly challenging cancer with high morbidity and mortality, largely due to the lack of early diagnosis and effective therapy. The selective tumor-killing effects of TRAIL and death receptor agonists make them promising avenues for treating many cancers, including pancreatic cancer. Several recombinant TRAIL or anti-human DR4 or DR5 monoclonal antibodies have been tested in phase I-III clinical trials. These agents are generally well-tolerated and low toxicity in patients, however, they have shown limited efficacy. Therefore, better understanding of basic mechanisms underlying resistance of cancer cells to TRAIL-induced apoptosis is warranted for the development of novel strategies for early diagnosis and therapy. Studies from our group and others have demonstrated that regulation of the apoptosis or survival mediators in the TRAIL-activated DISC could effectively promote TRAIL-induced apoptosis in resistant pancreatic cancer cells, thus, enhancing the efficacy of TRAIL therapy (Fig. 11.1). Literature also suggests that the expression of functional death receptors and the decoy receptors could be utilized as effective biomarkers for diagnosis and possibly targets for therapy. Decreased expression or mutation of the DR4 or DR5 death receptor, increased expression of the decoy receptors and upregulation of anti-apoptotic regulators such Bcl-2, Bcl-X_L, Mcl-1 and IAPs have been shown to increase TRAIL resistance in may tumors. As shown in the schematic Fig. 11.1, inhibition of the recruitment and activation of the key apoptotic mediator, caspase-8, by survival signals in the DISC, such as FLIP, CaM, Src and PARP-1, effectively sensitized resistant cancer cells to TRAIL-induced apoptosis. Therefore, using combination therapies of TRAIL agonists with the antagonists of these DISC survival regulators may represent novel strategies to enhance therapeutic efficacy for TRAIL-resistant pancreatic cancer.

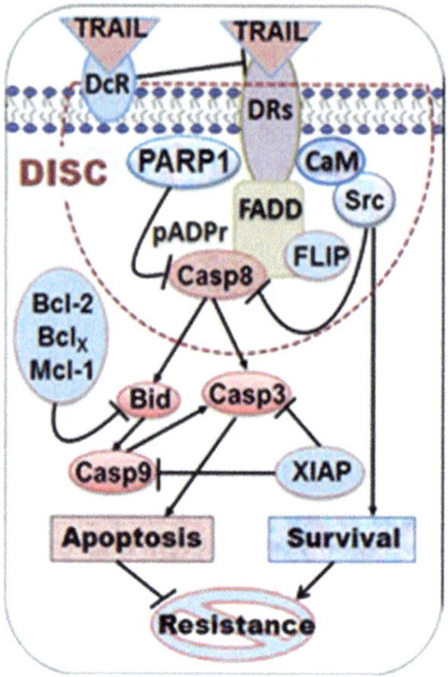

Fig. 11.1 The contribution of TRAIL receptors and regulators in the death-inducing signaling complex (DISC) to TRAIL resistance. Down regulation of TRAIL functional death receptors (DRs) and upregulation of the decoy receptors (DcR) render resistance of cancer cells to TRAIL-induced apoptosis, and enable cancer cells to escape from immune surveillance. TRAIL-activated DISC formation and recruitment determine the downstream apoptotic and survival signaling pathways. TRAIL-induced DISC recruitment and cleavage (activation) of caspase-8 by FADD are key to activating downstream the apoptotic effector caspase-3, directly or indirectly, via cleaving Bid in the mitochondria that leads to activation of caspase-9. The anti-apoptotic Bcl-2 family members, including Bcl-2, Bcl-X and Mcl-1, inhibit mitochondria-mediated caspase-8 activation, which decreases activation of downstream effectors. The increased expression of *i*nhibitor of *a*poptosis *p*roteins (IAPs), such as XIAP, have also been shown to inhibit activation of downstream effectors of caspase-8. The increased expression and recruitment of survival regulators in the TRAIL-induced DISC, such as FLIP, CaM/Src and PARP-1, block recruitment or cleavage of caspase-8, and thus mediating TRAIL-induced survival signals that lead to TRAIL resistance. The antagonists for CaM, Src and PARP-1 have been shown to enhance TRAIL-induced apoptosis and sensitize resistant cancer cells to TRAIL therapy. Therefore, combination therapy using TRAIL with antagonists for the survival signals in the DISC, including CaM, Src and PARP-1, may represent a novel strategy to enhance the efficacy of the TRAIL therapy

Acknowledgements The original research programs of the authors are supported by the Veterans Affairs Research Department Merit Review Awards, BX000311 (JMM) and BX002296 (YC).

References

1. Raimondi S, Maisonneuve P, Lowenfels AB. Epidemiology of pancreatic cancer: an overview. Nat Rev Gastroenterol Hepatol. 2009;6:699–708.
2. Hartman DJ, Krasinskas AM. Assessing treatment effect in pancreatic cancer. Arch Pathol Lab Med. 2012;136:100–9.

3. Klein AP, Brune KA, Petersen GM, Goggins M, Tersmette AC, Offerhaus GJ, Griffin C, Cameron JL, Yeo CJ, Kern S, Hruban RH. Prospective risk of pancreatic cancer in familial pancreatic cancer kindreds. Cancer Res. 2004;64:2634–8.
4. Amundadottir L, Kraft P, Stolzenberg-Solomon RZ, Fuchs CS, Petersen GM, Arslan AA, Bueno-de-Mesquita HB, Gross M, Helzlsouer K, Jacobs EJ, LaCroix A, Zheng W, Albanes D, Bamlet W, Berg CD, Berrino F, Bingham S, Buring JE, Bracci PM, Canzian F, Clavel-Chapelon F, Clipp S, Cotterchio M, de Andrade M, Duell EJ, Fox JW Jr, Gallinger S, Gaziano JM, Giovannucci EL, Goggins M, González CA, Hallmans G, Hankinson SE, Hassan M, Holly EA, Hunter DJ, Hutchinson A, Jackson R, Jacobs KB, Jenab M, Kaaks R, Klein AP, Kooperberg C, Kurtz RC, Li D, Lynch SM, Mandelson M, McWilliams RR, Mendelsohn JB, Michaud DS, Olson SH, Overvad K, Patel AV, Peeters PH, Rajkovic A, Riboli E, Risch HA, Shu XO, Thomas G, Tobias GS, Trichopoulos D, Van Den Eeden SK, Virtamo J, Wactawski-Wende J, Wolpin BM, Yu H, Yu K, Zeleniuch-Jacquotte A, Chanock SJ, Hartge P, Hoover RN. Genome-wide association study identifies variants in the ABO locus associated with susceptibility to pancreatic cancer. Nat Genet 2009;41:986–90.
5. Moore MJ, Goldstein D, Hamm J, Figer A, Hecht JR, Gallinger S, Au HJ, Murawa P, Walde D, Wolff RA, Campos D, Lim R, Ding K, Clark G, Voskoglou-Nomikos T, Ptasynski M, Parulekar W. Erlotinib plus gemcitabine compared with gemcitabine alone in patients with advanced pancreatic cancer: a phase III trial of the National Cancer Institute of Canada Clinical Trials Group. J Clin Oncol. 2007;25:1960–6.
6. Ojajarvi IA, Partanen TJ, Ahlbom A, Boffetta P, Hakulinen T, Jourenkova N, Kauppinen TP, Kogevinas M, Porta M, Vainio HU, Weiderpass E, Wesseling CH. Occupational exposures and pancreatic cancer: a meta-analysis. Occup Environ Med. 2000;57:316–24.
7. Saif MW. Controversies in the adjuvant treatment of pancreatic adenocarcinoma. JOP. 2007;8:545–52.
8. Conroy T, Desseigne F, Ychou M, Bouche O, Guimbaud R, Becouarn Y, Adenis A, Raoul JL, Gourgou-Bourgade S, de la Fouchardiere C, Bennouna J, Bachet JB, Khemissa-Akouz F, Pere-Verge D, Delbaldo C, Assenat E, Chauffert B, Michel P, Montoto-Grillot C, Ducreux M. FOLFIRINOX versus gemcitabine for metastatic pancreatic cancer. N Engl J Med. 2011;364:1817–25.
9. Chen Y, Budd RC, Kelm Jr RJ, Sobel BE, Schneider DJ. Augmentation of proliferation of vascular smooth muscle cells by plasminogen activator inhibitor type 1. Arterioscler Thromb Vasc Biol. 2006;26:1777–83.
10. Chen Y, Xu J, Jhala N, Pawar P, Zhu ZB, Ma L, Byon CH, McDonald JM. Fas-mediated apoptosis in cholangiocarcinoma cells is enhanced by 3,3′-diindolylmethane through inhibition of AKT signaling and FLICE-like inhibitory protein. Am J Pathol. 2006;169:1833–42.
11. Chen Y, Pawar P, Pan G, Ma L, Liu H, McDonald JM. Calmodulin binding to the Fas-mediated death-inducing signaling complex in cholangiocarcinoma cells. J Cell Biochem. 2008;103:788–99.
12. Jing G, Yuan K, Turk AN, Jhala NC, Arnoletti JP, Zhang K, McDonald JM, Chen Y. Tamoxifen enhances therapeutic effects of gemcitabine on cholangiocarcinoma tumorigenesis. Lab Invest. 2011;91:896–904.
13. Jing G, Yuan K, Liang Q, Sun Y, Mao X, McDonald JM, Chen Y. Reduced CaM/FLIP binding by a single point mutation in c-FLIP(L) modulates Fas-mediated apoptosis and decreases tumorigenesis. Lab Invest. 2012;92:82–90.
14. Pan G, Ahn EY, Chen Y, Feng G, Reddy V, Jhala NC, McDonald JM. Reciprocal co-expression of Fas and Fas ligand in human cholangiocarcinoma. Int J Oncol. 2007;31:843–50.
15. Pawar P, Ma L, Byon CH, Liu H, Ahn EY, Jhala N, Arnoletti JP, McDonald JM, Chen Y. Molecular mechanisms of tamoxifen therapy for cholangiocarcinoma: role of calmodulin. Clin Cancer Res. 2009;15:1288–96.
16. Pawar PS, Micoli KJ, Ding H, Cook WJ, Kappes JC, Chen Y, McDonald JM. Calmodulin binding to cellular FLICE-like inhibitory protein modulates Fas-induced signalling. Biochem J. 2008;412:459–68.

17. Yuan K, Jing G, Chen J, Liu H, Zhang K, Li Y, Wu H, McDonald JM, Chen Y. Calmodulin mediates Fas-induced FADD-independent survival signaling in pancreatic cancer cells via activation of Src-extracellular signal-regulated kinase (ERK). J Biol Chem. 2011;286: 24776–84.
18. Hanahan D, Weinberg RA. The hallmarks of cancer. Cell. 2000;100:57–70.
19. Schutze S, Tchikov V, Schneider-Brachert W. Regulation of TNFR1 and CD95 signalling by receptor compartmentalization. Nat Rev Mol Cell Biol. 2008;9:655–62.
20. Fulda S, Debatin KM. Extrinsic versus intrinsic apoptosis pathways in anticancer chemotherapy. Oncogene. 2006;25:4798–811.
21. Mahmood Z, Shukla Y. Death receptors: targets for cancer therapy. Exp Cell Res. 2010; 316:887–99.
22. Russo M, Mupo A, Spagnuolo C, Russo GL. Exploring death receptor pathways as selective targets in cancer therapy. Biochem Pharmacol. 2010;80:674–82.
23. Micheau O, Tschopp J. Induction of TNF receptor I-mediated apoptosis via two sequential signaling complexes. Cell. 2003;114:181–90.
24. Locksley RM, Killeen N, Lenardo MJ. The TNF and TNF receptor superfamilies: integrating mammalian biology. Cell. 2001;104:487–501.
25. Wajant H, Pfizenmaier K, Scheurich P. Tumor necrosis factor signaling. Cell Death Differ. 2003;10:45–65.
26. Hsu H, Shu HB, Pan MG, Goeddel DV. TRADD-TRAF2 and TRADD-FADD interactions define two distinct TNF receptor 1 signal transduction pathways. Cell. 1996;84:299–308.
27. Fulda S, Debatin KM. Exploiting death receptor signaling pathways for tumor therapy. Biochim Biophys Acta. 2004;1705:27–41.
28. Krammer PH. CD95's deadly mission in the immune system. Nature. 2000;407:789–95.
29. Ashkenazi A. Targeting death and decoy receptors of the tumour-necrosis factor superfamily. Nat Rev Cancer. 2002;2:420–30.
30. Kischkel FC, Lawrence DA, Chuntharapai A, Schow P, Kim KJ, Ashkenazi A. Apo2L/TRAIL-dependent recruitment of endogenous FADD and caspase-8 to death receptors 4 and 5. Immunity. 2000;12:611–20.
31. Merino D, Lalaoui N, Morizot A, Schneider P, Solary E, Micheau O. Differential inhibition of TRAIL-mediated DR5-DISC formation by decoy receptors 1 and 2. Mol Cell Biol. 2006;26:7046–55.
32. Kimberley FC, Screaton GR. Following a TRAIL: update on a ligand and its five receptors. Cell Res. 2004;14:359–72.
33. Wilson NS, Dixit V, Ashkenazi A. Death receptor signal transducers: nodes of coordination in immune signaling networks. Nat Immunol. 2009;10:348–55.
34. Yang A, Wilson NS, Ashkenazi A. Proapoptotic DR4 and DR5 signaling in cancer cells: toward clinical translation. Curr Opin Cell Biol. 2010;22:837–44.
35. Li H, Zhu H, Xu CJ, Yuan J. Cleavage of BID by caspase 8 mediates the mitochondrial damage in the Fas pathway of apoptosis. Cell. 1998;94:491–501.
36. Barnhart BC, Alappat EC, Peter ME. The CD95 type I/type II model. Semin Immunol. 2003;15:185–93.
37. Irmler M, Thome M, Hahne M, Schneider P, Hofmann K, Steiner V, Bodmer JL, Schroter M, Burns K, Mattmann C, Rimoldi D, French LE, Tschopp J. Inhibition of death receptor signals by cellular FLIP. Nature. 1997;388:190–5.
38. Scaffidi C, Schmitz I, Krammer PH, Peter ME. The role of c-FLIP in modulation of CD95-induced apoptosis. J Biol Chem. 1999;274:1541–8.
39. Pan D, Yan Q, Chen Y, McDonald JM, Song Y. Trifluoperazine regulation of calmodulin binding to Fas: a computational study. Proteins. 2011;79:2543–56.
40. Daniel D, Wilson NS. Tumor necrosis factor: renaissance as a cancer therapeutic? Curr Cancer Drug Targets. 2008;8:124–31.
41. Croft M, Benedict CA, Ware CF. Clinical targeting of the TNF and TNFR superfamilies. Nat Rev Drug Discov. 2013;12:147–68.

42. Costelli P, Aoki P, Zingaro B, Carbo N, Reffo P, Lopez-Soriano FJ, Bonelli G, Argiles JM, Baccino FM. Mice lacking TNFalpha receptors 1 and 2 are resistant to death and fulminant liver injury induced by agonistic anti-Fas antibody. Cell Death Differ. 2003;10:997–1004.
43. Ogasawara J, Watanabe-Fukunaga R, Adachi M, Matsuzawa A, Kasugai T, Kitamura Y, Itoh N, Suda T, Nagata S. Lethal effect of the anti-Fas antibody in mice. Nature. 1993;364: 806–9.
44. Papenfuss K, Cordier SM, Walczak H. Death receptors as targets for anti-cancer therapy. J Cell Mol Med. 2008;12:2566–85.
45. Eisele G, Roth P, Hasenbach K, Aulwurm S, Wolpert F, Tabatabai G, Wick W, Weller M. APO010, a synthetic hexameric CD95 ligand, induces human glioma cell death in vitro and in vivo. Neuro Oncol. 2011;13:155–64.
46. Verbrugge I, Maas C, Heijkoop M, Verheij M, Borst J. Radiation and anticancer drugs can facilitate mitochondrial bypass by CD95/Fas via c-FLIP downregulation. Cell Death Differ. 2010;17:551–61.
47. Verbrugge I, Wissink EH, Rooswinkel RW, Jongsma J, Beltraminelli N, Dupuis M, Borst J, Verheij M. Combining radiotherapy with APO010 in cancer treatment. Clin Cancer Res. 2009;15:2031–8.
48. Etter AL, Bassi I, Germain S, Delaloye JF, Tschopp J, Sordat B, Dupuis M. The combination of chemotherapy and intraperitoneal MegaFas ligand improves treatment of ovarian carcinoma. Gynecol Oncol. 2007;107:14–21.
49. Pitti RM, Marsters SA, Ruppert S, Donahue CJ, Moore A, Ashkenazi A. Induction of apoptosis by Apo-2 ligand, a new member of the tumor necrosis factor cytokine family. J Biol Chem. 1996;271:12687–90.
50. Wiley SR, Schooley K, Smolak PJ, Din WS, Huang CP, Nicholl JK, Sutherland GR, Smith TD, Rauch C, Smith CA. Identification and characterization of a new member of the TNF family that induces apoptosis. Immunity. 1995;3:673–82.
51. Kelley SK, Harris LA, Xie D, DeForge L, Totpal K, Bussiere J, Fox JA. Preclinical studies to predict the disposition of Apo2L/tumor necrosis factor-related apoptosis-inducing ligand in humans: characterization of in vivo efficacy, pharmacokinetics, and safety. J Pharmacol Exp Ther. 2001;299:31–8.
52. Pollack IF, Erff M, Ashkenazi A. Direct stimulation of apoptotic signaling by soluble Apo2l/tumor necrosis factor-related apoptosis-inducing ligand leads to selective killing of glioma cells. Clin Cancer Res. 2001;7:1362–9.
53. Gazitt Y. TRAIL is a potent inducer of apoptosis in myeloma cells derived from multiple myeloma patients and is not cytotoxic to hematopoietic stem cells. Leukemia. 1999;13: 1817–24.
54. Ashkenazi A, Pai RC, Fong S, Leung S, Lawrence DA, Marsters SA, Blackie C, Chang L, McMurtrey AE, Hebert A, DeForge L, Koumenis IL, Lewis D, Harris L, Bussiere J, Koeppen H, Shahrokh Z, Schwall RH. Safety and antitumor activity of recombinant soluble Apo2 ligand. J Clin Invest. 1999;104:155–62.
55. Walczak H, Miller RE, Ariail K, Gliniak B, Griffith TS, Kubin M, Chin W, Jones J, Woodward A, Le T, Smith C, Smolak P, Goodwin RG, Rauch CT, Schuh JC, Lynch DH. Tumoricidal activity of tumor necrosis factor-related apoptosis-inducing ligand in vivo. Nat Med. 1999;5:157–63.
56. Zeng Y, Wu XX, Fiscella M, Shimada O, Humphreys R, Albert V, Kakehi Y. Monoclonal antibody to tumor necrosis factor-related apoptosis-inducing ligand receptor 2 (TRAIL-R2) induces apoptosis in primary renal cell carcinoma cells in vitro and inhibits tumor growth in vivo. Int J Oncol. 2006;28:421–30.
57. Pukac L, Kanakaraj P, Humphreys R, Alderson R, Bloom M, Sung C, Riccobene T, Johnson R, Fiscella M, Mahoney A, Carrell J, Boyd E, Yao XT, Zhang L, Zhong L, von Kerczek A, Shepard L, Vaughan T, Edwards B, Dobson C, Salcedo T, Albert V. HGS-ETR1, a fully human TRAIL-receptor 1 monoclonal antibody, induces cell death in multiple tumour types in vitro and in vivo. Br J Cancer. 2005;92:1430–41.

58. Motoki K, Mori E, Matsumoto A, Thomas M, Tomura T, Humphreys R, Albert V, Muto M, Yoshida H, Aoki M, Tamada T, Kuroki R, Yoshida H, Ishida I, Ware CF, Kataoka S. Enhanced apoptosis and tumor regression induced by a direct agonist antibody to tumor necrosis factor-related apoptosis-inducing ligand receptor 2. Clin Cancer Res. 2005;11:3126–35.
59. Ichikawa K, Liu W, Zhao L, Wang Z, Liu D, Ohtsuka T, Zhang H, Mountz JD, Koopman WJ, Kimberly RP, Zhou T. Tumoricidal activity of a novel anti-human DR5 monoclonal antibody without hepatocyte cytotoxicity. Nat Med. 2001;7:954–60.
60. Chuntharapai A, Dodge K, Grimmer K, Schroeder K, Marsters SA, Koeppen H, Ashkenazi A, Kim KJ. Isotype-dependent inhibition of tumor growth in vivo by monoclonal antibodies to death receptor 4. J Immunol. 2001;166:4891–8.
61. Tolcher AW, Mita M, Meropol NJ, von Mehren M, Patnaik A, Padavic K, Hill M, Mays T, McCoy T, Fox NL, Halpern W, Corey A, Cohen RB. Phase I pharmacokinetic and biologic correlative study of mapatumumab, a fully human monoclonal antibody with agonist activity to tumor necrosis factor-related apoptosis-inducing ligand receptor-1. J Clin Oncol. 2007; 25:1390–5.
62. Herbst RS, Eckhardt SG, Kurzrock R, Ebbinghaus S, O'Dwyer PJ, Gordon MS, Novotny W, Goldwasser MA, Tohnya TM, Lum BL, Ashkenazi A, Jubb AM, Mendelson DS. Phase I dose-escalation study of recombinant human Apo2L/TRAIL, a dual proapoptotic receptor agonist, in patients with advanced cancer. J Clin Oncol. 2010;28:2839–46.
63. Younes A, Vose JM, Zelenetz AD, Smith MR, Burris HA, Ansell SM, Klein J, Halpern W, Miceli R, Kumm E, Fox NL, Czuczman MS. A phase 1b/2 trial of mapatumumab in patients with relapsed/refractory non-Hodgkin's lymphoma. Br J Cancer. 2010;103:1783–7.
64. Hotte SJ, Hirte HW, Chen EX, Siu LL, Le LH, Corey A, Iacobucci A, MacLean M, Lo L, Fox NL, Oza AM. A phase 1 study of mapatumumab (fully human monoclonal antibody to TRAIL-R1) in patients with advanced solid malignancies. Clin Cancer Res. 2008;14:3450–5.
65. Greco FA, Bonomi P, Crawford J, Kelly K, Oh Y, Halpern W, Lo L, Gallant G, Klein J. Phase 2 study of mapatumumab, a fully human agonistic monoclonal antibody which targets and activates the TRAIL receptor-1, in patients with advanced non-small cell lung cancer. Lung Cancer. 2008;61:82–90.
66. Herbst RS, Kurzrock R, Hong DS, Valdivieso M, Hsu CP, Goyal L, Juan G, Hwang YC, Wong S, Hill JS, Friberg G, LoRusso PM. A first-in-human study of conatumumab in adult patients with advanced solid tumors. Clin Cancer Res. 2010;16:5883–91.
67. Lynch HT, Boland CR, Rodriguez-Bigas MA, Amos C, Lynch JF, Lynch PM. Who should be sent for genetic testing in hereditary colorectal cancer syndromes? J Clin Oncol. 2007;25: 3534–42.
68. Forero-Torres A, Shah J, Wood T, Posey J, Carlisle R, Copigneaux C, Luo FR, Wojtowicz-Praga S, Percent I, Saleh M. Phase I trial of weekly tigatuzumab, an agonistic humanized monoclonal antibody targeting death receptor 5 (DR5). Cancer Biother Radiopharm. 2010; 25:13–9.
69. Plummer R, Attard G, Pacey S, Li L, Razak A, Perrett R, Barrett M, Judson I, Kaye S, Fox NL, Halpern W, Corey A, Calvert H, de Bono J. Phase 1 and pharmacokinetic study of lexatumumab in patients with advanced cancers. Clin Cancer Res. 2007;13:6187–94.
70. Camidge DR, Herbst RS, Gordon MS, Eckhardt SG, Kurzrock R, Durbin B, Ing J, Tohnya TM, Sager J, Ashkenazi A, Bray G, Mendelson D. A phase I safety and pharmacokinetic study of the death receptor 5 agonistic antibody PRO95780 in patients with advanced malignancies. Clin Cancer Res. 2010;16:1256–63.
71. Camidge DR. Apomab: an agonist monoclonal antibody directed against death receptor 5/ TRAIL-receptor 2 for use in the treatment of solid tumors. Expert Opin Biol Ther. 2008;8: 1167–76.
72. Kindler HL, Richards DA, Garbo LE, Garon EB, Stephenson Jr JJ, Rocha-Lima CM, Safran H, Chan D, Kocs DM, Galimi F, McGreivy J, Bray SL, Hei Y, Feigal EG, Loh E, Fuchs CS. A randomized, placebo-controlled phase 2 study of ganitumab (AMG 479) or conatumumab (AMG 655) in combination with gemcitabine in patients with metastatic pancreatic cancer. Ann Oncol. 2012;23:2834–42.

73. Rajeshkumar NV, Rasheed ZA, Garcia-Garcia E, Lopez-Rios F, Fujiwara K, Matsui WH, Hidalgo M. A combination of DR5 agonistic monoclonal antibody with gemcitabine targets pancreatic cancer stem cells and results in long-term disease control in human pancreatic cancer model. Mol Cancer Ther. 2010;9:2582–92.
74. Wiezorek J, Holland P, Graves J. Death receptor agonists as a targeted therapy for cancer. Clin Cancer Res. 2010;16:1701–8.
75. Wang S. TRAIL: a sword for killing tumors. Curr Med Chem. 2010;17:3309–17.
76. Holoch PA, Griffith TS. TNF-related apoptosis-inducing ligand (TRAIL): a new path to anti-cancer therapies. Eur J Pharmacol. 2009;625:63–72.
77. Merchant MS, Geller JI, Baird K, Chou AJ, Galli S, Charles A, Amaoko M, Rhee EH, Price A, Wexler LH, Meyers PA, Widemann BC, Tsokos M, Mackall CL. Phase I trial and pharmacokinetic study of lexatumumab in pediatric patients with solid tumors. J Clin Oncol. 2012; 30:4141–7.
78. Fuchs CS, Fakih M, Schwartzberg L, Cohn AL, Yee L, Dreisbach L, Kozloff MF, Hei YJ, Galimi F, Pan Y, Haddad V, Hsu CP, Sabin A, Saltz L. TRAIL receptor agonist conatumumab with modified FOLFOX6 plus bevacizumab for first-line treatment of metastatic colorectal cancer: a randomized phase 1b/2 trial. Cancer. 2013;119:4290–8.
79. Rocha Lima CM, Bayraktar S, Flores AM, MacIntyre J, Montero A, Baranda JC, Wallmark J, Portera C, Raja R, Stern H, Royer-Joo S, Amler LC. Phase Ib study of drozitumab combined with first-line mFOLFOX6 plus bevacizumab in patients with metastatic colorectal cancer. Cancer Invest. 2012;30:727–31.
80. Demetri GD, Le Cesne A, Chawla SP, Brodowicz T, Maki RG, Bach BA, Smethurst DP, Bray S, Hei YJ, Blay JY. First-line treatment of metastatic or locally advanced unresectable soft tissue sarcomas with conatumumab in combination with doxorubicin or doxorubicin alone: a phase I/II open-label and double-blind study. Eur J Cancer. 2012;48:547–63.
81. Soria JC, Mark Z, Zatloukal P, Szima B, Albert I, Juhasz E, Pujol JL, Kozielski J, Baker N, Smethurst D, Hei YJ, Ashkenazi A, Stern H, Amler L, Pan Y, Blackhall F. Randomized phase II study of dulanermin in combination with paclitaxel, carboplatin, and bevacizumab in advanced non-small-cell lung cancer. J Clin Oncol. 2011;29:4442–51.
82. Soria JC, Smit E, Khayat D, Besse B, Yang X, Hsu CP, Reese D, Wiezorek J, Blackhall F. Phase 1b study of dulanermin (recombinant human Apo2L/TRAIL) in combination with paclitaxel, carboplatin, and bevacizumab in patients with advanced non-squamous non-small-cell lung cancer. J Clin Oncol. 2010;28:1527–33.
83. Mom CH, Verweij J, Oldenhuis CN, Gietema JA, Fox NL, Miceli R, Eskens FA, Loos WJ, de Vries EG, Sleijfer S. Mapatumumab, a fully human agonistic monoclonal antibody that targets TRAIL-R1, in combination with gemcitabine and cisplatin: a phase I study. Clin Cancer Res. 2009;15:5584–90.
84. Leong S, Cohen RB, Gustafson DL, Langer CJ, Camidge DR, Padavic K, Gore L, Smith M, Chow LQ, von Mehren M, O'Bryant C, Hariharan S, Diab S, Fox NL, Miceli R, Eckhardt SG. Mapatumumab, an antibody targeting TRAIL-R1, in combination with paclitaxel and carboplatin in patients with advanced solid malignancies: results of a phase I and pharmacokinetic study. J Clin Oncol. 2009;27:4413–21.
85. Hinz S, Trauzold A, Boenicke L, Sandberg C, Beckmann S, Bayer E, Walczak H, Kalthoff H, Ungefroren H. Bcl-XL protects pancreatic adenocarcinoma cells against. Oncogene. 2000;19:5477–86.
86. Jacob D, Davis J, Zhu H, Zhang L, Teraishi F, Wu S, Marini III FC, Fang B. Suppressing orthotopic pancreatic tumor growth with a fiber-modified adenovector expressing the TRAIL gene from the human telomerase reverse transcriptase promoter. Clin Cancer Res. 2004;10:3535–41.
87. Jacob D, Davis JJ, Zhang L, Zhu H, Teraishi F, Fang B. Suppression of pancreatic tumor growth in the liver by systemic administration of the TRAIL gene driven by the hTERT promoter. Cancer Gene Ther. 2005;12:109–15.
88. Hylander BL, Pitoniak R, Penetrante RB, Gibbs JF, Oktay D, Cheng J, Repasky EA. The anti-tumor effect of Apo2L/TRAIL on patient pancreatic adenocarcinomas grown as xenografts in SCID mice. J Transl Med. 2005;3:22.

89. Matsuzaki H, Schmied BM, Ulrich A, Standop J, Schneider MB, Batra SK, Picha KS, Pour PM. Combination of tumor necrosis factor-related apoptosis-inducing ligand (TRAIL) and actinomycin D induces apoptosis even in TRAIL-resistant human pancreatic cancer cells. Clin Cancer Res. 2001;7:407–14.
90. Azijli K, Weyhenmeyer B, Peters GJ, de Jong S, Kruyt FA. Non-canonical kinase signaling by the death ligand TRAIL in cancer cells: discord in the death receptor family. Cell Death Differ. 2013;20:858–68.
91. Satoh K, Kaneko K, Hirota M, Masamune A, Satoh A, Shimosegawa T. Tumor necrosis factor-related apoptosis-inducing ligand and its receptor expression and the pathway of apoptosis in human pancreatic cancer. Pancreas. 2001;23:251–8.
92. Sheikh MS, Huang Y, Fernandez-Salas EA, El-Deiry WS, Friess H, Amundson S, Yin J, Meltzer SJ, Holbrook NJ, Fornace Jr AJ. The antiapoptotic decoy receptor TRID/TRAIL-R3 is a p53-regulated DNA damage-inducible gene that is overexpressed in primary tumors of the gastrointestinal tract. Oncogene. 1999;18:4153–9.
93. Sanlioglu AD, Koksal IT, Ciftcioglu A, Baykara M, Luleci G, Sanlioglu S. Differential expression of TRAIL and its receptors in benign and malignant prostate tissues. J Urol. 2007;177:359–64.
94. Aydin C, Sanlioglu AD, Karacay B, Ozbilim G, Dertsiz L, Ozbudak O, Akdis CA, Sanlioglu S. Decoy receptor-2 small interfering RNA (siRNA) strategy employing three different siRNA constructs in combination defeats adenovirus-transferred tumor necrosis factor-related apoptosis-inducing ligand resistance in lung cancer cells. Hum Gene Ther. 2007;18: 39–50.
95. Riccioni R, Pasquini L, Mariani G, Saulle E, Rossini A, Diverio D, Pelosi E, Vitale A, Chierichini A, Cedrone M, Foa R, Lo Coco F, Peschle C, Testa U. TRAIL decoy receptors mediate resistance of acute myeloid leukemia cells to TRAIL. Haematologica. 2005;90: 612–24.
96. Shivapurkar N, Toyooka S, Toyooka KO, Reddy J, Miyajima K, Suzuki M, Shigematsu H, Takahashi T, Parikh G, Pass HI, Chaudhary PM, Gazdar AF. Aberrant methylation of trail decoy receptor genes is frequent in multiple tumor types. Int J Cancer (Journal international du cancer). 2004;109:786–92.
97. van Noesel MM, van Bezouw S, Salomons GS, Voute PA, Pieters R, Baylin SB, Herman JG, Versteeg R. Tumor-specific down-regulation of the tumor necrosis factor-related apoptosis-inducing ligand decoy receptors DcR1 and DcR2 is associated with dense promoter hypermethylation. Cancer Res. 2002;62:2157–61.
98. Kong LN, Zuo PP, Mu L, Liu YY, Yang N. Gene expression profile of amyloid beta protein-injected mouse model for Alzheimer disease. Acta Pharmacol Sin. 2005;26:666–72.
99. Buneker C, Mohr A, Zwacka RM. The TRAIL-receptor-1: TRAIL-receptor-3 and -4 ratio is a predictor for TRAIL sensitivity of cancer cells. Oncol Rep. 2009;21:1289–95.
100. Bernard D, Quatannens B, Vandenbunder B, Abbadie C. Rel/NF-kappaB transcription factors protect against tumor necrosis factor (TNF)-related apoptosis-inducing ligand (TRAIL)-induced apoptosis by up-regulating the TRAIL decoy receptor DcR1. J Biol Chem. 2001; 276:27322–8.
101. Degli-Esposti MA, Smolak PJ, Walczak H, Waugh J, Huang CP, DuBose RF, Goodwin RG, Smith CA. Cloning and characterization of TRAIL-R3, a novel member of the emerging TRAIL receptor family. J Exp Med. 1997;186:1165–70.
102. Sheridan JP, Marsters SA, Pitti RM, Gurney A, Skubatch M, Baldwin D, Ramakrishnan L, Gray CL, Baker K, Wood WI, Goddard AD, Godowski P, Ashkenazi A. Control of TRAIL-induced apoptosis by a family of signaling and decoy receptors. Science. 1997;277:818–21.
103. Pan G, Ni J, Wei YF, Yu G, Gentz R, Dixit VM. An antagonist decoy receptor and a death domain-containing receptor for TRAIL. Science. 1997;277:815–8.
104. Marsters SA, Sheridan JP, Pitti RM, Huang A, Skubatch M, Baldwin D, Yuan J, Gurney A, Goddard AD, Godowski P, Ashkenazi A. A novel receptor for Apo2L/TRAIL contains a truncated death domain. Curr Biol. 1997;7:1003–6.

105. Zhang XD, Franco A, Myers K, Gray C, Nguyen T, Hersey P. Relation of TNF-related apoptosis-inducing ligand (TRAIL) receptor and FLICE-inhibitory protein expression to TRAIL-induced apoptosis of melanoma. Cancer Res. 1999;59:2747–53.
106. Griffith TS, Chin WA, Jackson GC, Lynch DH, Kubin MZ. Intracellular regulation of TRAIL-induced apoptosis in human melanoma cells. J Immunol. 1998;161:2833–40.
107. Sayers TJ, Murphy WJ. Combining proteasome inhibition with TNF-related apoptosis-inducing ligand (Apo2L/TRAIL) for cancer therapy. Cancer Immunol Immunother. 2006;55: 76–84.
108. Yuan K, Sun Y, Zhou T, McDonald J, Chen Y. PARP-1 regulates resistance of pancreatic cancer to TRAIL therapy. Clin Cancer Res. 2013;19:4750–9.
109. Mori T, Doi R, Toyoda E, Koizumi M, Ito D, Kami K, Kida A, Masui T, Kawaguchi Y, Fujimoto K. Regulation of the resistance to TRAIL-induced apoptosis as a new strategy for pancreatic cancer. Surgery. 2005;138:71–7.
110. Ozawa F, Friess H, Kleeff J, Xu ZW, Zimmermann A, Sheikh MS, Buchler MW. Effects and expression of TRAIL and its apoptosis-promoting receptors in human pancreatic cancer. Cancer Lett. 2001;163:71–81.
111. Petak I, Douglas L, Tillman DM, Vernes R, Houghton JA. Pediatric rhabdomyosarcoma cell lines are resistant to Fas-induced apoptosis and highly sensitive to TRAIL-induced apoptosis. Clin Cancer Res. 2000;6:4119–27.
112. Kim K, Fisher MJ, Xu SQ, El-Deiry WS. Molecular determinants of response to TRAIL in killing of normal and cancer cells. Clin Cancer Res. 2000;6:335–46.
113. Keane MM, Ettenberg SA, Nau MM, Russell EK, Lipkowitz S. Chemotherapy augments TRAIL-induced apoptosis in breast cell lines. Cancer Res. 1999;59:734–41.
114. MacFarlane M, Ahmad M, Srinivasula SM, Fernandes-Alnemri T, Cohen GM, Alnemri ES. Identification and molecular cloning of two novel receptors for the cytotoxic ligand TRAIL. J Biol Chem. 1997;272:25417–20.
115. Pineau P, Nagai H, Prigent S, Wei Y, Gyapay G, Weissenbach J, Tiollais P, Buendia MA, Dejean A. Identification of three distinct regions of allelic deletions on the short arm of chromosome 8 in hepatocellular carcinoma. Oncogene. 1999;18:3127–34.
116. Chen B, Liu S, Wang XL, Xu W, Li Y, Zhao WH, Wu JQ. TRAIL-R1 polymorphisms and cancer susceptibility: an evidence-based meta-analysis. Eur J Cancer. 2009;45:2598–605.
117. Fisher MJ, Virmani AK, Wu L, Aplenc R, Harper JC, Powell SM, Rebbeck TR, Sidransky D, Gazdar AF, El-Deiry WS. Nucleotide substitution in the ectodomain of trail receptor DR4 is associated with lung cancer and head and neck cancer. Clin Cancer Res. 2001;7:1688–97.
118. Pai SI, Wu GS, Ozoren N, Wu L, Jen J, Sidransky D, El-Deiry WS. Rare loss-of-function mutation of a death receptor gene in head and neck cancer. Cancer Res. 1998;58:3513–8.
119. Lee SH, Shin MS, Kim HS, Lee HK, Park WS, Kim SY, Lee JH, Han SY, Park JY, Oh RR, Jang JJ, Han JY, Lee JY, Yoo NJ. Alterations of the DR5/TRAIL receptor 2 gene in non-small cell lung cancers. Cancer Res. 1999;59:5683–6.
120. Shin MS, Kim HS, Lee SH, Park WS, Kim SY, Park JY, Lee JH, Lee SK, Lee SN, Jung SS, Han JY, Kim H, Lee JY, Yoo NJ. Mutations of tumor necrosis factor-related apoptosis-inducing ligand receptor 1 (TRAIL-R1) and receptor 2 (TRAIL-R2) genes in metastatic breast cancers. Cancer Res. 2001;61:4942–6.
121. Lee SH, Shin MS, Kim HS, Lee HK, Park WS, Kim SY, Lee JH, Han SY, Park JY, Oh RR, Kang CS, Kim KM, Jang JJ, Nam SW, Lee JY, Yoo NJ. Somatic mutations of TRAIL-receptor 1 and TRAIL-receptor 2 genes in non-Hodgkin's lymphoma. Oncogene. 2001;20: 399–403.
122. Jeng YM, Hsu HC. Mutation of the DR5/TRAIL receptor 2 gene is infrequent in hepatocellular carcinoma. Cancer Lett. 2002;181:205–8.
123. Park WS, Lee JH, Shin MS, Park JY, Kim HS, Kim YS, Park CH, Lee SK, Lee SH, Lee SN, Kim H, Yoo NJ, Lee JY. Inactivating mutations of KILLER/DR5 gene in gastric cancers. Gastroenterology. 2001;121:1219–25.
124. Langsenlehner T, Langsenlehner U, Renner W, Kapp KS, Krippl P, Hofmann G, Clar H, Pummer K, Mayer R. The Glu228Ala polymorphism in the ligand binding domain of death

receptor 4 is associated with increased risk for prostate cancer metastases. Prostate. 2008; 68:264–8.
125. Dick MG, Versmold B, Engel C, Meindl A, Arnold N, Varon-Mateeva R, Sutter C, Niederacher D, Deissler H, Preisler-Adams S, Kast K, Schafer D, Gadzicki D, Heinritz W, Wappenschmidt B, Schmutzler RK. Association of death receptor 4 variant (683A>C) with ovarian cancer risk in BRCA1 mutation carriers. Int J Cancer (Journal international du cancer). 2012;130:1314–8.
126. Bin L, Thorburn J, Thomas LR, Clark PE, Humphreys R, Thorburn A. Tumor-derived mutations in the TRAIL receptor DR5 inhibit TRAIL signaling through the DR4 receptor by competing for ligand binding. J Biol Chem. 2007;282:28189–94.
127. Wagner KW, Punnoose EA, Januario T, Lawrence DA, Pitti RM, Lancaster K, Lee D, von Goetz M, Yee SF, Totpal K, Huw L, Katta V, Cavet G, Hymowitz SG, Amler L, Ashkenazi A. Death-receptor O-glycosylation controls tumor-cell sensitivity to the proapoptotic ligand Apo2L/TRAIL. Nat Med. 2007;13:1070–7.
128. Rossin A, Derouet M, Abdel-Sater F, Hueber AO. Palmitoylation of the TRAIL receptor DR4 confers an efficient TRAIL-induced cell death signalling. Biochem J. 2009;419:185–92, 2.
129. Wu YH, Yang CY, Chien WL, Lin KI, Lai MZ. Removal of syndecan-1 promotes TRAIL-induced apoptosis in myeloma cells. J Immunol. 2012;188:2914–21.
130. Wu XX, Kakehi Y, Mizutani Y, Nishiyama H, Kamoto T, Megumi Y, Ito N, Ogawa O. Enhancement of TRAIL/Apo2L-mediated apoptosis by adriamycin through inducing DR4 and DR5 in renal cell carcinoma cells. Int J Cancer (Journal international du cancer). 2003; 104:409–17.
131. Gibson SB, Oyer R, Spalding AC, Anderson SM, Johnson GL. Increased expression of death receptors 4 and 5 synergizes the apoptosis response to combined treatment with etoposide and TRAIL. Mol Cell Biol. 2000;20:205–12.
132. Kannappan R, Ravindran J, Prasad S, Sung B, Yadav VR, Reuter S, Chaturvedi MM, Aggarwal BB. Gamma-tocotrienol promotes TRAIL-induced apoptosis through reactive oxygen species/extracellular signal-regulated kinase/p53-mediated upregulation of death receptors. Mol Cancer Ther. 2010;9:2196–207.
133. Gupta SC, Reuter S, Phromnoi K, Park B, Hema PS, Nair M, Aggarwal BB. Nimbolide sensitizes human colon cancer cells to TRAIL through reactive oxygen species- and ERK-dependent up-regulation of death receptors, p53, and Bax. J Biol Chem. 2011;286:1134–46.
134. Shenoy K, Wu Y, Pervaiz S. LY303511 enhances TRAIL sensitivity of SHEP-1 neuroblastoma cells via hydrogen peroxide-mediated mitogen-activated protein kinase activation and up-regulation of death receptors. Cancer Res. 2009;69:1941–50.
135. Sung B, Ravindran J, Prasad S, Pandey MK, Aggarwal BB. Gossypol induces death receptor-5 through activation of the ROS-ERK-CHOP pathway and sensitizes colon cancer cells to TRAIL. J Biol Chem. 2010;285:35418–27.
136. Earel Jr JK, VanOosten RL, Griffith TS. Histone deacetylase inhibitors modulate the sensitivity of tumor necrosis factor-related apoptosis-inducing ligand-resistant bladder tumor cells. Cancer Res. 2006;66:499–507.
137. Sprick MR, Weigand MA, Rieser E, Rauch CT, Juo P, Blenis J, Krammer PH, Walczak H. FADD/MORT1 and caspase-8 are recruited to TRAIL receptors 1 and 2 and are essential for apoptosis mediated by TRAIL receptor 2. Immunity. 2000;12:599–609.
138. Fulda S. Caspase-8 in cancer biology and therapy. Cancer Lett. 2009;281:128–33.
139. Scaffidi C, Medema JP, Krammer PH, Peter ME. FLICE is predominantly expressed as two functionally active isoforms, caspase-8/a and caspase-8/b. J Biol Chem. 1997;272:26953–8.
140. Degterev A, Boyce M, Yuan J. A decade of caspases. Oncogene. 2003;22:8543–67.
141. Mandruzzato S, Brasseur F, Andry G, Boon T, van der Bruggen P. A CASP-8 mutation recognized by cytolytic T lymphocytes on a human head and neck carcinoma. J Exp Med. 1997;186:785–93.
142. Soung YH, Lee JW, Kim SY, Jang J, Park YG, Park WS, Nam SW, Lee JY, Yoo NJ, Lee SH. CASPASE-8 gene is inactivated by somatic mutations in gastric carcinomas. Cancer Res. 2005;65:815–21.

143. Soung YH, Lee JW, Kim SY, Sung YJ, Park WS, Nam SW, Kim SH, Lee JY, Yoo NJ, Lee SH. Caspase-8 gene is frequently inactivated by the frameshift somatic mutation 1225_1226delTG in hepatocellular carcinomas. Oncogene. 2005;24:141–7.
144. Kim HS, Lee JW, Soung YH, Park WS, Kim SY, Lee JH, Park JY, Cho YG, Kim CJ, Jeong SW, Nam SW, Kim SH, Lee JY, Yoo NJ, Lee SH. Inactivating mutations of caspase-8 gene in colorectal carcinomas. Gastroenterology. 2003;125:708–15.
145. Liu J, Uematsu H, Tsuchida N, Ikeda MA. Association of caspase-8 mutation with chemoresistance to cisplatin in HOC313 head and neck squamous cell carcinoma cells. Biochem Biophys Res Commun. 2009;390:989–94.
146. Zuzak TJ, Steinhoff DF, Sutton LN, Phillips PC, Eggert A, Grotzer MA. Loss of caspase-8 mRNA expression is common in childhood primitive neuroectodermal brain tumour/medulloblastoma. Eur J Cancer. 2002;38:83–91.
147. Coffey DC, Kutko MC, Glick RD, Swendeman SL, Butler L, Rifkind R, Marks PA, Richon VM, LaQuaglia MP. Histone deacetylase inhibitors and retinoic acids inhibit growth of human neuroblastoma in vitro. Med Pediatr Oncol. 2000;35:577–81.
148. Grotzer MA, Eggert A, Zuzak TJ, Janss AJ, Marwaha S, Wiewrodt BR, Ikegaki N, Brodeur GM, Phillips PC. Resistance to TRAIL-induced apoptosis in primitive neuroectodermal brain tumor cells correlates with a loss of caspase-8 expression. Oncogene. 2000;19:4604–10.
149. Hopkins-Donaldson S, Bodmer JL, Bourloud KB, Brognara CB, Tschopp J, Gross N. Loss of caspase-8 expression in highly malignant human neuroblastoma cells correlates with resistance to tumor necrosis factor-related apoptosis-inducing ligand-induced apoptosis. Cancer Res. 2000;60:4315–9.
150. Hopkins-Donaldson S, Ziegler A, Kurtz S, Bigosch C, Kandioler D, Ludwig C, Zangemeister-Wittke U, Stahel R. Silencing of death receptor and caspase-8 expression in small cell lung carcinoma cell lines and tumors by DNA methylation. Cell Death Differ. 2003;10:356–64.
151. Hacker S, Dittrich A, Mohr A, Schweitzer T, Rutkowski S, Krauss J, Debatin KM, Fulda S. Histone deacetylase inhibitors cooperate with IFN-gamma to restore caspase-8 expression and overcome TRAIL resistance in cancers with silencing of caspase-8. Oncogene. 2009; 28:3097–110.
152. Zhang L, Zhu H, Teraishi F, Davis JJ, Guo W, Fan Z, Fang B. Accelerated degradation of caspase-8 protein correlates with TRAIL resistance in a DLD1 human colon cancer cell line. Neoplasia. 2005;7:594–602.
153. Jin Z, Li Y, Pitti R, Lawrence D, Pham VC, Lill JR, Ashkenazi A. Cullin3-based polyubiquitination and p62-dependent aggregation of caspase-8 mediate extrinsic apoptosis signaling. Cell. 2009;137:721–35.
154. Krueger A, Baumann S, Krammer PH, Kirchhoff S. FLICE-inhibitory proteins: regulators of death receptor-mediated apoptosis. Mol Cell Biol. 2001;21:8247–54.
155. Pop C, Oberst A, Drag M, Van Raam BJ, Riedl SJ, Green DR, Salvesen GS. FLIP(L) induces caspase 8 activity in the absence of interdomain caspase 8 cleavage and alters substrate specificity. Biochem J. 2011;433:447–57.
156. Micheau O, Lens S, Gaide O, Alevizopoulos K, Tschopp J. NF-kappaB signals induce the expression of c-FLIP. Mol Cell Biol. 2001;21:5299–305.
157. Okano H, Shiraki K, Inoue H, Kawakita T, Yamanaka T, Deguchi M, Sugimoto K, Sakai T, Ohmori S, Fujikawa K, Murata K, Nakano T. Cellular FLICE/caspase-8-inhibitory protein as a principal regulator of cell death and survival in human hepatocellular carcinoma. Lab Invest. 2003;83:1033–43.
158. Tepper CG, Seldin MF. Modulation of caspase-8 and FLICE-inhibitory protein expression as a potential mechanism of Epstein-Barr virus tumorigenesis in Burkitt's lymphoma. Blood. 1999;94:1727–37.
159. Hernandez A, Wang QD, Schwartz SA, Evers BM. Sensitization of human colon cancer cells to TRAIL-mediated apoptosis. J Gastrointest Surg. 2001;5:56–65.
160. Nam SY, Jung GA, Hur GC, Chung HY, Kim WH, Seol DW, Lee BL. Upregulation of FLIP(S) by Akt, a possible inhibition mechanism of TRAIL-induced apoptosis in human gastric cancers. Cancer Sci. 2003;94:1066–73.

161. Mathas S, Lietz A, Anagnostopoulos I, Hummel F, Wiesner B, Janz M, Jundt F, Hirsch B, Johrens-Leder K, Vornlocher HP, Bommert K, Stein H, Dorken B. c-FLIP mediates resistance of Hodgkin/Reed-Sternberg cells to death receptor-induced apoptosis. J Exp Med. 2004;199:1041–52.
162. Ricci MS, Jin Z, Dews M, Yu D, Thomas-Tikhonenko A, Dicker DT, El-Deiry WS. Direct repression of FLIP expression by c-myc is a major determinant of TRAIL sensitivity. Mol Cell Biol. 2004;24:8541–55.
163. Siegmund D, Hadwiger P, Pfizenmaier K, Vornlocher HP, Wajant H. Selective inhibition of FLICE-like inhibitory protein expression with small interfering RNA oligonucleotides is sufficient to sensitize tumor cells for TRAIL-induced apoptosis. Mol Med. 2002;8:725–32.
164. Sung B, Park B, Yadav VR, Aggarwal BB. Celastrol, a triterpene, enhances TRAIL-induced apoptosis through the down-regulation of cell survival proteins and up-regulation of death receptors. J Biol Chem. 2010;285:11498–507.
165. Murtaza I, Saleem M, Adhami VM, Hafeez BB, Mukhtar H. Suppression of cFLIP by lupeol, a dietary triterpene, is sufficient to overcome resistance to TRAIL-mediated apoptosis in chemoresistant human pancreatic cancer cells. Cancer Res. 2009;69:1156–65.
166. Bortul R, Tazzari PL, Cappellini A, Tabellini G, Billi AM, Bareggi R, Manzoli L, Cocco L, Martelli AM. Constitutively active Akt1 protects HL60 leukemia cells from TRAIL-induced apoptosis through a mechanism involving NF-kappaB activation and cFLIP(L) up-regulation. Leukemia. 2003;17:379–89.
167. Logan AE, Wilson TR, Fenning C, Cummins R, Kay E, Johnston PG, Longley DB. In vitro and in vivo characterisation of a novel c-FLIP-targeted antisense phosphorothioate oligonucleotide. Apoptosis. 2010;15:1435–43.
168. Youle RJ, Strasser A. The BCL-2 protein family: opposing activities that mediate cell death. Nat Rev Mol Cell Biol. 2008;9:47–59.
169. Kandasamy K, Srinivasula SM, Alnemri ES, Thompson CB, Korsmeyer SJ, Bryant JL, Srivastava RK. Involvement of proapoptotic molecules Bax and Bak in tumor necrosis factor-related apoptosis-inducing ligand (TRAIL)-induced mitochondrial disruption and apoptosis: differential regulation of cytochrome c and Smac/DIABLO release. Cancer Res. 2003;63:1712–21.
170. LeBlanc H, Lawrence D, Varfolomeev E, Totpal K, Morlan J, Schow P, Fong S, Schwall R, Sinicropi D, Ashkenazi A. Tumor-cell resistance to death receptor–induced apoptosis through mutational inactivation of the proapoptotic Bcl-2 homolog Bax. Nat Med. 2002;8:274–81.
171. Deng Y, Lin Y, Wu X. TRAIL-induced apoptosis requires Bax-dependent mitochondrial release of Smac/DIABLO. Genes Dev. 2002;16:33–45.
172. Burns TF, El-Deiry WS. Identification of inhibitors of TRAIL-induced death (ITIDs) in the TRAIL-sensitive colon carcinoma cell line SW480 using a genetic approach. J Biol Chem. 2001;276:37879–86.
173. Sinicrope FA, Penington RC, Tang XM. Tumor necrosis factor-related apoptosis-inducing ligand-induced apoptosis is inhibited by Bcl-2 but restored by the small molecule Bcl-2 inhibitor, HA 14-1, in human colon cancer cells. Clin Cancer Res. 2004;10:8284–92.
174. Fulda S, Meyer E, Debatin KM. Inhibition of TRAIL-induced apoptosis by Bcl-2 overexpression. Oncogene. 2002;21:2283–94.
175. Taniai M, Grambihler A, Higuchi H, Werneburg N, Bronk SF, Farrugia DJ, Kaufmann SH, Gores GJ. Mcl-1 mediates tumor necrosis factor-related apoptosis-inducing ligand resistance in human cholangiocarcinoma cells. Cancer Res. 2004;64:3517–24.
176. Okaro AC, Deery AR, Hutchins RR, Davidson BR. The expression of antiapoptotic proteins Bcl-2, Bcl-X(L), and Mcl-1 in benign, dysplastic, and malignant biliary epithelium. J Clin Pathol. 2001;54:927–32.
177. Clohessy JG, Zhuang J, de Boer J, Gil-Gomez G, Brady HJ. Mcl-1 interacts with truncated Bid and inhibits its induction of cytochrome c release and its role in receptor-mediated apoptosis. J Biol Chem. 2006;281:5750–9.
178. Dubrez L, Berthelet J, Glorian V. IAP proteins as targets for drug development in oncology. Onco Targets Ther. 2013;9:1285–304.

179. Deveraux QL, Takahashi R, Salvesen GS, Reed JC. X-linked IAP is a direct inhibitor of cell-death proteases. Nature. 1997;388:300–4.
180. Srinivasula SM, Hegde R, Saleh A, Datta P, Shiozaki E, Chai J, Lee RA, Robbins PD, Fernandes-Alnemri T, Shi Y, Alnemri ES. A conserved XIAP-interaction motif in caspase-9 and Smac/DIABLO regulates caspase activity and apoptosis. Nature. 2001;410:112–6.
181. Spee B, Jonkers MD, Arends B, Rutteman GR, Rothuizen J, Penning LC. Specific down-regulation of XIAP with RNA interference enhances the sensitivity of canine tumor cell-lines to TRAIL and doxorubicin. Mol Cancer. 2006;5:34.
182. Chawla-Sarkar M, Bae SI, Reu FJ, Jacobs BS, Lindner DJ, Borden EC. Downregulation of Bcl-2, FLIP or IAPs (XIAP and survivin) by siRNAs sensitizes resistant melanoma cells to Apo2L/TRAIL-induced apoptosis. Cell Death Differ. 2004;11:915–23.
183. Roa WH, Chen H, Fulton D, Gulavita S, Shaw A, Th'ng J, Farr-Jones M, Moore R, Petruk K. X-linked inhibitor regulating TRAIL-induced apoptosis in chemoresistant human primary glioblastoma cells. Clin Invest Med (Medecine clinique et experimentale). 2003;26:231–42.
184. Ng CP, Bonavida B. X-linked inhibitor of apoptosis (XIAP) blocks Apo2 ligand/tumor necrosis factor-related apoptosis-inducing ligand-mediated apoptosis of prostate cancer cells in the presence of mitochondrial activation: sensitization by overexpression of second mitochondria-derived activator of caspase/direct IAP-binding protein with low pl (Smac/DIABLO). Mol Cancer Ther. 2002;1:1051–8.
185. Jazirehi AR, Ng CP, Gan XH, Schiller G, Bonavida B. Adriamycin sensitizes the adriamycin-resistant 8226/Dox40 human multiple myeloma cells to Apo2L/tumor necrosis factor-related apoptosis-inducing ligand-mediated (TRAIL) apoptosis. Clin Cancer Res. 2001;7:3874–83.
186. Griffith TS, Kucaba TA, O'Donnell MA, Burns J, Benetatos C, McKinlay MA, Condon S, Chunduru S. Sensitization of human bladder tumor cells to TNF-related apoptosis-inducing ligand (TRAIL)-induced apoptosis with a small molecule IAP antagonist. Apoptosis. 2011;16:13–26.
187. Karikari CA, Roy I, Tryggestad E, Feldmann G, Pinilla C, Welsh K, Reed JC, Armour EP, Wong J, Herman J, Rakheja D, Maitra A. Targeting the apoptotic machinery in pancreatic cancers using small-molecule antagonists of the X-linked inhibitor of apoptosis protein. Mol Cancer Ther. 2007;6:957–66.
188. Schimmer AD, Welsh K, Pinilla C, Wang Z, Krajewska M, Bonneau MJ, Pedersen IM, Kitada S, Scott FL, Bailly-Maitre B, Glinsky G, Scudiero D, Sausville E, Salvesen G, Nefzi A, Ostresh JM, Houghten RA, Reed JC. Small-molecule antagonists of apoptosis suppressor XIAP exhibit broad antitumor activity. Cancer Cell. 2004;5:25–35.
189. Bertrand MJ, Milutinovic S, Dickson KM, Ho WC, Boudreault A, Durkin J, Gillard JW, Jaquith JB, Morris SJ, Barker PA. cIAP1 and cIAP2 facilitate cancer cell survival by functioning as E3 ligases that promote RIP1 ubiquitination. Mol Cell. 2008;30:689–700.
190. Ahn EY, Pan G, Oh JH, Tytler EM, McDonald JM. The combination of calmodulin antagonists and interferon-gamma induces apoptosis through caspase-dependent and -independent pathways in cholangiocarcinoma cells. Am J Pathol. 2003;163:2053–63.
191. Vickers SM, Jhala NC, Ahn EY, McDonald JM, Pan G, Bland KI. Tamoxifen (TMX)/Fas induced growth inhibition of human cholangiocarcinoma (HCC) by gamma interferon (IFN-gamma). Ann Surg. 2002;235:872–8.
192. Williams JP, Blair HC, McKenna MA, Jordan SE, McDonald JM. Regulation of avian osteoclastic H+ -ATPase and bone resorption by tamoxifen and calmodulin antagonists. Effects independent of steroid receptors. J Biol Chem. 1996;271:12488–95.
193. Moser MJ, Lee SY, Klevit RE, Davis TN. Ca2+ binding to calmodulin and its role in Schizosaccharomyces pombe as revealed by mutagenesis and NMR spectroscopy. J Biol Chem. 1995;270:20643–52.
194. Hait WN, Lazo JS. Calmodulin: a potential target for cancer chemotherapeutic agents. J Clin Oncol. 1986;4:994–1012.
195. Ito H, Wang JZ, Shimura K. Inhibition of lung metastasis by a calmodulin antagonist, N-(6-aminohexyl)-5-chloro-1-naphthalenesulfonamide (W-7), in mice bearing Lewis lung carcinoma. Anticancer Res. 1991;11:249–52.

196. Yang BF, Xiao C, Roa WH, Krammer PH, Hao C. Calcium/calmodulin-dependent protein kinase II regulation of c-FLIP expression and phosphorylation in modulation of Fas-mediated signaling in malignant glioma cells. J Biol Chem. 2003;278:7043–50.
197. Song JH, Bellail A, Tse MC, Yong VW, Hao C. Human astrocytes are resistant to Fas ligand and tumor necrosis factor-related apoptosis-inducing ligand-induced apoptosis. J Neurosci. 2006;26:3299–308.
198. Ahn EY, Lim ST, Cook WJ, McDonald JM. Calmodulin binding to the Fas death domain. Regulation by Fas activation. J Biol Chem. 2004;279:5661–6.
199. Wu X, Ahn EY, McKenna MA, Yeo H, McDonald JM. Fas binding to calmodulin regulates apoptosis in osteoclasts. J Biol Chem. 2005;280:29964–70.
200. Zhang XH, Wang Q, Gerald W, Hudis CA, Norton L, Smid M, Foekens JA, Massague J. Latent bone metastasis in breast cancer tied to Src-dependent survival signals. Cancer Cell. 2009;16:67–78.
201. De Toni EN, Kuntzen C, Gerbes AL, Thasler WE, Sonuc N, Mucha SR, Camaj P, Bruns C, Goke B, Eichhorst ST. P60-c-src suppresses apoptosis through inhibition of caspase 8 activation in hepatoma cells, but not in primary hepatocytes. J Hepatol. 2007;46:682–91.
202. Song JJ, Kim JH, Sun BK, Alcala Jr MA, Bartlett DL, Lee YJ. c-Cbl acts as a mediator of Src-induced activation of the PI3K-Akt signal transduction pathway during TRAIL treatment. Cell Signal. 2010;22:377–85.
203. Van SS, Kelly DM, Kyula J, Stokesberry S, Fennell DA, Johnston PG, Longley DB. Src and ADAM-17-mediated shedding of transforming growth factor-alpha is a mechanism of acute resistance to TRAIL. Cancer Res. 2008;68:8312–21.
204. Cursi S, Rufini A, Stagni V, Condo I, Matafora V, Bachi A, Bonifazi AP, Coppola L, Superti-Furga G, Testi R, Barila D. Src kinase phosphorylates caspase-8 on Tyr380: a novel mechanism of apoptosis suppression. EMBO J. 2006;25:1895–905.
205. Wu X, Balu N, Li W, Chen Y, Shi X, Kummitha CM, Yu X, Yuan C, Lu ZR. Molecular MRI of atherosclerotic plaque progression in an ApoE(−/−) mouse model with a CLT1 peptide targeted macrocyclic Gd(III) chelate. Am J Nucl Med Mol Imaging. 2013;3:446–55.
206. Rouleau M, Patel A, Hendzel MJ, Kaufmann SH, Poirier GG. PARP inhibition: PARP1 and beyond. Nat Rev Cancer. 2010;10:293–301.
207. Sodhi RK, Singh N, Jaggi AS. Poly(ADP-ribose) polymerase-1 (PARP-1) and its therapeutic implications. Vascul Pharmacol. 2010;53:77–87.
208. Gibson BA, Kraus WL. New insights into the molecular and cellular functions of poly(ADP-ribose) and PARPs. Nat Rev Mol Cell Biol. 2012;13:411–24.
209. de Murcia JM, Niedergang C, Trucco C, Ricoul M, Dutrillaux B, Mark M, Oliver FJ, Masson M, Dierich A, LeMeur M, Walztinger C, Chambon P, de Murcia MG. Requirement of poly(ADP-ribose) polymerase in recovery from DNA damage in mice and in cells. Proc Natl Acad Sci U S A. 1997;94:7303–7.
210. Samper E, Goytisolo FA, Menissier-de Murcia J, Gonzalez-Suarez E, Cigudosa JC, de Murcia G, Blasco MA. Normal telomere length and chromosomal end capping in poly(ADP-ribose) polymerase-deficient mice and primary cells despite increased chromosomal instability. J Cell Biol. 2001;154:49–60.
211. Trucco C, Oliver FJ, de Murcia G, Menissier-de Murcia J. DNA repair defect in poly(ADP-ribose) polymerase-deficient cell lines. Nucl Acids Res. 1998;26:2644–9.
212. Vodenicharov MD, Sallmann FR, Satoh MS, Poirier GG. Base excision repair is efficient in cells lacking poly(ADP-ribose) polymerase 1. Nucleic Acids Res. 2000;28:3887–96.
213. Prasad SC, Thraves PJ, Bhatia KG, Smulson ME, Dritschilo A. Enhanced poly(adenosine diphosphate ribose) polymerase activity and gene expression in Ewing's sarcoma cells. Cancer Res. 1990;50:38–43.
214. Tomoda T, Kurashige T, Moriki T, Yamamoto H, Fujimoto S, Taniguchi T. Enhanced expression of poly(ADP-ribose) synthetase gene in malignant lymphoma. Am J Hematol. 1991;37:223–7.
215. Quiles-Perez R, Munoz-Gamez JA, Ruiz-Extremera A, O'Valle F, Sanjuan-Nunez L, Martin-Alvarez AB, Martin-Oliva D, Caballero T, Munoz de Rueda P, Leon J, Gonzalez R, Muntane

J, Oliver FJ, Salmeron J. Inhibition of poly adenosine diphosphate-ribose polymerase decreases hepatocellular carcinoma growth by modulation of tumor-related gene expression. Hepatology. 2010;51:255–66.
216. Ossovskaya V, Koo IC, Kaldjian EP, Alvares C, Sherman BM. Upregulation of poly (ADP-ribose) polymerase-1 (PARP1) in triple-negative breast cancer and other primary human tumor types. Genes Cancer. 2010;1:812–21.
217. Goncalves A, Finetti P, Sabatier R, Gilabert M, Adelaide J, Borg JP, Chaffanet M, Viens P, Birnbaum D, Bertucci F. Poly(ADP-ribose) polymerase-1 mRNA expression in human breast cancer: a meta-analysis. Breast Cancer Res Treat. 2011;127:273–81.
218. Yelamos J, Farres J, Llacuna L, Ampurdanes C, Martin-Caballero J. PARP-1 and PARP-2: new players in tumour development. Am J Cancer Res. 2011;1:328–46.
219. Csete B, Lengyel Z, Kadar Z, Battyani Z. Poly(adenosine diphosphate-ribose) polymerase-1 expression in cutaneous malignant melanomas as a new molecular marker of aggressive tumor. Pathol Oncol Res. 2009;15:47–53.
220. Mangerich A, Burkle A. How to kill tumor cells with inhibitors of poly(ADP-ribosyl)ation. Int J Cancer. 2011;128:251–65.
221. Fogelman DR, Wolff RA, Kopetz S, Javle M, Bradley C, Mok I, Cabanillas F, Abbruzzese JL. Evidence for the efficacy of Iniparib, a PARP-1 inhibitor, in BRCA2-associated pancreatic cancer. Anticancer Res. 2011;31:1417–20.
222. Porcelli L, Quatrale AE, Mantuano P, Leo MG, Silvestris N, Rolland JF, Carioggia E, Lioce M, Paradiso A, Azzariti A. Optimize radiochemotherapy in pancreatic cancer: PARP inhibitors a new therapeutic opportunity. Mol Oncol. 2013;7:308–22.
223. Melisi D, Ossovskaya V, Zhu C, Rosa R, Ling J, Dougherty PM, Sherman BM, Abbruzzese JL, Chiao PJ. Oral poly(ADP-ribose) polymerase-1 inhibitor BSI-401 has antitumor activity and synergizes with oxaliplatin against pancreatic cancer, preventing acute neurotoxicity. Clin Cancer Res. 2009;15:6367–77.
224. Fong PC, Boss DS, Yap TA, Tutt A, Wu P, Mergui-Roelvink M, Mortimer P, Swaisland H, Lau A, O'Connor MJ, Ashworth A, Carmichael J, Kaye SB, Schellens JH, de Bono JS. Inhibition of poly(ADP-ribose) polymerase in tumors from BRCA mutation carriers. N Engl J Med. 2009;361:123–34.
225. Zhao Y, Sui X, Ren H. From procaspase-8 to caspase-8: revisiting structural functions of caspase-8. J Cell Physiol. 2010;225:316–20.
226. Lavrik IN, Krammer PH. Regulation of CD95/Fas signaling at the DISC. Cell Death Differ. 2012;19:36–41.

Chapter 12
Epithelial Mesenchymal Transition Influence on CTL Activity

Wilfried Engl, Virgile Viasnoff, and Jean Paul Thiery

Abstract Epithelial-mesenchymal transition (EMT) is a fundamental process orchestrating embryonic morphogenesis that also operates during carcinoma progression to promote invasion and metastasis. This review critically assesses whether EMT confers stemness, resistance to chemo- and targeted therapeutics, and immune escape. EMT inducers share common targets that alter apico-basal polarity, intercellular adhesion and the actin cytoskeleton, events that also contribute to the transdifferentiation of epithelial into mesenchymal cells. The considerable genomic heterogeneity exhibited by tumors, concomitant with their rapidly evolving subclones, is a major caveat in the success of targeted therapeutics. With the recent spectacular progress in immunotherapy for some solid tumors, one can now envision expanding upon this strategy for other tumors, pending the improved efficacy of T lymphocyte-mediated cytotoxicity. This review explores how the immunological synapse can be affected by EMT and posits how EMT reversal by kinase inhibitors could help restore a functional immunological synapse, in cooperation with antibodies abrogating immune suppression.

Keywords Epithelial-mesenchymal transition • Immunological synapse • Actin cytoskeleton

No potential conflicts of interest were disclosed.

W. Engl • V. Viasnoff
Mechanobiology Institute, National University of Singapore, Singapore, Singapore

J.P. Thiery (✉)
Department of Biochemistry, Yong Loo Lin School of Medicine, National University of Singapore, MD7, 8 Medical Drive, Singapore 117597, Singapore

Cancer Science Institute of Singapore, National University of Singapore, Singapore, Singapore

Institute of Molecular and Cell Biology, A*STAR (Agency for Science, Technology and Research), Singapore, Singapore
e-mail: bchtjp@nus.edu.sg

B. Bonavida, S. Chouaib (eds.), *Resistance of Cancer Cells to CTL-Mediated Immunotherapy*, Resistance to Targeted Anti-Cancer Therapeutics 7,
DOI 10.1007/978-3-319-17807-3_12

Abbreviations

ALDH1	Aldehyde dehydrogenase-1
APC	Antigen presenting cell
CK1	Casein kinase 1
cSMAC	Central supra-molecular activation cluster
CT	Computed tomography
CTL	Cytotoxic T lymphocyte
CTLA-4	Cytotoxic T lymphocyte associated protein 4
dSMAC	Distal supramolecular activation cluster
EGF	Epidermal growth factors
EGFR	Epidermal growth factor receptor
EMT	Epithelial-mesenchymal Transition
ERBB2	Receptor tyrosine-protein kinase
FGF	Fibroblast growth factor
GSK3b	Glycogen synthase 1
HGF	Hepatocyte growth factor
HMLE	Human mammary epithelial cell line
h-TERT	Human telomerase reverse transcriptase
ICAM-1	Intercellular adhesion molecule-1
IGF	Insulin-like growth factor
LFA-1	Lymphocyte function associated antigen-1
MAPK	Mitogen activated protein kinase
MCF7	Epithelial mammary adenocarcinoma cell line
MHC	Major histocompatibility antigen
miRNA	MicroRNAs
MRI	Magnetic resonance imaging
NSCLC	Non-small cell lung cancer
PD-1	Programmed death-1 protein
PD-1 L	Programmed death-1 protein ligand
PET	Positron emission tomography
PI3K	phosphoinositide 3-kinase
pMHCs	Peptide-bound major histocompatibility complex
PRC	Polycomb repressor complex
pSMAC	Peripheral supra-molecular activation cluster
SHP2	Tyrosine-protein phosphatase non-receptor type 11
TCR	T-cell surface receptors
TGF-β	Transforming growth factor beta
TNF-α	Tumor necrosis factor alpha
T_{reg}	Regulatory T cell
WISP2	Wnt1-inducible signaling pathway protein 2
ZAP70	Zeta-chain-associated protein kinase 70

12.1 Introduction

Carcinoma—the most predominant form of malignancy—derives from the transformation of epithelial cells; yet, decades can separate an initial oncogenic event and the formation of a clinically detectable mass. Recent deep-sequencing studies have shown that carcinomas accumulate thousands of point mutations and considerable genomic alterations [1]. Although the concept of clonal evolution is well accepted today, it now appears that primary carcinoma comprises multiple, independent clones and that metastases also exhibit considerable heterogeneity and evolve independently from the primary carcinoma; this knowledge therefore puts into question the value and validity of prognoses and therapeutic interventions that are implemented based on the histopathology and expression of markers and mutational profiles at the primary site. In addition, the number of potential driver mutations far exceeds the number of targeted therapeutics that can be used in combination to circumvent the progression of primary and metastatic tumors. The outstanding responses observed in some advanced cancers, such a melanoma and lung cancer, with B-RAF and epidermal growth factor receptor (EGFR) kinase inhibitors are not long-lasting in the majority of patients due to multiple resistance mechanisms, including de novo mutations and the activation of alternate pathways [2]. We are thus facing a considerable dilemma as to how to effectively treat the primary carcinoma, aside from surgery and radiotherapy, not-withstanding the even much more demanding treatment of the metastases.

In the neo-adjuvant setting, clinicians can explore a combination of conventional and targeted therapeutics but complete pathological is not frequently observed and a residual tumor mass needs to be surgically removed. The lines of treatment in adjuvant therapies remain more difficult to adjust since one cannot follow responses in apparently diseased-free patients based on margin-free surgical specimens and the lack of detection of disease extension by imaging. Minimal residual disease of less than 5 mm in diameter cannot be detected today even by the most advanced combined CT-PET and MRI imaging even though such a tumor mass actually represents more than 100 million carcinoma cells. Strategies to combat these rapidly evolving molecular heterogeneities must be equally effective to target all cancer cells, whatever their genetic and epigenetic statuses.

Promising results have recently been obtained in restoring the immune response in patients. In particular, one of the now well-studied mechanisms of immune modulation of cytotoxic T lymphocytes (CTLs) is initially triggered by the programmed death protein 1 (PD1), a cell surface receptor of the Ig superfamily, which, upon binding to its PD1-L ligand, becomes phosphorylated in the immunoreceptor tyrosine-based switch motif in the cytoplasmic domain. Phosphorylated PD-1 can then recruit the tyrosine phosphatase SHP-2, which deactivates the T-cell receptor (TCR)/co-receptor complex-associated tyrosine kinase ZAP70, leading to the inhibition of cytokine production and CTL clonal expansion [3]. Clinical trials based on the use of PD1 or PD1-L antibodies have shown promising clinical results for patients with cutaneous melanoma [4] as well as for those with non-small cell lung cancer (NSCLC) and renal carcinoma [5]. These patient responses have prompted multiple studies to further understand the extraordinary complexity of the immune network, which, once perturbed, unfortunately leads to major toxicities and side effects, such fatigue, rash, pruritus, diarrhea and, oftentimes, autoimmune diseases. Altering PD1-mediating tolerance has major consequences in promoting the aggressiveness of CTLs and other immune cells within the normal tissues [3, 6]. Nevertheless, knowing that all other cancer treatments exhibit serious side effects, the immunology community remains engaged in defining and undertaking more advanced preclinical studies and clinical trials to manage these side effects, which are fortunately reversible.

Aside from inhibiting T-cell responses through surface molecules, such as CTL-associated protein 4 (CTLA-4) and PD-1, numerous other mechanisms can intervene to energize the cytotoxic responses of T-lymphocytes, some of which can be intrinsic to carcinoma cells. Indeed, the cells may not present adequately the tumor antigens due to the lack of expression of the major histocompatibility complex (MHC) class 1 antigens or through defective intracellular processing of the tumor antigens [7]. Other mechanisms involve epithelial cell plasticity, which occurs in most carcinomas that have undergone dedifferentiation, a hallmark in the pathological grading system. This review briefly describes the role of Epithelial-Mesenchymal Transition (EMT) in development, a process that is likely hijacked by carcinoma cells to invade and disseminate. The review describes how EMT is induced and executed, and explores the functional consequences of EMT in carcinoma cells, particularly in terms of its effect on the functionality of the immunological synapse as a consequence of the acquisition of a mesenchymal-like phenotype. The hypothesis that carcinoma cells exhibiting a mesenchymal-like phenotype can escape immune response may result from altered dynamics of the actin cytoskeleton. Thus, the dynamic structure of the immunological synapse is reviewed, with attempts to envisage the potential mechanisms needed to restore cytotoxic functions in T-cells, possibly through an EMT reversal of mesenchymal-like carcinoma target cells.

12.2 EMT in Development

One of us previously proposed that carcinoma cells high-jack this process for their invasion and metastasis [8]. To understand the concept and significance of EMT in carcinoma, it is necessary to explain EMT in development and the predominant mechanisms involved in its induction and execution.

EMT is an evolutionarily conserved, fundamental process in embryogenesis [9] that allows immobilized epithelial cells to assume a migratory behavior as single cells and move to different territories to ultimately contribute to tissue morphogenesis. EMT is implicated in gastrulation, the most important morphogenetic step during which a primitive embryo, composed of hundreds to thousands of cells, forms the three germ layers—ectoderm, mesoderm and endoderm—to shape the body plan. The initial discoveries were made in *Drosophila*, where it was demonstrated that two transcription factors, Snail and Twist, played major roles in orchestrating these gastrulation events. Later, two orthologs of *dSnail* were linked with driving EMT during gastrulation in higher vertebrates. Snail is also implicated in the formation of the neural crest in vertebrates. Interestingly, the neural crest gives rise to various derivatives including the peripheral nervous system and melanocytes; the latter are notorious for becoming invasive and metastatic upon acquiring a malignant phenotype, resuming part of their embryonic program, which involves EMT.

12.3 EMT Inducers and Transducers

In numerous epithelial cell lines, ligands, such as hepatocyte growth factor (HGF), fibroblast growth factors (FGFs), epidermal growth factors (EGFs), insulin-like growth factors (IGFs) and transforming growth factor beta (TGF-β), have been shown to activate their cognate kinase surface receptors and promote EMT. Other factors, namely endothelin-1, interleukin 6 and tumor necrosis factor alpha (TNF-α), are also documented to initiate EMT. Activation of the canonical Ras/mitogen activated protein kinase (MAPK) pathway, Src kinase and phosphoinositide 3-kinase (PI3K) pathway have been described in multiple instances to promote the transcription of EMT drivers leading to modulation of E-cadherin-mediated intercellular adhesion and actin cytoskeleton remodeling [10]. In mammals, several classes of transcriptional repressors have been extensively described [11]. A prototypic example of the repression mechanism is provided by Snail1 and Snail2 binding to E-boxes in the E-cadherin proximal promoter, which is reinforced by the recruitment of the histone deacetylases as part of the Mi-2/nucleosome remodeling and deacetylase (NurD) complex. Snail also interacts with the histone methyltransferases, EZH2 and SUZ12, which are components of the polycomb repressor 2 (PRC2) complex and are involved in catalyzing trimethylate H3K27 repressive marks. The histone methyltransferase, G9a, can dimethylate H3K9, which is then additionally methylated by SUV39H1 to create a strong repressive mark. The recruitment of DNA methyl transferases (DNMTs) to sites of repressive H3K9me3 marks will further re-enforce E-cadherin repression. The PRC2 complex can then recruit the PRC1 complex, including BMI1, which contributes to the maintenance of the mesenchymal phenotype and stemness in carcinoma cells. Similar mechanisms operate for Zeb and Twist transcriptional repression.

Other epigenetic mechanisms include epithelial splicing regulatory proteins (ESPRs), which lead to splice variants. Furthermore, microRNAs (miRNA) offer another important layer of regulation. In particular, the miR-200 family directly inhibits EMT in a number of cell lines by targeting Zeb transcripts. miR-205 also targets Suz12 and BMI1 in addition to Zeb transcripts. Mir-34, a downstream gene of p53, can also inhibit EMT, whereas miR-9 targets E-cadherin and needs additional events to induce to EMT. Interestingly, this higher level of regulation of EMT is also subjected to epigenetic silencing. Finally, post-translational modification can affect the stability of repressors, such is the case for Snail1, which can be phosphorylated by casein kinase 1 (CK1) and by glycogen synthase 1 (GSK3b), promoting its ubiquitination and degradation [11].

12.4 How Is EMT Executed?

The signaling pathways described above induce drastic reorganization of the apico-basal polarity of normal epithelial cells as well as that of well-differentiated adenoma or in situ carcinomas, which still possess some degree of apico-basal polarity and retain intercellular adhesive structures. Tight junctions are the first structures affected at the onset of progression. These proteins are initially assembled at the apex of epithelial cells through the specific localization of the occludin and claudin tetraspan proteins, which are themselves connected with the cortical actin microfilaments through PDZ-containing adaptor proteins [12]. Most interestingly, tight junctions also recruit polarity genes and exhibit an indirect control of the Hippo pathway [13]. In one seminal study, EMT signaling, mediated by TGF-βRs localized at tight junctions, was shown to induce degradation of RhoA through the non-canonical Par6/Smurf-1 pathway and consequently destabilize the actin microfilaments [14–16]. Once an epithelial cell loses its tight junctions—especially in the context of oncogenic events such as that of p53 mutations—hyperplasia is triggered through a weakening of growth control, and this weakening has been linked to the dysregulation of the Hippo pathway and other control mechanisms of the cell cycle, ultimately inducing anoikis resistance [17].

Adherens junctions, the most critical E-cadherin mediated adhesion system in epithelial cells, are then rapidly affected, as EMT inducers target signaling nodes that affect actin microfilament dynamics [10]. Cells then lose their adherens junctions either through a direct downregulation event mediated by the aforementioned transcriptional repressors and/or through a network of newly activated kinases, such as Src kinase, which can suppress E-cadherin–actin cytoskeleton coupling and adhesion strengthening.

Finally, desmosomes, another landmark adhesive structure of epithelial cells, are destabilized, and evidence points to various mutations in essential components, such as the desmosomal cadherins and their associated cytoplasmic partners [12, 18], in hindering their reassembly.

12.5 What Are the Functional Consequences of EMT and When Does It Occurs in Carcinoma

One landmark study [19] showed that human mammary epithelial cells (HMLEs)—h-TERT (human telomerase reverse transcriptase) and SV40 large and small T antigen immortalized—can acquire stemness when induced to undergo EMT by the forced expression of Snail1 or Twist or by adding TGF-β. Most mesenchymally transitioned or 'EMTed' cells express normal mammary stem cell markers with high CD44 and low CD24 expression. Others have shown that H-RASV12-transformed HMLE cells readily acquire a mesenchymal phenotype with stem cell-like attributes [19, 20]. Fluorescence-activated cell sorted $CD44^{high}/CD24^{low}$

human breast carcinoma cells exhibit an EMTed phenotype, concomitant with a loss of E-cadherin expression, an increase in the transcriptional repressors Snail, Twist and Zeb, and expression of the classical EMT markers, Vimentin, N-cadherin and fibronectin. HMLE cells can spontaneously generate CD44^{high}/CD24^{low} stem cells from an initial population of CD44^{low}/CD24^{high} cells that lack any stem cell capacity, and it was this finding that helped to illustrate the potential for non-clonogenic mammary cells to generate stem cells under certain circumstances [21]. To further document the capacity of non-stem cells to acquire stemness, the forced expression of several combinations of transcription factors was investigated in epithelial mammary adenocarcinoma cell line (MCF7), and this, in turn, led to the discovery that the co-expression of Snail2 and Sox9 is sufficient to engender stem cell properties [22]. Recent investigations, however, have identified two types of stem cells in the normal mammary gland and in breast carcinoma [23]: one exhibits similar mesenchymal-like properties as those described above and are CD44^{high}/CD24^{low}, whereas another population exhibits an epithelial phenotype and expresses aldehyde dehydrogenase-1 (ALDH1), another stem cell marker. Remarkably, the two stem cell compartments can be interconverted, at least in vitro. These studies stress that stem cells exhibit remarkable plasticity and can be potentially generated from a non-stem cell compartment. Thus, the theory that stem cells form a stable population with low proliferative capacity and can accumulate more mutations than the rapidly cycling cancer cells with a finite life span may need to be revisited. This is a crucial issue with regard to therapeutic strategies that aim to eliminate stem cells specifically, as these cells appear capable of re-emerging from a non-stem cell population and therefore may not be completely eliminated during treatment.

Another note of caution is that EMT may not necessarily engender stemness but may only favor carcinoma cell dissemination. The transcription factor Prrx1, a homeobox protein expressed in the early embryonic stage, can affect EMT in the paraxial mesoderm in a manner that is independent of Snail activity [24]. Such transcription can promote invasion and the formation of micrometastases but it would need to be downregulated for secondary tumors to develop, indicating that EMT and the acquisition of stemness may be uncoupled. EMT reversal was hypothesized to allow for secondary carcinoma formation [8], and this hypothesis was vindicated in an experimental model analyzing the behavior of carcinogen-induced primary squamous skin carcinoma using a Twist-inducible system [25]. Thus, the spatiotemporal regulation of EMT is essential for squamous cell carcinoma metastasis.

12.6 EMT Confers Resistance to Chemotherapeutics and to Targeted Therapeutics

Multiple mechanisms have been described to confer drug resistance in cancer cells. Drug resistance can be elicited by rapid efflux, metabolic inactivation, mutations of the target, DNA damage repair, and escape from apoptosis [2]. EMT may also induce refractoriness in carcinoma acquiring a mesenchymal phenotype, as observed in sarcoma. Numerous studies have emphasized that EMT acquisition can account for resistance to targeted therapeutics, such as in NSCLC and prostate cancer [26]. However, the documentation that EMT will promote resistance is often circumstantial and not fully elucidated. Epithelial carcinoma cells that are chronically exposed to chemotherapeutic agents can progressively acquire a mesenchymal phenotype; however, in many established cell lines exhibiting a mesenchymal phenotype, the drug GI50 values do not always mirror an increase in resistance [27]. Tan and colleagues recently established a specific and generic EMT scoring method for tumors and their corresponding cell lines [28], wherein a systemic survey of the drug GI50 was undertaken to determine the extent to which the EMT score correlated with increased drug resistance. They showed a correlation in particular tumor types or molecular subtypes for certain drugs, but an anti-correlation was also found for other drugs in the same or other tumor types. This study, in addition to many other studies, reflects the extraordinary complexity of drug resistance, which is further compounded by the comparisons of innate or acquired resistance in these tumors.

12.7 EMT Can Induce Immune Escape

In 2009, a pioneering study by Kudo-Saito and colleagues showed that the forced expression of Snail1 could induce an EMT-like mechanism in B16F10 melanoma cells, which are not epithelial but express E-cadherin [29]. Co-culture of spleen cells with the B16F10 Snail-expressing cells revealed an induction of Foxp3 in the regulatory $CD4^{+}CD25^{-}$ T cell population (T_{reg}); this occurred as a result of the presence of impaired antigen-presenting dendritic cells (APCs) generated through direct contact with these Snail-expressing B16F10 cells. Similarly, in syngeneic mice, the primary tumors of mock-transfected B16F10 melanomas became infiltrated by CTLs following injection of dendritic cells whereas the Snail-expressing melanomas induced $CD4^{+}Foxp3^{+}$ T_{reg} cells and was thus able to abrogate dendritic cell responses.

CTL lysis is also inhibited in MCF7 cells that are rendered mesenchymal through the forced expression of wild-type, constitutively activated Snail1 or following long-term exposure to TNFα [30]. The immunological synapse of the mesenchymal-like MCF7 cell line seems defective, as shown by its morphology and phosphorylation status. Immune escape was also associated with activation of an autophagic program, which may contribute to promoting survival in these cells. Perturbing the secreted protein WISP2 (Wnt1-inducible signaling pathway protein 2) also leads to the acquisition of a mesenchymal phenotype, and WISP2 knockdown was shown to activate the TGFβR pathway, a much lower expression of miR-7-5b, and a higher expression of the stem cell transcription factor KLF4, one of its target genes. Carcinoma cells expressing KLF4, TGFβ, Smad2/3 and Twist have been detected in basal-like breast cancer, and the expression of these proteins possibly contributes to the immune escape in these cells [31]. The lack of a functional immunological synapse may be in part due to diminished antigen presentation, but it also likely results from defective cortical machinery in the post-synaptic cytoplasmic domain, reminiscent of the mechanism described above for Snail-expressing or TNFα-treated MCF7 cells [32].

12.8 Genesis of an EMT Phenotype in Primary Tumors

Tumors of different histotypes exhibit a wide spectrum of EMT scores [28], and this EMT spectrum has been broadly classified previously as four categories: epithelial, intermediate-epithelial, intermediate-mesenchymal and mesenchymal [33]. However, this scoring method provides only an average value of the EMT score of a particular carcinoma and its stroma. For example, laser-microdissection of specific breast tumor sections, of which there are known to be five molecular subtypes (Luminal A, Luminal B, ERBB2-positive, Claudin-low and Basal) was undertaken to eliminate this stromal cell component. The dissected tumors in the Luminal A, Luminal B and ERBB2 subtypes demonstrated relatively more epithelial-like scores as compared with those for their non-dissected counterparts, whereas the Basal subtype was more mesenchymal-like than the three other molecular subtypes. Remarkably, the Claudin-low subtype retained a very high EMT score after microdissection, with a high EMT score indicative of a more mesenchymal phenotype [28].

Nonetheless, these scores—microdissected or not—still only offer a global score of the tumor. To investigate EMT scoring at the level of single cells, tissue microarray analyses comprising 500 breast samples (representing all molecular subtypes) were performed using a panel of 28 epithelial and mesenchymal markers, and, more recently, in situ hybridization was carried out to identify cells potentially engaged in EMT. Together, the results of the two studies point toward the presence of approximately 3 % of intermediate-mesenchymal and mesenchymal-like carcinoma cells in Luminal-type tumors and 11 % in basal-like tumors [34, 35].

Also at the cellular level, studies have elucidated that a significantly high percentage of circulating tumors cells (CTCs) exhibit a mesenchymal-like phenotype [35, 36]. CTCs are derived from either primary or metastatic tumors as single cells or cell clusters, and these cells tend to display a partial or complete EMTed phenotype. The mechanisms by which EMT is induced prior to the release of CTCs into the blood stream may involve the local induction by stromal cells, such as macrophages [37] or bone marrow-derived cells [38], or hypoxic environmental conditions [7]. EMT can also occur in these cells while in the circulation, presumably through their interactions with platelets in microemboli [39, 40].

12.9 Immunological Synapse Biomechanics

T-cell activation and function require physical contact with APCs. T-cells are highly motile cells that are constantly in transit throughout the tissues. T-cell surface receptors (TCR) continually scan the APCs for antigenic peptides bound to the MHC (pMHC). As few as 10 pMHCs are capable of actuating a T-cell response [41]. The type and amount of information that is exchanged between T-cells and APCs is determined by the duration of the interaction, the identity of the receptors/signaling molecules engaged and recruited, the strength of the signals transmitted, and the presence or absence of secretion [42]. These diverse interaction modes might define a molecular code, in which the differences in timing, spacing and molecular composition of the signaling platform determine the outcome of T-cell–APC interactions.

12.9.1 Architecture of the Immunological Synapse

Formation of the immunological synapse results from a close coordination between the actin cytoskeleton, the pMHC–TCR interactions, and integrin-based adhesion signaling that occurs between LFA-1 (lymphocyte function associated antigen-1) on the T-cell and ICAM-1 (intercellular adhesion molecule-1) on the APC.

In a first phase, the T-cell must transform rapidly, changing from loosely adherent and highly motile to a tightly and arrested cell in a matter of seconds. The plasma membranes of both T-cells and APCs are coated with glycocalyx, a layer consisting of large glycoproteins and proteoglycans [43] that creates a repulsive barrier between these two cells. To counteract this steric hindrance, integrin-based adhesion must bring the two cell membranes within 40 nm of each other. Induction of invasive pseudopodia [44] can further reduce the distance between opposing membranes down to 15 nm and thus can promote TCR binding to the pMHC complex. In inactivated T-cells, LFA-1 is held in a state of low affinity with its ligand. However, during pMHC–TCR ligation, integrins undergo conformational changes mediated by cytoplasmic proteins that link integrins with the actin cytoskeleton. This process increases the affinity and avidity of integrins with their ligands [45].

TCR triggering leads to the rapid nucleation of F-actin, which is coupled to various adaptor molecules downstream of TCRs. In turn, this signaling favors the coalescence of TCRs into stable "microclusters" that are actively engaged in signaling [46, 47]. As a result, the actin cytoskeleton has a supportive role in promoting a continued signaling wherein the motile T-cell becomes sessile and engages the APC for a longer duration. Upon TCR signaling, a reduction in RhoA activity and an increase in Rac1 activity suppress the polarized state of the motile T-cell [48]. In addition, Ca^{2+} is released from endoplasmic reticulum [49, 50], and this induces Ca^{2+}-modulated actin-binding proteins to globally reduce the cortical tension and collapse the uropod-like structure.

At this stage, the T-cell is spreading and a mature immunological synapse appears within approximately 30 min for naïve T cells and 1–3 min for T-cell blasts after initial T-cell-APC contact [51]; this synapse might persist for as long as 20 h depending on the nature of the T-cell [52]. Various cell surface receptors, including TCR and LFA-1, are ultimately segregated. The TCR microclusters translocate centripetally and fuse into the zone of central supra-molecular activation cluster (cSMAC). Interestingly, PD-1 is associated with these microclusters and it thus very effectively transduces inhibitory signals through a SHP2-mediated dephosphorylation of the proximal TCR-associated transducers [53]. LFA-1 clusters, on the other hand, are organized around the cSMAC to form a highly contractile zone, known as the peripheral SMAC (pSMAC).

Immunological synapse formation is concomitant with the dramatic induction of polarization of several organelles, such as the Golgi apparatus (GA), mitochondria and the endoplasmic reticulum. A key event is the movement of the centrosome right up to the membrane at the edge of the cSMAC [54–56]. The centrosome rapidly polymerizes α/β tubulin dimers in microtubules [57], and these organize a profuse radial network of microtubules at the T-cell–APC contact area [57, 58]. This dynamic network provides a platform for intracellular transport [59] and promotes TCR microcluster translocation towards the cSMAC in a dynein-dependent manner. The reorientation of the GA and associated vesicles depends on the correct localization of the centrosome at the immunological synapse, thereby favoring the polarized secretion of cytokines and microvesicles. In cSMAC, receptors are targeted for degradation [47] and the immunological synapse will then be terminated when its symmetry is destroyed [60].

12.9.2 Actin Dynamics, Force Generation and Mechanosensing

Dynamic rearrangements of the actin cytoskeleton are necessary for the various effective functions of immune cells (Fig. 12.1). They provide powerful mechanical forces by which immune cells can migrate, polarize, and exert effector functions.

During immunological synapse formation, cells must overcome the repulsion that is present as a result of the negative charges on their surface as well as the protective layer of glycocalyx that hinders the interaction of relatively small surface molecules, such as TCR or pMHC. This ability to overcome repulsion is achieved by invasive pseudopodia. Using high-resolution microscopy on T-helper cells, Ueda and co-workers visualized pseudopodia that penetrated deeply into the APC and almost reaching the nuclear envelope; this penetration occurred without damaging either of the cell membranes [52]. This event may involve considerable force and might help to increase the surface area between the two cells. This allows more TCR-pMHC conjugates to form and a full response to be initiated.

Upon engagement of the TCR, the T-cell starts to reorganize its actin cytoskeleton. The radial actin polymerization forms a lamellipodia over the APC increasing the contact area. In many cases, actin regulation is overlapped between different

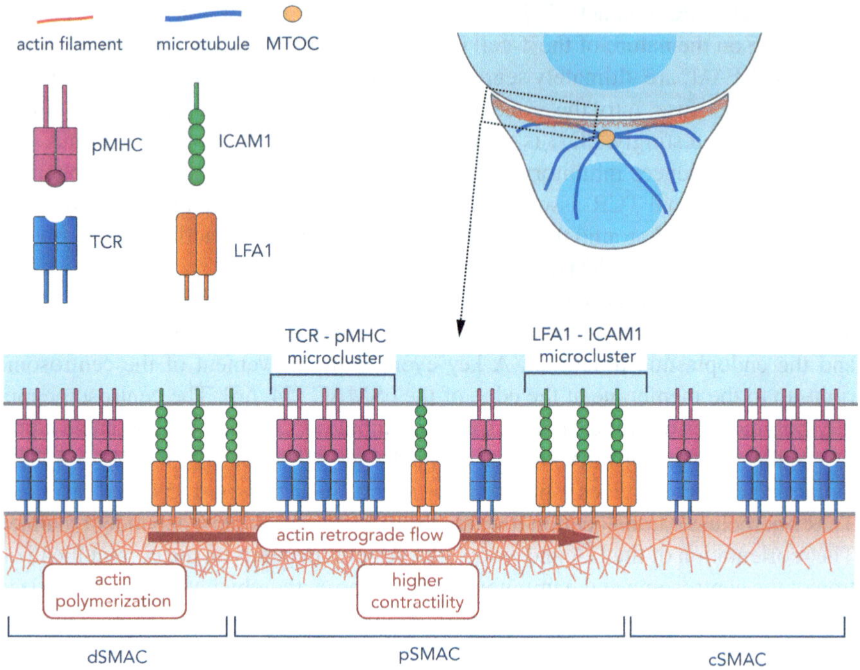

Fig. 12.1 Initiation and maturation of the immunological synapse. Localization of the different F-actin structures with a predominance of actomyosin in the peripheral supra-molecular activation cluster (pSMAC) and the actin-rich distal supramolecular activation cluster dSMAC [76]. Both of the pMHC–TCR (peptide-bound major histocompatibility complex–T cell receptor) and LFA1–ICAM1 (lymphocyte function associated antigen-1–intercellular adhesion molecule-1) complexes are carried centripetally by the actin retrograde flow. The formation of the immunological synapse induces polarization of several organelles, such as the Golgi apparatus, mitochondria, the endoplasmic reticulum, and the centrosome

processes in the cell. Here, both the formation of lamellipodia during rapid migration and actin reorganization at the T cell-APC interface are similar processes in terms of cytoskeletal rearrangements, as common actin regulators are recruited [61, 62]. After the area reaches its maximal size, the F-actin layer beneath the contact zone continues to undergo polymerization at the edge, which results in centripetal actin flow driving TCR microcluster migration. Genetic manipulation of the actin polymerization effectors yields significantly affects T cell activation, and F-actin severing proteins have also been reported to be crucial for T-cell function [63]. Thus, actin dynamics at the T-cell synapse are tightly regulated to achieve optimal T-cell function.

An increasing number of models propose that biomechanical processes are the driving forces behind T cell activation. Using a biomembrane force probe, Husson et al. [64] demonstrated that, upon engagement of TCR alone, T-cells generate a reproducible sequence of pushing and pulling forces, with the pushing phase supported by actin polymerization. The pulling phase, by comparison, might constitute an additional level for the cell to evaluate the "quality" of the contact formed. It is also now accepted [65, 66] that force loads modulate the molecular interactions, in particular, through exponentially shifting dissociation constants. Indeed, several studies by different groups have shown that applying mechanical forces to the TCR can activate T-cells and that the TCR can act as a mechanosensor: Lateral forces applied to the TCR were able to trigger an elevation in cytoplasmic Ca^{2+} [67] whereas axial forces applied by micro-manipulation were able to rescue T-cell stimulating defects associated with elongated pMHCs [68]. Moreover, in mouse [69] and human [70] studies, T-cells displayed correlations between substrate stiffness and T-cell response.

12.9.3 Mesenchymal-Like Carcinoma Can Alter the Cortical Actin Dynamics of CTL During the Ontogeny of the Immunological Synapse

As described above, following initial recognition by the TCR, adhesive contact in an immunological synapse is initiated, in part, by the heterophilic interaction between LFA-1 and ICAM-1, which is, in turn, strengthened by the subsequent coupling of this complex with a stable actin network. LFA-1 can interact indirectly with cortical actin microfilaments through Talin, and I-CAM through Ezrin. This adhesive structure, which assembles at the periphery of the immunological synapse, can constitute a platform for ensuring the subsequent maturation events of the immunological synapse. The external ring of adhesion is reminiscent of the cadherin-mediated adhesion structure that assembles in cell doublets in suspension [71]. These E-cadherin microclusters that are assembling at the onset of cell-cell contact rapidly migrate to the periphery of the contact area and develop into tight cadherin clusters equally spaced on a ring-like structure. This process is entirely dependent on acto-myosin contractility.

To form a stable ring, the two cells should be equally effective in their ability to form cadherin microclusters that are appropriately linked and stabilized with actin microfilaments. Indeed, the ring structure cannot form when one of these cell partners expresses a defective, truncated cadherin that is unable to engage into adhesion strengthening; this has been clearly shown by measuring the force of separation of cells [72]. Thus, we hypothesize that if the target carcinoma has a more mesenchymal-like morphology, the cells could be refractory to establishing a pSMAC ring when interacting with a CTL, and this, consequently, could affect the formation of the cSMAC and its lysis of the target. Clearly, this hypothesis needs to take into account the many other features of the immunological synapse and, in particular, the polarization of organelles. It is noteworthy that epithelial cells transform their putative adhesive rings as a circumferential belt promoting the final stage of polarization of their basal polarity plasma membrane domains and organelles.

Further studies will allow us to address the quality and dynamics of critical actin cytoskeleton-associated proteins [73], ascertain the associated molecular machinery that could become partially defective in carcinoma cells undergoing EMT, and how this defect can prevent the maturation of the immunological synapse.

12.10 Conclusion

This brief review emphasizes the critical role of EMT is the progression of carcinoma and the potential to improve the functional activity through EMT reversal drug-mediated strategies [74]. On-going experiments in breast, lung and ovarian carcinoma cell lines show the potential of kinase inhibitors to revert partially the EMT phenotype, which is hoped to reduce the invasion and clonogenic properties of these cells [28, 31, 33, 75].

Acknowledgements The authors would like to thank Rebecca Anne Jackson for her excellent editing. JP Thiery is supported by core grants from IMCB and NUS.

References

1. Nik-Zainal S, Van Loo P, Wedge DC, Alexandrov LB, Greenman CD, Lau KW, Raine K, Jones D, Marshall J, Ramakrishna M, Shlien A, Cooke SL, Hinton J, Menzies A, Stebbings LA, Leroy C, Jia M, Rance R, Mudie LJ, Gamble SJ, Stephens PJ, McLaren S, Tarpey PS, Papaemmanuil E, Davies HR, Varela I, McBride DJ, Bignell GR, Leung K, Butler AP, Teague JW, Martin S, Jonsson G, Mariani O, Boyault S, Miron P, Fatima A, Langerod A, Aparicio SA, Tutt A, Sieuwerts AM, Borg A, Thomas G, Salomon AV, Richardson AL, Borresen-Dale AL, Futreal PA, Stratton MR, Campbell PJ, Breast Cancer Working Group of the International Cancer Genome C. The life history of 21 breast cancers. Cell. 2012;149:994–1007.
2. Holohan C, Van Schaeybroeck S, Longley DB, Johnston PG. Cancer drug resistance: an evolving paradigm. Nat Rev Cancer. 2013;13:714–26.
3. Okazaki T, Chikuma S, Iwai Y, Fagarasan S, Honjo T. A rheostat for immune responses: the unique properties of PD-1 and their advantages for clinical application. Nat Immunol. 2013; 14:1212–8.
4. Eggermont AM, Spatz A, Robert C. Cutaneous melanoma. Lancet. 2014;383:816–27.
5. Topalian SL, Hodi FS, Brahmer JR, Gettinger SN, Smith DC, McDermott DF, Powderly JD, Carvajal RD, Sosman JA, Atkins MB, Leming PD, Spigel DR, Antonia SJ, Horn L, Drake CG, Pardoll DM, Chen L, Sharfman WH, Anders RA, Taube JM, McMiller TL, Xu H, Korman AJ, Jure-Kunkel M, Agrawal S, McDonald D, Kollia GD, Gupta A, Wigginton JM, Sznol M. Safety, activity, and immune correlates of anti-PD-1 antibody in cancer. N Engl J Med. 2012;366:2443–54.
6. Gangadhar TC, Vonderheide RH. Mitigating the toxic effects of anticancer immunotherapy. Nat Rev Clin Oncol. 2014;11:91–9.
7. Noman MZ, Messai Y, Muret J, Hasmim M, Chouaib S. Crosstalk between CTC, immune system and hypoxic tumor microenvironment. Cancer Microenviron. 2014;7:153–60.
8. Thiery JP. Epithelial-mesenchymal transitions in tumour progression. Nat Rev Cancer. 2002;2:442–54.

9. Lim J, Thiery JP. Epithelial-mesenchymal transitions: insights from development. Development. 2012;139:3471–86.
10. Thiery JP, Sleeman JP. Complex networks orchestrate epithelial-mesenchymal transitions. Nat Rev Mol Cell Biol. 2006;7:131–42.
11. De Craene B, Berx G. Regulatory networks defining EMT during cancer initiation and progression. Nat Rev Cancer. 2013;13:97–110.
12. Huang RY, Guilford P, Thiery JP. Early events in cell adhesion and polarity during epithelial-mesenchymal transition. J Cell Sci. 2012;125:4417–22.
13. Gumbiner BM, Kim NG. The Hippo-YAP signaling pathway and contact inhibition of growth. J Cell Sci. 2014;127:709–17.
14. Barrios-Rodiles M, Brown KR, Ozdamar B, Bose R, Liu Z, Donovan RS, Shinjo F, Liu Y, Dembowy J, Taylor IW, Luga V, Przulj N, Robinson M, Suzuki H, Hayashizaki Y, Jurisica I, Wrana JL. High-throughput mapping of a dynamic signaling network in mammalian cells. Science. 2005;307:1621–5.
15. Ozdamar B, Bose R, Barrios-Rodiles M, Wang HR, Zhang Y, Wrana JL. Regulation of the polarity protein Par6 by TGFbeta receptors controls epithelial cell plasticity. Science. 2005;307:1603–9.
16. Thiery JP, Huang R. Linking epithelial-mesenchymal transition to the well-known polarity protein Par6. Dev Cell. 2005;8:456–8.
17. Zhao B, Li L, Wang L, Wang CY, Yu J, Guan KL. Cell detachment activates the Hippo pathway via cytoskeleton reorganization to induce anoikis. Genes Dev. 2012;26:54–68.
18. Thomason HA, Scothern A, McHarg S, Garrod DR. Desmosomes: adhesive strength and signalling in health and disease. Biochem J. 2010;429:419–33.
19. Mani SA, Guo W, Liao MJ, Eaton EN, Ayyanan A, Zhou AY, Brooks M, Reinhard F, Zhang CC, Shipitsin M, Campbell LL, Polyak K, Brisken C, Yang J, Weinberg RA. The epithelial-mesenchymal transition generates cells with properties of stem cells. Cell. 2008;133:704–15.
20. Morel AP, Lievre M, Thomas C, Hinkal G, Ansieau S, Puisieux A. Generation of breast cancer stem cells through epithelial-mesenchymal transition. PLoS One. 2008;3:e2888.
21. Chaffer CL, Brueckmann I, Scheel C, Kaestli AJ, Wiggins PA, Rodrigues LO, Brooks M, Reinhardt F, Su Y, Polyak K, Arendt LM, Kuperwasser C, Bierie B, Weinberg RA. Normal and neoplastic nonstem cells can spontaneously convert to a stem-like state. Proc Natl Acad Sci U S A. 2011;108:7950–5.
22. Guo W, Keckesova Z, Donaher JL, Shibue T, Tischler V, Reinhardt F, Itzkovitz S, Noske A, Zurrer-Hardi U, Bell G, Tam WL, Mani SA, van Oudenaarden A, Weinberg RA. Slug and Sox9 cooperatively determine the mammary stem cell state. Cell. 2012;148:1015–28.
23. Liu S, Cong Y, Wang D, Sun Y, Deng L, Liu Y, Martin-Trevino R, Shang L, McDermott SP, Landis MD, Hong S, Adams A, D'Angelo R, Ginestier C, Charafe-Jauffret E, Clouthier SG, Birnbaum D, Wong ST, Zhan M, Chang JC, Wicha MS. Breast cancer stem cells transition between epithelial and mesenchymal states reflective of their normal counterparts. Stem Cell Rep. 2014;2:78–91.
24. Ocana OH, Corcoles R, Fabra A, Moreno-Bueno G, Acloque H, Vega S, Barrallo-Gimeno A, Cano A, Nieto MA. Metastatic colonization requires the repression of the epithelial-mesenchymal transition inducer Prrx1. Cancer Cell. 2012;22:709–24.
25. Tsai JH, Donaher JL, Murphy DA, Chau S, Yang J. Spatiotemporal regulation of epithelial-mesenchymal transition is essential for squamous cell carcinoma metastasis. Cancer Cell. 2012;22:725–36.
26. Lackner MR, Wilson TR, Settleman J. Mechanisms of acquired resistance to targeted cancer therapies. Future Oncol. 2012;8:999–1014.
27. Miow QH, Tan TZ, Ye J, Lau JA, Yokomizo T, Thiery JP, Mori S. Epithelial-mesenchymal status renders differential responses to cisplatin in ovarian cancer. Oncogene. 2015;34:1899–907. doi:10.1038/onc.2014.136.
28. Tan TZ, Miow QH, Miki Y, Noda T, Mori S, Huang RY, Thiery JP. Epithelial-mesenchymal transition spectrum quantification and its efficacy in deciphering survival and drug responses of cancer patients. EMBO Mol Med. 2014;6:1279–93.

29. Kudo-Saito C, Shirako H, Takeuchi T, Kawakami Y. Cancer metastasis is accelerated through immunosuppression during Snail-induced EMT of cancer cells. Cancer Cell. 2009;15: 195–206.
30. Akalay I, Janji B, Hasmim M, Noman MZ, Andre F, De Cremoux P, Bertheau P, Badoual C, Vielh P, Larsen AK, Sabbah M, Tan TZ, Keira JH, Hung NT, Thiery JP, Mami-Chouaib F, Chouaib S. Epithelial-to-mesenchymal transition and autophagy induction in breast carcinoma promote escape from T-cell-mediated lysis. Cancer Res. 2013;73:2418–27.
31. Akalay I, Tan TZ, Kumar P, Janji B, Mami-Chouaib F, Charpy C, Vielh P, Larsen AK, Thiery JP, Sabbah M, Chouaib S. Targeting WNT1-inducible signaling pathway protein 2 alters human breast cancer cell susceptibility to specific lysis through regulation of KLF-4 and miR-7 expression. Oncogene. 2014;0. doi: 10.1038/onc.2014.151.
32. Chouaib S, Janji B, Tittarelli A, Eggermont A, Thiery JP. Tumor plasticity interferes with anti-tumor immunity. Crit Rev Immunol. 2014;34:91–102.
33. Huang RY, Wong MK, Tan TZ, Kuay KT, Ng AH, Chung VY, Chu YS, Matsumura N, Lai HC, Lee YF, Sim WJ, Chai C, Pietschmann E, Mori S, Low JJ, Choolani M, Thiery JP. An EMT spectrum defines an anoikis-resistant and spheroidogenic intermediate mesenchymal state that is sensitive to e-cadherin restoration by a src-kinase inhibitor, saracatinib (AZD0530). Cell Death Dis. 2013;4:e915.
34. Sarrio D, Rodriguez-Pinilla SM, Hardisson D, Cano A, Moreno-Bueno G, Palacios J. Epithelial-mesenchymal transition in breast cancer relates to the basal-like phenotype. Cancer Res. 2008;68:989–97.
35. Yu M, Bardia A, Wittner BS, Stott SL, Smas ME, Ting DT, Isakoff SJ, Ciciliano JC, Wells MN, Shah AM, Concannon KF, Donaldson MC, Sequist LV, Brachtel E, Sgroi D, Baselga J, Ramaswamy S, Toner M, Haber DA, Maheswaran S. Circulating breast tumor cells exhibit dynamic changes in epithelial and mesenchymal composition. Science. 2013;339:580–4.
36. Khoo BL, Lee SC, Kumar P, Tan TZ, Warkiani ME, Ow SG, Nandi S, Lim CT, Thiery JP. Expansion of breast circulating cancer cells predicts response to anti-cancer therapy. EMBO Mol Med. 2014 (in press).
37. Goswami S, Sahai E, Wyckoff JB, Cammer M, Cox D, Pixley FJ, Stanley ER, Segall JE, Condeelis JS. Macrophages promote the invasion of breast carcinoma cells via a colony-stimulating factor-1/epidermal growth factor paracrine loop. Cancer Res. 2005;65:5278–83.
38. Toh B, Wang X, Keeble J, Sim WJ, Khoo K, Wong WC, Kato M, Prevost-Blondel A, Thiery JP, Abastado JP. Mesenchymal transition and dissemination of cancer cells is driven by myeloid-derived suppressor cells infiltrating the primary tumor. PLoS Biol. 2011;9:e1001162.
39. Labelle M, Hynes RO. The initial hours of metastasis: the importance of cooperative host-tumor cell interactions during hematogenous dissemination. Cancer Discov. 2012;2:1091–9.
40. Thiery JP, Lim CT. Tumor dissemination: an EMT affair. Cancer Cell. 2013;23:272–3.
41. Irvine DJ, Purbhoo MA, Krogsgaard M, Davis MM. Direct observation of ligand recognition by T cells. Nature. 2002;419:845–9.
42. Kumari S, Curado S, Mayya V, Dustin ML. T cell antigen receptor activation and actin cyto-skeleton remodeling. Biochim Biophys Acta. 1838;2014:546–56.
43. Cyster JG, Shotton DM, Williams AF. The dimensions of the T lymphocyte glycoprotein leu-kosialin and identification of linear protein epitopes that can be modified by glycosylation. EMBO J. 1991;10:893–902.
44. Sage PT, Varghese LM, Martinelli R, Sciuto TE, Kamei M, Dvorak AM, Springer TA, Sharpe AH, Carman CV. Antigen recognition is facilitated by invadosome-like protrusions formed by memory/effector T cells. J Immunol. 2012;188:3686–99.
45. Hogg N, Patzak I, Willenbrock F. The insider's guide to leukocyte integrin signalling and function. Nat Rev Immunol. 2011;11:416–26.
46. Campi G, Varma R, Dustin ML. Actin and agonist MHC-peptide complex-dependent T cell receptor microclusters as scaffolds for signaling. J Exp Med. 2005;202:1031–6.
47. Varma R, Campi G, Yokosuka T, Saito T, Dustin ML. T cell receptor-proximal signals are sustained in peripheral microclusters and terminated in the central supramolecular activation cluster. Immunity. 2006;25:117–27.

48. Cernuda-Morollon E, Millan J, Shipman M, Marelli-Berg FM, Ridley AJ. Rac activation by the T-cell receptor inhibits T cell migration. PLoS One. 2010;5:e12393.
49. Bhakta NR, Oh DY, Lewis RS. Calcium oscillations regulate thymocyte motility during positive selection in the three-dimensional thymic environment. Nat Immunol. 2005;6:143–51.
50. Skokos D, Shakhar G, Varma R, Waite JC, Cameron TO, Lindquist RL, Schwickert T, Nussenzweig MC, Dustin ML. Peptide-MHC potency governs dynamic interactions between T cells and dendritic cells in lymph nodes. Nat Immunol. 2007;8:835–44.
51. Lee KH, Holdorf AD, Dustin ML, Chan AC, Allen PM, Shaw AS. T cell receptor signaling precedes immunological synapse formation. Science. 2002;295:1539–42.
52. Iezzi G, Karjalainen K, Lanzavecchia A. The duration of antigenic stimulation determines the fate of naive and effector T cells. Immunity. 1998;8:89–95.
53. Yokosuka T, Takamatsu M, Kobayashi-Imanishi W, Hashimoto-Tane A, Azuma M, Saito T. Programmed cell death 1 forms negative costimulatory microclusters that directly inhibit T cell receptor signaling by recruiting phosphatase SHP2. J Exp Med. 2012;209:1201–17.
54. Stinchcombe JC, Majorovits E, Bossi G, Fuller S, Griffiths GM. Centrosome polarization delivers secretory granules to the immunological synapse. Nature. 2006;443:462–5.
55. Stinchcombe JC, Salio M, Cerundolo V, Pende D, Arico M, Griffiths GM. Centriole polarisation to the immunological synapse directs secretion from cytolytic cells of both the innate and adaptive immune systems. BMC Biol. 2011;9:45.
56. Ueda H, Morphew MK, McIntosh JR, Davis MM. CD4+ T-cell synapses involve multiple distinct stages. Proc Natl Acad Sci U S A. 2011;108:17099–104.
57. Martin-Cofreces NB, Baixauli F, Lopez MJ, Gil D, Monjas A, Alarcon B, Sanchez-Madrid F. End-binding protein 1 controls signal propagation from the T cell receptor. EMBO J. 2012; 31:4140–52.
58. Lasserre R, Cuche C, Blecher-Gonen R, Libman E, Biquand E, Danckaert A, Yablonski D, Alcover A, Di Bartolo V. Release of serine/threonine-phosphorylated adaptors from signaling microclusters down-regulates T cell activation. J Cell Biol. 2011;195:839–53.
59. Lasserre R, Charrin S, Cuche C, Danckaert A, Thoulouze MI, de Chaumont F, Duong T, Perrault N, Varin-Blank N, Olivo-Marin JC, Etienne-Manneville S, Arpin M, Di Bartolo V, Alcover A. Ezrin tunes T-cell activation by controlling Dlg1 and microtubule positioning at the immunological synapse. EMBO J. 2010;29:2301–14.
60. Dustin ML. T-cell activation through immunological synapses and kinapses. Immunol Rev. 2008;221:77–89.
61. Hamon M, Bierne H, Cossart P. Listeria monocytogenes: a multifaceted model. Nat Rev Microbiol. 2006;4:423–34.
62. Veiga E, Cossart P. Listeria hijacks the clathrin-dependent endocytic machinery to invade mammalian cells. Nat Cell Biol. 2005;7:894–900.
63. Eibert SM, Lee KH, Pipkorn R, Sester U, Wabnitz GH, Giese T, Meuer SC, Samstag Y. Cofilin peptide homologs interfere with immunological synapse formation and T cell activation. Proc Natl Acad Sci U S A. 2004;101:1957–62.
64. Husson J, Chemin K, Bohineust A, Hivroz C, Henry N. Force generation upon T cell receptor engagement. PLoS One. 2011;6:e19680.
65. Bell GI. Models for the specific adhesion of cells to cells. Science. 1978;200:618–27.
66. Evans E. Probing the relation between force–lifetime–and chemistry in single molecular bonds. Annu Rev Biophys Biomol Struct. 2001;30:105–28.
67. Kim ST, Takeuchi K, Sun ZY, Touma M, Castro CE, Fahmy A, Lang MJ, Wagner G, Reinherz EL. The alphabeta T cell receptor is an anisotropic mechanosensor. J Biol Chem. 2009;284:31028–37.
68. Li YC, Chen BM, Wu PC, Cheng TL, Kao LS, Tao MH, Lieber A, Roffler SR. Cutting edge: mechanical forces acting on T cells immobilized via the TCR complex can trigger TCR signaling. J Immunol. 2010;184:5959–63.
69. Judokusumo E, Tabdanov E, Kumari S, Dustin ML, Kam LC. Mechanosensing in T lymphocyte activation. Biophys J. 2012;102:L5–7.

70. O'Connor RS, Hao X, Shen K, Bashour K, Akimova T, Hancock WW, Kam LC, Milone MC. Substrate rigidity regulates human T cell activation and proliferation. J Immunol. 2012; 189:1330–9.
71. Engl W, Arasi B, Yap LL, Thiery JP, Viasnoff V. Actin dynamics modulate mechanosensitive immobilization of E-cadherin at adherens junctions. Nat Cell Biol. 2014;16:587–94.
72. Chu YS, Thomas WA, Eder O, Pincet F, Perez E, Thiery JP, Dufour S. Force measurements in E-cadherin-mediated cell doublets reveal rapid adhesion strengthened by actin cytoskeleton remodeling through Rac and Cdc42. J Cell Biol. 2004;167:1183–94.
73. Gomez TS, Billadeau DD. T cell activation and the cytoskeleton: you can't have one without the other. Adv Immunol. 2008;97:1–64.
74. Chua KN, Sim WJ, Racine V, Lee SY, Goh BC, Thiery JP. A cell-based small molecule screening method for identifying inhibitors of epithelial-mesenchymal transition in carcinoma. PLoS One. 2012;7:e33183.
75. Aref AR, Huang RY, Yu W, Chua KN, Sun W, Tu TY, Bai J, Sim WJ, Zervantonakis IK, Thiery JP, Kamm RD. Screening therapeutic EMT blocking agents in a three-dimensional microenvironment. Integr Biol (Camb). 2013;5:381–9.
76. Kaizuka Y, Douglass AD, Varma R, Dustin ML, Vale RD. Mechanisms for segregating T cell receptor and adhesion molecules during immunological synapse formation in Jurkat T cells. Proc Natl Acad Sci U S A. 2007;104:20296–301.

Part IV
Future Directions and Challenges

Chapter 13
Cancer Induced Immunosuppression and Its Modulation by Signal Inhibitors

Yutaka Kawakami, Li Qian, Naoshi Kawamura, Junichiro Miyazaki, Kinya Tsubota, Tomonari Kinoshita, Kenta Nakamura, Gaku Ohmura, Ryosuke Satomi, Juri Sugiyama, Hiroshi Nishio, Taeko Hayakawa, Boryana Popivanova, Sunthamala Nuchsupha, Tracy Hsin-ju Liu, Hajime Kamijuku, Chie Kudo-Saito, Nobuo Tsukamoto, Toshiharu Sakurai, Tomonobu Fujita, and Tomonori Yaguchi

Abstract Although cancer immunotherapy has recently demonstrated durable responses even in patients with advanced cancer, not all patients or cancer types respond to the therapy. Pretreatment immune status varies among cancer patients and is correlated with responses to immunotherapy. Immune conditions may be defined by the balance of positive and negative pathways in the anti-tumor immune responses, which are regulated by both cancer cell characteristics and patients' immune-reactivity along with various environmental factors. Gene alterations and signal activation define the immunological characteristics of cancer cells; tumor specific peptides derived from passenger mutations induce anti-tumor T-cells and oncogene activation (e.g. driver mutations, overexpression: MAPK, STAT3, NF-κB, β-catenin) rather promote immunosuppression. Oncogene/signal activation in cancer cells triggers multiple immunosuppressive cascades involving various immunosuppressive molecules and cells (e.g. TGF-β, IL10, IL6, VEGF, Treg, MDSC). Signal inhibitors are able to augment anti-tumor T-cell responses through multiple mechanisms including inhibition of cancer-induced immunosuppression, immunogenic cancer cell death, and enhancement of immune cell functions. Since the oncogene-signal activation status is different among patients, personalized immunotherapy combined with appropriate signal inhibitors may be considered for the development of effective immunotherapy.

No potential conflicts of interest were disclosed.

Y. Kawakami (✉) • L. Qian • N. Kawamura • J. Miyazaki • K. Tsubota • T. Kinoshita
K. Nakamura • G. Ohmura • R. Satomi • J. Sugiyama • H. Nishio • T. Hayakawa
B. Popivanova • S. Nuchsupha • T.H.-j. Liu • H. Kamijuku • C. Kudo-Saito • N. Tsukamoto
T. Sakurai • T. Fujita • T. Yaguchi
Division of Cellular Signaling, Institute for Advanced Medical Research, Keio University School of Medicine, 35 Shinanomachi, Shinjuku, Tokyo, Japan
e-mail: yutakawa@z5.keio.jp

B. Bonavida, S. Chouaib (eds.), *Resistance of Cancer Cells to CTL-Mediated Immunotherapy*, Resistance to Targeted Anti-Cancer Therapeutics 7,
DOI 10.1007/978-3-319-17807-3_13

Keywords Tumor immunoenvironment • Immunosuppression • Oncogenes • Signal inhibitors • Immunotherapy

Abbreviations

ACT	Adoptive cell therapy
CAF	Cancer associated fibroblast
CAR	Chimeric antigen receptor
CTL	Cytotoxic T lymphocyte
DC	Dendritic cell
EMT	Epithelial to mesenchymal transition
MDSC	Myeloid derived suppressor cells
MSI	Microsatellite instability
pDC	Plasmacytoid DC
TCR	T-cell receptor
Tfh	Follicular helper T-cells
TIL	Tumor infiltrating T-cells
Treg	Regulatory T-cells

13.1 Introduction

Human cancer cells acquire immunoresistance through multiple mechanisms during long developmental processes and evade from immune-defense systems (Immune-editing) [1]. Thus, immunological elimination of cancer is relatively difficult. However, recent cancer immunotherapies including immune checkpoint blockade (PD-1/PD-L1, CTLA-4 blockade) and adoptive cell therapy (ACT) using anti-tumor T-cells (tumor infiltrating T-cells, T-cell receptor (TCR) or chimeric antigen receptor (CAR) gene transduced T-cells) have shown clear anti-tumor effects in clinical trials for patients with various advanced cancers [2–6] However, these are still patients and cancer types not responding to these immunotherapies. Therefore, their improvement is needed possibly by combination of immune-interventions targeting multiple key regulating points (e.g. reversal of cancer induced immune-suppression) in the anti-tumor immune responses through the understanding of human immunopathology particularly in the tumor microenvironments.

13.2 Differences of the T-Cell Immune Status in the Tumor Microenvironments

Anti-tumor T-cells appear to be essential for the clinical effects of the immune-checkpoint blockade therapies and ACTs. In the anti-PD-1 Ab therapy, patients with cancer cells expressing PD-L1, which appears to be induced by IFN-γ produced by tumor infiltrating $CD8^+$ T-cells, are highly responsive to the therapy, indicating that preexisting anti-tumor T-cell responses is essential for the anti-PD-1 Ab therapy to work [7]. In addition, T-cell infiltrations in tumors were reported to correlate with prognosis after various cancer therapies, including surgery, radiation, chemotherapy, and immunotherapy in patients with various cancers (e.g. colon cancer, lung cancer, ovarian cancer, head and neck cancer, melanoma) [8]. High infiltrations of $CD3^+$ T-cells, $CD8^+$ T-cells, $FOXP3^+$ T-cells, and $CD20^+$ B-cells in tumors are correlated with favorable prognosis after curative surgery in Japanese patients with colon cancer. An international collaboration was organized by the Society for Immunotherapy of Cancer (SITC) (initiated by Jerome Galon, INSERM) to confirm the prognostic role of the tumor infiltrating $CD3^+$ T-cells and $CD8^+$ T-cells (Immunoscore) in large numbers of colon cancer patients by using a customized analytic software [9]. The inclusion of immunological status into the current prognostic TNM staging criteria may improve clinical management of colon cancer patients. Peripheral blood immune status also varies in cancer patients and correlates with responses to various cancer therapies including immunotherapy. High plasma IL6 or IL8, but not other cytokines such as TNF-α and IL1β, were found to correlate with poor prognosis of patients with various cancers including colon cancer, prostate cancer, and liver cancer after various cancer vaccines (e.g. peptide vaccine, dendritic cell vaccine) (Fig. 13.1).

13.3 Positive and Negative Immune Pathways for Anti-Tumor T-Cell Responses

The heterogeneity of the immune-status in cancer patients may be defined by a balance of positive and negative pathways in the anti-tumor T-cell responses. Various environmental factors including intestinal microbiota, which have recently been reported to influence on the systemic anti-tumor immune responses, diet which causes obesity and promotes chronic inflammation, and smoking which introduces various chemicals affecting the immune system, may also influence the immune status. We have previously reported that tumor infiltrating T-cells (TILs) in melanoma recognize not only shared tumor antigens, but also tumor specific peptides (one amino acid difference from corresponding self-peptides) derived from genomic DNA missense mutations [10–14]. It has recently been demonstrated that melanoma TILs often recognize patients' unique peptides derived from passenger mutations by evaluating TIL responses to the mutations identified by whole exomic DNA

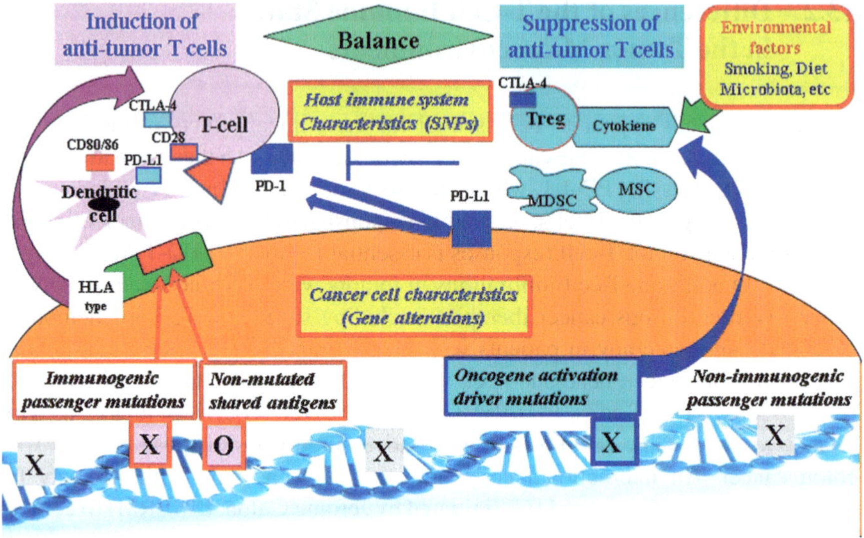

Fig. 13.1 Mechanisms defining the immune status of cancer patients. The immune status of cancer patients may be defined by a balance of positive and negative pathways in the anti-tumor T-cell response along with environmental factors. Passenger mutations may induce anti-tumor T-cells, while driver mutations and oncogene activation rather trigger immunosuppressive cascades

sequencing [15]. In particular, UV-related melanoma and smoking-related lung cancer were found to have more DNA mutations than other cancers, and they are relatively responsive cancers to anti-PD-1 Ab therapy, suggesting that spontaneous T-cell responses against mutated antigens are involved in the anti-tumor effects of the anti-PD-1 Ab therapy. High $CD8^+$ T-cell infiltration was observed in MSI (microsatellite instability) $^+$ colon cancer, and the patients have relatively good prognosis after surgery even though with pathologically malignant appearance. Immune responses to frameshift mutations caused by dysfunction of DNA mismatch repair enzymes such as MLH1 were detected [16], suggesting that MSI^+ colon cancer may be a good candidate for the anti-PD-1 Ab therapy. Therefore, quantity and quality of DNA mutations in cancer cells may be one of the factors defining the T-cell immune status of cancer patients. Other DNA alterations also affect T-cell infiltration in tumors. Deletion of DNA-encoding the chemokine CXCL13, which may recruit $CXCR5^+$ follicular helper T-cells (Tfh) and induce subsequent IL-21-dependent support of memory $CD8^+$ T-cells and B-cells, and deletion of DNA encoding the cytokine IL15 which may expand TILs, were reported to cause less T- cell infiltration in colon cancers [17, 18]. In addition to these cancer cell's gene alterations, difference in patients' immune-reactivity partly defined by polymorphism of immunoregulating molecules including HLA, may influence the anti-tumor T-cell induction pathway (Fig. 13.2).

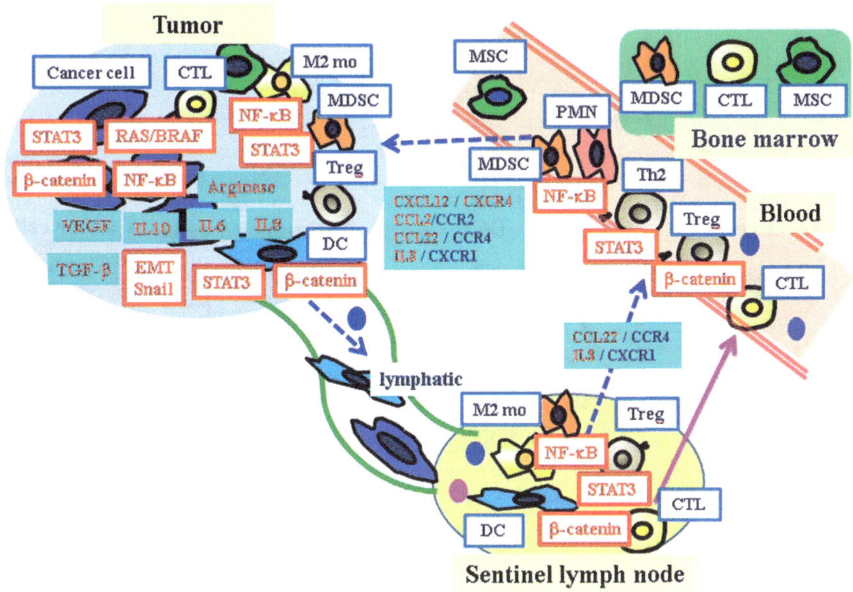

Fig. 13.2 Gene alterations in cancer cells trigger multiple immunosuppressive cascades. Activation of oncogenes and subsequent signaling trigger multiple immunosuppressive cascades involving various immunosuppressive molecules and cells in tumor-associated microenvironments, including tumors, sentinel lymph nodes, and bone marrow. Personalized use of signal inhibitors may reverse the cancer-induced immunosuppression

13.4 Immunosuppressive Cascades Triggered by Cancer Cell's Oncogenes and Signal Activation

In a negative immunosuppressive pathway, overproduction of immunosuppressive molecules such as TGF-β in the tumor microenvironments triggers a series of immunosuppressive cascades and consequent inhibition of anti-tumor T-cell induction and accumulation into tumors. For example, TGF-β not only impairs T-cell stimulatory function of dendritic cells (DCs) through decrease of CD80/CD86 and MHC expressions, but also recruits immunosuppressive regulatory T-cells (Treg), and myeloid derived suppressor cells (MDSCs) in tumors and sentinel lymph nodes [19]. TGF-β also induces epithelial to mesenchymal transition (EMT) which promotes invasion and metastasis of cancer cells via a decrease of the adhesion molecule E-cadherin and an increase of protease MMPs. Interestingly, one of the EMT-inducing transcription factors, snail, induces multiple immunosuppressive cytokines such as IL10, TGF-β and TSP−1, and chemokines such as CCL2. IL10, TGF-β and TSP−1 have abilities to impair DC functions and subsequent induction of Tregs, and CCL2 recruits $CCR2^+$ immunosuppressive MDSCs. These EMT-related immunosuppressions may further promote metastasis of cancer cells [20, 21].

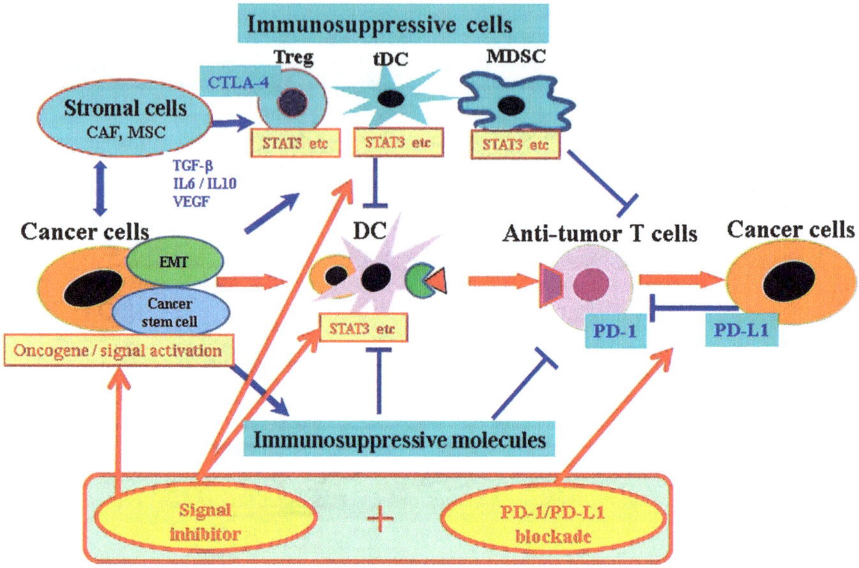

Fig. 13.3 Combination of signal inhibitors and other immune-interventions. Signal inhibitors may augment the induction of anti-tumor T-cells by acting on both the cancer cells and the various immune cells, and enhance anti-tumor effects of immunotherapy including immune-checkpoint blockades

M2-like macrophages which produce abundant CCL22 were also generated in tumors and sentinel lymph nodes, and recruit $CCR4^+$ Tregs into tumors and sentinel lymph nodes, resulting in immunosuppressive conditions in the tumor associated microenvironments [22]. TGF-β is produced by cancer cells via genetic alterations and various infiltrated immune cells. In contrast to the involvement of passenger DNA mutations the in anti-tumor T-cell induction pathway, driver mutations of oncogenes appear to rather promote the negative immunosuppressive pathway in the anti-tumor immune responses. Because oncogene and subsequent signaling activation status are different among cancer types and patients even with the same histology, immunosuppression mechanisms triggered by each oncogene should be investigated, and in a therapeutic view, personalized use of appropriate signal inhibitors should be considered [23] (Fig. 13.3).

13.5 Immunosuppression Induced by the MAPK Signaling Pathway and Its Modulation

One of the reasons we began the research on oncogene-associated immunosuppression is based on the findings of the possible involvement of constitutively activated MAPK signaling in human melanoma-induced immunosuppression. The common BRAF mutation dependent MAPK signal activation was found to not only augment cell proliferation and invasion of melanoma cells, but also induce production of multiple cytokines, IL-6, IL-10, and VEGF, which have an ability to suppress T-cell stimulatory function of DCs through inhibition of IL-12 and TNF-α production and augmentation of IL-10 production [24, 25]. Treatment of human melanoma cells by either lentiviral BRAF (V600E) specific shRNAs or MEK inhibitors decreased the immunosuppressive activity of human melanoma cells. MEK inhibitors were also reported to increase the susceptibility of melanoma cells to cytotoxic T cell (CTL) lysis partly due to increased expression of melanocyte differentiation antigens such as MART-1/melan-A and gp100 [26].

Mutant BRAF selective inhibitors have recently been developed, and their administration resulted in strong clinical responses. Dramatic tumor reduction by the BRAF inhibitors indicated the cytolysis of melanoma cells, which may release multiple endogenous tumor antigens including mutated antigens and trigger anti-tumor T-cell responses via antigen presentation by DC (Immunogenic cancer cell death). In addition, decrease of tumor cell numbers, decreased production of multiple immunosuppressive cytokines, increased susceptibility of cancer cells to CTLs partly via increased tumor antigen expression, and less inhibition of T-cell activation (T-cells also use wild type BRAF signaling), altogether may promote induction of anti-tumor T-cells. Interestingly, the administration of mutant BRAF selective inhibitors did not suppress the general immune responses [27, 28], and actually increased the infiltration of granzyme positive $CD8^+$ T cells in tumors, in regressing tumors with necrosis but not in progressing tumors [29]. This T-cell infiltration appears to be not a simple scavenger phenomenon, rather an active induction and recruitment of tumor antigen-specific T-cells. These observations suggest that the combined use of BRAF inhibitors may enhance the current immunotherapy for melanoma patients, including cancer vaccines, immune-checkpoint blockers and T-cell based ACT. The clinical trials of these combination immunotherapies have already begun. "Avoiding immune destruction" is now recognized as one of the hallmarks of cancer [30], and targeting a common signaling pathway such as the BRAF (N-RAS)-MAPK axis involved in the multiple hallmarks of cancer, including immunosuppression, proliferation and invasion, may be an attractive strategy for cancer treatment. Inhibitors for EGF-R, which is upstream of MAPK signaling, were also found to inhibit production of immunosuppressive cytokines such as IL-6 and VEGF from human lung cancer cells with EGF-R mutations. The administration of the EGF-R inhibitors showed synergistic anti-tumor effects when combined with cancer vaccines or immune-checkpoint blockades. Therefore, MAPK signal inhibitors may be useful for immunotherapy for patients with various cancers.

13.6 Immunosuppression Induced by the JAK/STAT3 Signaling Pathway and Its Modulation

During analysis of the immunological role of mutant BRAF in the cancer-induced immunosuppression, STAT3 activation in some melanoma cell lines was also found to induce similar immunosuppression. STAT3 depletion by lentiviral shRNAs resulted in the inhibition of production of multiple immunosuppressive cytokines including IL-6, IL-10, and VEGF, and the reduction of the immunosuppressive activity of STAT3-activated human melanoma cells [25]. Interestingly, these immunosuppressive cytokines activated STAT3 in various immune cells, including DCs, MDSCs, and Tregs, and rendered them immunosuppressive phenotypes. STAT3 activation in DCs generated high IL-10 and low IL-12, thus, producing tolerogenic DCs in vitro, which have less T-cell stimulatory activity and Treg-inducing ability. In a mouse model, STAT3 depleted DCs had enhanced T-cell stimulatory activity and relatively resistant to tumor-derived immunosuppressive factors including IL6, IL10 and VEGF. Injection of the STAT3-depleted DCs into tumors which are under an immunosuppressed condition, induced better anti-tumor effects accompanied by high IFN-γ producing tumor antigen specific Th1 responses compared to control DCs [31]. Similarly, generation of immunosuppressive macrophages and MDSCs by tumor-derived immunosuppressive factors were partially inhibited by STAT3 depletion of these myeloid cells. STAT3 was also involved in the expansion of MDSCs [32]. Increased STAT3 activation was observed in $CD14^{+}HLA\text{-}DR^{negative/low}$ MDSCs in peripheral blood of cancer patients [33]. STAT3 was also reported to be involved in the immunosuppressive Treg and anti-tumor $CD8^{+}$T cells in which STAT3 depletion enhanced anti-tumor activity when adoptively transferred [34, 35]. The importance of STAT3 activation by tumor-derived factors such as IL6 in tumor-promoting cancer-associated fibroblasts (CAFs) was also indicated. These observations indicate that the constitutive activation of STAT3 in cancer cells triggers the production of multiple immunosuppressive cytokines and the induction of various immunosuppressive and tumor promoting cells, including tolerogenic DCs, MDSCs, Tregs, and CAFs, partly through the activation of STAT3 in these cells [36]. Therefore, STAT3 inhibitors may be useful for the reversal of the cancer-induced immunosuppression through acting on both cancer cells and various immune cells and stromal cells.

Clinical trials of STAT3 inhibitors have been being conducted for patients with various cancers for which direct inhibition of cancer growth is expected. In addition to the direct STAT3 inhibitors, drugs inhibiting STAT3 signaling at upstream or downstream may also be useful for reversal of immunosuppression and their combined use with immunotherapy. Inhibitors of JAK2, which is a direct upstream of STAT3 signaling, have been shown to augment anti-tumor immunity and enhance anti-tumor effects of immunotherapies such as IL-12 administration [37]. Administration of a multikinase inhibitor Sunitinib, which also suppresses downstream STAT3 signaling, decreased MDSCs and Tregs along with increase of IFN-γ-producing T-cells in peripheral blood of patients with kidney cancer [38]. Another multikinase inhibitor Dasatinib increasedthe response rate in about half of the patients with $Ph1^{+}$CML and $Ph1^{+}$ ALL accompanied by LGL lymphocytosis and autoimmune-like syndrome such as pleuritis. Dasatinib was reported to inhibit STAT3 signaling in peripheral blood leukocytes in these leukemia patients [39]. One of the natural compounds contained in the Japanese traditional medicines was found to have an activity by inhibiting both STAT3 and MAPK signaling and to inhibit production of immunosuppressive cytokines from human cancer cells.

The administration of this compound augmented tumor specific T-cells accompanied by a decrease of Tregs in tumor-bearing mice. Therefore, there may be various ways to inhibit the STAT3-associated immunosuppression.

13.7 Immunosuppression Induced by the NF-κB Signaling Pathway and Its Modulation

High plasma IL-6 and IL-8, which are correlated with poor prognosis after various cancer immunotherapies, were observed in patients with ovarian cancer. The correlation between NF-kB p65 and IL6 staining in the tumor microenvironment was observed by immunohistochemial analysis. An NF-κB inhibitor such as DHMEQ inhibited production of these immunosuppressive cytokines and chemokines (e.g. IL6, IL8, CCL2) by human ovarian cancer cells [40]. DHMEQ also inhibited the generation of immunosuppressive macrophages from human peripheral blood monocytes in the presence of human ovarian cancer cell-derived factors. In nude mice implanted with human ovarian cancer cell lines, impairment of T-cell stimulatory activity of murine DCs and accumulation of murine MDSCs in the spleen and tumors were observed partly due to increase of mouse compatible human IL6 produced by human ovarian cancer cells. Administration of DHMEQ reversed these immunosuppressive effects accompanied by decrease of hIL6. When mouse naïve T-cells were transferred into these mice, xenogeneic anti-tumor T-cells were induced and regressed human ovarian cancer cells. Administration of DHMEQ to these mice further enhanced T-cell dependent regression of human ovarian cancer cells. Thus, appropriate doses of NF-κB inhibitors may augment T-cell mediated anti-tumor activity via reversal of the cancer induced immunosuppression, although NF-κB is also involved in the T-cell induction pathway. Recently, various compounds that have an activity to inhibit NF-kB signaling were found in Japanese traditional medicines and drugs which already are used for other diseases (drug repositioning), and their administration enhanced the induction of anti-tumor T-cells, and augmented anti-tumor effects of the immune-checkpoint blockade in a syngeneic NF-κB-dependent IL6 producing murine tumor model.

Type 1 IFNs were recently found to be important for the induction of anti-tumor T-cells. Plasmacytoid DCs (pDC) are one of the significant producers of IFN-α, however, pDC functions such as type 1 IFN production was reported to be impaired in the tumor microenvironment. The ILT7 ligand (ILT7L) expressed on human cancer cells was found to inhibits IFN-α production by ILT7 expressing pDCs and is possibly involved in the immunosuppression. NF-κB inhibitors inhibit the intrinsic expression of ILT7L in some of human renal cell cancer (RCC) cells, suggesting that NF-kB inhibitors may be useful for the cancer-induced immunosuppression in various ways [41]. Some cancer cells intrinsically express PD-L1 through activation of the AKT signaling in human glioma and the MAPK signaling in some cancer cells [42], although the main mechanism of PD-L1 expression appears to be the adaptive resistance induced by cytokines produced by tumor infiltrating T-cells. Therefore, signal inhibitors may also be useful for the reversal of the immunosuppression by intrinsically expressed immunosuppressive membrane molecules (e.g., ILT7L and PD-L1).

13.8 Immunosuppression Induced by the Wnt/β-Catenin Signaling Pathway and Its Modulation

Activation of the Wnt/β-catenin signaling detected by nuclear staining of β-catenin was observed in various human cancers including about 30 % of melanoma which produce IL10. IL10 gene expression was found to be directly regulated by β-catenin signaling. Melanoma culture supernatants induced high IL-10 and low IL-12-producing DCs with low T-cell stimulatory activity in vitro in an IL-10-dependent manner, and these DCs had an ability to induce immunosuppressive FOXP3^{+} Tregs. Depletion of β-catenin by specific shRNAs reduced the immunosuppressive activity of human melanoma cells [43]. The melanoma supernatants also had β-catenin-dependent immunosuppressive activity on the effector function of melanoma specific CTLs. T-cell stimulatory activity of murine DCs was impaired possibly via increased mouse compatible hIL10, when human melanoma cell lines were implanted in immunodeficient SCID mice. The administration of a β-catenin inhibitor restored murine DC's T-cell stimulatory activity along with a decrease of hIL-10. Interestingly, the β-catenin inhibitor had an ability to directly enhance T-cell stimulatory activity of human DCs partly due to decreased IL-10 production by the DC themselves [44, 45]. β-catenin was also reported to be involved in the generation of regulatory DCs and survival of Tregs [46]. Therefore, β-catenin inhibitors may also be useful for the reversal of the immunosuppression induced by cancer cells with activated Wnt/β-catenin signaling.

13.9 Personalized Combination of Immune-Modulators Targeting Multiple Key Points in the Anti-Tumor T-Cell Responses for Effective Cancer Immunotherapy

Two T-cell based immune-interventions, the immune-checkpoint blockade and T-cell based ACT, were shown to be effective for some of the advanced cancer patients, but they still need further improvement possibly by combination therapies. For development of effective cancer immunotherapy, based on the detailed immunological analyses in various clinical trials of tumor antigen specific immunotherapies [47, 48], we have previously proposed the importance of combination of the following immune-interventions; (1) use of tumor antigens involved in cancer cell proliferation and survival, and expressed in cancer initiating cells [49], (2) in situ tumor destruction methods to induce immune responses to endogenous tumor antigens including unique mutated peptides (immunogenic cancer cell death) (e.g. chemotherapy, molecular targeted drugs, anti-tumor Ab, radiation, cryoablation, radiofrequency ablation, oncolytic viruses) [50, 51], (3) methods to augment antigen presenting DC functions (e.g. adjuvants (TLR/STING stimulators), cytokines (IL12, TNF-α), agonistic antibodies (anti-CD40 Ab)) [52], (4) in vivo anti-tumor T-cell activation and expansion (e.g. cytokines (IL2, IL7, IL15, IL21), agonistic Abs for co-stimulatory molecules on T-cells (anti-CD134, CD137 Ab), T-cell based ACT), and (5) methods to reverse the immunosuppression (neutralizing and depleting Abs (e.g. TGF-β, Treg), immune-checkpoint blockers (e.g. anti-CTLA-4, anti-PD-1/PD-L1, anti-LAG3, anti-TIM3 Abs), chemotherapy, and molecular targeted drugs (e.g. signal inhibitors)) [53].

The patients with less T-cell tumor infiltrations and high levels of some cytokines (IL6, IL8) were shown to be of poor prognosis after various immunotherapies. Thus, one of the intriguing strategies is the use of above mentioned signal inhibitors for the immunosuppression inducing signaling. In addition to direct inhibition of cancer cell growth and invasion, signal inhibitors have activities to augment endogenous tumor antigen specific T-cell induction through causing immunogenic cancer cell death, enhancing DC functions, and decreasing immunosuppressive factors. In murine tumor models, combination of signal inhibitors and various immunotherapies including cancer vaccine and immune-checkpoint blockade has already been shown to be more effective. Clinical trials of combination immunotherapy has currently begun. One of the problems in the combination immunotherapy is the increase of adverse effects such as liver toxicity as observed in the combination of anti-CTLA-4 Ab and chemotherapy/molecular target therapy.

Since the oncogene-signaling activation status in cancer cells are different among patients, the personalized use of appropriate signal inhibitors is essential. In addition, treatment strategies should be designed based on the pretreatment immune status of patients. For instance, immune-checkpoint blockades such as the PD-1/PD-L1 blockade may be sufficient for the patients with preexisting anti-tumor T-cell immunity. If immunosuppression mechanisms other than PD-1/PD-L1 interaction are dominant, methods to reverse such mechanism should be combined. If anti-tumor T-cell induction is not enough, combination of strong T-cell inducing methods including immunogenic cancer cell death inducers, strong cancer vaccines, and DC stimulating agents, should be considered. If the immunogenicity of cancer cells is too low (no presence of good immunogenic antigens), artificial anti-tumor T-cells such as tumor antigen recognizing TCR/CAR gene-transduced T cells could be used.

13.10 Concluding Remarks

Cancer cell characteristics defined by gene alterations (immunogenicity and immunosuppression ability) are the major factors for both positive and negative regulation of the anti-tumor immune responses. Inhibitors targeting activated oncogene-signaling not only directly inhibit cancer cell growth and invasion, but also improve the tumor immunoenvironment through multiple mechanisms acting on both the cancer cells and the immune cells, resulting in enhanced anti-tumor T-cell responses. Based on the patients' immune status, personalized immune-interventions on multiple key regulating points, including reversal of the cancer-induced immune suppression, will lead to a more effective cancer control.

Acknowledgements This studies were supported by Grants-in-Aid for Scientific Research (23240128, 26221005) from the Japan Society for Promotion of Science, a research program of the Project for Development of Innovative Research on Cancer Therapeutics (P-Direct) from the Ministry of Education, Culture, Sports, Science and Technology of Japan, a Grant-in-Aid for Cancer Research (23-A-22, 19-14) from the Ministry of Health, Labour, and Welfare, Japan. We also thank technical support and editorial assistance of Ms. Misako Sakamoto and Ms. Ryoko Suzuki.

References

1. Schreiber RD, Old LJ, Smyth MJ. Cancer immunoediting: integrating immunity's roles in cancer suppression and promotion. Science. 2011;331:1565–70.
2. Hodi FS, O'Day SJ, McDermott DF, Weber RW, Sosman JA, Haanen JB, Gonzalez R, Robert C, Schadendorf D, Hassel JC, Akerley W, van den Eertwegh AJ, Lutzky J, Lorigan P, Vaubel JM, Linette GP, Hogg D, Ottensmeier CH, Lebbé C, Peschel C, Quirt I, Clark JI, Wolchok JD, Weber JS, Tian J, Yellin MJ, Nichol GM, Hoos A, Urba WJ. Improved survival with ipilimumab in patients with metastatic melanoma. N Engl J Med. 2010;363:711–23.
3. Brahmer JR, Tykodi SS, Chow LQ, Hwu WJ, Topalian SL, Hwu P, Drake CG, Camacho LH, Kauh J, Odunsi K, Pitot HC, Hamid O, Bhatia S, Martins R, Eaton K, Chen S, Salay TM, Alaparthy S, Grosso JF, Korman AJ, Parker SM, Agrawal S, Goldberg SM, Pardoll DM, Gupta A, Wigginton JM. Safety, activity, and immune correlates of anti-PD-1 antibody in cancer. N Engl J Med. 2012;366:2455–65.
4. Rosenberg SA, Yang JC, Sherry RM, Kammula US, Hughes MS, Phan GQ, Citrin DE, Restifo NP, Robbins PF, Wunderlich JR, Morton KE, Laurencot CM, Steinberg SM, White DE, Dudley ME. Durable complete responses in heavily pretreated patients with metastatic melanoma using T-cell transfer immunotherapy. Clin Cancer Res. 2011;17:4550–7.
5. Robbins PF, Morgan RA, Feldman SA, Yang JC, Sherry RM, Dudley ME, Wunderlich JR, Nahvi AV, Helman LJ, Mackall CL, Kammula US, Hughes MS, Restifo NP, Raffeld M, Lee CC, Levy CL, Li YF, El-Gamil M, Schwarz SL, Laurencot C, Rosenberg SA. Tumor regression in patients with metastatic synovial cell sarcoma and melanoma using genetically engineered lymphocytes reactive with NY-ESO-1. J Clin Oncol. 2011;29:917–24.
6. Kalos M, Levine BL, Porter DL, Katz S, Grupp SA, Bagg A, June CH. T cells with chimeric antigen receptors have potent antitumor effects and can establish memory in patients with advanced leukemia. Sci Transl Med. 2011;3:95.
7. Taube JM, Anders RA, Young GD, Xu H, Sharma R, McMiller TL, Chen S, Klein AP, Pardoll DM, Topalian SL, Chen L. Colocalization of inflammatory response with B7-h1 expression in human melanocytic lesions supports an adaptive resistance mechanism of immune escape. Sci Transl Med. 2012;4:127.
8. Fridman WH, Pagès F, Sautès-Fridman C, Galon J. The immune contexture in human tumours: impact on clinical outcome. Nat Rev Cancer. 2012;12:298–306.
9. Galon J, Mlecnik B, Bindea G, Angell HK, Berger A, Lagorce C, Lugli A, Zlobec I, Hartmann A, Bifulco C, Nagtegaal ID, Palmqvist R, Masucci GV, Botti G, Tatangelo F, Delrio P, Maio

M, Laghi L, Grizzi F, Asslaber M, D'Arrigo C, Vidal-Vanaclocha F, Zavadova E, Chouchane L, Ohashi PS, Hafezi-Bakhtiari S, Wouters BG, Roehrl M, Nguyen L, Kawakami Y, Hazama S, Okuno K, Ogino S, Gibbs P, Waring P, Sato N, Torigoe T, Itoh K, Patel PS, Shukla SN, Wang Y, Kopetz S, Sinicrope FA, Scripcariu V, Ascierto PA, Marincola FM, Fox BA, Pagès F. Towards the introduction of the 'Immunoscore' in the classification of malignant tumours. J Pathol. 2014;232:199–209.

10. Kawakami Y, Rosenberg SA. Human tumor antigens recognized by T cells. Immunol Res. 1997;16:313–39.
11. Kawakami Y, Fujita T, Matsuzaki Y, Sakurai T, Tsukamoto M, Toda M, Sumimoto H. Identification of human tumor antigens and its implications for diagnosis and treatment of cancer. Cancer Sci. 2004;95:784–91.
12. Kawakami Y, Eliyahu S, Delgado CH, Robbins PF, Rivoltini L, Topalian SL, Miki T, Rosenberg SA. Cloning of the gene coding for a shared human melanoma antigen recognized by autologous T cells infiltrating into tumor. Proc Natl Acad Sci U S A. 1994;91:3515–9.
13. Robbins PF, El-Gamil M, Li YF, Kawakami Y, Loftus D, Appella E, Rosenberg SA. A mutated b2-catenin gene encodes a melanoma – specific antigen recognized by tumor infiltrating lymphocytes. J Exp Med. 1996;183:1185–92.
14. Kawakami Y, Wang X, Shofuda T, Sumimoto H, Tupesis J, Fitzgerald E, Rosenberg S. Isolation of a new melanoma antigen, MART-2, containing a mutated epitope recognized by autologous tumor infiltrating T lymphocytes. J Immunol. 2001;166:2871–7.
15. Robbins PF, Lu YC, El-Gamil M, Li YF, Gross C, Gartner J, Lin JC, Teer JK, Cliften P, Tycksen E, Samuels Y, Rosenberg SA. Mining exomic sequencing data to identify mutated antigens recognized by adoptively transferred tumor-reactive T cells. Nat Med. 2013;19: 747–52.
16. Ishikawa T, Fujita T, Suzuki Y, Okabe S, Yuasa Y, Iwai T, Kawakami Y. Tumor-specific immunological recognition of frameshift-mutated peptides in colon cancer with microsatellite instability. Cancer Res. 2003;63:5564–72.
17. Bindea G, Mlecnik B, Tosolini M, Kirilovsky A, Waldner M, Obenauf AC, Angell H, Fredriksen T, Lafontaine L, Berger A, Bruneval P, Fridman WH, Becker C, Pagès F, Speicher MR, Trajanoski Z, Galon J. Spatiotemporal dynamics of intratumoral immune cells reveal the immune landscape in human cancer. Immunity. 2013;39:782–95.
18. Mlecnik B, Bindea G, Angell HK, Sasso MS, Obenauf AC, Fredriksen T, Lafontaine L, Bilocq AM, Kirilovsky A, Tosolini M, Waldner M, Berger A, Fridman WH, Rafii A, Valge-Archer V, Pagès F, Speicher MR, Galon J. Functional network pipeline reveals genetic determinants associated with in situ lymphocyte proliferation and survival of cancer patients. Sci Transl Med. 2014;6:228.
19. Nakamura S, Yaguchi T, Kawamura N, Kobayashi A, Sakurai T, Higuchi H, Takaishi H, Hibi T, Kawakami Y. TGF-β1 in tumor microenvironments induces immunosuppression in the tumors and sentinel lymph nodes and promotes tumor progression. J Immunother. 2014;37: 63–72.
20. Kudo-Saito C, Shirako H, Takeuchi T, Kawakami Y. Cancer metastasis is accelerated through immunosuppression during EMT of cancer cell. Cancer Cell. 2009;15:195–206.
21. Kudo-Saito C, Shirako H, Ohike M, Tsukamoto N, Kawakami Y. CCL2 is critical for immunosuppression to promote cancer metastasis. Clin Exp Metastasis. 2013;30:393–405.
22. Tsujikawa T, Yaguchi T, Ohmura G, Ohta S, Kobayashi A, Kawamura N, Fujita T, Nakano H, Shimada T, Takahashi T, Nakao R, Yanagisawa A, Hisa Y, Kawakami Y. Autocrine and paracrine loops between cancer cells and macrophages promote lymph node metastasis via CCR4/ CCL22 in head and neck squamous cell carcinoma. Int J Cancer. 2012;132:2755–66.
23. Yaguchi T, Sumimoto H, Kudo-Saito C, Tsukamoto N, Ueda R, Iwata-Kajihara T, Nishio H, Kawamura N, Kawakami Y. The mechanisms of cancer immunoescape and development of overcoming strategies. Int J Hematol. 2011;93:294–300.
24. Sumimoto H, Miyagishi M, Miyoshi H, Yamagata S, Shimizu A, Taira K, Kawakami Y. Inhibition of growth and invasive ability of melanoma by inactivation of mutated BRAF with lentivirus-mediated RNA interference. Oncogene. 2004;23:6031–9.

25. Sumimoto H, Imabayashi F, Iwata T, Kawakami Y. The BRAF-MAPK signaling pathway is essential for cancer immune evasion in human melanoma cells. J Exp Med. 2006;203:1651–6.
26. Kono M, Dunn IS, Durda PJ, Butera D, Rose LB, Haggerty TJ, Benson EM, Kurnick JT. Role of the mitogen-activated protein kinase signaling pathway in the regulation of human melanocytic antigen expression. Mol Cancer Res. 2006;4:779–92.
27. Hong DS, Vence L, Falchook G, Radvanyi LG, Liu C, Goodman V, Legos JJ, Blackman S, Scarmadio A, Kurzrock R, Lizee G, Hwu P. BRAF(V600) inhibitor GSK2118436 targeted inhibition of mutant BRAF in cancer patients does not impair overall immune competency. Clin Cancer Res. 2012;18:2326–35.
28. Boni A, Cogdill AP, Dang P, Udayakumar D, Njauw CN, Sloss CM, Ferrone CR, Flaherty KT, Lawrence DP, Fisher DE, Tsao H, Wargo JA. Selective BRAFV600E inhibition enhances T-cell recognition of melanoma without affecting lymphocyte function. Cancer Res. 2010;70:5213–9.
29. Wilmott JS, Long GV, Howle JR, Haydu LE, Sharma RN, Thompson JF, Kefford RF, Hersey P, Scolyer RA. Selective BRAF inhibitors induce marked T-cell infiltration into human metastatic melanoma. Clin Cancer Res. 2012;18:1386–94.
30. Hanahan D, Weinberg RA. Hallmarks of cancer: the next generation. Cell. 2011;144:646–74.
31. Iwata-Kajihara T, Sumimoto H, Kawamura N, Ueda R, Takahashi T, Mizuguchi H, Miyagishi M, Takeda K, Kawakami Y. Enhanced cancer immunotherapy using STAT3-depleted dendritic cells with high Th1-inducing ability and resistance to cancer cell-derived inhibitory factors. J Immunol. 2011;187:27–36.
32. Wu L, Du H, Li Y, Qu P, Yan C. Signal transducer and activator of transcription 3 (Stat3C) promotes myeloid-derived suppressor cell expansion and immune suppression during lung tumorigenesis. Am J Pathol. 2011;179:2131–41.
33. Poschke I, Mougiakakos D, Hansson J, Masucci GV, Kiessling R. Immature immunosuppressive CD14+HLA-DR-/low cells in melanoma patients are Stat3hi and overexpress CD80, CD83, and DC-sign. Cancer Res. 2010;70:4335–45.
34. Pallandre JR, Brillard E, Créhange G, Radlovic A, Remy-Martin JP, Saas P, Rohrlich PS, Pivot X, Ling X, Tiberghien P, Borg C. Role of STAT3 in CD4+CD25+FOXP3+ regulatory lymphocyte generation: implications in graft-versus-host disease and antitumor immunity. J Immunol. 2007;179:7593–604.
35. Kujawski M, Zhang C, Herrmann A, Reckamp K, Scuto A, Jensen M, Deng J, Forman S, Figlin R, Yu H. Targeting STAT3 in adoptively transferred T cells promotes their in vivo expansion and antitumor effects. Cancer Res. 2010;70:9599–610.
36. Lee H, Pal SK, Reckamp K, Figlin RA, Yu H. STAT3: a target to enhance antitumor immune response. Curr Top Microbiol Immunol. 2011;344:41–59.
37. Burdelya L, Catlett-Falcone R, Levitzki A, Cheng F, Mora LB, Sotomayor E, Coppola D, Sun J, Sebti S, Dalton WS, Jove R, Yu H. Combination therapy with AG-490 and interleukin 12 achieves greater antitumor effects than either agent alone. Mol Cancer Ther. 2002;1:893–9.
38. Ko JS, Zea AH, Rini BI, Ireland JL, Elson P, Cohen P, Golshayan A, Rayman PA, Wood L, Garcia J, Dreicer R, Bukowski R, Finke JH. Sunitinib mediates reversal of myeloid-derived suppressor cell accumulation in renal cell carcinoma patients. Clin Cancer Res. 2009;15:2148–57.
39. Jalkanen SE, Vakkila J, Kreutzman A, Nieminen JK, Porkka K, Mustjoki S. Poor cytokine-induced phosphorylation in chronic myeloid leukemia patients at diagnosis is effectively reversed by tyrosine kinase inhibitor therapy. Exp Hematol. 2011;39:102–13.
40. Nishio H, Yaguchi T, Sugiyama J, Sumimoto H, Umezawa K, Iwata T, Susumu N, Fujii T, Kawamura N, Kobayashi A, Park J, Aoki D, Kawakami Y. Immunosuppression through constitutively activated NF-κB signaling in human ovarian cancer and its reversal by a NF-κB inhibitor. Br J Cancer. 2014;110:2965–74.
41. Tsukamoto N, Okada S, Onami Y, Sasaki Y, Umezawa K, Kawakami Y. Impairment of plasmacytoid dendritic cells for IFN production by the ligand for immunoglobulin-like transcript 7 expressed on human cancer cells. Clin Cancer Res. 2009;15:5733–43.

42. Parsa AT, Waldron JS, Panner A, Crane CA, Parney IF, Barry JJ, Cachola KE, Murray JC, Tihan T, Jensen MC, Mischel PS, Stokoe D, Pieper RO. Loss of tumor suppressor PTEN function increases B7-H1 expression and immunoresistance in glioma. Nat Med. 2007;13:84–8.
43. Yaguchi T, Goto Y, Kido K, Mochimaru H, Sakurai T, Tsukamoto N, Kudo-Saito C, Fujita T, Sumimoto H, Kawakami Y. Immune suppression and resistance mediated by constitutive activation of Wnt/β-catenin signaling in human melanoma cells. J Immunol. 2012;189:2110–7.
44. Fu C, Jiang A. Generation of tolerogenic dendritic cells via the E-cadherin/β-catenin-signaling pathway. Immunol Res. 2010;46:72–8.
45. Manicassamy S, Reizis B, Ravindran R, Nakaya H, Salazar-Gonzalez RM, Wang YC, Pulendran B. Activation of β-catenin in dendritic cells regulates immunity versus tolerance in the intestine. Science. 2010;329:849–53.
46. Ding Y, Shen S, Lino AC, Curotto de Lafaille MA, Lafaille JJ. Beta-catenin stabilization extends regulatory T cell survival and induces anergy in nonregulatory T cells. Nat Med. 2008;14:162–9.
47. Rosenberg SA, Yang JC, Schwartzentruber DJ, Hwu P, Marincola FM, Topalian SL, Restifo NP, Dudley ME, Schwarz SL, Spiess PJ, Wunderlich JR, Parkhurst MR, Kawakami Y, Seipp CA, Einhorn JH, White DE. Immunologic and therapeutic evaluation of a synthetic peptide vaccine for the treatment of patients with metastatic melanoma. Nat Med. 1998;4:321–7.
48. Salgaller ML, Afshar A, Marincola FM, Rivoltini L, Kawakami Y, Rosenberg SA. Recognition of multiple epitopes in the human melanoma antigen gp100 by antigen specific peripheral blood lymphocytes stimulated with synthetic peptides. Cancer Res. 1995;55:4972–9.
49. Ueda R, Ohkusu-Tsukada K, Fusaki N, Soeda A, Kawase T, Kawakami Y, Toda M. Identification of HLA-A2- and A24-restricted T-cell epitopes derived from SOX6 expressed in glioma stem cells for immunotherapy. Int J Cancer. 2010;126:919–29.
50. Toda M, Iizuka Y, Kawase T, Uyemura K, Kawakami Y. Immuno-viral therapy of brain tumors by combination of viral therapy with cancer vaccination using a replication-conditional HSV. Cancer Gene Ther. 2002;9:356–64.
51. Ohkusu-Tsukada K, Ohta S, Kawakami Y, Toda M. Adjuvant effects of formalin-inactivated HSV through activation of dendritic cells and inactivation of myeloid-derived suppressor cells in cancer immunotherapy. Int J Cancer. 2011;128:119–31.
52. Udagawa M, Kudo-Saito C, Hasegawa G, Yano K, Yamamoto A, Yaguchi M, Toda M, Azuma I, Iwai T, Kawakami Y. Enhancement of immunologic tumor regression by intratumoral administration of dendritic cells in combination with cryoablative tumor pretreatment and Bacillus Calmette-Guerin Cell Wall Skeleton Stimulation. Clin Cancer Res. 2006;12: 7465–75.
53. Kawakami Y, Yaguchi T, Sumimoto H, Kudo-Saito C, Iwata-Kajihara T, Nakamura S, Tsujikawa T, Park JH, Popivanova BK, Miyazaki J, Kawamura N. Improvement of cancer immunotherapy by combining molecular targeted therapy. Front Oncol. 2013;3:136.

Chapter 14
Quality of CTL Therapies: A Changing Landscape

Krishnamurthy Thyagarajan, Shilpak Chatterjee, Pravin Kesarwani, Michael I. Nishimura, and Shikhar Mehrotra

Abstract The identification and cloning of tumor-associated antigens (TAA) has led to clinical trials using vaccines designed to boost the host anti-tumor immune response. Impressive clinical responses have also been documented in melanoma patients treated with these tumor-reactive T cells. These studies and others indicate the potential of T cells for their use in the adoptive therapy of cancer. However, technical issues related to the generation of a large number of tumor-specific T cells have significantly restricted the use of this promising approach. Moreover, only limited success has been achieved in terms of tumor regression or patient survival in numerous other immunotherapy trials. Evidences suggest that various tumor-escape strategies such as defects in antigen presentation, tumor-induced immunosuppression, induction of T-cell death, T-cell receptor dysfunction, the presence of tolerogenic dendritic cells and regulatory T cells undermine the effectiveness of adoptively transferred T cells. Thus, a better understanding for eliciting effective anti-tumor immunity that leads to cancer regression in all patients is needed. Herein, we discuss the recent developments aimed at overcoming the constraints that exist and are changing the landscape for effectively employing adoptive T cell therapy to treat cancer.

Keywords Immunotherapy • Th1 • Th9 • Th17 • CD73 • Metabolism • Melanoma

---

Conflict of interest: The authors declare no conflict of interest.

K. Thyagarajan • S. Chatterjee • P. Kesarwani • S. Mehrotra (✉)
Department of Surgery, Hollings Cancer Center (HO 512H), Medical University of South Carolina, 86 Jonathan Lucas Street, Charleston, SC 29425, USA
e-mail: mehrotr@musc.edu

M.I. Nishimura
Department of Surgery, Loyola University, Maywood, IL 60153, USA

B. Bonavida, S. Chouaib (eds.), *Resistance of Cancer Cells to CTL-Mediated Immunotherapy*, Resistance to Targeted Anti-Cancer Therapeutics 7,
DOI 10.1007/978-3-319-17807-3_14

Abbreviations

2-DG	2-Deoxy-D-glucose
ACT	Adoptive cell therapy
AG	Antigen
AICD	Activation induced cell death
AMPK	Adenosine monophosphate-activated protein kinase
APC	Antigen presenting cell
BiTE	Bi-specific antibody T cell engager
BTLA-4	B and T lymphocyte attenuator 4
cAMP	Cyclic AMP
CAR	Chimeric antigen receptors
CMV	Cytomegalovirus
COX-2	Cyclooxygenase-2
c-SH	Cell surface thiols
CTL	Cytotoxic T lymphocyte
CTLA-4	Cytotoxic T-lymphocyte-associated protein 4
DC	Dendritic cells
GAPDH	Glyceraldehyde-3-phosphate dehydrogenase
GITR	Glucocorticoid-induced TNFR family related gene
GLUT-1	Glucose transporter 1
GM-CSF	Granulocyte-macrophage colony-stimulating factor
GzmB	Granzyme B
HAART	Highly active antiretroviral therapy
HIF-1α	Hypoxia-inducible factor 1-alpha
HIV	Human immunodeficiency virus
HLA	Human lymphocyte antigen
ICOS	Inducible T-cell costimulator
IFNγ	Interferon gamma
iGSH	Intracellular glutathione
IL	Interleukin
iNOS	Inducible nitric oxide synthase
KO	Knockout
LAG-3	Lymphocyte-activation gene 3
MDSC	Myeloid-derived suppressor cell
MHC	Major histocompatibility complex
miRNA	MicroRNA
mTOR	Mammalian target of rapamycin
NKT	Natural killer T cells
NO	Nitric oxide
PBL	Peripheral blood lymphocytes
PD-1	Programmed death receptor-1
PGE2	Prostaglandin E2
RIPK	Receptor interacting kinases

RNS	Reactive nitrogen species
ROS	Reactive oxygen species
TAA	Tumor associated antigens
TAM	Tumor-associated macrophages
TCA	Tricarboxylic acid
T_{CM}	T central memory
TCR	T cell receptor
Teff	T effector cell
T_{EM}	T effector memory
TGFβ	Transforming growth factor beta
TIL	Tumor infiltrating lymphocytes
TIM-3	T cell immunoglobulin mucin-3
TNFα	Tumor necrosis factor alpha
Treg	T regulatory cell
T_{SCM}	*T* memory stem cells

14.1 Introduction

Treatment of cancer has been a challenge despite the advances in therapeutic regimens. Although evidences exist that immunosurveillance processes keep the tumor in check, however, the immune cells or factors can still facilitate tumor progression. Chemotherapy, radiation therapy and immunotherapy have all shown promise in the treatment of cancer and in extending the life span of patients [1]. Since the identification of tumor-associated antigens (TAA), significant advances have been made in adopting immunotherapeutic approaches that target the tumor—either by using antigen-presenting dendritic cells (DC) to stimulate the tumor-antigen reactive cytolytic $CD8^+$ T cells (CTLs) [2], or directly expand tumor-reactive CTLs ex vivo before infusing back to the patients [3]. Adoptive immunotherapy, which involves the isolation of antigen-specific T cells, followed by their ex vivo expansion, and subsequent infusion into autologous tumor bearing hosts has developed as a promising approach for inducing objective responses and sometimes even cures in patients with advanced malignancies [4]. Several novel strategies to improve adoptive immunotherapy are emerging; such as blocking inhibitory molecules (*CTLA-4, PD1, LAG-3, Tim-3, BTLA-4*) [5, 6], engaging secondary costimulatory molecules (*4-1BB, OX-40, ICOS, VISTA*) [5, 7, 8], expanding T cells in different cytokines (*IL-2, IL-15, IL-12, IL-21*) [9–11], or using recently identified T cell subsets (*Th9, Th17*) [12, 13]. Although novel means for enhancing the quality of tumor-specific T cells in vitro have been discovered, how immunosuppressive elements produced by the tumor microenvironment impact the engraftment potential, function and anti-tumor activity of T cells in vivo are unknown. Though the therapeutic efficacy of CTLs is dependent on multiple factors, we limit our discussion to inter-twined aspects of survival, suppression, aging, and metabolism. We believe that these key aspects are interconnected tightly and control the extrinsic factors

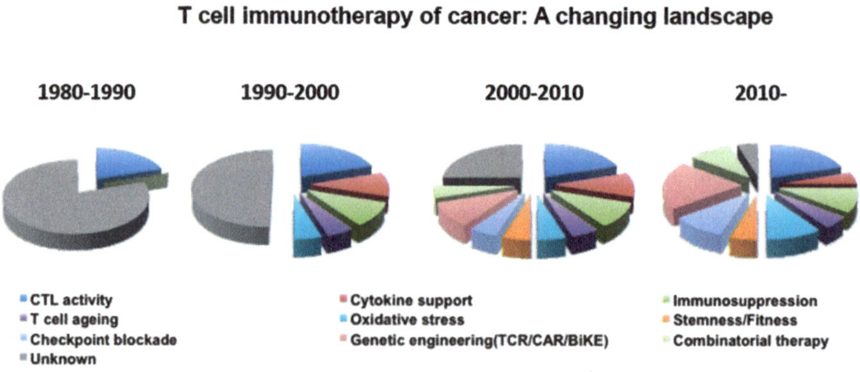

Fig. 14.1 Breaking up the 'gray' areas in T cell responses in cancer. A schematic representation of the different approaches that have been employed over the years to improve CTL responses, leading to better therapeutic potential as well as better survival. These strategies have helped us better harness the T cell 'powerhouse' and direct it against cancer. This has also improved our understanding of the underlying biology of how T cell activation, memory generation and persistence

(as cytokines in the microenvironment or during ex vivo expansion) to modulate the CTLs intrinsically (as survival, effector function, metabolic commitment), which result in differences in outcome. Figure 14.1 summarizes various strategies that have evolved with time due to our increased understanding of the innate and adaptive arms of the immune system and how they could be modulated to control the tumor progression. We discuss below in various sections some of the key changes that hold promise for current and future usages of CTLs in adoptive cell therapy (ACT) of cancer.

14.2 CTL Type

The maintenance of immunity to combat any disease is primarily dependent on the presence of a robust immune system. The adaptive immune system is responsible for elimination of disease-causing agents from the body so as to keep it disease-free [14]. Immunologic approaches for treating cancer patients have so far been partially successful, mainly due to their inability to elicit an effective long-term anti-tumor immunity [15]. Immunologic tolerance to antigens expressed by the tumors is a likely explanation for the difficulty in eliciting an effective anti-tumor immunity to self-antigens expressed by cancer cells. In order to break the immunological tolerance and mount anti-tumor T cell responses, various strategies such as repeated vaccination with antigen-pulsed DCs, expanding the T cells ex vivo, or inhibiting the action of inhibitory molecules/factors are employed [16–21]. Such therapeutic strategies based on stimulating the patient's immune system represent an important treatment modality, but much remains to be discovered to optimize their use, e.g. a number of associated factors as cell death due to repeated vaccination, replicative senescence of ex vivo expanded CTLs or susceptibility to autoimmunity that co-exist with these strategies. Another important question that needs to be addressed is the type of the CTL that should be used in ACT (Adoptive Cell Therapy) to achieve long-term tumor control.

14.2.1 CD8 vs. CD4 CTL

T cells either express the CD8 co-receptor on their cell surface and recognize 8–10 amino acid peptide fragments that are bound to MHC class I molecules, or the CD4 co-receptor on their cell surface which recognizes 10–15 amino acid peptide fragments bound to MHC class II molecules [22]. While CD8$^+$ T cells have cytolytic capacity and represent the effector arm of T cell-mediated immunity, CD4$^+$ T cells are primarily considered as helper T cells that secrete cytokines and initiate or augment the function of cytotoxic T lymphocytes (CTLs) and B cells. Despite earlier reports about the capability of CD4$^+$ T cells to control tumor growth, their use was abandoned due to the poor understanding of the origin of regulatory T cells after various reports highlighted that CD4$^+$ T cells can also be potential suppressors [23, 24]. A recent study, however, tried to readdress this issue using class II restricted CD4$^+$ transgenic T cells and concluded that CD4$^+$ T cells can be more efficient at tumor rejection than CD8$^+$ T cells [25]. In addition, other studies have argued for the potential of using the class I restricted CD4$^+$ T cells to generate cognate 'help' along with exploiting its potential to control tumor growth [26, 27]. It is, thus, believed that the efficacy of adoptive immunotherapy could be substantially improved if both CD8$^+$ T cells and CD4$^+$ T cells could be engaged in an anti-tumor immune response directed at the same tumor-associated epitope. Thus, the fact that CD4$^+$ T cells could be central to the function of the immune system and have a key role in tumor immunity remain under-appreciated. We have recently developed a novel transgenic strain using a human tyrosinase epitope-reactive CD8 independent TCR TIL3183I isolated from MHC class-I restricted CD4$^+$ T cells [28]. In these mice (referred hereafter as h3T –*h*uman *T*IL derived *T*yrosinase *T*CR), this HLA-A2 restricted, high affinity TCR is expressed on both CD4$^+$ and CD8$^+$ T cells. Our preliminary data show that a comparable numbers of class I restricted CD4$^+$ and CD8$^+$ T cells from the h3T mice are equally potent in controlling growth of human melanoma in a xenograft model. Thus, methodologies that induce the robust stimulation of lytic properties of both CD8$^+$ and CD4$^+$ in parallel, in turn, might lead to a direct attack on tumor cells as well as an efficient establishment of T cell memory.

Interestingly, CD4 T cells can also behave as CTLs depending on the conditions of activation. The CTL activity associated with CD4 T cells gets initiated upon repeated stimulation after which CD4 T cells show an increase in cytolytic molecules such as perforin and granzyme [29]. Reports have shown that the initiation of a cytolytic program is associated with concordant changes in transcription factors, which are responsible for regulating this switch. Primarily, CD4 and CD8 T cells develop in the thymus under the control of two key transcription factors, namely ThPOK and Runx3 [30]. ThPOK is responsible for the generation of CD4 T cells and Runx3 is responsible for CD8 T cells. Runx3 has also been shown to be responsible for regulating genes associated with the CTL developmental program. CD4 T cells that are stimulated repeatedly by a cognate antigen lose ThPOK and upregulate Runx3, thereby diverting the classical 'helper' T cells to cytotoxic CD4 T cells. The cytotoxic CD4 T cells also acquire a surface phenotype of markers that are associated with natural killer cells and CD8 T cells. Cell surface receptors such as CRTAM [31, 32] and CD244 [33] are also upregulated and IFNγ production is boosted. These cytotoxic CD4 T cells are capable of controlling infections as well as tumors. Transfer of CD4 T cells into tumor-bearing mice was reported to cause an increased expansion of T cells in vivo, differentiation and reduction in tumor burden in a mouse model of melanoma [34]. The transferred CD4 T cells acquire cytotoxic abilities on encounter with antigen and then mediate tumor clearance. Further, CD4 T cells have been shown to increase tumor infiltration and proliferation of CD8 T cells, thus enhancing Class-I-mediated tumor rejection. There has also been a single case report in which a patient treated with ex vivo generated autologous $CD4^+$ T cell clones, that recognize the tumor-associated antigen NY-ESO-1 [35], remained disease-free two years later with the persistence of the transferred cells. Importantly, the patient had not received any lymphodepleting conditioning that is usually administered before adoptive immunotherapy with the intention of augmenting homeostatic proliferation and persistence of effector cells [36, 37]. Moreover, IL-2 was not administered after the transfer. This study indicates the potential of tumor epitope-specific $CD4^+$ T cells in immunotherapy. Despite the above-mentioned attributes, CD4 T cells only cause Class II-mediated tumor rejection and since most solid tumors express MHC class I and not MHC class II [38] the use of CD4 T cells as direct mediators of tumor killing is limited. However, the ability of CD4 T cells to enhance CD8 T cell responses to tumor may be an important area to explore for the use of CD4 T cells in immunotherapy.

14.2.2 Quality of the CTL Response

The primary premise of ex vivo expansion is to selectively enrich the tumor antigen-specific T cells and, at the same time, improve the quality of the T cell response. We further discuss below the two important parameters that crucially determine the quality of anti-tumor T cells, namely: *a)* strong effector functions and *b)* ability to persist longer in the tumor-bearing host.

14.2.2.1 Role of Cytokine Preconditioning in CTL Function

Cytokines play an important role in the homeostasis as well as the proliferation of T cells in vivo. For optimal T cell activation and proliferation, T cells require three signals [39]. Signaling through the TCR and the co-stimulatory receptors constitute the first two signals while engagement of the cytokine receptors by appropriate cytokines makes up the third signal [40]. Since signals mediated through cytokine receptors are required for T cell proliferation and homeostasis, cytokine supplementation is important while administration of T cells to patients. Also, gene transfer studies have suggested that the expression of cytokine genes in tumor cells increases their immunogenicity and thus makes them more susceptible to killing by the CTLs [41–45]. Cytokines such as IL2 are supplemented with autologous T cells transfer and have been shown to increase the in vivo function and persistence. However, careful evaluation of the role of cytokines is necessary, prior to administration, as these may have either adverse effects such as lymphodepletion when administered in higher doses [46] or potential toxicities associated with them, as in the case of IL12 [47]. Similarly, other studies have shown that expanding anti-tumor T cells in IL15 or IL21 can result in a better persistence and an improved anti-tumor outcome [48, 49]

While toxic effects of IL12 were noted at high concentrations [47], when used at low concentration, it can be used for preconditioning T cells towards Th1 cells, which have the ability to produce high amount of IFN-γ. Mescher's group has shown that IL12 can act as third signal for clonal expansion [40]. It was also shown that IL12 can also impart the memory phenotype to the T cells after antigen encounter and clonal expansion [50]. Recently, several groups have shown the potential role of IL12 in tumor immunotherapy. These studies show that $CD8^+$ T cells activated in the presence of IL12 exhibit a better tumor treatment [51, 52]. The mechanisms of IL12 anti-tumor function are intricate and may be attributed to either higher expression of CD25 [53], or other co-stimulatory molecules such as ICOS or OX-40 [52]. A recent study shows that IL12 induces up regulation as several cell cycle proteins mediating robust cell division, prolongs CD25 expression, and therefore making cells more sensitive/responsive to IL2 [54]. Similarly, other studies have shown that preconditioning anti-tumor T cells in the presence of IL15 or IL21 can result in their better persistence and an improved anti-tumor outcome. Klebanoff et al. have shown that exogenous IL15 can improve the T cell efficacy [9], primarily by increasing the anti-apoptotic phenotype and expression of CD62L on T cells that aid in homing. Recently, our group has also shown that IL15 may act by increasing the antioxidant capacity and cell surface thiol levels of T cells, therefore these cells may have an edge over cells cultured in IL2 in a rich oxidative tumor microenvironment [55]. Similarly, the presence of IL21 during priming also enhances tumor immunotherapy [49], by decreasing the transcription factor *EOMES*, increasing the expression of CD62L (L-selectin) and imparting T cells with a central memory-like phenotype. Another study suggests that IL21 may act by giving CD8 T cells a unique effector phenotype of $CD44^{high}PD1^{low}CD25^{low}CD134^{low}CD137^{low}$ [56]. One of the groups has also shown that IL21 acts synergistically with IL15 and IL7 for proliferation of $CD8^+$ T cells and exhibits a better anti-tumor response [48]. Moreover, reports suggest that IL21 increases degranulation and expression of IFNγ by tumor infiltrating CD8 T cells [57]. In addition to enhancing cytotoxicity of T cells, IL21 was also shown to augment the production of other inflammatory cytokines like IFNγ, IL2, TNFα, GM-CSF, IL1β and IL6 that can in turn potentiate the anti-tumor response of the T cells [58]. Thus, preconditioning with some of these cytokines alone or in combination can increase the efficacy of CTLs for adoptive cell therapy.

14.2.2.2 Effector Cytokine Secretion by CTLs

The effector functions of anti-tumor T cells are usually characterized by their ability to secrete various cytokines and cytolytic molecules following the recognition of its target antigen. Among various cytokines, the ability to secret IFNγ by anti-tumor T cells has been shown to be indispensable for tumor rejection. The crucial role of IFNγ-mediating anti-tumor response was originally highlighted by the study showing that neutralization of IFNγ, but not TNFα, abrogates the LPS-mediated rejection of Meth A cells (3-methylcholanthrene (MCA)-induced fibrosarcoma cells of BALB/c mice) [59]. This observation was further supported by the fact that deficiency of IFNγ in tumor antigen specific transgenic T cells significantly impaired their anti-tumor potential [60]. Studies have shown that IFNγ can increase the immunogenicity of tumor cells by up-regulating their MHC expression and thus making them more susceptible to CTL-mediated lysis [61–63]. Moreover, IFNγ also has a direct pro-apoptotic and anti-angiogenic effect on tumor cells and can activate the tumor-resident APCs towards a pro-immunogenic type [64]. Evidences suggest that the co-operation of other cytokines with IFNγ is required for effective eradication of tumor. The study by Nagoshi et al. showed that production of GM-CSF along with IFNγ determined the efficacy of adoptive cellular immunotherapy since neutralization of GM-CSF with a specific monoclonal antibody increased the tumor burden [65]. It was speculated that production of GM-CSF by the T cells resulted in the activation of macrophages and dendritic cells, which in turn actively participated in the induction of profound anti-tumor responses [66]. Another study showed that IL3 also plays an important role in anti-tumor immunity along with IFNγ and GM-CSF. Mice deficient in IL3, IFNγ and GM-CSF (IL-$3^{-/-}$GM-$CSF^{-/-}$IFN$\gamma^{-/-}$) developed lymphomas and non-lymphoid solid tumors at a higher rate than mice deficient in IFNγ alone or both IL3 and GM-CSF or GM-CSF alone [67]. Similarly, some other studies have shown the role of TNFα as an important cytokine in controlling tumor growth [68]. Of late, a number of studies have established that rather than one dominant individual cytokine; a cumulative effect of many different cytokines imparts a much efficient and long-lasting 'polyfunctional' phenotype that has an improved ability to control tumor growth [69].

In addition to the Th1 category of cytokines mentioned above, recent studies have implicated the involvement of IL9 (previously considered to be a type-2 cytokine), and IL17 in controlling tumor progression. With advancements in the availability of various recombinant cytokines and antibodies, it has now become feasible to ex vivo program several conditions that promote the differentiation of the T cell subsets (Th1/Tc1, Th9/Tc9, Th17/Tc17) for use in the ACT protocol. Recent pre-clinical studies that utilize these strategies are discussed below.

Th1/Tc1

The primary cellular subsets that have been shown to be important for immunotherapy have been the T cells that can initiate an IFNγ response [70, 71]. Both CD4 and CD8 T cells have shown potential, for treatment of tumors when cultured in the presence of IL12 to become polarized as either Th1 or Tc1 cells [72]. These T cell subsets express high levels of cytolytic molecules such as perforin and granzyme, which make them excellent candidates for anti-tumor effectors. The induction of the cytolytic program is also accompanied by an increase in the levels of transcription factors like *T-bet* and *IRF4* which are responsible for the effector functions of these T cells [73]. These T cells upregulate CD25 that make them dependent on IL2 and induce STAT5. Signaling through the IL12 receptor enhanced the STAT4 levels, which regulate T-bet, and thus IFNγ production [74].

However, Th1 or Tc1 cells are unable to provide long-term protection against tumors because of their effector-like phenotypes. There are conflicting reports regarding this phenomenon. Some studies argue that due to the faster expansion of T cells and increased proliferation, the Th1/Tc1 cells become exhausted and cannot persist for prolonged immune surveillance [75]. Other reports suggests that Tc1 cells are able to persist as long-term homeostatic proliferating memory cells, which are able to retain function and mediate tumor growth suppression and metastasis [76]. With the identification of different T cell subsets (i.e. Th9/Tc9, Th17/Tc17), that also exhibit anti-tumor potential when co-secreting IFNγ, the Th1/Tc1 cells that primarily secrete IFNγ have lost their prominence—but further studies that design the ex vivo culture conditions to program the T cell subsets with best features from all the subsets in building a potent hybrid CTL may improve immunotherapy.

Th17/Tc17

Intensive investigation has been focused on Th17 cells and indicates that this T helper subset is capable of mediating an anti-tumor effect [77–79]. Studies have shown that adoptive transfer of tumor antigen-specific T cells committed to produce IL17 swiftly eradicates large established tumors in mice [60]. The efficacy of tumor-specific type-17 responses has also been reported in murine CD8 T cells (Tc17) and genetically engineered human CD4 T cells [80, 81]. Although Th17/Tc17 cells are committed to produce IL-17, however, their anti-tumor response depends on their ability to secret IFNγ, the absence of which significantly dampens the anti-tumor response of Th17 cells [60]. However, the question remains that if IFNγ is crucial in mounting an effective anti-tumor response, then why the Th1/Tc1 cells that are committed to produce IFNγ are unable to provide a prolonged anti-tumor immunity. It is, thus, likely that the ability to mount a protective anti-tumor response depends not only on the cytokine response but also on the ability of the anti-tumor T cells to persist and develop long-term memory.

Studies have shown that although Th1 cells possess an effector phenotype ($IFN\gamma^{hi}$ and $GzmB^{hi}$), however, their inability to persist longer in the tumor-bearing recipients restrains their usefulness in anti-tumor immunotherapy. On the contrary, Th17 cells exhibit reduced effector functions as compared to Th1 cells, but possess stem cell-like characteristics [77, 79], which allows them to persist longer in the tumor-bearing host and thus mount protective anti-tumor responses [77]. Genetic analysis of ex vivo polarized Th17 cells unveiled that they have overexpression of *Tcf7* and some other genes in the downstream pathway of the Wnt/β -catenin signalling pathway [77]. The overexpression of *Tcf7* is generally found in naïve T cells and gradually decreases following activation. Thus, the overexpression of *Tcf7* and stemness-associated genes in Th17 might be responsible for the maintenance of their "young" phenotype and self-renewal capacity, which are necessary for their long term persistence in the host.

Another issue that needs to be considered when using Th17 cells is that of 'plasticity' [82], that refers to changing the phenotype with the dynamic microenvironment. It has been noticed that Th17 cells are not stable as they can also convert into an IL-17^{+}FoxP3^{+} regulatory T cell (Treg) phenotype [83], or an effector IL-17^{-}IFNγ^{+} phenotype under inflammatory conditions in the tumor microenvironment [84–87]. This 'plasticity' or skew in the effector phenotype by Th17 cells may be responsible for decreased longevity in the anti-tumor activity of these cells. Further, IL17 has also been shown to be pro-tumorogenic in certain scenarios [88]. Thus, in order to promote the anti-tumor activity of Th17 cells, it may be crucial to understand the factors that are responsible for regulating its pro- vs. anti-tumorogenic properties. Our recent study has shown that while TGFβ and IL-6 help ex vivo differentiation to Th17^{TGF}β cells, they were also responsible for upregulation of the ectonucleotidase CD73 on Th17^{TGF}β cells. CD73 (along with CD39) sequentially cleaves ATP to produce adenosine, which is immunosuppressive [89]. Thus, an alternative strategy to generate Th17 cells in the presence of IL-1βIL-6 (i.e. Th17^{IL1}β) was more efficient in controlling the tumor due to a reduced CD73 expression and a highly polyfunctional phenotype (as IFN-γ^{hi}, CD107a^{hi}, T-bet^{hi}, Granzyme B^{hi}, HIF-1α^{hi}). Although Th17^{IL1}β cells lacked the expression of key stem cell genes (as *β-catenin*, *TCF-6*, *Lef-1*) that have been attributed to the increased persistence of conventional Th17^{TGF}β cells, adding a trace amount of TGFβ to Th17^{IL1}β cells not only restored the expression of stem cell genes and increased persistence, but also reduced activation-induced cell death [89]. Our data also show that Th17^{TGF}β and Th17^{IL1}β are the two spectrums of the T cell response—with Th17^{TGF}β being less glycolytic (discussed in detail later) than Th17^{IL1}β. The higher effector response associated with higher glycolytic Th17^{IL1}β is also correlated to increased susceptibility to cell death. Our data also shows that including TGFβ at lower concentrations drops glycolysis and increases the stemness feature with reduced susceptibility to AICD as well. Thus, a comprehensive understanding of the factors that control long-term and stable anti-tumor T cell function is needed for improving ACT of cancer. Figure 14.2 show how the understanding of the Th17^{TGF}β and Th17^{IL1}β cells led us to devise ex vivo culture conditions to achieve long-term tumor control using Th17 cells with a hybrid Th1 + Th17 phenotype.

Interestingly, a recent report has suggested that the ability of Tc17 to control tumors is poorer than Tc1 cells. This enhanced ability of Tc1 cells has been attributed

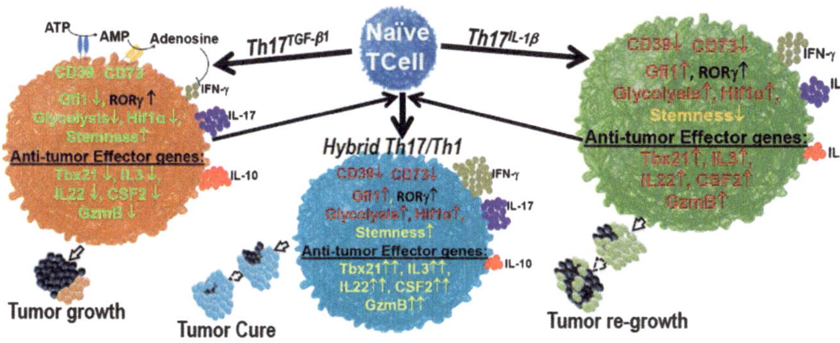

Fig. 14.2 A schematic figure highlighting the differences in effector molecules, stem cell associated genes, and metabolic commitment between the Th17 cells generated ex vivo using either TGFβ ($Th17^{TGF}β$) or IL1β ($Th17^{IL1}β$) programming conditions. The key useful traits of these two type of Th17 cells used to generate hybrid Th17/Th1 cells result in improved immunotherapeutic control of the tumor growth

to IFNγ signaling in the tumor cells [90]. The abrogation of IFNγ signaling in tumor cells completely blocks the effect of Tc1 cells. Further, transcription factors, especially T-bet, RORγ and IRF4 play an important role in regulating the ability of Th17/Tc17 cells in mediating tumor regression and need to be considered when designing optimal culture conditions for CTL generation [91, 92].

Th9/Tc9

IL9, originally discovered as p40 in human T cell growth factor, has been shown to have pleiotropic roles on both myeloid and lymphoid cells [93]. Though understudied for a long time, recent studies have focused on the role of IL9 and its effects on anti-tumor immunity [94]. T cells can be programmed to produce IL9 using TGFβ and IL4. Early studies have associated the IL9-producing T cells as a subset of the Th2 type cells. However, it has been observed that Th9 cells do not produce the classical Th2 cytokines [95, 96]. Instead, the production of IL9 leads to the suppression of Th2 cytokines. Further, the production of IL9 is also responsible for reduced IL12 production by APCs, thus blunting any possible Th1 type response [97]. Therefore, IL9 acts as both positive and negative regulator of immune responses. The majority work in the field of IL9-producing T cells has shown the usefulness of CD4 T cells. Th9 cells have been shown to clear established melanoma in a mouse model [12, 98]. It was clearly demonstrated that IL9 was responsible for this effect using an IL9-blocking antibody. Administration of recombinant IL9 also led to reduction in tumor burden. The observed tumor regression was found to be dependent on the interaction of IL9 and IL9R and signaling mediated through the IL9R. Further investigation revealed that the effect of IL-9 in inhibiting tumor growth is primarily mediated through mast cells, since deficiency of mast cells failed to control tumor growth [98]. The anti-tumor potential of IL-9 is only restricted to non-lymphoid tumors since they potentiate the growth and survival of lymphomas that express the IL-9R [98].

Recently, there has also been interest in IL9-producing CD8 T cells and their ability to mediate tumor killing. IL9-producing CD8 T cells or Tc9 cells were recently studied and have been shown to be effective in mediating tumor regression while maintaining their signature cytokine profiles for an extended period of time [99, 100]. However, IL9 has been shown to have detrimental effects as well. IL9 has been reported to be involved in atopic dermatitis [101], and airway inflammation [102]. Further, it has been shown that the expression of IL9 T cells is exclusive of IFNγ and is inhibited by IFNγ [103]. IFNγ is a key cytokine, which assists in tumor killing and also makes the tumors more susceptible to T cell killing. Since IL9-producing cells do not produce IFNγ, it may be of concern to use these cells for immunotherapy. Further, Th9 cells in vitro have been shown to retain IL9 production for a short period of time, thereby, contradicting the findings of Tc9 cells, which maintain IL9 production even after retrieval from the tumor- bearing mice. Nevertheless, further studies using IL9 are essential before these cells can be used as a potential therapy for different types of tumors.

14.2.2.3 CTL Persistence

The persistence of transferred CTLs is important to mediate immunosurveillance against cancer. In addition, for adoptively transferred ex vivo expanded autologous T cells, it is imperative that T cells persist in the host and are, not only able to mediate tumor killing, but also able to prevent recurrence of tumor growth. Survival of transferred T cells requires the availability of accessible niches that can be used by the T cell to engraft, ability to self-renew whereas death of transferred CTLs in the tumor microenvironment can be caused by repeated antigenic restimulation or activation-induced cell death (AICD), apoptosis and hypoxia among other factors. Other factors affecting T cell survival include oxidative stress in the microenvironment of tumor; inhibitory molecules expressed by tumors and suppressive cells which mediate immune suppression under the aegis of the tumor. In addition, the niche available in vivo to the CTL for engraftment in tumor milieu could also affect the outcome of a T cell response and will be discussed below.

T Cell Death

There are various ways cell death occurs. One of the most common ways of T cell death is caspase-dependent cell death, commonly known as apoptosis [104]. T cells upon antigen challenge undergo clonal expansion. However, if antigen is present in abundance then T cells upon chronic re-stimulation undergo cell death commonly known as AICD [105, 106]. Snow et al. demonstrated that in the X-linked lymphoproliferative disease, patients have a defective AICD machinery that leads to a fatal increase in the number of lymphocytes [107]. Therefore, AICD is an important mechanism for the immune system to get rid of extra inflammation. Earlier studies have shown that AICD requires caspase 3, and in some cases could be independent of activator caspases such as caspase 8 and caspase 9 [108]. Other groups have also shown that AICD is independent of granzyme and perforin-induced cell death and can be inhibited by blocking TNFα [109]. AICD can also be inhibited by blocking FasL or Fas receptor along with TNFα [110].

With reference to T cell immunotherapy, it may be important to interfere with the death/contraction/AICD of the tumor-epitope reactive T cells to increase their persistence in the tumor microenvironment in order to achieve a meaningful and sustained tumor regression. Thus, an understanding of the kind of cell death that an effector T cell subset may undergo upon encountering TCR restimulation by TAA will be important, and has also been the focus of our group [111, 112]. Peter Kramer's group has shown that AICD can be reduced in T cells by glucocorticoids by decreasing the FasL expression in T cells [113]. Several groups have utilized different cytokines during polarization, which may reduce AICD. One such strategy is the use of IL-15 during T cell activation [114]. We have shown that cells cultured in IL15 show less death in comparison to those cultured in IL2, as IL15 increases antioxidant levels and cell surface thiols on the T cells [55]. Another recent study shows that IL15 cultured cells show reduced caspase 3 activity by nitrosylating caspase 3 at cys163 site [115].

One other common form of T cell death is caspase 1-mediated cell death, which is commonly referred to as pyroptosis [116, 117]. Pyroptosis mainly occurs during a chronic microbial or viral inflammation. It is a form of programmed cell death orchestrated by caspase 1, which was known for its function to cleave pro-IL-1β and therefore known as IL1β converting enzyme (ICE) [118]. Recently, it has been demonstrated that CD4⁺T cell death occurring in HIV infection is through the caspase-1/ IL-1 β-mediated pathway [119]. T cells could be rescued by inhibiting caspase -1. One of the caspase-1 inhibitors, VX-765, which has already been validated for treating epilepsy [120], also has the potential to rescue T cells from pyroptosis induced by HIV [119]. One other less known form of cell death is necroptosis. Necrosis was found to occur in a programmed manner and therefore termed as necroptosis [121]. Necroptosis is a caspase independent form of cell death, which requires the activation of receptor interacting kinases 1 and 3 (RIPK1 and RIPK3). Degterev et al. have also identified a compound (necrostatin-1), which can inhibit the RIPK1 [121]. Another group has recently shown that T cells deficient in caspase 8 do not undergo classical cell death and instead may be undergoing Ripk1-mediated cell death which is not induced by TNF-α [122]. A recent study shows that some of the $CD4^+$ T cells infected with HIV may undergo necroptosis [123]. One other form of recently identified cell death is ferroptosis. It is a non-apoptotic form of cell death, which is an iron-dependent form of cell death [124]. This type of cell death occurs due to iron-dependent accumulation of reactive oxygen species (ROS). Expression signature of ferroptosis is different for other types of cell death such as apoptosis or pyroptosis. A small molecule inhibitor known as ferrostatin 1 can inhibit ferroptosis [124]. While necroptosis as well as ferroptosis have not been yet identified as prominent pathways for T cell death, it is likely that under different physiological conditions in vivo such death pathways may ensue the death/contraction of certain subsets of CTLs. If so, the inhibitors as Necrostatin-1 or ferrostatin-1 may be used for rescuing the T cells from such forms of cell death. Thus, further studies are needed to comprehensively understand if there are any differences in the type of cell death at various stages of the CTL life-span, so that the longevity of anti-tumor effector T cells can be accordingly modulated. We believe that using one of these approaches or a combination of these approaches may rescue the T cells from AICD and increase the efficacy of immunotherapy [55, 108–110, 113–119, 121, 124].

Availability of Niches

The transfer of autologous T cells into patients helps in bolstering the immune response to cancer and also in killing the tumor cells [35, 125, 126]. The long-term goal of adoptive immunotherapy has been that after the clearance of the tumor, the transferred T cells persist as memory cells to prevent any further recurrence [127, 128]. However, for this to happen, the T cells must reside in the secondary lymphoid organs as memory T cells so as to provide a rapid secondary immune response on re-encountering the tumor antigen. Since the host homeostatic mechanisms are involved in equilibrating the number of T cells, by balancing out T cell expansion and death, it is only possible to transiently increase the available niche for transferred the T cells. It has been reported that the persistence or long-term survival of adoptively transferred T cells is dependent on the availability of spaces for engraftment of these cells [129]. This is important for the continued presence of increased frequency of tumor-specific T cells and suppression of tumor growth [130]. Various reports have suggested the beneficial effects of radiation therapy in improving the immunotherapy of cancer [131–133]. It has been suggested that the use of radiation therapy enhances T cell therapy in various ways. Firstly, radiation therapy directly causes a dent in the tumor growth. Secondly, radiation has been shown to enhance the immunogenicity of cancer cells, which is essential for their recognition by T cells. Finally and most importantly, it has been shown that radiation causes the death of host T cells and regulatory T cells (Treg) that can act as barriers to effective CTL therapy [36, 37]. The deletion of host T cells enhances the availability of cytokines to transferred CTLs [134], and Treg death leads to lower suppression of transferred T cells. Recent reports have suggested that low dose radiation enhances T cell stimulation leading to an increase in the production of IFNγ as well as lowering the threshold for T cell activation [135, 136]. Another study suggested that low dose radiation affects macrophage polarization, which in turn enhances the efficacy of T cell immunotherapy [137]. Therefore, the ability of CTL therapy in controlling tumors depends on the ability of T cells to proliferate, persist and retain functionality, for which radiation therapy is an important tool in improving success.

Ability to Self-Renew

One fundamental insight borne out of various clinical and adoptive T cell therapy studies is that the objective response is directly related to the long-term persistence of the adoptively transferred T cells into the host. The primary prerequisite for the long-term persistence of T cells is their ability to express various stem cell-like characteristics, which endows longevity, self-renewal capacity, and lesser susceptibility to activation-induced death. Recent studies describe a novel subset of memory T cells termed as memory stem cells (T_{SCM}) which display stem-cell like features and can be identified by the expression of $CD62^{hi}$, $CCR7^{hi}$, $CD44^{lo}$, $SCA\text{-}1^{hi}$ and $Bcl2^{hi}$ cells. Studies by Gattinoni et al. suggest that the Wnt/β-catenin pathway is highly operational in T_{SCM} cells as described for other self-renewing populations [138]. Indeed, stabilization of β-catenin by constitutive degradation of GSK3β during antigenic stimulation of CD8 cells enhances T_{SCM} formation. Emerging evidences suggest that since T_{SCM} cells do not achieve a full terminal differentiation in vitro, they are more effective than terminally differentiated effector T cells in eradicating the tumor in vivo. One potential reason behind this phenomenon is that although effector T cells are highly cytotoxic in vitro, they lose the ability to secrete IL2 and up-regulate KLRG-1 and are very sensitive to replicative senescence.

A recent study has also shown that the frequency of $CD8^+$ T_{SCM} is decreased in individuals with chronic, untreated HIV-1 infection, and that HAART has a restorative effect on this subset [139]. In contrast, natural controllers of HIV-1 had the highest absolute number of $CD4^+$ T_{SCM} cells among all the infected groups. Therefore, the $CD8^+$ T_{SCM} population may represent a correlate of protection in chronic HIV-1 infection that is directly relevant to the design of T cell-based vaccines, adoptive immunotherapy approaches or the pharmacologic induction of T_{SCM}. Also, T cell expansion after encountering bacterial infection shows that the $CD62L^{hi}$ cells have a stem cell like property and these cells can expand to provide protection. The same has also been shown to be the case in ultra-low dose CMV infections [140]. From these reports it is evident that a small pool of T cells that are similar to stem cells are able to provide protection against various ailments and that this might be the key to improve immunotherapy of cancer [141]. Further, harnessing the capability of these cells to self-renew may be another important step to mediate long-lived anti-tumor immunity.

Susceptibility to Tumor Microenvironment Stress

Various activation and inhibitory receptors on the tumor cell may mediate apoptosis of CTLs by inducing pro-apoptotic signaling. Tumors are known to express high levels of FasL, which causes apoptosis of CTLs that express Fas on their surface, due to their activation status [142]. Tumor-infiltrating macrophages respond to IFNγ by producing TNFα and nitric oxide that induces the apoptosis of T cells. In order to make T cells resistant to these mechanisms of apoptosis, researchers have introduced siRNA to Fas in CTLs, which led to decreased apoptosis of the transferred

T cells via the Fas-FasL interaction [143]. Downstream inhibition of signaling molecules such as c-jun N-terminal kinases (JNK) leads to poorer activation of the apoptosis inducing factor (AIF) and effector caspases, thus leading to reduced AICD of T cells [144, 145]. Further, CTLs in the tumor microenvironment are subject to oxidative and metabolic stress. The tumor microenvironment is an oxidative environment, which reduces the ability of T cells to function as well as induces apoptosis. The presence of ROS, RNS and superoxide's induces oxidative stress that in turn could affect the T cell function and its ability to control tumor growth. Various reports show that the use of antioxidants during cancer therapy, especially vitamins as supplements, increases the potential for tumor regression [146, 147]. Antioxidants help reduce the free radicals which cause damage to cells. As prophylactic agents, these may be helpful in reducing the initiation of cancer. Further there is a possibility that these antioxidants may help reduce the oxidative environment in the tumors and make them more susceptible to killing by CTLs. However, the role of anti-oxidant enzymes in various T cell subsets is not clearly established. We have recently shown that TCR restimulation results in a decrease in the reductive state of actively dividing cells, rendering them more sensitive to oxidative stress [148]. We also show that a subset of T cells with central memory-like phenotype (T_{CM} cells) show increased expression of cell surface sulfhydryl groups (thiols; c-SH), a key target of redox regulation and other antioxidant protein molecules as compared to the effector memory-like phenotype (T_{EM} cells) [148].

Cells use thiols such as glutathione and thioredoxin for protection against the detrimental effects of oxidants. It has also been documented that the overall level of reduced thiols on cell surface molecules differs on individual subsets of peripheral blood mononuclear cells and that these levels can be manipulated in vitro by altering the level of intracellular glutathione (iGSH). Glutathione (GSH), a cysteine-containing tripeptide (γ-glutamylcysteinylglycine) and its oxidized dimer GSSG, plays a key role in regulating the intracellular redox balance and the status of –SH groups on proteins and other molecules. Via GSSG, thioredoxin, glutaredoxin, glutathione peroxidases, and other enzymes in the GSH system, GSH regulates the activity of enzymes and transcription factors by controlling whether the –SH group remains reduced and, hence, free or whether it is covalently coupled to GSH (or NO) [149]. Depletion of GSH is an early hallmark observed in apoptosis and the relationship between GSH depletion, generation of ROS, and progression of apoptosis has been recently addressed. Simultaneous single cell analysis of changes in the GSH content and ROS formation by multi-parametric flow-cytometry revealed that the loss of intracellular GSH was paralleled by the generation of different ROS including hydrogen peroxide, superoxide anion, hydroxyl radical, and lipid peroxides. iGSH levels also tend to decrease as HIV disease progresses and low GSH levels in subjects with advanced HIV disease predict poor survival and impact T cell function [150, 151].

The role of ROS in determining T cell susceptibility to arthritis has also been shown recently [152]. These studies showed that the lower capacity to produce ROS is associated with an increased number of reduced thiol groups (–SH) on the T cell membrane surfaces. Our recent data also show that in adoptive cell therapy, the increased expression of thiols on T cells could be directly correlated to increased efficacy of the transferred CTLs [148]. CTLs with higher cell surface thiols were better in mediating rejection of tumors as compared to those having lower levels of thiol. Further, the persistence of T cells with higher cell surface thiols was also enhanced. T cells with higher cell surface thiols showed a $CD62L^{hi}CD44^{hi}$ memory T cell-like phenotype. These data suggested that promoting the reductive cellular environment could result in the long-term maintenance of $CD8^{+}$ T cells, and may have implications in T cell adoptive immunotherapy protocols.

14.2.3 Immunosuppression and CTL Response

Despite the major advances being made to improve the quality of tumor immunotherapy, a plethora of immunosuppressive mechanisms operating at the tumor site are considered to be the major obstacle for successful immunotherapy of cancer. Thus, increased understanding of these immunosuppressive mechanisms might open up new avenues to overcome the tolerizing conditions employed by the tumor microenvironment and, thus, dramatically increase the objective response of anti-tumor T cells. Compelling evidences suggest that the growing tumor can employ a myriad of immunosuppressive strategies to evade the anti-tumor T cell response. It has been widely accepted that tumor-mediated immunosuppression is not merely the property of tumor cells, rather, it crucially depends on its microenvironment. The tumor microenvironment is a dynamic network of various immunosuppressive cell populations that may act in concert to thwart anti-tumor T cell responses. We discuss briefly different immunosuppressive strategies that affect the CTL responses:

14.2.3.1 Immunosuppressive Cytokines

Secretion of various immunosuppressive cytokines and growth factors by the tumor cells and the associated stromal cells is an important mechanism dampening the effector T cell response. Among various immunosuppressive cytokines, TGFβ is the extensively studied cytokine that has shown to impair effector T cells function and proliferation. Historically, TGFβ has been considered as a growth promoting factor for the tumor cells. However, Ranges et al. [153] showed that apart from promoting the tumor growth, TGFβ may also play an important role in mediating tumor escape from host immune surveillance. Later on, Gorelik and Flavell confirmed this finding by demonstrating that tumor evasion from immune response can be overcome by T cells specific blockade of TGFβ that results in the generation of robust the anti-tumor CTL response even against poorly immunogenic tumors [154]. Further study by Thomas et al. demonstrated that TGFβ can suppress various cytotoxic gene expressions namely perforin, GzmA, GzmB, FasL and IFN-γ in T cells and thus block the generation of anti-tumor CTL response. The study also indicated that neutralization of TGFβ can be of a potential therapeutic approach in restoring the cytotoxic gene expression in tumor specific CTL, leading to tumor clearance.

In combination with TGFβ, the cytokine IL-13 has also shown to impair the generation of tumor specific CTL response. In a study by Terabe et al. showed that CD1d restricted NKT cells can repress the CTL response by mechanism involving production of IL-13 and TGFβ and activation of IL-4R/STAT-6 signaling pathway [155]. Thus, it is important to point out that blocking of TGFβ not only improves the quality of anti-tumor CTL therapy but also can overcome the NKT cell-mediated immunosuppression. Several strategies have been explored to inhibit the TGFβ signaling including the administration of antisense TGFβ oligonucleotides that bind to the TGFβ mRNA resulting in the reduction of TGFβ secretion [156], use of different TGFβ receptor kinase inhibitors, therefore, preventing the phosphorylation of downstream effectors such as SMADs [157–160], use of monoclonal antibodies to neutralize TGFβ depending on tumor localization and administration of monoclonal antibody to TGFβRII to interrupt the binding of TGFβ to its receptor [161]. Studies indicate that IL10 can also suppress the generation of a tumor-specific CTL response. It has been reported that tumor-associated macrophages (TAMs) and tumor-induced regulatory T cells (iTreg) secrete an elevated level of IL10 and protect the tumor cells by suppressing the functionality of cytotoxic T cells at the tumor site [162, 163].

14.2.3.2 Ectonucleotidases

Recent studies suggest that accumulation of adenosine in the tumor microenvironment is an important mechanism of suppressing the effector function of anti-tumor T cells [164, 165]. The accumulation of adenosine at the tumor site is thought to be mediated by the sequential cleavage of ATP that is present at a very high level in the tumor milieu [166], by ectonucleotidases namely CD39 and CD73 [167]. The ectonucleotidase CD39 is involved in the breakdown of ATP to form AMP and CD73 cleaves AMP to form adenosine [167]. Studies have shown that tumor cells including melanoma, breast carcinoma, and HNSCC co-express CD39 and CD73 and contribute to adenosine at the tumor site [168, 169]. Several studies have shown that Tregs also express enzymatically active CD39 and CD73 on their cell surface [167, 170]. It has been shown extensively that expression of CD39 and CD73 on Tregs is crucial for exerting their immunosuppressive function [167, 170]. Effector T cells cultured in the presence of CD39 and CD73 co-expressing suppressive cells fail to secrete various effector cytokines. A recent study from our group also reported that tumor-specific Th17 cells differentiated in the presence of TGFβ failed to control melanoma tumor growth since they co-express CD39 and CD73 which caused diminished IFNγ secretion by these cells at the tumor site [89]. Studies have shown that adenosine generated by the cleavage of ATP by CD39 and CD73 binds with A2AR and A2BR receptors, resulting in the concomitant activation of adenylyl cyclase (AC) and upregulation of cAMP which causes the suppression of effector cytokine production by T cells [171, 172]. Several attempts are currently being made to counteract the adenosine-mediated suppression of anti-tumor T cells by inhibiting CD73 and, thereby, disrupt the sequential cleavage of ATP leading to the generation of adenosine. The study by Stagg et al. showed that administration of monoclonal antibody to CD73 significantly inhibits the tumor growth and spontaneous metastasis in mice model [173]. A recent study has also shown that blocking of CD73 can increase the therapeutic potential of anti-PD1 and anti-CTLA-4 and, thus, can be used in combination with the checkpoint blockers for cancer immunotherapy [174].

Similarly, prostaglandin E2 (PGE2) has an important role in the suppression of anti-tumor T cell response. PGE2 is the product of cyclooxygenase-2 (COX-2) activity that has been reported to be elevated in various tumors [175]. PGE2 binds to G-protein coupled receptors (EP1–EP4) on the cell surface and leads to an increase in the intracellular c-AMP levels resulting in the suppression of proliferation and the effector response of the T cells [176].

14.2.3.3 Negative Co-stimulation

Emerging evidences suggest that signaling through the negative co-stimulatory pathways is one of the major confounding factors in mounting an adequate anti-tumor CTL response. Several strategies have been tested to block the negative co-stimulatory pathways to improve the effector response of anti-tumor T cells. One of the best studied negative immunological checkpoints is CTLA-4, which has been shown to inhibit T cell activation and function through its engagement with the co-stimulatory molecule B7.1 [177]. Allison and his group first showed that blocking of the CTLA-4-B7 interaction significantly increases the anti-tumor immune responses [177]. Further studies by this group showed that blockade of CTLA-4 in combination with a GM-CSF-transduced vaccine could eradicate poorly immunogenic tumors by enhancing the efficacy of tumor-reactive T cells and altering the intratumor balance of effector and regulatory T cells [178].

Another immunological checkpoint that contributes to the tumor evasion of immune response is the interaction between programmed death receptor-1 (PD-1) and its ligand (PD-L1) [179]. It has been shown that PD-1 expression on the T cells, following its activation upon engagement with its ligand PD-L1 or PD-L2 leads to the inhibition of T cell proliferation and effector cytokine production [180]. An interesting study by Dong et al. showed that the majority of the human tumors including breast cancer, lung cancer, melanoma, ovarian cancer, and adenocarcinoma expressed PD-L1 and its expression is enhanced in the presence of IFNγ [181]. The expression of PD-L1 on tumor cells blocks the CTL response but induces apoptosis of the tumor antigen-specific T cells via induction of FasL and IL-10 [181]. It has also been shown that monoclonal antibody-mediated blocking of PD-L1 can enhance the CTL response by reducing the death of tumor specific T cells, resulting in a heightened objective response in various tumor models. In addition to blocking PD-L1, a recent study disclosed that an effective CTL response can also be generated by antibody-mediated blocking of PD1 [181, 182]. A clinical study by Topalian et al. demonstrated that administration of anti-PD1 monoclonal antibody elicited a significant objective response in a substantial proportion of patients with non–small-cell lung cancer, melanoma, or renal-cell cancer and in various sites of metastasis, including the liver, lung, lymph nodes, and bone [183].

Emerging evidences indicated that another impediment for an effective anti-tumor CTL response is LAG-3, an immunological checkpoint which can restrain an anti-tumor T cells response [184]. Compelling evidences suggest that Lag-3 can be up-regulated on both CD4 and CD8 T cells following their activation and can be further stimulated by IL12 [185]. The expression of LAG-3 on T cells has been shown to negatively regulate T cells function by inhibiting their proliferation and cytokines secretion. Study by Grosso et al. [186] showed that by either genetic ablation or by antibody-mediated blockade of LAG-3 significantly increased the accumulation and effector function of anti-tumor CD8 T cells at the tumor site. In particular, dual blockade of LAG-3 and PD-1 exerted a synergistic effect in reversing the anergy among anti-tumor CD8 T cells [187]. Substantial evidences suggest that an augmented CTL response against the tumor can also be achieved by blocking TIM-3, which has been shown to negatively regulate the T cell function. Zarour and colleagues convincingly showed that blockade of TIM-3 along with other checkpoint blocks like PD-1 could reverse the tumor-induced T cell exhaustion in patients with advanced melanoma [188]. This finding was further confirmed by the study of Ngiow et al. [189] who showed that antibody-mediated blockade of TIM-3 has significant therapeutic potential in eradicating large and established tumor growth by eliciting an effective anti-tumor CTL response.

14.2.3.4 Myeloid Derived Suppressor Cells (MDSC)

Myeloid-derived suppressor cells (MDSCs), a heterogeneous population of immature monocytes, macrophages, neutrophils and DCs, accumulate in the blood, bone marrow, spleen and within the primary and metastatic tumor site of a tumor-bearing individual and expand dramatically as the tumor progresses [190] In mice, MDSCs can be identified by the surface expression of the myeloid lineage differentiation antigen Gr1 (Ly6G and LyGC) and the α_M integrin CD11b. Like murine MDSCs, in cancer patients, MDSCs can be identified primarily on the basis of $CD11b^+CD33^+CD34^+HLA\text{-}DR^-$ along with CD14 predominantly for monocytic-MDSCs (m-MDSCs) and CD15 for granulocyte-MDSCs (g-MDSCs) [191]. The hallmark of MDSCs is their ability to suppress the anti-tumor T cell response. Studies have shown that MDSCs can induce tolerance to the antigen-specific $CD8^+$ T cells and inhibit their IFNγ production [192]. Kusmartsev et al. showed that MDSCs can take up soluble antigens, process and present then to their surface and induce antigen-specific T cells anergy [193]. Further studies revealed MDSC- mediated secretion of ROS and NO, which are predominantly used by g-MDSCs and m-MDSCs, respectively, suppress the T cell function. It has been shown that higher expressions of the NADPH oxidase subunit p47phox and gp91phox are associated with the production of ROS whereas the elevated expression of iNOS is responsible for NO generation by the MDSCs [194–196]. Reports suggest that NO can itself inhibit anti-tumor T cell responses using a variety of different pathways including the induction of T cell apoptosis, inhibition of the activation of JAK3/STAT5 signaling pathway [197], and inhibition of the MHC class II expression [198]. However, the inhibition becomes robust when the MDSC-mediated hyper-production of NO and ROS combines with each other to form peroxynitrite [199]. Accumulation of peroxynitrite causes nitration of the TCR-CD8 complex and, thus, induces unresponsiveness of the CD8 T cells to antigen-specific stimulation by affecting the conformational flexibility of the TCR/CD8 and its interaction with the peptide-loaded MHC [199]. Moreover, peroxynitrite can also lead to the nitration of MHC class I on tumor cells and inhibits their ability to present processed tumor antigens, thus rendering the tumor cells resistant to an antigen-specific CTL response [200]. A recent study also suggests that MDSC-derived peroxynitrite not only induces an unresponsiveness to antigen specific CTLs but also blocks their recruitment to the tumor site by causing nitration of the chemokine CCL2 [201]. In addition, MDSCs by secreting IL10 and TGFβ can induce the generation of Tregs, which in turn can block the anti-tumor CTL responses [202].

Targeting signaling pathways underlying the suppressive potential of MDSCs in combination with ACT would be a promising approach in eradicating cancer. Several attempts are currently being made to inhibit the suppressive property of MDSCs. One convincing approach is to use the pharmacological inhibitor of ROS and NO to block peroxynitrite generation, since it plays an immense role in suppressing the anti-tumor CTL response. Indeed, Molon et al. reported that attenuating RNS generation by a novel NO-donating drug AT38 dramatically improves the efficacy of ACT protocols by inducing a massive increase in the intratumoral T cell infiltration leading to inhibition of MDSC-mediated nitration of the chemokine CCL2, generally involved in the migration of CTLs to the tumor site [201]. Various agents that deplete or interfere with the generation of MDSCs can be used in combination with ACT to increase their functionality. For instance, the tyrosine kinase inhibitor sunitinib, which interferes with the generation and suppressive function of $CD33^+HLADR^-$ and $CD15^+CD14^-$ MDSCs could be a good candidate to test in a combinatorial immunotherapy of cancer [203].

14.2.3.5 Regulatory T Cells (Treg)

Regulatory T cells (Tregs), a subset of $CD4^+$ T cells characterized by the high surface expression of CD25 and the lineage specific transcription factor FoxP3, suppress the effector functions of conventional T cells and play an important role in maintaining peripheral tolerance. Tregs were originally identified as a small population (>5 %) of naturally occurring $CD4^+$ T cells, and have a role in preventing autoimmunity by curtailing the autoreactive T cells [204]. However, significant interest on Tregs affecting the anti-tumor T cell response has arisen since they accumulated in many human tumors. Studies have shown that $CD4^+CD35^+FoxP3^+$ cells are highly abundant at both the tumor site and in the circulation of patients with head-neck, lung, liver, breast, ovary, pancreatic, and skin cancers and inversely correlates with the survival of patients [205–208]. This observation was further supported by the study of Curiel et al. which shows that specific accumulation of Tregs at the tumor site but not in the draining lymph nodes directly correlates with the reduced survival of patients with malignant ovarian carcinoma [209]. The authors have also shown that the migration of Tregs to the tumor site is mediated by the chemokine CCL22 that is secreted by tumor cells and the micro-environmental macrophages. However, other studies suggest that inflammation might be a factor for the recruitment of Tregs to the tumor site [210]. It is also believed that the high amount of self-antigens generated from the dying tumor cells get recognized by Tregs and recruit them to the tumor site. Subsets of Tregs (iTregs) present at the tumor site are different from the thymus derived conventional Tregs (nTregs) required for the maintenance of peripheral tolerance. It has been shown that iTregs are induced by cytokines and soluble factors secreted by the tumor cells and are highly suppressive in nature. Reports have shown that the tumor cell-derived TGFβ plays a decisive role in the preferential generation and recruitment of iTregs to the tumor site since blocking TGFβ selectively impairs the function of iTregs without affecting nTregs [211]. It has been reported that in addition to the high surface expression of CD25 and the transcription factor FoxP3, iTregs can be identified by the expression of various surface markers including CTLA-4, GITR, LAG-3, CD39 and CD73, which are required for the suppressive function of Tregs [212, 213].

Pioneering studies revealed that depletion of Tregs by administration of the anti-CD25 monoclonal antibody heightened T cell-mediated rejection of tumor growth. Study by Turk et al. [214] demonstrated that depletion of Tregs in tumor-bearing mice results in concomitant immunity to poorly immunogenic tumors. Another potential therapeutic approach for depletion of Tregs is the use of Denileukin diftitox (Ontak), a ligand toxin fusion consisting of full-length IL2 fused to the enzymatically active and translocating domains of diphtheria toxin [215]. The drug is specifically internalized by the $CD25^+$ T cells where the ADP-ribosyltransferase activity of diphtheria toxin is cleaved in the endosome, resulting in their translocation into the cytosol, where it inhibits protein synthesis, leading to apoptosis. Ontak has been approved by FDA for treating patients with cutaneous T-cell leukaemia/lymphoma. But this drug can be used in other tumor models in order to decrease the frequency of Tregs so that anti-tumor CTL response can be generated. Furthermore, several other approaches thwarting the immunosuppressiveness of Tregs have been explored including the use of anti-GITR agonistic antibody to attenuate the suppressive activity of Tregs and engagement of TLR-8 to reverse the function of Tregs. Heeger and his group have also shown that signaling through the C3aR/C5aR negatively regulates the function of Tregs [216], and thus, the use of anti-C3aR/C5aR agonistic antibody could be exploited as a therapeutic target to manipulate the functionality of Tregs so as to increase the anti-tumor CTL response.

14.3 T Cell Metabolism

The nutrient requirements of any cell are linked with the metabolic pathways that are required for the cell to carry out its functionality. The energy machinery, therefore, drives either anabolic or catabolic processes depending on the needs of the cell. The main source of energy, adenosine triphosphate or ATP, is generated in the cell by two major processes viz. (1) glycolysis and (2) oxidative phosphorylation. Carbohydrates, especially glucose, are the main source of energy in the cell. Amino acids and lipids are also utilized but the intermediates enter the tricarboxylic acid (TCA) cycle directly from where they subsequently follow similar pathways of oxidative phosphorylation. T cell activation leads to dramatic shifts in cell metabolism in order to make the building blocks for daughter cells [217]. Quiescent T cells require predominantly ATP-generating processes, whereas proliferating effector T cells require high metabolic flux through growth-promoting pathways. Further, functionally distinct T cell subsets require distinct energetic and biosynthetic pathways to support their specific functional needs. Pathways that control immune cell function and metabolism are intimately linked, and changes in cell metabolism at both the cell and system levels have been shown to enhance or suppress specific T cell functions. As a result of these findings, cell metabolism is now appreciated as a key regulator of T cell function specification and fate [218, 219]. It is now apparent that activation of T cells leads to an increase in the glucose uptake as well as production of lactate. Recent studies have shown that activated T cells increase the breakdown of glucose and glutamine in order to meet the requirements of production of structural constituents prior to division. There is also a concomitant increase in the uptake of glucose by up-regulation of a soluble carrier family receptor, Glut-1 [220]. Apart from proliferation, T cells differentiate on activation to become effectors, whose main function is the production of effector cytokines for initiating the resolution of disease state [218]. It has been recently shown that CD4 T cells depend on glycolysis for the production of effector cytokines like interferon gamma (IFNγ) [221]. Further it has also been demonstrated that the initial activation phase requires the generation of reactive-oxygen species from the mitochondria [222]. It is therefore evident that energy metabolism plays an important role in regulating the function of T cells [217–219].

The control of T cell function by metabolism and therefore, the disease outcome is a field of active study and emerging studies in this field have led to slow but comprehensive understanding of the energetics of T cell biology. Proliferating T cells as well as the tumors that they are being used to treat are inherently glycolytic in nature. Therefore, reduction in glucose availability for either the effector or the target is detrimental. Since the tumor cells are already established prior to immunotherapy, they have the ability to decrease the availability of glucose to the CTLs. Another requirement is for the CTLs to have the ability to form long-lived memory cells efficiently. Complicating the matter further is the fact that T cells encounter lower levels of oxygen i.e. hypoxic conditions within the tumor microenvironment, which leads to the upregulation of a key regulatory molecule, HIF-1α, that causes an increase in the glycolytic rate. This balance between the extrinsic factors and its affect on T cell function and metabolism is depicted in Fig. 14.3. Thus, ways to manipulate the bioenergetics of T cells in order for it to adapt to the glycolytically active tumor microenvironment will be a useful strategy to increase the life-span and function of the anti-tumor T cell effectors.

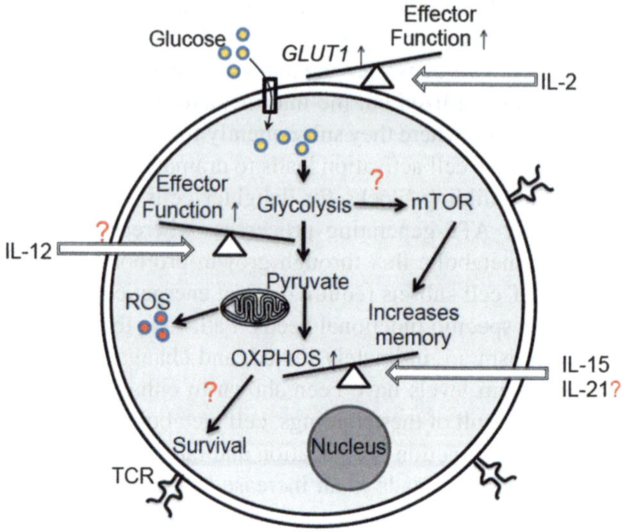

Fig. 14.3 A schematic diagram illustrating how extrinsic factors can synergize or affect T cell intrinsic pathways that influences CTL fate. T cells utilize glucose as a primary carbon source for generating energy. Glucose is transported inside the cell by glucose transporter (*GLUT1*). Glucose (*yellow dots*) is converted to pyruvate in process known as glycolysis. Pyruvate may enter into mitochondria for generating ATP through oxidative phosphorylation (OXPHOS). OXPHOS or mitochondrial respiration produces reactive oxygen species (ROS—*red dots*). Increase in GLUT1 may suggest higher glucose uptake. Increased glycolysis and increased glucose uptake have been associated with increased T cell effector functions. On the other hand increase in OXPHOS is associated with memory generation. It is also suggested that increased OXPHOS may increase longevity/survival of T cells. However, this is not yet completely understood (*red question mark*). There may exist a crosstalk between mTOR pathway, glycolysis and OXPHOS. It is known that blocking mTOR increases memory generation. However crosstalk between mTOR and glycolysis is still under investigation (*red question mark*). Extrinsic factors such as IL2, IL12, IL15 and IL21 may affect one of these pathways, thereby effecting effector function or memory T cell generation

A recent study has suggested that the use of the glucose analog 2-DG that limits glycolysis can improve long term T cell functionality by preserving the generation of long-term memory T cells. The report suggests that the inherent glycolytic nature of proliferating T cells leads them to become exhausted and terminally differentiated, which makes them unsuitable for mediating long-term immune surveillance. Inhibition of glycolysis by using 2-deoxyglucose leads to activated T cells forming long-lived memory cells. Additionally and more importantly, this leads to the T cells being less susceptible to apoptosis due to the withdrawal of glucose by tumor cells in vivo [223]. The functionality of CTLs is a key factor that determines the efficacy of therapy i.e. the effector molecules and cytokines secreted by the anti-tumor T cells determine the therapeutic potential of T cells. A recent study showed a link between the metabolic state of a T cell and the ability of T cells to metabolize glucose [221]. The study showed that IFNγ produced by T cells is dependent on the ability of T cells to utilize glucose and induce a key glycolytic enzyme, glyceraldehyde-3-phosphate dehydrogenase (GAPDH), which regulates the translation of IFNγ. Therefore, it is evident that T cells require glucose for their anti-tumor functionality but inhibiting their glycolysis for a short time during the effector phase enhances long-term anti-tumor immunity.

Different polarized T cells such as Th1, Th2, and Th17 among others, have shown promise for anti-tumor therapy. These T cells differ in their cytokine production patterns and consequently, in their metabolic states as well [218]. The cytokine-induced polarization also modulates the metabolic signaling within the T cells. A recent study has shown that Teff and Tregs require distinct metabolic programs to support these functions. Th1, Th2, and Th17 cells express high surface levels of the glucose transporter Glut1 and are highly glycolytic. Tregs, in contrast, expressed low levels of Glut1 and have high lipid oxidation rates [218]. The mTOR and AMPK pathways are important regulators of the balance of energy metabolism in T cells. mTOR regulates glycolysis whereas AMPK promotes oxidative phosphorylation and lipid oxidation. Data suggests that the effector T cell subsets are preferentially glycolytic and activate mTOR to various degrees for energy generation [224]. A recent study has also dissected the requirement of fatty acid oxidation in memory T cells [225]. The study also shows that there is a transition (to what?) of the metabolic state when memory T cells generate an effector response. Inhibitors of glycolysis such as rapamycin have also been shown to enhance the memory-like phenotype without affecting the efficacy of T cells [148]. In essence, the role of metabolism in regulating T cell responses is very important and different avenues of modulating the metabolic state are being studied so as to improve T cell responses and get a better therapeutic efficacy.

14.4 T Cell Aging

Age has been a factor that is closely associated with the occurrence of cancer. The accumulation of somatic mutations, telomeric instability and epigenetic dysregulation increases with age leading to the phenomenon of cellular senescence [226]. The breakdown of internal regulatory mechanisms in the cell leads to genomic instability that finally initiates tumorigenesis. Another consequence of this dysregulation is degeneration of the ability of the immune system to maintain proper immunosurveillance. This is an additional factor that leads to increase in chances of tumorigenesis. More importantly, age is a major hurdle in the immunotherapy of cancer. Aging is a natural process that leads to a decrease in functionality and effectiveness of the immune system. Specifically, there is a decrease in the number of hematopoietic progenitor cells and involution of the thymus that leads to a reduction in the naïve pool of T cells. CD4 T cells in an aging individual lose their ability to get stimulated adequately because of their inability to form stable, functional synapses and, therefore, are not able to proliferate and differentiate. Further defects in the B cell compartment also lead to a poorer differentiation of Th cell subsets [227, 228]. CD8 T cells, on the other hand, show a shift in the available repertoire of TCR Vβ due to the variety of infections encountered during an individuals' lifetime and hence, may not be able to respond adequately to the different tumor antigens [229]. Additionally, there is also an increase in the regulatory populations such as Treg's that retard the generation of a potent immune reaction. All of these factors lead to a poorer immune response to tumor antigens in an aged individual.

The goal of CTL therapy is to be able to engineer the T cells from a patient and then infuse them back, such that there is an increase in the efficiency of T cells in recognizing and eliminating tumor cells. The underlying assumption is that the T cells that are isolated from patients are functional and are amenable to manipulations that are done ex vivo before infusion. Another issue of concern is the ability of the infused cells to persist in the patient and perform the cytolytic activity. T cells in an individual progressively lose their function and become deregulated by a process known as immunosenescence. At a single cell level, T cells lose their ability to respond effectively to stimuli due to various factors such as changes in signal transduction, costimulatory molecules, membrane fluidity and/or the formation of the T cell receptor complex itself. It has been suggested that the membrane fluidity in T cells from aged individuals is compromised, which leads to poorer formation of the TCR complex [230]. This has been attributed to an increased level of membrane cholesterol that is associated with ageing [231, 232]. Further downregulation of costimulatory molecules such as CD28 also leads to poorer ability of T cells to initiate a T cell signaling cascade [233]. The loss of such receptors leads to changes in signaling efficiencies between young and old individuals which results in differences in the cellular outcome i.e. activation, proliferation and apoptosis. Reports studying T cell clones at different passage stages suggest a global change in the gene expression of molecules involved in signal transduction and apoptosis [234]. Further, there is also evidence to suggest that T cells from aged individuals show poorer activation of the Src family kinase, Lck, during activation of T cells [235].

The apparent problems in ageing, therefore, need to be overcome in order to improve the immunotherapy using an aged immune system. Aging also leads to reduction in the telomere length. However, a recent study shows that substituting a glucose rich diet can increase the lifespan of telomerase knockout (KO) mice with a dysfunctional telomere [236]. High glucose diet also rescued a dysfunctional mitochondrial metabolism in telomerase knockout (KO) mice. This study showed that blocking mTOR by rapamycin may reduce the rescue of mitochondrial biogenesis [236]. However, this study does not account for the energy metabolism in T cells, however, we have recently reported that using rapamycin reduces mitochondrial respiration in anti-tumor T cells [148], and improves in vivo CTL's survival. Therefore, regulating the metabolism in aged T cell may be helpful for T cell adoptive therapy. Reports suggest that the hematopoietic progenitor cells, which have the capability to self-renew, can be used to generate T cells, which would be similar to those from a young individual [237, 238]. Further thymic involution, which is the main reason for loss of young cells, can be reversed by the use of IL7, growth hormones or keratinocyte growth factors [238]. The signal strength to activate T cells can be boosted by using adjuvants that can activate other receptors whose signaling cross talks with that of the TCR [237, 239]. Further, recent advances have also improved the potential for personalized medicine, which can be used to identify T cells that have the potential to mediate tumor regression in aged individuals so as to achieve improved specificities. Overall, rejuvenation of the aged immune system will involve identifying different pathways that cause T cells to lose functionality and targeting these pathways will be the key to a better immunotherapy in these individuals.

14.5 Future Strategies

14.5.1 Genetic Modification of T Cells for Immunotherapy

With the development of retroviral gene transfer technology, it is now possible to efficiently endow T cells with antigen-specific receptors. Recently, two clinical trials successfully used this approach to show that normal autologous T lymphocytes transduced ex vivo with anti-TAA–TCR genes and re-infused in cancer patients can persist and express the transgene for a prolonged time in vivo and mediate the durable regression of large established tumors [240, 241]. Thus, genetic modification of T cells, prior to adoptive transfer, has provided a potential means to overcome many other obstacles and enhance the efficacy of T-cell therapy. We have been able to retrovirally transduce an antioxidant enzyme, catalase in human T cells and protect them from oxidative stress [242]. The T cells thus obtained with high catalase, expression were able to better overcome the hydrogen peroxide (H_2O_2)-mediated oxidative stress and retain functionality (Fig. 14.4). We foresee that combining TCR transductions with molecules that could rescue CTLs from cell death and increase persistence could improve immunotherapy.

14.5.2 TCR Gene Transfer for the Immunotherapy of Cancer

The ultimate goal of cancer immunotherapy is to manipulate the immune system of cancer patients to eliminate malignant cells. Research has mainly focused on the generation of effective, antigen-specific T-cell responses because of the general belief that T-cell immunity is essential in controlling tumor growth and protection against viral infections. However, the isolation of antigen-specific T cells for therapeutic application is laborious, and it is often impossible to isolate and expand autologous, tumor-specific T cells for adoptive immunotherapy. Therefore, strategies are being developed to genetically transfer tumor-specific immune receptors into patients' T cells. This alternative gene therapy approach that can provide antitumor immunity to any cancer patient, regardless of their immune status, has been described in the literature [243]. Since TAAs are recognized by the TCR on the T lymphocyte surface, which is composed of the TCR α and β chains, this approach involves identifying and cloning the TCR genes from tumor-reactive T cells,

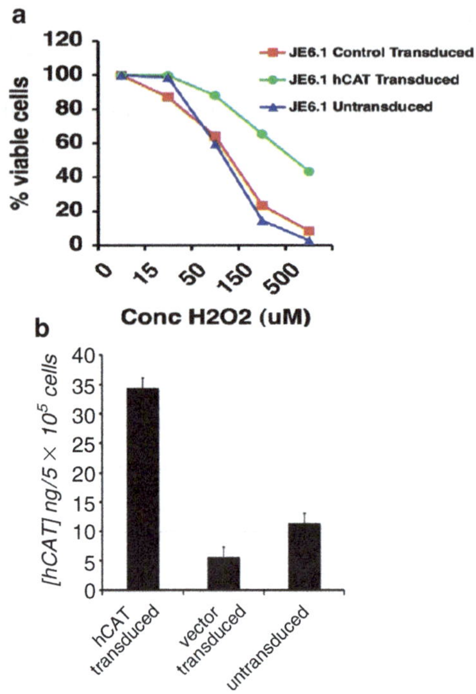

Fig. 14.4 Engineering anti-oxidant overexpression in T cells reduces susceptibility to oxidative stress. (**a**) Catalase transduced Jurkat T cells (JE6.1) were exposed to hydrogen peroxide (H_2O_2) at various concentration for 48 h and viability was determined using Annexin/PI staining. (**b**) Catalase ELISA using Jurkat cells that were used in the A, confirming the differences in catalase expression in T cells with or without transduction

constructing a vector capable of introducing these genes into normal T cells, thereby genetically modifying the patients T cells ex vivo, and returning these TCR gene-modified T cells to the patient. The genes encoding the TCR that are specific for a variety of TAA have now been cloned, including the TCR-recognizing MART-1 and gp100 melanoma/melanocyte differentiation antigens, the NYESO-1 cancer-testis antigen that is present on many common epithelial cancers, and an epitope from the p53 molecule, which is expressed on the surface of approximately 50 % of cancers of common epithelial origin [244, 245].

In each case, these antigens were detected by the TCR when they were presented as peptides by molecules encoded by the major histocompatibility complex (MHC) protein human lymphocyte antigen (HLA)-A2. Thus, initial studies validated this approach to use a TCR reactive with the HLA-A2-restricted MART-1_{27-35} epitope and subsequently, TCR reactive to other tumor antigens as gp-100, p53, HCV, WT1 were isolated, cloned and characterized in in vitro and in vivo models, which strengthened the case for their subsequent use in human trials [240, 246–248]. With the development of retroviral gene transfer technology, it is now possible to efficiently endow T cells with antigen-specific receptors and use this powerful approach to rapidly generate large number of tumor-specific T lymphocytes for adoptive transfer to cancer patients. Recently, two clinical trials successfully used this approach of genetically engineering T cell specificity by TCR gene transfer. Results from these studies proved that normal autologous T lymphocytes, transduced ex vivo with anti-TAA–TCR genes and reinfused in cancer patients, can persist and express the transgene for a prolonged time in vivo and mediate durable regression of large established tumors. Although the response rate was lower than that achieved by the infusion of autologous tumor infiltrating lymphocytes (TILs) (50 %) [68], this method has the potential for use in patients for whom TILs are not available. These trials also ameliorated toxicity concerns related to gene-modified T cells—the multitude of divisions required to obtain a billion T cells does not lead to transformation of T cells that can possibly adversely affect patients. Thus, engineering PBLs to express high-affinity TCRs enables in vitro recognition of TAAs expressed on a variety of common cancers, even in immuno-compromised individuals.

14.5.2.1 Strategies for Improving TCR Gene Transfer for Immunotherapy

Various investigators are now improving this new technological advancement by focusing on a common goal of either increased TCR surface expression or increasing TCR affinity to enhance the biological responses (that translates functionally as tumor regression). To this end, adding a single cysteine on each receptor chain to promote the formation of an additional inter-chain disulfide bond has been recently shown to improve TCR gene transfer [249]. This approach overcomes a major limitation resulting from mispairing of the introduced chains with the endogenous TCR subunits, which leads to reduced TCR surface expression and subsequently, to lower biological activity. The expression of cysteine-modified receptors was higher on the surface of human lymphocytes compared with their wild-type counterparts and showed larger amounts of cytokine secretion and specific lysis when cocultured with specific tumor cell lines. Enhanced anti-tumor activity associated with improved pairing and TCR/CD3 stability has also been found in human lymphocytes, when transduced with murine-human hybrid TCR created by swapping the original constant regions with either human or mouse ones, respectively [250]. Furthermore, it has also been shown that high-affinity, peptide-specific TCR can be generated by mutations in CDR1, CDR2, or CDR3 without altering T-cell specificity [251, 252]. A recent study has compared the response of high- and low-affinity TCRs towards a comprehensive set of peptides containing single substitutions at each TCR contact residue, and this specificity analysis suggested that the increase in affinity also results in a dramatic increase in the number of stimulatory peptides [75]. Thus, efforts are directed at either improving TCR affinity of already existing low-affinity TCR or isolating naturally occurring, high-affinity TCRs to improve TCR gene transfer immunotherapy.

14.5.2.2 Strategies to Improve Tumor Targeting by T Cells for Immunotherapy

Apart from different strategies to improve tumor antigen recognition by T cells and expression of high affinity TCRs, researchers have been developing methodologies for improving TCR independent tumor recognition by T cells. These include molecules such as chimeric antigen receptors (CARs) and bi-specific antibody T cell engager (BiTE). CARs are artificial T cell receptors that are recombinant proteins consisting of an extracellular domain conferring antibody-like specificity to tumor cell-surface antigen and an intracellular domain for amplifying TCR signals [253]. Different iterations of CARs have been generated, each enhancing the signal strength and downstream functionality of T cells. The first generation CAR incorporated the intracellular domain of CD3ξ chain, thus amplifying the TCR signal. Second generation CARs provide for the intracellular domain of co-stimulatory molecules like CD28 [254], 4-1BB [255, 256], OX-40 [257] or ICOS [258], to name a few. The more recent third generation CAR includes intracellular domains for both CD3ξ as well as co-stimulatory molecules to further increase the potency of therapy. Expression of this molecule on the T cell surface reduces off target effect as well as improves the specificity of T cell activity. Also signaling through the co-stimulatory, CARs lead to improved functionality and persistence of the transferred T cells [254–258]. Further signaling through the CAR has also been shown to reduce AIED in T cells [259–262], thereby, further enhancing the ability of T cell to persist in the host.

Another modality for treatment that has been promising is the use of monoclonal bi-specific antibodies along with T cell therapy to improve tumor targeting by T cells. Bi-specific T cell engagers or BiTEs mediate stronger interactions between T cell and target cells by binding both to the CD3 on T cells and tumor-specific epitope on the tumor cell [263]. When BiTEs are used along with T cell therapy, there is no requirement for T cell to engage MHC on tumor cell and, therefore, BiTEs mediate MHC independent but TCR signaling dependent activation of T cells in close proximity of the tumor cells. Treatment of B cell malignancies by using CD3–CD19 BiTE has shown to improve the efficacy of T cells in clearing tumor B cells. Further, it has also been shown to be better than the use of to tandem antibodies [264–266]. Similar approaches have also been used along with NK cell therapy and the antibody used therein is called bi-specific killer cell engager (BiKE). These BiKEs have a CD16 binding antibody domain along with the antibody domain binding to specific tumors, thus, leading to the activation of NK cells and mediating tumor killing [267, 268]. Further, with the increased understanding of the molecular regulators of T cells at the level of microRNAs (miRNAs), which small endogenously processed RNAs regulating key gene expression and controlling cellular functioning, several novel strategies to improve CTL response by targeting miRNA (or other coding and non-coding RNA, RNA binding proteins) could be envisioned. Several thousands of miRNAs exist in the human genome and each has more than one mRNA target [269]. In T cells, miRNAs play a crucial role in differentiation of various effector T cells subtypes and, thus, maintain the balance between effector and regulatory T cells [270, 271]. Recent evidence suggests that miRNAs can regulate the activation of mTOR signaling in T cells resulting in the determination of the effector function of the T cells. It has been shown that miRNAs can be of potential targets to override anergy induction in T cells and, thus, would be very useful in T cells therapy of cancer. Recent combinatorial approach with CAR-transduced T cells with co-transduction of miRNA-17-92 have shown improved therapeutic potency in patients with glioblastoma [272]. It is evident from these studies that miRNAs would be an important area to investigate in order to improve the efficacy of T cells immunotherapy of cancer. Therefore, with the evolution of gene engineering techniques, improvements in T cell therapy would eventually lead to a better future for cancer patients.

14.6 Conclusion

Cancer therapies based on stimulating the patient's immune system represent an important treatment modality, but much remains to be discovered to optimize their use. Naive T lymphocytes, following activation with antigen (Ag), differentiate into short-lived effector cells and long-lived memory T cells [12]. Vaccine efficacy might be improved by strategies that are designed to modulate the expansion and contraction of the effector T-cell response [273]. A careful evaluation of the immunotherapeutic protocols and innovative strategies that would help the persistence of T cell subsets are needed [274]. The multiplicity of cell death pathways, targeting positive and negative co-stimulation, cytokines, metabolic commitment and relevant proteins in CTL provides additional opportunities to develop new strategies for therapeutically increasing effector T cell persistence and function (Fig. 14.5).

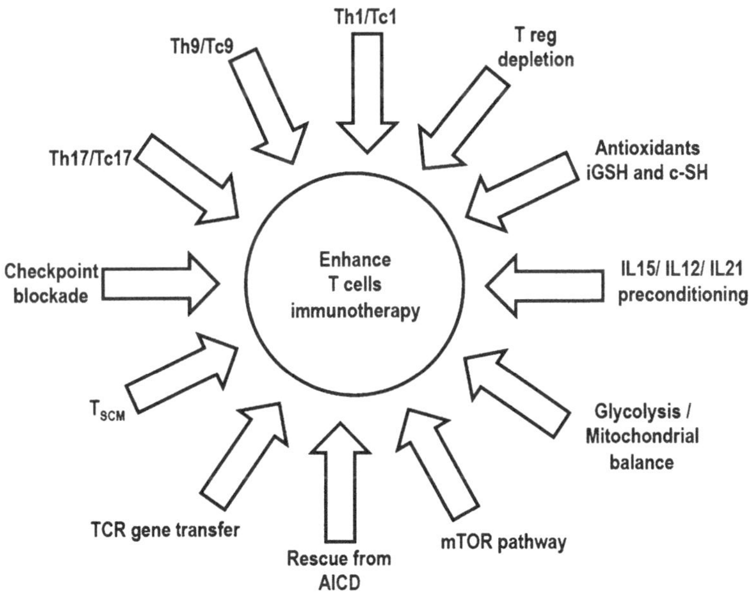

Fig. 14.5 A summary of multiple approaches and the factors that could result in differences in quality of the CTL employed for adoptive T cell therapy of cancer. Skewing any of the marked conditions is likely to integrate and influence other listed parameters and modulate the eventual outcome of CTL function or persistence in immunotherapy

Acknowledgement Authors acknowledge help from Dr. Radhika Gudi at MUSC for critical reading of this manuscript and help in preparing this manuscript. We also apologize to our colleagues for not citing all primary research articles owing to space restrictions. This work was supported in part by funds from the Department of Surgery (MUSC) and NIH R01CA138930, R01AR057643 and PO1 CA154778.

References

1. Baskar R, Lee KA, Yeo R, Yeoh KW. Cancer and radiation therapy: current advances and future directions. Int J Med Sci. 2012;9:193–9.
2. Schuler PJ, Harasymczuk M, Visus C, Deleo A, Trivedi S, Lei Y, Argiris A, Gooding W, Butterfield LH, Whiteside TL, Ferris RL. Phase I dendritic cell p53 peptide vaccine for head and neck cancer. Clin Cancer Res. 2014;20:2433–44.
3. Kochenderfer JN, Dudley ME, Kassim SH, Somerville RP, Carpenter RO, Stetler-Stevenson M, Yang JC, Phan GQ, Hughes MS, Sherry RM, Raffeld M, Feldman S, Lu L, Li YF, Ngo LT, Goy A, Feldman T, Spaner DE, Wang ML, Chen CC, Kranick SM, Nath A, Nathan DA, Morton KE, Toomey MA, Rosenberg SA. Chemotherapy-refractory diffuse large B-cell lymphoma and indolent B-cell malignancies can be effectively treated with autologous T cells expressing an anti-CD19 chimeric antigen receptor. J Clin Oncol. 2015;33:540–9.
4. Corrigan-Curay J, Kiem HP, Baltimore D, O'Reilly M, Brentjens RJ, Cooper L, Forman S, Gottschalk S, Greenberg P, Junghans R, Heslop H, Jensen M, Mackall C, June C, Press O, Powell D, Ribas A, Rosenberg S, Sadelain M, Till B, Patterson AP, Jambou RC, Rosenthal E, Gargiulo L, Montgomery M, Kohn DB. T-cell immunotherapy: looking forward. Mol Ther. 2014;22:1564–74.
5. Ward RC, Kaufman HL. Targeting costimulatory pathways for tumor immunotherapy. Int Rev Immunol. 2007;26:161–96.
6. Ngiow SF, Teng MW, Smyth MJ. Prospects for TIM3-targeted antitumor immunotherapy. Cancer Res. 2011;71:6567–71.
7. Capece D, Verzella D, Fischietti M, Zazzeroni F, Alesse E. Targeting costimulatory molecules to improve antitumor immunity. J Biomed Biotechnol. 2012;2012:926321.
8. Wang L, Rubinstein R, Lines JL, Wasiuk A, Ahonen C, Guo Y, Lu LF, Gondek D, Wang Y, Fava RA, Fiser A, Almo S, Noelle RJ. VISTA, a novel mouse Ig superfamily ligand that negatively regulates T cell responses. J Exp Med. 2011;208:577–92.
9. Klebanoff CA, Finkelstein SE, Surman DR, Lichtman MK, Gattinoni L, Theoret MR, Grewal N, Spiess PJ, Antony PA, Palmer DC, Tagaya Y, Rosenberg SA, Waldmann TA, Restifo NP. IL-15 enhances the in vivo antitumor activity of tumor-reactive CD8+ T cells. Proc Natl Acad Sci U S A. 2004;101:1969–74.
10. Moroz A, Eppolito C, Li Q, Tao J, Clegg CH, Shrikant PA. IL-21 enhances and sustains CD8+ T cell responses to achieve durable tumor immunity: comparative evaluation of IL-2, IL-15, and IL-21. J Immunol. 2004;173:900–9.
11. Waldmann TA, Dubois S, Tagaya Y. Contrasting roles of IL-2 and IL-15 in the life and death of lymphocytes: implications for immunotherapy. Immunity. 2001;14:105–10.
12. Lu Y, Hong S, Li H, Park J, Hong B, Wang L, Zheng Y, Liu Z, Xu J, He J, Yang J, Qian J, Yi Q. Th9 cells promote antitumor immune responses in vivo. J Clin Invest. 2012;122: 4160–71.
13. Martin-Orozco N, Muranski P, Chung Y, Yang XO, Yamazaki T, Lu S, Hwu P, Restifo NP, Overwijk WW, Dong C. T helper 17 cells promote cytotoxic T cell activation in tumor immunity. Immunity. 2009;31:787–98.
14. Dempsey PW, Vaidya SA, Cheng G. The art of war: innate and adaptive immune responses. Cell Mol Life Sci. 2003;60:2604–21.

15. Chaudhuri D, Suriano R, Mittelman A, Tiwari RK. Targeting the immune system in cancer. Curr Pharm Biotechnol. 2009;10:166–84.
16. Vieweg J, Jackson A. Modulation of antitumor responses by dendritic cells. Springer Semin Immunopathol. 2005;26:329–41.
17. Berry LJ, Moeller M, Darcy PK. Adoptive immunotherapy for cancer: the next generation of gene-engineered immune cells. Tissue Antigens. 2009;74:277–89.
18. Stewart TJ, Smyth MJ. Improving cancer immunotherapy by targeting tumor-induced immune suppression. Cancer Metastasis Rev. 2011;30:125–40.
19. Palucka K, Banchereau J. Dendritic-cell-based therapeutic cancer vaccines. Immunity. 2013;39:38–48.
20. Dougan M, Dranoff G. Immune therapy for cancer. Annu Rev Immunol. 2009;27:83–117.
21. Yee C. Adoptive T-cell therapy of cancer. Hematol Oncol Clin North Am. 2006;20:711–33.
22. Castellino F, Germain RN. Cooperation between CD4+ and CD8+ T cells: when, where, and how. Annu Rev Immunol. 2006;24:519–40.
23. North RJ, Bursuker I. Generation and decay of the immune response to a progressive fibrosarcoma. I. Ly-1 + 2- suppressor T cells down-regulate the generation of Ly-1-2+ effector T cells. J Exp Med. 1984;159:1295–311.
24. Mills CD, North RJ. Ly-1 + 2- suppressor T cells inhibit the expression of passively transferred antitumor immunity by suppressing the generation of cytolytic T cells. Transplantation. 1985;39:202–8.
25. Perez-Diez A, Joncker NT, Choi K, Chan WF, Anderson CC, Lantz O, Matzinger P. CD4 cells can be more efficient at tumor rejection than CD8 cells. Blood. 2007;109:5346–54.
26. Morris EC, Tsallios A, Bendle GM, Xue SA, Stauss HJ. A critical role of T cell antigen receptor-transduced MHC class I-restricted helper T cells in tumor protection. Proc Natl Acad Sci U S A. 2005;102:7934–9.
27. Chhabra A, Yang L, Wang P, Comin-Anduix B, Das R, Chakraborty NG, Ray S, Mehrotra S, Yang H, Hardee CL, Hollis R, Dorsky DI, Koya R, Kohn DB, Ribas A, Economou JS, Baltimore D, Mukherji B. CD4 + CD25- T cells transduced to express MHC class I-restricted epitope-specific TCR synthesize Th1 cytokines and exhibit MHC class I-restricted cytolytic effector function in a human melanoma model. J Immunol. 2008;181:1063–70.
28. Nishimura MI, Avichezer D, Custer MC, Lee CS, Chen C, Parkhurst MR, Diamond RA, Robbins PF, Schwartzentruber DJ, Rosenberg SA. MHC class I-restricted recognition of a melanoma antigen by a human CD4+ tumor infiltrating lymphocyte. Cancer Res. 1999;59: 6230–8.
29. Mucida D, Husain MM, Muroi S, van Wijk F, Shinnakasu R, Naoe Y, Reis BS, Huang Y, Lambolez F, Docherty M, Attinger A, Shui JW, Kim G, Lena CJ, Sakaguchi S, Miyamoto C, Wang P, Atarashi K, Park Y, Nakayama T, Honda K, Ellmeier W, Kronenberg M, Taniuchi I, Cheroutre H. Transcriptional reprogramming of mature CD4(+) helper T cells generates distinct MHC class II-restricted cytotoxic T lymphocytes. Nat Immunol. 2013;14:281–9.
30. Cheroutre H, Husain MM. CD4 CTL: living up to the challenge. Semin Immunol. 2013; 25:273–81.
31. Kennedy J, Vicari AP, Saylor V, Zurawski SM, Copeland NG, Gilbert DJ, Jenkins NA, Zlotnik A. A molecular analysis of NKT cells: identification of a class-I restricted T cell-associated molecule (CRTAM). J Leukoc Biol. 2000;67:725–34.
32. Boles KS, Barchet W, Diacovo T, Cella M, Colonna M. The tumor suppressor TSLC1/NECL-2 triggers NK-cell and CD8+ T-cell responses through the cell-surface receptor CRTAM. Blood. 2005;106:779–86.
33. Boles KS, Stepp SE, Bennett M, Kumar V, Mathew PA. 2B4 (CD244) and CS1: novel members of the CD2 subset of the immunoglobulin superfamily molecules expressed on natural killer cells and other leukocytes. Immunol Rev. 2001;181:234–49.
34. Quezada SA, Simpson TR, Peggs KS, Merghoub T, Vider J, Fan X, Blasberg R, Yagita H, Muranski P, Antony PA, Restifo NP, Allison JP. Tumor-reactive CD4(+) T cells develop cytotoxic activity and eradicate large established melanoma after transfer into lymphopenic hosts. J Exp Med. 2010;207:637–50.

35. Hunder NN, Wallen H, Cao J, Hendricks DW, Reilly JZ, Rodmyre R, Jungbluth A, Gnjatic S, Thompson JA, Yee C. Treatment of metastatic melanoma with autologous CD4+ T cells against NY-ESO-1. N Engl J Med. 2008;358:2698–703.
36. Gattinoni L, Finkelstein SE, Klebanoff CA, Antony PA, Palmer DC, Spiess PJ, Hwang LN, Yu Z, Wrzesinski C, Heimann DM, Surh CD, Rosenberg SA, Restifo NP. Removal of homeostatic cytokine sinks by lymphodepletion enhances the efficacy of adoptively transferred tumor-specific CD8+ T cells. J Exp Med. 2005;202:907–12.
37. Klebanoff CA, Khong HT, Antony PA, Palmer DC, Restifo NP. Sinks, suppressors and antigen presenters: how lymphodepletion enhances T cell-mediated tumor immunotherapy. Trends Immunol. 2005;26:111–7.
38. Wang LX, Shu S, Disis ML, Plautz GE. Adoptive transfer of tumor-primed, in vitro-activated, CD4+ T effector cells (TEs) combined with CD8+ TEs provides intratumoral TE proliferation and synergistic antitumor response. Blood. 2007;109:4865–76.
39. Curtsinger JM, Schmidt CS, Mondino A, Lins DC, Kedl RM, Jenkins MK, Mescher MF. Inflammatory cytokines provide a third signal for activation of naive CD4+ and CD8+ T cells. J Immunol. 1999;162:3256–62.
40. Valenzuela J, Schmidt C, Mescher M. The roles of IL-12 in providing a third signal for clonal expansion of naive CD8 T cells. J Immunol. 2002;169:6842–9.
41. Tepper RI, Mule JJ. Experimental and clinical studies of cytokine gene-modified tumor cells. Hum Gene Ther. 1994;5:153–64.
42. Blankenstein T, Rowley DA, Schreiber H. Cytokines and cancer: experimental systems. Curr Opin Immunol. 1991;3:694–8.
43. Colombo MP, Forni G. Cytokine gene transfer in tumor inhibition and tumor therapy: where are we now? Immunol Today. 1994;15:48–51.
44. Dranoff G, Jaffee E, Lazenby A, Golumbek P, Levitsky H, Brose K, Jackson V, Hamada H, Pardoll D, Mulligan RC. Vaccination with irradiated tumor cells engineered to secrete murine granulocyte-macrophage colony-stimulating factor stimulates potent, specific, and long-lasting anti-tumor immunity. Proc Natl Acad Sci U S A. 1993;90:3539–43.
45. Colombo MP, Parmiani G. Tumor-cell-targeted cytokine gene therapy. Immunol Today. 1991;12:249–50.
46. Dudley ME, Wunderlich JR, Robbins PF, Yang JC, Hwu P, Schwartzentruber DJ, Topalian SL, Sherry R, Restifo NP, Hubicki AM, Robinson MR, Raffeld M, Duray P, Seipp CA, Rogers-Freezer L, Morton KE, Mavroukakis SA, White DE, Rosenberg SA. Cancer regression and autoimmunity in patients after clonal repopulation with antitumor lymphocytes. Science. 2002;298:850–4.
47. Colombo MP, Trinchieri G. Interleukin-12 in anti-tumor immunity and immunotherapy. Cytokine Growth Factor Rev. 2002;13:155–68.
48. Zeng R, Spolski R, Finkelstein SE, Oh S, Kovanen PE, Hinrichs CS, Pise-Masison CA, Radonovich MF, Brady JN, Restifo NP, Berzofsky JA, Leonard WJ. Synergy of IL-21 and IL-15 in regulating CD8+ T cell expansion and function. J Exp Med. 2005;201:139–48.
49. Hinrichs CS, Spolski R, Paulos CM, Gattinoni L, Kerstann KW, Palmer DC, Klebanoff CA, Rosenberg SA, Leonard WJ, Restifo NP. IL-2 and IL-21 confer opposing differentiation programs to CD8+ T cells for adoptive immunotherapy. Blood. 2008;111:5326–33.
50. Xiao Z, Casey KA, Jameson SC, Curtsinger JM, Mescher MF. Programming for CD8 T cell memory development requires IL-12 or type I IFN. J Immunol. 2009;182:2786–94.
51. Gerner MY, Heltemes-Harris LM, Fife BT, Mescher MF. Cutting edge: IL-12 and type I IFN differentially program CD8 T cells for programmed death 1 re-expression levels and tumor control. J Immunol. 2013;191:1011–5.
52. Rubinstein MP, Cloud CA, Garrett TE, Moore CJ, Schwartz KM, Johnson CB, Craig DH, Salem ML, Paulos CM, Cole DJ. Ex vivo interleukin-12-priming during CD8(+) T cell activation dramatically improves adoptive T cell transfer antitumor efficacy in a lymphodepleted host. J Am Coll Surg. 2012;214:700–7. discussion 707–708.
53. Nguyen T, Wang R, Russell JH. IL-12 enhances IL-2 function by inducing CD25 expression through a p38 mitogen-activated protein kinase pathway. Eur J Immunol. 2000;30:1445–52.

54. Starbeck-Miller GR, Xue HH, Harty JT. IL-12 and type I interferon prolong the division of activated CD8 T cells by maintaining high-affinity IL-2 signaling in vivo. J Exp Med. 2014;211:105–20.
55. Kaur N, Naga OS, Norell H, Al-Khami AA, Scheffel MJ, Chakraborty NG, Voelkel-Johnson C, Mukherji B, Mehrotra S. T cells expanded in presence of IL-15 exhibit increased antioxidant capacity and innate effector molecules. Cytokine. 2011;55:307–17.
56. Casey KA, Mescher MF. IL-21 promotes differentiation of naive CD8 T cells to a unique effector phenotype. J Immunol. 2007;178:7640–8.
57. Sondergaard H, Galsgaard ED, Bartholomaeussen M, Straten PT, Odum N, Skak K. Intratumoral interleukin-21 increases antitumor immunity, tumor-infiltrating CD8+ T-cell density and activity, and enlarges draining lymph nodes. J Immunother. 2010;33:236–49.
58. Liu S, Lizee G, Lou Y, Liu C, Overwijk WW, Wang G, Hwu P. IL-21 synergizes with IL-7 to augment expansion and anti-tumor function of cytotoxic T cells. Int Immunol. 2007;19:1213–21.
59. Dighe AS, Richards E, Old LJ, Schreiber RD. Enhanced in vivo growth and resistance to rejection of tumor cells expressing dominant negative IFN gamma receptors. Immunity. 1994;1:447–56.
60. Muranski P, Boni A, Antony PA, Cassard L, Irvine KR, Kaiser A, Paulos CM, Palmer DC, Touloukian CE, Ptak K, Gattinoni L, Wrzesinski C, Hinrichs CS, Kerstann KW, Feigenbaum L, Chan CC, Restifo NP. Tumor-specific Th17-polarized cells eradicate large established melanoma. Blood. 2008;112:362–73.
61. Propper DJ, Chao D, Braybrooke JP, Bahl P, Thavasu P, Balkwill F, Turley H, Dobbs N, Gatter K, Talbot DC, Harris AL, Ganesan TS. Low-dose IFN-gamma induces tumor MHC expression in metastatic malignant melanoma. Clin Cancer Res. 2003;9:84–92.
62. Yang I, Kremen TJ, Giovannone AJ, Paik E, Odesa SK, Prins RM, Liau LM. Modulation of major histocompatibility complex class I molecules and major histocompatibility complex-bound immunogenic peptides induced by interferon-alpha and interferon-gamma treatment of human glioblastoma multiforme. J Neurosurg. 2004;100:310–9.
63. Bohm W, Thoma S, Leithauser F, Moller P, Schirmbeck R, Reimann J. T cell-mediated, IFN-gamma-facilitated rejection of murine B16 melanomas. J Immunol. 1998;161:897–908.
64. Wigginton JM, Gruys E, Geiselhart L, Subleski J, Komschlies KL, Park JW, Wiltrout TA, Nagashima K, Back TC, Wiltrout RH. IFN-gamma and Fas/FasL are required for the antitumor and antiangiogenic effects of IL-12/pulse IL-2 therapy. J Clin Invest. 2001;108:51–62.
65. Nagoshi M, Goedegebuure PS, Burger UL, Sadanaga N, Chang MP, Eberlein TJ. Successful adoptive cellular immunotherapy is dependent on induction of a host immune response triggered by cytokine (IFN-gamma and granulocyte/macrophage colony-stimulating factor) producing donor tumor-infiltrating lymphocytes. J Immunol. 1998;160:334–44.
66. Nagoshi M, Sadanaga N, Joo HG, Goedegebuure PS, Eberlein TJ. Tumor-specific cytokine release by donor T cells induces an effective host anti-tumor response through recruitment of host naive antigen presenting cells. Int J Cancer. 1999;80:308–14.
67. Zarei S, Schwenter F, Luy P, Aurrand-Lions M, Morel P, Kopf M, Dranoff G, Mach N. Role of GM-CSF signaling in cell-based tumor immunization. Blood. 2009;113:6658–68.
68. van Horssen R, Ten Hagen TL, Eggermont AM. TNF-alpha in cancer treatment: molecular insights, antitumor effects, and clinical utility. Oncologist. 2006;11:397–408.
69. Koup RA, Roederer M, Lamoreaux L, Fischer J, Novik L, Nason MC, Larkin BD, Enama ME, Ledgerwood JE, Bailer RT, Mascola JR, Nabel GJ, Graham BS, Team VRCS, Team VRCS. Priming immunization with DNA augments immunogenicity of recombinant adenoviral vectors for both HIV-1 specific antibody and T-cell responses. PLoS One. 2010;5:e9015.
70. Lugade AA, Sorensen EW, Gerber SA, Moran JP, Frelinger JG, Lord EM. Radiation-induced IFN-gamma production within the tumor microenvironment influences antitumor immunity. J Immunol. 2008;180:3132–9.
71. Raez LE, Cassileth PA, Schlesselman JJ, Padmanabhan S, Fisher EZ, Baldie PA, Sridhar K, Podack ER. Induction of CD8 T-cell-IFN-gamma response and positive clinical outcome

after immunization with gene-modified allogeneic tumor cells in advanced non-small-cell lung carcinoma. Cancer Gene Ther. 2003;10:850–8.

72. Emtage PC, Clarke D, Gonzalo-Daganzo R, Junghans RP. Generating potent Th1/Tc1 T cell adoptive immunotherapy doses using human IL-12: harnessing the immunomodulatory potential of IL-12 without the in vivo-associated toxicity. J Immunother. 2003;26:97–106.
73. Zhu Y, Ju S, Chen E, Dai S, Li C, Morel P, Liu L, Zhang X, Lu B. T-bet and eomesodermin are required for T cell-mediated antitumor immune responses. J Immunol. 2010;185: 3174–83.
74. Thieu VT, Yu Q, Chang HC, Yeh N, Nguyen ET, Sehra S, Kaplan MH. Signal transducer and activator of transcription 4 is required for the transcription factor T-bet to promote T helper 1 cell-fate determination. Immunity. 2008;29:679–90.
75. Luckey CJ, Weaver CT. Stem-cell-like qualities of immune memory; CD4+ T cells join the party. Cell Stem Cell. 2012;10:107–8.
76. Dobrzanski MJ, Reome JB, Hollenbaugh JA, Dutton RW. Tc1 and Tc2 effector cell therapy elicit long-term tumor immunity by contrasting mechanisms that result in complementary endogenous type 1 antitumor responses. J Immunol. 2004;172:1380–90.
77. Muranski P, Borman ZA, Kerkar SP, Klebanoff CA, Ji Y, Sanchez-Perez L, Sukumar M, Reger RN, Yu Z, Kern SJ, Roychoudhuri R, Ferreyra GA, Shen W, Durum SK, Feigenbaum L, Palmer DC, Antony PA, Chan CC, Laurence A, Danner RL, Gattinoni L, Restifo NP. Th17 cells are long lived and retain a stem cell-like molecular signature. Immunity. 2011;35: 972–85.
78. Wei S, Zhao E, Kryczek I, Zou W. Th17 cells have stem cell-like features and promote long-term immunity. Oncoimmunology. 2012;1:516–9.
79. Kryczek I, Zhao E, Liu Y, Wang Y, Vatan L, Szeliga W, Moyer J, Klimczak A, Lange A, Zou W. Human TH17 cells are long-lived effector memory cells. Sci Transl Med. 2011; 3:104ra100.
80. Paulos CM, Carpenito C, Plesa G, Suhoski MM, Varela-Rohena A, Golovina TN, Carroll RG, Riley JL, June CH. The inducible costimulator (ICOS) is critical for the development of human T(H)17 cells. Sci Transl Med. 2010;2:55ra78.
81. Hinrichs CS, Kaiser A, Paulos CM, Cassard L, Sanchez-Perez L, Heemskerk B, Wrzesinski C, Borman ZA, Muranski P, Restifo NP. Type 17 CD8+ T cells display enhanced antitumor immunity. Blood. 2009;114:596–9.
82. Muranski P, Restifo NP. Essentials of Th17 cell commitment and plasticity. Blood. 2013; 121:2402–14.
83. Beriou G, Costantino CM, Ashley CW, Yang L, Kuchroo VK, Baecher-Allan C, Hafler DA. IL-17-producing human peripheral regulatory T cells retain suppressive function. Blood. 2009;113:4240–9.
84. Tartar DM, VanMorlan AM, Wan X, Guloglu FB, Jain R, Haymaker CL, Ellis JS, Hoeman CM, Cascio JA, Dhakal M, Oukka M, Zaghouani H. FoxP3+RORgammat+T helper intermediates display suppressive function against autoimmune diabetes. J Immunol. 2010; 184:3377–85.
85. Kaufmann SH, Kuchroo VK. Th17 cells. Microbes Infect. 2009;11:579–83.
86. Korn T, Bettelli E, Oukka M, Kuchroo VK. IL-17 and Th17 cells. Annu Rev Immunol. 2009;27:485–517.
87. Annunziato F, Romagnani S. The transient nature of the Th17 phenotype. Eur J Immunol. 2010;40:3312–6.
88. Kryczek I, Wei S, Szeliga W, Vatan L, Zou W. Endogenous IL-17 contributes to reduced tumor growth and metastasis. Blood. 2009;114:357–9.
89. Chatterjee S, Thyagarajan K, Kesarwani P, Song JH, Soloshchenko M, Fu J, Bailey SR, Vasu C, Kraft AS, Paulos CM, Yu XZ, Mehrotra S. Reducing CD73 Expression by IL1beta-Programmed Th17 Cells Improves Immunotherapeutic Control of Tumors. Cancer Res. 2014;74:6048–59.

90. Yu Y, Cho HI, Wang D, Kaosaard K, Anasetti C, Celis E, Yu XZ. Adoptive transfer of Tc1 or Tc17 cells elicits antitumor immunity against established melanoma through distinct mechanisms. J Immunol. 2013;190:1873–81.
91. Wang Y, Godec J, Ben-Aissa K, Cui K, Zhao K, Pucsek AB, Lee YK, Weaver CT, Yagi R, Lazarevic V. The transcription factors T-bet and Runx are required for the ontogeny of pathogenic interferon-gamma-producing T helper 17 cells. Immunity. 2014;40:355–66.
92. Duhen R, Glatigny S, Arbelaez CA, Blair TC, Oukka M, Bettelli E. Cutting edge: the pathogenicity of IFN-gamma-producing Th17 cells is independent of T-bet. J Immunol. 2013;190:4478–82.
93. Goswami R, Kaplan MH. A brief history of IL-9. J Immunol. 2011;186:3283–8.
94. Kaplan MH. Th9 cells: differentiation and disease. Immunol Rev. 2013;252:104–15.
95. Schmitt E, Germann T, Goedert S, Hoehn P, Huels C, Koelsch S, Kuhn R, Muller W, Palm N, Rude E. IL-9 production of naive CD4+ T cells depends on IL-2, is synergistically enhanced by a combination of TGF-beta and IL-4, and is inhibited by IFN-gamma. J Immunol. 1994;153:3989–96.
96. Veldhoen M, Uyttenhove C, van Snick J, Helmby H, Westendorf A, Buer J, Martin B, Wilhelm C, Stockinger B. Transforming growth factor-beta 'reprograms' the differentiation of T helper 2 cells and promotes an interleukin 9-producing subset. Nat Immunol. 2008;9: 1341–6.
97. Grohmann U, Van Snick J, Campanile F, Silla S, Giampietri A, Vacca C, Renauld JC, Fioretti MC, Puccetti P. IL-9 protects mice from Gram-negative bacterial shock: suppression of TNF-alpha, IL-12, and IFN-gamma, and induction of IL-10. J Immunol. 2000;164:4197–203.
98. Purwar R, Schlapbach C, Xiao S, Kang HS, Elyaman W, Jiang X, Jetten AM, Khoury SJ, Fuhlbrigge RC, Kuchroo VK, Clark RA, Kupper TS. Robust tumor immunity to melanoma mediated by interleukin-9-producing T cells. Nat Med. 2012;18:1248–53.
99. Lu Y, Hong B, Li H, Zheng Y, Zhang M, Wang S, Qian J, Yi Q. Tumor-specific IL-9-producing CD8+ Tc9 cells are superior effector than type-I cytotoxic Tc1 cells for adoptive immunotherapy of cancers. Proc Natl Acad Sci U S A. 2014;111:2265–70.
100. Lu Y, Wang Q, Yi Q. Anticancer Tc9 cells: long-lived tumor-killing T cells for adoptive therapy. Oncoimmunology. 2014;3:e28542.
101. Ma L, Xue HB, Guan XH, Shu CM, Zhang JH, Yu J. Possible pathogenic role of T helper type 9 cells and interleukin (IL)-9 in atopic dermatitis. Clin Exp Immunol. 2014;175:25–31.
102. Visekruna A, Ritter J, Scholz T, Campos L, Guralnik A, Poncette L, Raifer H, Hagner S, Garn H, Staudt V, Bopp T, Reuter S, Taube C, Loser K, Huber M. Tc9 cells, a new subset of CD8(+) T cells, support Th2-mediated airway inflammation. Eur J Immunol. 2013;43: 606–18.
103. Wong MT, Ye JJ, Alonso MN, Landrigan A, Cheung RK, Engleman E, Utz PJ. Regulation of human Th9 differentiation by type I interferons and IL-21. Immunol Cell Biol. 2010;88: 624–31.
104. Elmore S. Apoptosis: a review of programmed cell death. Toxicol Pathol. 2007;35:495–516.
105. Lenardo MJ. Interleukin-2 programs mouse alpha beta T lymphocytes for apoptosis. Nature. 1991;353:858–61.
106. Russell JH, White CL, Loh DY, Meleedy-Rey P. Receptor-stimulated death pathway is opened by antigen in mature T cells. Proc Natl Acad Sci U S A. 1991;88:2151–5.
107. Snow AL, Marsh RA, Krummey SM, Roehrs P, Young LR, Zhang K, van Hoff J, Dhar D, Nichols KE, Filipovich AH, Su HC, Bleesing JJ, Lenardo MJ. Restimulation-induced apoptosis of T cells is impaired in patients with X-linked lymphoproliferative disease caused by SAP deficiency. J Clin Invest. 2009;119:2976–89.
108. Chen L, Woo M, Hakem R, Miller RG. Perforin-dependent activation-induced cell death acts through caspase 3 but not through caspases 8 or 9. Eur J Immunol. 2003;33:769–78.
109. Speiser DE, Sebzda E, Ohteki T, Bachmann MF, Pfeffer K, Mak TW, Ohashi PS. Tumor necrosis factor receptor p55 mediates deletion of peripheral cytotoxic T lymphocytes in vivo. Eur J Immunol. 1996;26:3055–60.

110. Sytwu HK, Liblau RS, McDevitt HO. The roles of Fas/APO-1 (CD95) and TNF in antigen-induced programmed cell death in T cell receptor transgenic mice. Immunity. 1996;5:17–30.
111. Norell H, Martins da Palma T, Lesher A, Kaur N, Mehrotra M, Naga OS, Spivey N, Olafimihan S, Chakraborty NG, Voelkel-Johnson C, Nishimura MI, Mukherji B, Mehrotra S. Inhibition of superoxide generation upon T-cell receptor engagement rescues Mart-1(27–35)-reactive T cells from activation-induced cell death. Cancer Res. 2009;69:6282–9.
112. Mehrotra S, Chhabra A, Chattopadhyay S, Dorsky DI, Chakraborty NG, Mukherji B. Rescuing melanoma epitope-specific cytolytic T lymphocytes from activation-induced cell death, by SP600125, an inhibitor of JNK: implications in cancer immunotherapy. J Immunol. 2004;173:6017–24.
113. Baumann S, Dostert A, Novac N, Bauer A, Schmid W, Fas SC, Krueger A, Heinzel T, Kirchhoff S, Schutz G, Krammer PH. Glucocorticoids inhibit activation-induced cell death (AICD) via direct DNA-dependent repression of the CD95 ligand gene by a glucocorticoid receptor dimer. Blood. 2005;106:617–25.
114. Marks-Konczalik J, Dubois S, Losi JM, Sabzevari H, Yamada N, Feigenbaum L, Waldmann TA, Tagaya Y. IL-2-induced activation-induced cell death is inhibited in IL-15 transgenic mice. Proc Natl Acad Sci U S A. 2000;97:11445–50.
115. Saligrama PT, Fortner KA, Secinaro MA, Collins CC, Russell JQ, Budd RC. IL-15 maintains T-cell survival via S-nitrosylation-mediated inhibition of caspase-3. Cell Death Differ. 2014;21:904–14.
116. Boise LH, Collins CM. Salmonella-induced cell death: apoptosis, necrosis or programmed cell death? Trends Microbiol. 2001;9:64–7.
117. Sansonetti PJ, Phalipon A, Arondel J, Thirumalai K, Banerjee S, Akira S, Takeda K, Zychlinsky A. Caspase-1 activation of IL-1beta and IL-18 are essential for Shigella flexneri-induced inflammation. Immunity. 2000;12:581–90.
118. Thornberry NA, Bull HG, Calaycay JR, Chapman KT, Howard AD, Kostura MJ, Miller DK, Molineaux SM, Weidner JR, Aunins J, et al. A novel heterodimeric cysteine protease is required for interleukin-1 beta processing in monocytes. Nature. 1992;356:768–74.
119. Doitsh G, Galloway NL, Geng X, Yang Z, Monroe KM, Zepeda O, Hunt PW, Hatano H, Sowinski S, Munoz-Arias I, Greene WC. Cell death by pyroptosis drives CD4 T-cell depletion in HIV-1 infection. Nature. 2014;505:509–14.
120. Boxer MB, Quinn AM, Shen M, Jadhav A, Leister W, Simeonov A, Auld DS, Thomas CJ. A highly potent and selective caspase 1 inhibitor that utilizes a key 3-cyanopropanoic acid moiety. ChemMedChem. 2010;5:730–8.
121. Degterev A, Huang Z, Boyce M, Li Y, Jagtap P, Mizushima N, Cuny GD, Mitchison TJ, Moskowitz MA, Yuan J. Chemical inhibitor of nonapoptotic cell death with therapeutic potential for ischemic brain injury. Nat Chem Biol. 2005;1:112–9.
122. Ch'en IL, Tsau JS, Molkentin JD, Komatsu M, Hedrick SM. Mechanisms of necroptosis in T cells. J Exp Med. 2011;208:633–41.
123. Pan T, Wu S, He X, Luo H, Zhang Y, Fan M, Geng G, Ruiz VC, Zhang J, Mills L, Bai C, Zhang H. Necroptosis takes place in human immunodeficiency virus type-1 (HIV-1)-infected CD4+ T lymphocytes. PLoS One. 2014;9:e93944.
124. Dixon SJ, Lemberg KM, Lamprecht MR, Skouta R, Zaitsev EM, Gleason CE, Patel DN, Bauer AJ, Cantley AM, Yang WS, Morrison 3rd B, Stockwell BR. Ferroptosis: an iron-dependent form of nonapoptotic cell death. Cell. 2012;149:1060–72.
125. Rosenberg SA, Dudley ME. Adoptive cell therapy for the treatment of patients with metastatic melanoma. Curr Opin Immunol. 2009;21:233–40.
126. Yee C, Thompson JA, Byrd D, Riddell SR, Roche P, Celis E, Greenberg PD. Adoptive T cell therapy using antigen-specific CD8+ T cell clones for the treatment of patients with metastatic melanoma: in vivo persistence, migration, and antitumor effect of transferred T cells. Proc Natl Acad Sci U S A. 2002;99:16168–73.
127. Chapuis AG, Thompson JA, Margolin KA, Rodmyre R, Lai IP, Dowdy K, Farrar EA, Bhatia S, Sabath DE, Cao J, Li Y, Yee C. Transferred melanoma-specific CD8+ T cells persist,

mediate tumor regression, and acquire central memory phenotype. Proc Natl Acad Sci U S A. 2012;109:4592–7.

128. Butler MO, Friedlander P, Milstein MI, Mooney MM, Metzler G, Murray AP, Tanaka M, Berezovskaya A, Imataki O, Drury L, Brennan L, Flavin M, Neuberg D, Stevenson K, Lawrence D, Hodi FS, Velazquez EF, Jaklitsch MT, Russell SE, Mihm M, Nadler LM, Hirano N. Establishment of antitumor memory in humans using in vitro-educated CD8+ T cells. Sci Transl Med. 2011;3:80ra34.
129. Muranski P, Boni A, Wrzesinski C, Citrin DE, Rosenberg SA, Childs R, Restifo NP. Increased intensity lymphodepletion and adoptive immunotherapy—how far can we go? Nat Clin Pract Oncol. 2006;3:668–81.
130. Dummer W, Niethammer AG, Baccala R, Lawson BR, Wagner N, Reisfeld RA, Theofilopoulos AN. T cell homeostatic proliferation elicits effective antitumor autoimmunity. J Clin Invest. 2002;110:185–92.
131. Hodge JW, Guha C, Neefjes J, Gulley JL. Synergizing radiation therapy and immunotherapy for curing incurable cancers. Opportunities and challenges. Oncology (Williston Park). 2008;22:1064–70; discussion 1075, 1080–1061, 1084.
132. Demaria S, Bhardwaj N, McBride WH, Formenti SC. Combining radiotherapy and immunotherapy: a revived partnership. Int J Radiat Oncol Biol Phys. 2005;63:655–66.
133. Formenti SC, Demaria S. Combining radiotherapy and cancer immunotherapy: a paradigm shift. J Natl Cancer Inst. 2013;105:256–65.
134. Dudley ME, Yang JC, Sherry R, Hughes MS, Royal R, Kammula U, Robbins PF, Huang J, Citrin DE, Leitman SF, Wunderlich J, Restifo NP, Thomasian A, Downey SG, Smith FO, Klapper J, Morton K, Laurencot C, White DE, Rosenberg SA. Adoptive cell therapy for patients with metastatic melanoma: evaluation of intensive myeloablative chemoradiation preparative regimens. J Clin Oncol. 2008;26:5233–9.
135. Spary LK, Al-Taei S, Salimu J, Cook AD, Ager A, Watson HA, Clayton A, Staffurth J, Mason MD, Tabi Z. Enhancement of T cell responses as a result of synergy between lower doses of radiation and T cell stimulation. J Immunol. 2014;192:3101–10.
136. Lerret NM, Marzo AL. Adoptive T-cell transfer combined with a single low dose of total body irradiation eradicates breast tumors. Oncoimmunology. 2013;2:e22731.
137. Klug F, Prakash H, Huber PE, Seibel T, Bender N, Halama N, Pfirschke C, Voss RH, Timke C, Umansky L, Klapproth K, Schakel K, Garbi N, Jager D, Weitz J, Schmitz-Winnenthal H, Hammerling GJ, Beckhove P. Low-dose irradiation programs macrophage differentiation to an iNOS(+)/M1 phenotype that orchestrates effective T cell immunotherapy. Cancer Cell. 2013;24:589–602.
138. Gattinoni L, Lugli E, Ji Y, Pos Z, Paulos CM, Quigley MF, Almeida JR, Gostick E, Yu Z, Carpenito C, Wang E, Douek DC, Price DA, June CH, Marincola FM, Roederer M, Restifo NP. A human memory T cell subset with stem cell-like properties. Nat Med. 2011;17:1290–7.
139. Ribeiro SP, Milush JM, Cunha-Neto E, Kallas EG, Kalil J, Somsouk M, Hunt PW, Deeks SG, Nixon DF, SenGupta D. The CD8+ memory stem T cell (TSCM) subset is associated with improved prognosis in chronic HIV-1 infection. J Virol. 2014;88:13836–44.
140. Stemberger C, Graef P, Odendahl M, Albrecht J, Dossinger G, Anderl F, Buchholz VR, Gasteiger G, Schiemann M, Grigoleit GU, Schuster FR, Borkhardt A, Versluys B, Tonn T, Seifried E, Einsele H, Germeroth L, Busch DH, Neuenhahn M. Lowest numbers of primary CD8(+) T cells can reconstitute protective immunity upon adoptive immunotherapy. Blood. 2014;124:628–37.
141. Restifo NP. Big bang theory of stem-like T cells confirmed. Blood. 2014;124:476–7.
142. Zeytun A, Hassuneh M, Nagarkatti M, Nagarkatti PS. Fas-Fas ligand-based interactions between tumor cells and tumor-specific cytotoxic T lymphocytes: a lethal two-way street. Blood. 1997;90:1952–9.
143. Dotti G, Savoldo B, Pule M, Straathof KC, Biagi E, Yvon E, Vigouroux S, Brenner MK, Rooney CM. Human cytotoxic T lymphocytes with reduced sensitivity to Fas-induced apoptosis. Blood. 2005;105:4677–84.

144. Chhabra A, Mehrotra S, Chakraborty NG, Dorsky DI, Mukherji B. Activation-induced cell death of human melanoma specific cytotoxic T lymphocytes is mediated by apoptosis-inducing factor. Eur J Immunol. 2006;36:3167–74.
145. Mehrotra S, Chhabra A, Hegde U, Chakraborty NG, Mukherji B. Inhibition of c-Jun N-terminal kinase rescues influenza epitope-specific human cytolytic T lymphocytes from activation-induced cell death. J Leukoc Biol. 2007;81:539–47.
146. Ladas EJ, Jacobson JS, Kennedy DD, Teel K, Fleischauer A, Kelly KM. Antioxidants and cancer therapy: a systematic review. J Clin Oncol. 2004;22:517–28.
147. Velicer CM, Ulrich CM. Vitamin and mineral supplement use among US adults after cancer diagnosis: a systematic review. J Clin Oncol. 2008;26:665–73.
148. Kesarwani P, Al-Khami AA, Scurti G, Thyagarajan K, Kaur N, Husain S, Fang Q, Naga OS, Simms P, Beeson G, Voelkel-Johnson C, Garrett-Mayer E, Beeson CC, Nishimura MI, Mehrotra S. Promoting thiol expression increases the durability of antitumor T-cell functions. Cancer Res. 2014;74:6036–47.
149. Trachootham D, Lu W, Ogasawara MA, Nilsa RD, Huang P. Redox regulation of cell survival. Antioxid Redox Signal. 2008;10:1343–74.
150. De Rosa SC, Zaretsky MD, Dubs JG, Roederer M, Anderson M, Green A, Mitra D, Watanabe N, Nakamura H, Tjioe I, Deresinski SC, Moore WA, Ela SW, Parks D, Herzenberg LA, Herzenberg LA. N-acetylcysteine replenishes glutathione in HIV infection. Eur J Clin Invest. 2000;30:915–29.
151. Herzenberg LA, De Rosa SC, Dubs JG, Roederer M, Anderson MT, Ela SW, Deresinski SC, Herzenberg LA. Glutathione deficiency is associated with impaired survival in HIV disease. Proc Natl Acad Sci U S A. 1997;94:1967–72.
152. Gelderman KA, Hultqvist M, Pizzolla A, Zhao M, Nandakumar KS, Mattsson R, Holmdahl R. Macrophages suppress T cell responses and arthritis development in mice by producing reactive oxygen species. J Clin Invest. 2007;117:3020–8.
153. Ranges GE, Figari IS, Espevik T, Palladino Jr MA. Inhibition of cytotoxic T cell development by transforming growth factor beta and reversal by recombinant tumor necrosis factor alpha. J Exp Med. 1987;166:991–8.
154. Gorelik L, Flavell RA. Immune-mediated eradication of tumors through the blockade of transforming growth factor-beta signaling in T cells. Nat Med. 2001;7:1118–22.
155. Terabe M, Khanna C, Bose S, Melchionda F, Mendoza A, Mackall CL, Helman LJ, Berzofsky JA. CD1d-restricted natural killer T cells can down-regulate tumor immunosurveillance independent of interleukin-4 receptor-signal transducer and activator of transcription 6 or transforming growth factor-beta. Cancer Res. 2006;66:3869–75.
156. Hau P, Jachimczak P, Bogdahn U. Treatment of malignant gliomas with TGF-beta2 antisense oligonucleotides. Expert Rev Anticancer Ther. 2009;9:1663–74.
157. Anido J, Saez-Borderias A, Gonzalez-Junca A, Rodon L, Folch G, Carmona MA, Prieto-Sanchez RM, Barba I, Martinez-Saez E, Prudkin L, Cuartas I, Raventos C, Martinez-Ricarte F, Poca MA, Garcia-Dorado D, Lahn MM, Yingling JM, Rodon J, Sahuquillo J, Baselga J, Seoane J. TGF-beta receptor inhibitors target the CD44(high)/Id1(high) glioma-initiating cell population in human glioblastoma. Cancer Cell. 2010;18:655–68.
158. Fu K, Corbley MJ, Sun L, Friedman JE, Shan F, Papadatos JL, Costa D, Lutterodt F, Sweigard H, Bowes S, Choi M, Boriack-Sjodin PA, Arduini RM, Sun D, Newman MN, Zhang X, Mead JN, Chuaqui CE, Cheung HK, Zhang X, Cornebise M, Carter MB, Josiah S, Singh J, Lee WC, Gill A, Ling LE. SM16, an orally active TGF-beta type I receptor inhibitor prevents myofibroblast induction and vascular fibrosis in the rat carotid injury model. Arterioscler Thromb Vasc Biol. 2008;28:665–71.
159. Halder SK, Beauchamp RD, Datta PK. A specific inhibitor of TGF-beta receptor kinase, SB-431542, as a potent antitumor agent for human cancers. Neoplasia. 2005;7:509–21.
160. Haritunians T, Gueller S, O'Kelly J, Ilaria Jr R, Koeffler HP. Novel acyl sulfonamide LY573636-sodium: effect on hematopoietic malignant cells. Oncol Rep. 2008;20:1237–42.
161. Zhong Z, Carroll KD, Policarpio D, Osborn C, Gregory M, Bassi R, Jimenez X, Prewett M, Liebisch G, Persaud K, Burtrum D, Wang S, Surguladze D, Ng S, Griffith H, Balderes P,

Doody J, Schwartz JD, Youssoufian H, Rowinsky EK, Ludwig DL, Witte L, Zhu Z, Wu Y. Anti-transforming growth factor beta receptor II antibody has therapeutic efficacy against primary tumor growth and metastasis through multieffects on cancer, stroma, and immune cells. Clin Cancer Res. 2010;16:1191–205.

162. Chatterjee S, Mookerjee A, Basu JM, Chakraborty P, Ganguly A, Adhikary A, Mukhopadhyay D, Ganguli S, Banerjee R, Ashraf M, Biswas J, Das PK, Sa G, Chatterjee M, Das T, Choudhuri SK. A novel copper chelate modulates tumor associated macrophages to promote anti-tumor response of T cells. PLoS One. 2009;4:e7048.

163. Jarnicki AG, Lysaght J, Todryk S, Mills KH. Suppression of antitumor immunity by IL-10 and TGF-beta-producing T cells infiltrating the growing tumor: influence of tumor environment on the induction of CD4+ and CD8+ regulatory T cells. J Immunol. 2006;177: 896–904.

164. Hoskin DW, Mader JS, Furlong SJ, Conrad DM, Blay J. Inhibition of T cell and natural killer cell function by adenosine and its contribution to immune evasion by tumor cells (Review). Int J Oncol. 2008;32:527–35.

165. Blay J, White TD, Hoskin DW. The extracellular fluid of solid carcinomas contains immunosuppressive concentrations of adenosine. Cancer Res. 1997;57:2602–5.

166. Pellegatti P, Raffaghello L, Bianchi G, Piccardi F, Pistoia V, Di Virgilio F. Increased level of extracellular ATP at tumor sites: in vivo imaging with plasma membrane luciferase. PLoS One. 2008;3:e2599.

167. Deaglio S, Dwyer KM, Gao W, Friedman D, Usheva A, Erat A, Chen JF, Enjyoji K, Linden J, Oukka M, Kuchroo VK, Strom TB, Robson SC. Adenosine generation catalyzed by CD39 and CD73 expressed on regulatory T cells mediates immune suppression. J Exp Med. 2007;204:1257–65.

168. Suchard MS, Mayne E, Green VA, Shalekoff S, Donninger SL, Stevens WS, Gray CM, Tiemessen CT. FOXP3 expression is upregulated in CD4T cells in progressive HIV-1 infection and is a marker of disease severity. PLoS One. 2010;5:e11762.

169. Dzhandzhugazyan KN, Kirkin AF, thor Straten P, Zeuthen J. Ecto-ATP diphosphohydrolase/CD39 is overexpressed in differentiated human melanomas. FEBS Lett. 1998;430:227–30.

170. Schuler PJ, Saze Z, Hong CS, Muller L, Gillespie DG, Cheng D, Harasymczuk M, Mandapathil M, Lang S, Jackson EK, Whiteside TL. Human CD4+ CD39+ regulatory T cells produce adenosine upon co-expression of surface CD73 or contact with CD73+ exosomes or CD73+ cells. Clin Exp Immunol. 2014;177:531–43.

171. Mandapathil M, Whiteside TL. Targeting human inducible regulatory T cells (Tr1) in patients with cancer: blocking of adenosine-prostaglandin E(2) cooperation. Expert Opin Biol Ther. 2011;11:1203–14.

172. Zhang H, Conrad DM, Butler JJ, Zhao C, Blay J, Hoskin DW. Adenosine acts through A2 receptors to inhibit IL-2-induced tyrosine phosphorylation of STAT5 in T lymphocytes: role of cyclic adenosine 3′,5′-monophosphate and phosphatases. J Immunol. 2004;173:932–44.

173. Stagg J, Divisekera U, McLaughlin N, Sharkey J, Pommey S, Denoyer D, Dwyer KM, Smyth MJ. Anti-CD73 antibody therapy inhibits breast tumor growth and metastasis. Proc Natl Acad Sci U S A. 2010;107:1547–52.

174. Allard B, Pommey S, Smyth MJ, Stagg J. Targeting CD73 enhances the antitumor activity of anti-PD-1 and anti-CTLA-4 mAbs. Clin Cancer Res. 2013;19:5626–35.

175. Singh B, Cook KR, Vincent L, Hall CS, Berry JA, Multani AS, Lucci A. Cyclooxygenase-2 induces genomic instability, BCL2 expression, doxorubicin resistance, and altered cancer-initiating cell phenotype in MCF7 breast cancer cells. J Surg Res. 2008;147:240–6.

176. Yaqub S, Tasken K. Role for the cAMP-protein kinase A signaling pathway in suppression of antitumor immune responses by regulatory T cells. Crit Rev Oncog. 2008;14:57–77.

177. Leach DR, Krummel MF, Allison JP. Enhancement of antitumor immunity by CTLA-4 blockade. Science. 1996;271:1734–6.

178. Quezada SA, Peggs KS, Curran MA, Allison JP. CTLA4 blockade and GM-CSF combination immunotherapy alters the intratumor balance of effector and regulatory T cells. J Clin Invest. 2006;116:1935–45.

179. Ishida Y, Agata Y, Shibahara K, Honjo T. Induced expression of PD-1, a novel member of the immunoglobulin gene superfamily, upon programmed cell death. EMBO J. 1992;11: 3887–95.
180. Williams MA, Bevan MJ. Immunology: exhausted T cells perk up. Nature. 2006;439: 669–70.
181. Dong H, Strome SE, Salomao DR, Tamura H, Hirano F, Flies DB, Roche PC, Lu J, Zhu G, Tamada K, Lennon VA, Celis E, Chen L. Tumor-associated B7-H1 promotes T-cell apoptosis: a potential mechanism of immune evasion. Nat Med. 2002;8:793–800.
182. Iwai Y, Ishida M, Tanaka Y, Okazaki T, Honjo T, Minato N. Involvement of PD-L1 on tumor cells in the escape from host immune system and tumor immunotherapy by PD-L1 blockade. Proc Natl Acad Sci U S A. 2002;99:12293–7.
183. Topalian SL, Sznol M, McDermott DF, Kluger HM, Carvajal RD, Sharfman WH, Brahmer JR, Lawrence DP, Atkins MB, Powderly JD, Leming PD, Lipson EJ, Puzanov I, Smith DC, Taube JM, Wigginton JM, Kollia GD, Gupta A, Pardoll DM, Sosman JA, Hodi FS. Survival, durable tumor remission, and long-term safety in patients with advanced melanoma receiving nivolumab. J Clin Oncol. 2014;32:1020–30.
184. Workman CJ, Dugger KJ, Vignali DA. Cutting edge: molecular analysis of the negative regulatory function of lymphocyte activation gene-3. J Immunol. 2002;169:5392–5.
185. Angevin E, Kremer F, Gaudin C, Hercend T, Triebel F. Analysis of T-cell immune response in renal cell carcinoma: polarization to type 1-like differentiation pattern, clonal T-cell expansion and tumor-specific cytotoxicity. Int J Cancer. 1997;72:431–40.
186. Grosso JF, Kelleher CC, Harris TJ, Maris CH, Hipkiss EL, De Marzo A, Anders R, Netto G, Getnet D, Bruno TC, Goldberg MV, Pardoll DM, Drake CG. LAG-3 regulates CD8+ T cell accumulation and effector function in murine self- and tumor-tolerance systems. J Clin Invest. 2007;117:3383–92.
187. Woo SR, Turnis ME, Goldberg MV, Bankoti J, Selby M, Nirschl CJ, Bettini ML, Gravano DM, Vogel P, Liu CL, Tangsombatvisit S, Grosso JF, Netto G, Smeltzer MP, Chaux A, Utz PJ, Workman CJ, Pardoll DM, Korman AJ, Drake CG, Vignali DA. Immune inhibitory molecules LAG-3 and PD-1 synergistically regulate T-cell function to promote tumoral immune escape. Cancer Res. 2012;72:917–27.
188. Fourcade J, Sun Z, Benallaoua M, Guillaume P, Luescher IF, Sander C, Kirkwood JM, Kuchroo V, Zarour HM. Upregulation of Tim-3 and PD-1 expression is associated with tumor antigen-specific CD8+ T cell dysfunction in melanoma patients. J Exp Med. 2010;207: 2175–86.
189. Ngiow SF, von Scheidt B, Akiba H, Yagita H, Teng MW, Smyth MJ. Anti-TIM3 antibody promotes T cell IFN-gamma-mediated antitumor immunity and suppresses established tumors. Cancer Res. 2011;71:3540–51.
190. Gabrilovich DI, Nagaraj S. Myeloid-derived suppressor cells as regulators of the immune system. Nat Rev Immunol. 2009;9:162–74.
191. Lindau D, Gielen P, Kroesen M, Wesseling P, Adema GJ. The immunosuppressive tumour network: myeloid-derived suppressor cells, regulatory T cells and natural killer T cells. Immunology. 2013;138:105–15.
192. Gabrilovich DI, Velders MP, Sotomayor EM, Kast WM. Mechanism of immune dysfunction in cancer mediated by immature Gr-1+ myeloid cells. J Immunol. 2001;166:5398–406.
193. Kusmartsev S, Su Z, Heiser A, Dannull J, Eruslanov E, Kubler H, Yancey D, Dahm P, Vieweg J. Reversal of myeloid cell-mediated immunosuppression in patients with metastatic renal cell carcinoma. Clin Cancer Res. 2008;14:8270–8.
194. Kusmartsev S, Nagaraj S, Gabrilovich DI. Tumor-associated CD8+ T cell tolerance induced by bone marrow-derived immature myeloid cells. J Immunol. 2005;175:4583–92.
195. Schmielau J, Finn OJ. Activated granulocytes and granulocyte-derived hydrogen peroxide are the underlying mechanism of suppression of t-cell function in advanced cancer patients. Cancer Res. 2001;61:4756–60.
196. Corzo CA, Condamine T, Lu L, Cotter MJ, Youn JI, Cheng P, Cho HI, Celis E, Quiceno DG, Padhya T, McCaffrey TV, McCaffrey JC, Gabrilovich DI. HIF-1alpha regulates function and

differentiation of myeloid-derived suppressor cells in the tumor microenvironment. J Exp Med. 2010;207:2439–53.
197. Bingisser RM, Tilbrook PA, Holt PG, Kees UR. Macrophage-derived nitric oxide regulates T cell activation via reversible disruption of the Jak3/STAT5 signaling pathway. J Immunol. 1998;160:5729–34.
198. Harari O, Liao JK. Inhibition of MHC II gene transcription by nitric oxide and antioxidants. Curr Pharm Des. 2004;10:893–8.
199. Nagaraj S, Gupta K, Pisarev V, Kinarsky L, Sherman S, Kang L, Herber DL, Schneck J, Gabrilovich DI. Altered recognition of antigen is a mechanism of CD8+ T cell tolerance in cancer. Nat Med. 2007;13:828–35.
200. Lu T, Ramakrishnan R, Altiok S, Youn JI, Cheng P, Celis E, Pisarev V, Sherman S, Sporn MB, Gabrilovich D. Tumor-infiltrating myeloid cells induce tumor cell resistance to cytotoxic T cells in mice. J Clin Invest. 2011;121:4015–29.
201. Molon B, Ugel S, Del Pozzo F, Soldani C, Zilio S, Avella D, De Palma A, Mauri P, Monegal A, Rescigno M, Savino B, Colombo P, Jonjic N, Pecanic S, Lazzarato L, Fruttero R, Gasco A, Bronte V, Viola A. Chemokine nitration prevents intratumoral infiltration of antigen-specific T cells. J Exp Med. 2011;208:1949–62.
202. Huang B, Pan PY, Li Q, Sato AI, Levy DE, Bromberg J, Divino CM, Chen SH. Gr-1+CD115+ immature myeloid suppressor cells mediate the development of tumor-induced T regulatory cells and T-cell anergy in tumor-bearing host. Cancer Res. 2006;66:1123–31.
203. Ko JS, Zea AH, Rini BI, Ireland JL, Elson P, Cohen P, Golshayan A, Rayman PA, Wood L, Garcia J, Dreicer R, Bukowski R, Finke JH. Sunitinib mediates reversal of myeloid-derived suppressor cell accumulation in renal cell carcinoma patients. Clin Cancer Res. 2009;15:2148–57.
204. Sakaguchi S, Yamaguchi T, Nomura T, Ono M. Regulatory T cells and immune tolerance. Cell. 2008;133:775–87.
205. Schaefer C, Kim GG, Albers A, Hoermann K, Myers EN, Whiteside TL. Characteristics of CD4+CD25+ regulatory T cells in the peripheral circulation of patients with head and neck cancer. Br J Cancer. 2005;92:913–20.
206. Wolf AM, Wolf D, Steurer M, Gastl G, Gunsilius E, Grubeck-Loebenstein B. Increase of regulatory T cells in the peripheral blood of cancer patients. Clin Cancer Res. 2003;9:606–12.
207. Ormandy LA, Hillemann T, Wedemeyer H, Manns MP, Greten TF, Korangy F. Increased populations of regulatory T cells in peripheral blood of patients with hepatocellular carcinoma. Cancer Res. 2005;65:2457–64.
208. Ichihara F, Kono K, Takahashi A, Kawaida H, Sugai H, Fujii H. Increased populations of regulatory T cells in peripheral blood and tumor-infiltrating lymphocytes in patients with gastric and esophageal cancers. Clin Cancer Res. 2003;9:4404–8.
209. Curiel TJ, Coukos G, Zou L, Alvarez X, Cheng P, Mottram P, Evdemon-Hogan M, Conejo-Garcia JR, Zhang L, Burow M, Zhu Y, Wei S, Kryczek I, Daniel B, Gordon A, Myers L, Lackner A, Disis ML, Knutson KL, Chen L, Zou W. Specific recruitment of regulatory T cells in ovarian carcinoma fosters immune privilege and predicts reduced survival. Nat Med. 2004;10:942–9.
210. Pardoll D. Does the immune system see tumors as foreign or self? Annu Rev Immunol. 2003;21:807–39.
211. Sakaguchi S, Wing K, Onishi Y, Prieto-Martin P, Yamaguchi T. Regulatory T cells: how do they suppress immune responses? Int Immunol. 2009;21:1105–11.
212. Sakaguchi S. Naturally arising CD4+ regulatory t cells for immunologic self-tolerance and negative control of immune responses. Annu Rev Immunol. 2004;22:531–62.
213. Zou W. Immunosuppressive networks in the tumour environment and their therapeutic relevance. Nat Rev Cancer. 2005;5:263–74.
214. Turk MJ, Guevara-Patino JA, Rizzuto GA, Engelhorn ME, Sakaguchi S, Houghton AN. Concomitant tumor immunity to a poorly immunogenic melanoma is prevented by regulatory T cells. J Exp Med. 2004;200:771–82.

215. Foss FM. DAB(389)IL-2 (ONTAK): a novel fusion toxin therapy for lymphoma. Clin Lymphoma. 2000;1:110–6. discussion 117.
216. Kwan WH, van der Touw W, Paz-Artal E, Li MO, Heeger PS. Signaling through C5a receptor and C3a receptor diminishes function of murine natural regulatory T cells. J Exp Med. 2013;210:257–68.
217. Michalek RD, Rathmell JC. The metabolic life and times of a T-cell. Immunol Rev. 2010;236:190–202.
218. Michalek RD, Gerriets VA, Jacobs SR, Macintyre AN, MacIver NJ, Mason EF, Sullivan SA, Nichols AG, Rathmell JC. Cutting edge: distinct glycolytic and lipid oxidative metabolic programs are essential for effector and regulatory CD4+ T cell subsets. J Immunol. 2011;186:3299–303.
219. van der Windt GJ, Everts B, Chang CH, Curtis JD, Freitas TC, Amiel E, Pearce EJ, Pearce EL. Mitochondrial respiratory capacity is a critical regulator of CD8+ T cell memory development. Immunity. 2012;36:68–78.
220. Jacobs SR, Herman CE, Maciver NJ, Wofford JA, Wieman HL, Hammen JJ, Rathmell JC. Glucose uptake is limiting in T cell activation and requires CD28-mediated Akt-dependent and independent pathways. J Immunol. 2008;180:4476–86.
221. Chang CH, Curtis JD, Maggi Jr LB, Faubert B, Villarino AV, O'Sullivan D, Huang SC, van der Windt GJ, Blagih J, Qiu J, Weber JD, Pearce EJ, Jones RG, Pearce EL. Posttranscriptional control of T cell effector function by aerobic glycolysis. Cell. 2013;153:1239–51.
222. Sena LA, Li S, Jairaman A, Prakriya M, Ezponda T, Hildeman DA, Wang CR, Schumacker PT, Licht JD, Perlman H, Bryce PJ, Chandel NS. Mitochondria are required for antigen-specific T cell activation through reactive oxygen species signaling. Immunity. 2013;38: 225–36.
223. Sukumar M, Liu J, Ji Y, Subramanian M, Crompton JG, Yu Z, Roychoudhuri R, Palmer DC, Muranski P, Karoly ED, Mohney RP, Klebanoff CA, Lal A, Finkel T, Restifo NP, Gattinoni L. Inhibiting glycolytic metabolism enhances CD8+ T cell memory and antitumor function. J Clin Invest. 2013;123:4479–88.
224. Xu J, Ji J, Yan XH. Cross-talk between AMPK and mTOR in regulating energy balance. Crit Rev Food Sci Nutr. 2012;52:373–81.
225. van der Windt GJ, O'Sullivan D, Everts B, Huang SC, Buck MD, Curtis JD, Chang CH, Smith AM, Ai T, Faubert B, Jones RG, Pearce EJ, Pearce EL. CD8 memory T cells have a bioenergetic advantage that underlies their rapid recall ability. Proc Natl Acad Sci U S A. 2013;110:14336–41.
226. DePinho RA. The age of cancer. Nature. 2000;408:248–54.
227. Lefebvre JS, Haynes L. Aging of the CD4 T cell compartment. Open Longev Sci. 2012;6:83–91.
228. Kilpatrick RD, Rickabaugh T, Hultin LE, Hultin P, Hausner MA, Detels R, Phair J, Jamieson BD. Homeostasis of the naive CD4+ T cell compartment during aging. J Immunol. 2008;180:1499–507.
229. Goronzy JJ, Weyand CM. Aging, autoimmunity and arthritis: T-cell senescence and contraction of T-cell repertoire diversity – catalysts of autoimmunity and chronic inflammation. Arthritis Res Ther. 2003;5:225–34.
230. Rivnay B, Bergman S, Shinitzky M, Globerson A. Correlations between membrane viscosity, serum cholesterol, lymphocyte activation and aging in man. Mech Ageing Dev. 1980;12: 119–26.
231. Larbi A, Dupuis G, Khalil A, Douziech N, Fortin C, Fulop Jr T. Differential role of lipid rafts in the functions of CD4+ and CD8+ human T lymphocytes with aging. Cell Signal. 2006; 18:1017–30.
232. Larbi A, Grenier A, Frisch F, Douziech N, Fortin C, Carpentier AC, Fulop T. Acute in vivo elevation of intravascular triacylglycerol lipolysis impairs peripheral T cell activation in humans. Am J Clin Nutr. 2005;82:949–56.
233. Effros RB, Boucher N, Porter V, Zhu X, Spaulding C, Walford RL, Kronenberg M, Cohen D, Schachter F. Decline in CD28+ T cells in centenarians and in long-term T cell cultures: a

possible cause for both in vivo and in vitro immunosenescence. Exp Gerontol. 1994;29: 601–9.
234. Mazzatti DJ, White A, Forsey RJ, Powell JR, Pawelec G. Gene expression changes in long-term culture of T-cell clones: genomic effects of chronic antigenic stress in aging and immunosenescence. Aging Cell. 2007;6:155–63.
235. Tewari K, Walent J, Svaren J, Zamoyska R, Suresh M. Differential requirement for Lck during primary and memory CD8+ T cell responses. Proc Natl Acad Sci U S A. 2006; 103:16388–93.
236. Missios P, Zhou Y, Guachalla LM, von Figura G, Wegner A, Chakkarappan SR, Binz T, Gompf A, Hartleben G, Burkhalter MD, Wulff V, Gunes C, Sattler RW, Song Z, Illig T, Klaus S, Bohm BO, Wenz T, Hiller K, Rudolph KL. Glucose substitution prolongs maintenance of energy homeostasis and lifespan of telomere dysfunctional mice. Nat Commun. 2014;5:4924.
237. Haynes L, Maue AC. Effects of aging on T cell function. Curr Opin Immunol. 2009;21: 414–7.
238. Holland AM, van den Brink MR. Rejuvenation of the aging T cell compartment. Curr Opin Immunol. 2009;21:454–9.
239. McElhaney JE, Effros RB. Immunosenescence: what does it mean to health outcomes in older adults? Curr Opin Immunol. 2009;21:418–24.
240. Morgan RA, Dudley ME, Yu YY, Zheng Z, Robbins PF, Theoret MR, Wunderlich JR, Hughes MS, Restifo NP, Rosenberg SA. High efficiency TCR gene transfer into primary human lymphocytes affords avid recognition of melanoma tumor antigen glycoprotein 100 and does not alter the recognition of autologous melanoma antigens. J Immunol. 2003;171:3287–95.
241. Hughes MS, Yu YY, Dudley ME, Zheng Z, Robbins PF, Li Y, Wunderlich J, Hawley RG, Moayeri M, Rosenberg SA, Morgan RA. Transfer of a TCR gene derived from a patient with a marked antitumor response conveys highly active T-cell effector functions. Hum Gene Ther. 2005;16:457–72.
242. Ando T, Mimura K, Johansson CC, Hanson MG, Mougiakakos D, Larsson C, Martins da Palma T, Sakurai D, Norell H, Li M, Nishimura MI, Kiessling R. Transduction with the antioxidant enzyme catalase protects human T cells against oxidative stress. J Immunol. 2008; 181:8382–90.
243. Roszkowski JJ, Lyons GE, Kast WM, Yee C, Van Besien K, Nishimura MI. Simultaneous generation of CD8+ and CD4+ melanoma-reactive T cells by retroviral-mediated transfer of a single T-cell receptor. Cancer Res. 2005;65:1570–6.
244. Morgan RA, Dudley ME, Wunderlich JR, Hughes MS, Yang JC, Sherry RM, Royal RE, Topalian SL, Kammula US, Restifo NP, Zheng Z, Nahvi A, de Vries CR, Rogers-Freezer LJ, Mavroukakis SA, Rosenberg SA. Cancer regression in patients after transfer of genetically engineered lymphocytes. Science. 2006;314:126–9.
245. Vermeij R, Daemen T, de Bock GH, de Graeff P, Leffers N, Lambeck A, ten Hoor KA, Hollema H, van der Zee AG, Nijman HW. Potential target antigens for a universal vaccine in epithelial ovarian cancer. Clin Dev Immunol. 2010;2010.
246. Cohen CJ, Zheng Z, Bray R, Zhao Y, Sherman LA, Rosenberg SA, Morgan RA. Recognition of fresh human tumor by human peripheral blood lymphocytes transduced with a bicistronic retroviral vector encoding a murine anti-p53 TCR. J Immunol. 2005;175:5799–808.
247. Schaft N, Willemsen RA, de Vries J, Lankiewicz B, Essers BW, Gratama JW, Figdor CG, Bolhuis RL, Debets R, Adema GJ. Peptide fine specificity of anti-glycoprotein 100 CTL is preserved following transfer of engineered TCR alpha beta genes into primary human T lymphocytes. J Immunol. 2003;170:2186–94.
248. Tsuji T, Yasukawa M, Matsuzaki J, Ohkuri T, Chamoto K, Wakita D, Azuma T, Niiya H, Miyoshi H, Kuzushima K, Oka Y, Sugiyama H, Ikeda H, Nishimura T. Generation of tumor-specific, HLA class I-restricted human Th1 and Tc1 cells by cell engineering with tumor peptide-specific T-cell receptor genes. Blood. 2005;106:470–6.
249. Cohen CJ, Li YF, El-Gamil M, Robbins PF, Rosenberg SA, Morgan RA. Enhanced antitumor activity of T cells engineered to express T-cell receptors with a second disulfide bond. Cancer Res. 2007;67:3898–903.

250. Cohen CJ, Zhao Y, Zheng Z, Rosenberg SA, Morgan RA. Enhanced antitumor activity of murine-human hybrid T-cell receptor (TCR) in human lymphocytes is associated with improved pairing and TCR/CD3 stability. Cancer Res. 2006;66:8878–86.
251. Chlewicki LK, Holler PD, Monti BC, Clutter MR, Kranz DM. High-affinity, peptide-specific T cell receptors can be generated by mutations in CDR1, CDR2 or CDR3. J Mol Biol. 2005;346:223–39.
252. Bowerman NA, Crofts TS, Chlewicki L, Do P, Baker BM, Christopher Garcia K, Kranz DM. Engineering the binding properties of the T cell receptor:peptide:MHC ternary complex that governs T cell activity. Mol Immunol. 2009;46:3000–8.
253. Maus MV, Grupp SA, Porter DL, June CH. Antibody-modified T cells: CARs take the front seat for hematologic malignancies. Blood. 2014;123:2625–35.
254. Kowolik CM, Topp MS, Gonzalez S, Pfeiffer T, Olivares S, Gonzalez N, Smith DD, Forman SJ, Jensen MC, Cooper LJ. CD28 costimulation provided through a CD19-specific chimeric antigen receptor enhances in vivo persistence and antitumor efficacy of adoptively transferred T cells. Cancer Res. 2006;66:10995–1004.
255. Hernandez-Chacon JA, Li Y, Wu RC, Bernatchez C, Wang Y, Weber JS, Hwu P, Radvanyi LG. Costimulation through the CD137/4-1BB pathway protects human melanoma tumor-infiltrating lymphocytes from activation-induced cell death and enhances antitumor effector function. J Immunother. 2011;34:236–50.
256. Song DG, Ye Q, Carpenito C, Poussin M, Wang LP, Ji C, Figini M, June CH, Coukos G, Powell Jr DJ. In vivo persistence, tumor localization, and antitumor activity of CAR-engineered T cells is enhanced by costimulatory signaling through CD137 (4-1BB). Cancer Res. 2011;71:4617–27.
257. Hombach AA, Heiders J, Foppe M, Chmielewski M, Abken H. OX40 costimulation by a chimeric antigen receptor abrogates CD28 and IL-2 induced IL-10 secretion by redirected CD4(+) T cells. Oncoimmunology. 2012;1:458–66.
258. Guedan S, Chen X, Madar A, Carpenito C, McGettigan SE, Frigault MJ, Lee J, Posey Jr AD, Scholler J, Scholler N, Bonneau R, June CH. ICOS-based chimeric antigen receptors program bipolar TH17/TH1 cells. Blood. 2014;124:1070–80.
259. Starck L, Scholz C, Dorken B, Daniel PT. Costimulation by CD137/4-1BB inhibits T cell apoptosis and induces Bcl-xL and c-FLIP(short) via phosphatidylinositol 3-kinase and AKT/protein kinase B. Eur J Immunol. 2005;35:1257–66.
260. Hurtado JC, Kim YJ, Kwon BS. Signals through 4-1BB are costimulatory to previously activated splenic T cells and inhibit activation-induced cell death. J Immunol. 1997;158: 2600–9.
261. Saoulli K, Lee SY, Cannons JL, Yeh WC, Santana A, Goldstein MD, Bangia N, DeBenedette MA, Mak TW, Choi Y, Watts TH. CD28-independent, TRAF2-dependent costimulation of resting T cells by 4-1BB ligand. J Exp Med. 1998;187:1849–62.
262. Tan JT, Whitmire JK, Ahmed R, Pearson TC, Larsen CP. 4-1BB ligand, a member of the TNF family, is important for the generation of antiviral CD8 T cell responses. J Immunol. 1999;163:4859–68.
263. Wickramasinghe D. Tumor and T cell engagement by BiTE. Discov Med. 2013;16:149–52.
264. Hoffman LM, Gore L. Blinatumomab, a bi-specific anti-CD19/CD3 BiTE((R)) antibody for the treatment of acute lymphoblastic leukemia: perspectives and current pediatric applications. Front Oncol. 2014;4:63.
265. Molhoj M, Crommer S, Brischwein K, Rau D, Sriskandarajah M, Hoffmann P, Kufer P, Hofmeister R, Baeuerle PA. CD19-/CD3-bispecific antibody of the BiTE class is far superior to tandem diabody with respect to redirected tumor cell lysis. Mol Immunol. 2007;44: 1935–43.
266. Zimmerman Z, Maniar T, Nagorsen D. Unleashing the clinical power of T cells: CD19/CD3 bi-specific T cell engager (BiTE(R)) antibody construct blinatumomab as a potential therapy. Int Immunol. 2015;27:31–7.
267. Gleason MK, Ross JA, Warlick ED, Lund TC, Verneris MR, Wiernik A, Spellman S, Haagenson MD, Lenvik AJ, Litzow MR, Epling-Burnette PK, Blazar BR, Weiner LM,

Weisdorf DJ, Vallera DA, Miller JS. CD16xCD33 bispecific killer cell engager (BiKE) activates NK cells against primary MDS and MDSC CD33+ targets. Blood. 2014;123: 3016–26.

268. Wiernik A, Foley B, Zhang B, Verneris MR, Warlick E, Gleason MK, Ross JA, Luo X, Weisdorf DJ, Walcheck B, Vallera DA, Miller JS. Targeting natural killer cells to acute myeloid leukemia in vitro with a CD16 x 33 bispecific killer cell engager and ADAM17 inhibition. Clin Cancer Res. 2013;19:3844–55.
269. Baumjohann D, Ansel KM. MicroRNA-mediated regulation of T helper cell differentiation and plasticity. Nat Rev Immunol. 2013;13:666–78.
270. Cobb BS, Hertweck A, Smith J, O'Connor E, Graf D, Cook T, Smale ST, Sakaguchi S, Livesey FJ, Fisher AG, Merkenschlager M. A role for Dicer in immune regulation. J Exp Med. 2006;203:2519–27.
271. Muljo SA, Ansel KM, Kanellopoulou C, Livingston DM, Rao A, Rajewsky K. Aberrant T cell differentiation in the absence of Dicer. J Exp Med. 2005;202:261–9.
272. Ohno M, Ohkuri T, Kosaka A, Tanahashi K, June CH, Natsume A, Okada H. Expression of miR-17-92 enhances anti-tumor activity of T-cells transduced with the anti-EGFRvIII chimeric antigen receptor in mice bearing human GBM xenografts. J Immunother Cancer. 2013;1:21.
273. Kaech SM, Wherry EJ, Ahmed R. Effector and memory T-cell differentiation: implications for vaccine development. Nat Rev Immunol. 2002;2:251–62.
274. Robert-Tissot C, Nguyen LT, Ohashi PS, Speiser DE. Mobilizing and evaluating anticancer T cells: pitfalls and solutions. Expert Rev Vaccines. 2013;12:1325–40.

Index

B. Bonavida, S. Chouaib (eds.), *Resistance of Cancer Cells to CTL-Mediated Immunotherapy*, Resistance to Targeted Anti-Cancer Therapeutics 7,
DOI 10.1007/978-3-319-17807-3

T

Y

CPSIA information can be obtained at www.ICGtesting.com
Printed in the USA
LVOW01*1403100815

449512LV00001B/42/P